The Brilliant Book of
BABY NAMES

Also by **Pamela Redmond Satran** & **Linda Rosenkrantz**

The Brilliant Book of
BABY NAMES

What's Best, What's Hot & What's Not

Pamela Redmond Satran
Linda Rosenkrantz

Collins

HarperCollins Publishers Ltd
77–85 Fulham Palace Road
London
W6 8JB

www.collins.co.uk

Collins is a registered trademark of HarperCollins Publishers Ltd

First published in the USA in 2007 by St Martin's Press
Text © 2007 by Pamela Redmond Satran and Linda Rosenkrantz

13 12 11
7 6 5 4 3

ISBN:978-0-00-725889-5

Collins uses papers that are natural, renewable and recyclable products made from wood grown in sustainable forests. The manufacturing processes conform to the environmental regulations of the country of origin.

Printed and bound in China by South China Printing Co. Ltd

For our wonderful husbands:

Dick Satran,
my partner in real-life baby naming, and

Christopher Finch,
who, as always, helped with everything

Contents

contents

Boys' Names A–Z 303

with lists of

Acknowledgments

There are many people we must thank for their help in producing this tome. For almost twenty years, our editor, Hope Dellon, has been unfailingly helpful, supportive, enthusiastic and wise. Thanks, too, to all the others on the terrific team at St Martin's Press, in particular Matthew Shear, John Karle, Colleen Schwartz, Shannon Twomey, Kris Kamikawa, Susan Caplan and Tracy Martin. Others who helped gather and process information were Willa Beckman, Liz Dean, Linda Federico-O'Murchu, Mark Ludas (who brought calm and a great eye for detail to every storm), the impeccable Wendy Maring (whose contributions included wrestling with and conquering those pesky Slavic accents), Joe Satran, Rory Satran, Emily Shapiro (for her prescient reports on new naming trends) and Lisa Sisler. And very important, we owe a very special debt of gratitude to our sagacious and savvy agent, Brian de Fiore, and to his able associate Kate Garrick.

Introduction

Choosing the right name can seem daunting these days, with so many choices to sift through, so much new information about the importance of names, such creative baby naming in Hollywood and on the Web. How can you tell if a name is too popular or not mainstream enough, wonderfully creative or just plain weird? How can you find the name that is perfect for you and your baby?

We can help. In fact, we've been helping parents find the perfect name for their babies for two decades. We helped launch this wide – and wild – new world of names with our book *Beyond Jennifer & Jason,* first published in the pre–Baby Gap, pre-starbaby 1980s, back when everybody just named their babies after themselves or picked one of the trendy names of the day. *Please,* we urged parents: Look beyond the obvious choices. Consider using your mother's maiden name as your daughter's first, or dust off Grandpa's name for your son. Look to your cultural heritage for a name or pluck one from a map.

Now that Jennifer and Jason are all grown up and naming babies of their own, it's time for a new kind of book. The baby-naming shelves have become engorged with dozens of name dictionaries on steroids, most of them stuffed with ridiculous names and misleading, often made-up definitions and copycat lists. One, for example, lists Seth under 'Names Teachers Can't Pronounce,' while another informs us that the definition of Goddess is 'gorgeous'. You and your baby deserve a lot better than that.

And that's why we wrote *The Brilliant Book of Baby Names*. As the United States' foremost experts on style and names – we also wrote the bestselling *Cool Names for Babies* and have been interviewed about baby naming by everyone from *The New York Times* to *Us Weekly* to *The Today Show* and *Oprah* – we found ourselves in a position to create a unique baby-naming resource as authoritative, stylish and original as our other books, to provide the name information needed to make the all-important choice both you and your child will be happy with forever.

The crowning achievement of our twenty years' experience researching and writing about names in eight other books that have sold millions of copies, *The Brilliant Book of Baby Names:*

- Offers more than 50,000 terrific names from around the world, including a multitude of creative choices found nowhere else. References to the Top 100 names are UK government statistics for England and Wales.
- Includes real and accurate information on where the names come from and what they mean in their original language, as well as how they're perceived in the modern world.
- Guides you through the maze of style and image considerations by giving you expert enlightened and enlightening commentary on every name in the book.
- Helps you make the perfect name decision via the kind of specialised lists that we invented and still do best. Here are more than two hundred lists of beautiful names and strong names, names stars are giving their kids and names that would shock your grandma, lists of French names and African names and names you should consider if you like Emily but want to move beyond it.
- Keeps you entertained while you're making your momentous choice, with writing that's as sharp as it is illuminating.

Traditionally, name books start with tips for parents on choosing a name – make sure the first name goes with your last and that you don't give your kid the initials P.I.G. –

things you wouldn't have much trouble figuring out for yourself. Instead, as you embark on the great baby-naming adventure in this enlightened age, we offer a new level of advice on choosing a name:

TODAY'S ESSENTIAL TOP-10 OF BABY NAMING

1. **Aim to fall in love with a name.** Remember falling in love with your partner? Swooning the first time you heard your baby's heartbeat? That's the kind of emotional reaction you should go for with a name, too. Look for one that you love so much it makes your heart pound, that you can't stop thinking about, that you keep loving no matter what anybody says.

2. **Don't pay too much attention to what other people think.** It's lots of fun talking about names with your spouse, your friends, your family. Everyone will ask which names you're considering – and then they'll do their best to convince you that those names are stupid, ugly, ridiculous choices, and that you should pick the names *they* like instead. The problem is, these people are only giving their subjective opinions. Your parents' ideas are several decades out of style, your childless friends are clueless and the grocer and the postman – yes, everyone wants to get into the act – know even less. Talk about it if you like. Then tune out all those other opinions and make the big decision yourself – along with your partner.

3. **Remember, it's more about your child than about you.** Love aside, it's important to keep in mind that your child is the one who's going to live with your name choice – not just when he's a baby, oblivious in your arms, but in the playground and in the school canteen and on job interviews and at his fortieth birthday party and as an old man. The point is, it doesn't matter whether your friends think a name is cool or what kind of attention you get on your favourite baby-naming notice board for your ideas. Your child will be the one perspiring in his interview suit or hobbling around the nursing home, thinking, 'Crikey! Why did they have to name me Harley?'

4. But know that Harley isn't the same name it was when you were a child. Names have changed in a big way, so that the names that would have been considered strange or that would have gotten you teased in the playground when you were in school are now accepted as completely normal. Interchangeable names for boys and girls? Totally standard – though you still don't want to name your son Sue. (You probably don't want to name your daughter Sue either, but for different reasons.) Ethnic names? Found in many cities throughout the country. Unconventional spellings and invented names? Often, the traditional spelling is now the exception, and the girl down the road is more likely to be named Nevaeh than Nancy. It's a whole new baby-naming world out there.

5. Expand your view of creativity. Consistent with this new world of baby naming is the pressure lots of parents feel to be creative in their choices. Inventing a name or varying a spelling is great if that's your style, but there are lots of other ways to be creative, and this book can help you explore them. Try a fresh international twist on a familiar name. Consider names you never even knew existed; you'll find a wide menu of choices here that have never appeared in any name book before.

6. Look for a name with meaning. A name's meaning these days extends far beyond the original 'spear carrier' or 'God is gracious'. You'll want to consider what a name means in terms of your family history, your individual experience, your personal style. Can you find a name that relates to your family tree? Your cultural background? How about a place name or a word name or an occupational name that signals something with personal significance to you? Explore what different names mean in relation to your sense of style, of history, of yourself and your partner. A name that connects deeply on several levels will resonate into the future for both you and your child.

7. Do your own research. Everything you need from a book may be here, but you might also want to gather your own intelligence. Visit your local playground or read the birth announcements to familiarise yourself with the naming trends in your neighbourhood.

Find the most current popularity lists of baby names for both girls and boys at the British government's website www.statistics.gov.uk. Depending on your needs and tastes, you might also want to look at our style-oriented books, *Beyond Jennifer & Jason, Madison and Montana,* and *Cool Names for Babies* and our ethnic baby-naming guides, *Beyond Shannon & Sean* or *Beyond Sarah & Sam.*

8. Put baby naming in perspective. Of course, we believe names are important. They telegraph messages about a person's class, family, ethnicity, gender, creativity, intelligence – messages that you, as a conscientious parent, want to control. You want to do everything you can to choose the best possible name. And yet, let's not get carried away. Books that tell you that a name controls your child's destiny or holds the key to success are just trying to persuade you to buy something with little validity.

9. Have fun. Yes, choosing a name is a serious, long-term decision, but it can and should be fun and exciting. We want this to be the book you stay up late into the night reading. The subject of laugh-filled dinners and under-the-covers heart-to-hearts. There's so much that's frightening and out of your control about becoming a parent, you should enjoy this one aspect that has so much potential for pleasure.

10. Let us be your guides. Parents often ask us, 'How do I know whether a name I like is going to get too popular? How can I find a name that's distinctive without being too strange?' Such difficult questions are at the heart of most parents' search for the perfect name, and that's exactly where we come in. You don't have to somehow figure out or guess these things for yourself: Through our decades of research and experience, we know which names are coming into style and which are heading out, which old favourites are worth dusting off and which should stay in mothballs, what's cool and what's just freaky. That's exactly the kind of information you'll find throughout this book, leading you to a name you'll love even more through the years than you do today, the name your wonderful child deserves.

How to Use This Book

Symbols

The symbols in the book are designed to make it easy and quick for you to identify certain names.

★ The stars identify the names that are our recommended Best Bets – names we find to be particularly appealing in a wide range of styles.

♀ A unisex symbol means the name can be used for both boys and girls, so that you may find a choice in the boys' section that works for a daughter or vice versa.

Derivations and Meanings

There is much conflict and misinformation over the background and meaning of names, but what you'll find here is the most authoritative material available. We simplified derivations, saying Scottish and English and French, for instance, rather than getting into such fine points as Middle English and Old French. We do identify African and Native American tribal derivations, when accessible. For consistency, names that are related to other names are all called 'variations', while shortened forms are labelled 'diminutives'.

Spellings

The main entry is usually the classic spelling of the name, with variations, short forms and international versions listed beneath. When there is a spelling variation that is commonly found – for example, the popular KAITLYN for the original CAITLIN – that has an individual entry as well.

Lists

Rather than segregating our lists, we've woven them throughout the book. If you're looking for a name that sounds creative or one that means 'strong', if you want an inventive nickname for Elizabeth or a substitute for Dylan, you'll find them all in one place. A guide to the lists is in the Contents. Within each letter, there is a selective listing of recent choices of celebrity parents under the heading Stellar Starbabies.

Armed with all this information and advice, we're sure you will arrive at the best possible baby-naming decision for your baby, finding the one perfect name that you and your child will love forever.

The Brilliant Book of
BABY NAMES

A girls

AALIYAH. *Variation of* **ALIYA,** *Arabic, 'highborn'.* The most complicated and popular spelling of this once-obscure name. Aahliyah, Aailiyah, Aailyah, Aalaiya, Aaleah, Aalia, Aalieyha, Aaliya, Aaliyaha, Aaliyha, Aalliah, Aalyah, Aalyiah, Alia, Aliah, Alliyah.

ABBIE, ABBY. *Diminutive of* **ABIGAIL.** Gently old-fashioned nickname name that owes its popularity to Abigail, but it has been slipping down the Top 100 in recent years. Aabbee, Abbe, Abbea, Abbee, Abbeigh, Abbey, Abbi, Abbye, Abee, Abeey, Abey, Abi, Abia, Abie, Aby.

♂ **ABBOTT.** *Aramaic, Hebrew, 'father'.* Traditionally male surname that may find new life for girls thanks to its similarity to the popular Abby and Abigail. **Abbot.** International: **Abboid** *(Gaelic),* **Abad** *(Spanish),* **Abt** *(German).*

ABELIA. *Hebrew, 'sigh, breath'.* This feminine form of Abel makes a distinctive alternative to the widely used Abigail. International: **Abélia, Abelle, Abella** *(French).*

♂ **ABERDEEN.** *Scottish place name.* A much more modern choice than unfashionable Irish *een*-ending names like Noreen and Doreen.

ABIA. *Arabic, 'great'.* Simple plus unusual is a winning combination. **Abbia, Abbiah, Abiah, Abya, Abyah.**

ABIELA. *Hebrew, 'God is my father'.* More than the sum of Abby and Ella. **Abielah, Aviela.**

ABIGAIL. *Hebrew, 'my father is joyful'.* Old Testament name – Abigail was the wife of David – that became a term for a maid in the early nineteenth century and subsequently fell from favour. Now, it's back in a big way, liked for its proper vintage charm. **Abagael, Abagail, Abagale, Abagil, Abaigeal, Abbagail, Abbe, Abbey, Abbi, Abbie, Abbiegail, Abbiegayle, Abbigael, Abbigail, Abbigal, Abbigale, Abbigayl, Abbigayle, Abby, Abbye, Abbygael, Abbygail, Abbygale, Abegail, Abegale, Abgail, Abgale, Abgayle, Abichayil, Abihail, Abigael, Abigal, Abigaile, Abigaill, Abigal, Abigale, Abigayil, Abigayl, Abigayle, Abigel, Abigial, Abigil, Abigayle, Abugail, Abygail, Avichayil, Avigail, Avihail, Gael, Gail, Gaila, Gal, Gale, Gayel, Gayle.**

♂ **ABIJAH.** *Hebrew, 'God is my father'.* Abigail with rhythm. **Abeedja, Abeeja, Abeesha, Abija, Abisha, Abishah.**

ABILENE. *English from Hebrew, 'grass'; also American place name.* Here is a spiced-up spunky version of the popular Abbie nickname. **Abalene, Abalina, Abilena, Abiline.**

♂ **ABITAL.** *Hebrew, 'my father is dew'.* Although it's popular for boys as well as girls in Israel, we don't see it happening here. **Abeetal, Avital.**

ABRA. *Feminine variation of* **ABRAHAM.** Soft, sensitive feminine form of Abraham – but there is the risk that it could too often be followed by 'cadabra'. **Abame, Abarrane, Abbrienna, Abbryana, Abrahana, Abréa, Abrea, Abreana,**

Abreanna, Abreanne, Abree, Abreeana, Abreia, Abreona, Abreonia, Abri, Abria, Abriah, Abriann, Abrianna, Abriannah, Abrianne, Abriéa, Abrieana, Abrielle, Abrien, Abrienna, Abrienne, Abrietta, Abrion, Abrionée, Abrionne, Abriunna, Abryann, Abryanna, Abryona, Abrya. International: Abriana *(Italian)*.

ABRIAL. *French, 'open, secure, protected'.* Stronger, more distinctive than April or Avril. Aabriella, Abrail, Abreal, Abreale, Abriale, Abriel, Abriell, Abrielle, Abrilla, Abrille, Abryell.

ACACIA. *Greek nature name.* Attractive, rarely-used Greek nature name of a flowering shrub that symbolises resurrection and immortality, especially good for an Easter baby. Acasha, Acasia, Acasiya, Acasya, Acatia, Acaysha, Accacia, Accasie, Accassia, Acey, Acie, Akacia, Akakia, Akaysha, Caci, Cacia, Cacie, Casey, Casha, Casi, Casia, Casie, Cassie, Cassy, Caysha, Kacey, Kaci, Kacia, Kakia, Kakie, Kasi, Kasie, Kasia, Kassja, Kassi, Kassie, Kassya, Kassy.

ACADIA. *Place name.* The French name for Nova Scotia – and the name of a gorgeous American national park in Maine – makes a fresh, rhythmic choice for your little girl. Acadiah, Acadya, Acadyah, Cadi, Cadia, Cadie, Cady.

ADA. *German, 'noble, nobility'.* A favourite at the end of the nineteenth century that hasn't come back. . . . yet. But with the new trend towards simple, old-fashioned names beginning with a vowel – Ava, Ella – you may consider being one of the first to revive it. Adabella, Adabelle, Adah, Adalee, Adan, Adaya, Adda, Adette, Addi, Addie, Addiah, Addy, Adey, Adi, Adia, Adiah, Adie, Aida, Aidah, Auda.

ADAH. *Hebrew, 'beautiful, adorned'.* Pronounced *AH-dah,* this unusual biblical name – the first female name in Genesis after Eve – is a softer Ada equivalent. Ada, Addah.

♂ **ADAIR.** *Scottish and Irish, 'oak tree ford'.* Has lots of flair; consider it in place of the overused Aidan. Adaire, Adare, Adayre.

ADALIA. *Hebrew, 'God is my refuge'; German, 'noble one'.* Luxurious and distinctive. Adal, Adala, Adalane, Adalea, Adaleah, Adalee, Adalene, Adali, Adalie, Adaliah, Adalin, Adalina, Adaline, Adalinn, Adalley, Adaly, Adalya, Adalyah, Adalyn, Adalynn, Adalynne, Addal, Addala, Addaly, Addalyn, Addalynn.

ADAMINA. *Hebrew, 'child of the red earth'.* This feminine form of Adam (Adama is another one) has none of the simple elegance of the original. Try Eve. Ada, Adama, Adamah, Adameena, Adamine, Adaminna, Addie, Ademina, Ademeena, Mina, Minna.

ADARA. *Arabic, 'virgin'; Hebrew, 'noble, exalted'.* Perfect name for a Virgo baby. Adair, Adaira, Adaora, Adar, Adarah, Adare, Adaria, Adarra, Adasha, Adauré, Adra.

ADDIE. *Diminutive of* **ADELAIDE** *or* **ADELINE.** Old-fashioned nickname with sweet turn-of-the-last-century charm that could work today. Aday, Adde, Addee, Addey, Addi, Addia,

Addy, Ade, Adee, Adei, Adey, Adeye, Adi, Adie, Ady, Atti, Attie, Atty.

♂ **ADDISON.** *English, 'son of Adam'.* Rapidly moving in on Madison. **Addis, Addisen, Addisson, Addyson, Adis, Adisa, Adisen, Adison, Adisynne, Adysen.**

ADELAIDE. *German, 'noble, nobility'.* Best known as the German princess who married the British King William in the 1830s, inspiring the name of the Australian city and a craze for her name. Recently chosen by Aussie actress Rachel Griffiths. **Ada, Adalaide, Adalayde, Addala, Addalla, Addey, Addi, Addie, Addy, Adel, Adela, Adelade, Adelaid, Adelaida, Adelais, Adele, Adelei, Adelheid, Adeliade, Adelina, Adeline, Adelice, Adelicia, Adelis, Adelita, Adeliza, Adelka, Adelle, Adelvice, Adelvicia, Adey, Adi, Adlin, Adline, Ado, Ady, Aley, Aline, Aliosha, Alline, Alyosha, Del, Delia, Delle, Delli, Delly, Edeline, Eline, Heidi, Lady, Laidey, Laidy.** International: **Ailis** *(Irish),* **Adélaïde (a-day-la-EED)** *(French),* **Alida** *(Hungarian).*

ADELE. *German, 'noble, nobility'.* In fashion-limbo. **Adel, Adela, Adelia, Adelie, Adell, Adella, Adellah, Adelle, Adile, Edelle.**

ADELIA. *Variation of* **ADELAIDE.** Much more accessible and rarely-used form, worth consideration. **Adeliah, Adelya, Adelya.**

★**ADELINE.** *French, diminutive of* **ADELE.** Many contemporary parents like this name's old-fashioned 'Sweet Adeline' charm, perhaps seeing it as a less-used cousin of the ultratrendy Madeline. **Adalina, Adaline, Adallina, Adelaine, Adelin, Adelind, Adelita, Adeliya, Adella, Adellah, Adelle, Adelyn, Adelynn, Adelynne, Adilene, Adlin, Adlina, Adline, Adlyn, Adlynn, Ahdella, Aline, Dahlina, Dalina, Daline, Dallina, Delina, Deline, Dellina, Delly, Delyne, Edelie, Lina.** International: **Adelina, Adette** *(French),* **Adelina** *(Slavic).*

ADELPHA. *Greek, 'beloved sister'.* Seriously classic name with lovely meaning. **Adelfa, Adelfia, Adelphia, Delpha.**

ADINA. *Hebrew, 'slender, delicate'.* Name of an Old Testament soldier that can theoretically be used for either sex – but sounds overwhelmingly feminine. **Adena, Adinah, Adine, Aideen, Aidena, Aidina, Aidine, Aydeen, Aydeena, Aydina.**

ADOLPHA. *German, 'noble wolf'.* Nein. **Adolfa, Adollfa.**

ADORA. *Latin, 'adored'.* Better to lavish your child with adoration than give her this spoiled-girl name. **Adorabelle, Adorae, Adoray, Adore, Adoree, Adoria, Adorlee, Dora, Dorae, Dori, Dorie, Dorri, Dorne, Dorry, Dory.**

ADRIANA. *Latin, feminine variation of* **ADRIAN.** This *a*-ending feminine form of Adrian, from the northern Italian city of Adria, is a soft and lovely Italian choice. **Addie, Adrea, Adreana, Adreanna, Adreea, Adria, Adriah, Adrian, Adrianah, Adriane, Adrianna, Adriannah, Adrianne, Adrie, Adrieanne, Adrien, Adriena, Adrienah, Adriene, Adrienna, Adrina, Adriyanna, Aydrian, Aydrienne, Hadria, Hadrienne.**

ADRIENNE. *Latin, feminine variation of* **ADRIAN.** Earlier feminine form of Adrian, now knocked aside by the versions ending in *a.*

AERIN. *Tolkien Middle Earth invention, or variation of* **ERIN.** In Tolkien's world, the derivation of this airy name is Elvish. Regular folks might consider it an artsier form of Erin, borne by cosmetics heiress and socialite Aerin Lauder.

AERON. *Welsh mythology name.* Tolkien may have been inspired by this name of a Celtic goddess of war. **Aeronwen, Aeronwy.**

AFFINITY. *Word name.* Sympathetic new twist on a Puritan virtue name.

AFRA. *Arabic, 'colour of earth'; Hebrew, 'dust'.* Earthier version of the name of England's first female professional writer, Aphra Behn. **Affera, Affery, Affra, Affrey, Affrie, Afraa, Aphra.**

AFRICA. *Place name.* Most Africas today would be named for the continent, but the name actually existed in Scotland in medieval times, where there was a Celtic queen named Affrica. **Affrica, Affricah, Affrika, Affrikah, Afric, Africah, African, Africaya, Africia, Africiana, Afrika, Afrikah, Aifric, Aifrica, Aphria, Aphfrica, Apirka, Apirkah. International: Aifric** *(Scottish).*

♂ **AFTERNOON.** *Word name.* An early day name, found on slave rolls, and worthy of consideration today for someone seeking a truly unusual name.

♂ **AFTON.** *Place name.* Name of a town in Scotland that has a feminine strength. **Affton, Aftan, Aften, Aftin, Aftine, Aftinn, Aftonn, Aftonne, Aftyn, Aftynn.**

AGAPI. *Greek, 'love, affection'.* Sweet meaning, but clunky name.

AGATE. *French, a semiprecious stone, or variation of* **AGATHA.** The *Ag-* sound grates on the modern ear. **Aggie.**

AGATHA. *Greek, 'good'.* Agatha still summons up visions of martyred saints, mauve silk dresses and high lace collars, but some dauntless excavators have begun to resurrect it. **Ag, Agace, Agacia, Agata, Agatah, Agathe, Agathi, Agatta, Agetha, Aggi, Aggie, Aggy, Aggye, Agi, Agie, Agueda, Agy, Agye, Atka. International: Agathe** *(French, German),* **Agueda** *(Portuguese),* **Agata** *(Scandinavian),* **Agatá** *(Slavic),* **Atka** *(Polish),* **Agi, Agota, Agotha** *(Hungarian),* **Agafia, Agasha, Ganya, Gasha, Gashka** *(Russian)* **Agathe** *(Greek).*

AGNES. *Greek, 'pure, virginal'.* Though it was the third most common English girls' name for four hundred years, Agnes has long been stuck in the attic. But maybe it's so far out it's almost ready to come back in. French pronounciation – *ahn-YEZ* – helps, and Thom Yorke of Radiohead chose it for his daughter. **Ag, Aggi, Aggie, Aggye, Agi, Agie, Agna, Agnesse, Agnessina, Agnis, Agnus, Agy, Agye, Anais, Anees, Aneesha, Aneska, Anessa, Anesse, Anice, Anissa, Anisha, Annais, Anneyce, Annice, Annis, Annisah, Annise, Annisha, Anson, Ina, Inah, Nevsa, Nevesah, Nesa, Nesi, Nessa, Nessi, Nessie, Nessy, Nesta, Neysa, Oona, Oonagh, Oonah, Senga.** International: **Aignéis** *(Irish Gaelic),* **Nesta** *(Welsh),* **Ynes, Ynez** *(French, Spanish),* **Oanez** *(Breton),* **Agne, Agnella, Agnesca, Agnese, Agnesina, Agnola, Anete, Hagne** *(Italian),* **Agnese, Inesa** *(Spanish),* **Ines, Inez** *(Spanish, Portuguese),* **Anneke** *(Dutch),* **Agna, Agnethe, Anke, Antje** *(German),* **Agnethe, Agne, Agnek, Agneta** *(Scandinavian),* **Agnesa, Agneska, Anezka, Anka** *(Czech),* **Agnessa, Agnia, Inessa, Nessa** *(Russian)* **Neza** *(Slavic).*

AGRIPPINA. *Latin, 'born feet-first'.* Sister of Caligula and mother of Nero, who had her murdered. The original male version, Agrippa, can also used for girls – but who would want to? **Agrafina, Agrippa, Agrippine.**

AIBHILIN. *(ev-lin) Irish variation of* EVELYN. Makes Evelyn more exotic, but ultimately too difficult.

AIDA. *(eye-EE-da) Arabic, 'reward, present'.* Operatic. **Aeeda, Aidah, Aidan, Aide, Aidee, Aiden, Ayeeda, Ieeda, Iyeeda.**

♂ **AIDAN.** *Irish, 'little and fiery'.* Ancient Irish saint's name that's popular for boys and is taking off with girls as well. **Adan, Adann, Adanne, Aden, Adin, Adon, Adyn, Adynn, Adynne, Aidana, Aidann, Aidanna, Aidanne, Aiden, Aidin, Aidon, Aidyn, Aidynn, Aidynne, Aydan, Ayden, Aydenn, Aydin, Aydon, Aydyn, Aydynn, Aydynne, Edan.**

AIKO. *(ah-ee-ko) Japanese, 'love child'.* Very common Japanese name that is rarely heard outside the Asian community.

AILANI. *Hawaiian, 'chief'.* Lilting and lovely. **Aelani, Ailana.**

AILBHE. *(al-va) Irish, 'noble, bright'.* While Irish Gaelic spellings add intrigue to a name, they'll prove endlessly confusing. **Alva, Alvy, Elvy.**

AILEEN. *Irish variation of* HELEN. Never as popular as Eileen, and now both are out. **Aila, Ailean, Ailec, Aileena, Ailen, Ailene, Alley, Ailli, Aili, Ailie, Ailina, Ailine, Ailinn, Aillen, Aleen, Alene, Aline, Alline, Eileen, Eleen, Ellene, Ileana, Ileane, Ileanna, Ileen, Ilene, Iliana, Iliane, Ilianna, Illeanne, Illene, Leana, Leanah, Leanna, Leannah, Lena, Lenah, Liana, Lianna, Liannah, Lina, Linah.** International: **Ailinn** *(Portuguese),* **Aili** *(Finnish).*

AILSA. *(AYL-suh) Scottish place name.* Traditionally Scottish name – after the island called Ailsa Craig – that might make a good alternative to the overused Ashley or Ella. **Ailis, Ailse, Ailsha, Allasa Elsa, Elsha, Elshe.**

Irish Names That Aren't Overused

Áine

Aislinn

Aoife

Bidelia

Caoimhe

Ciara

Clodagh

Eimear

Fionnuala

Grainne

Juno

Maeve

Niamh

Orla

Roisin

Saoirse

Sinead

Sorcha

AIMÉE. *French, 'beloved'.* Whether you pronounce it like the original Amy or the Frenchified Ay-may, this form adds considerable élan to an old favourite. **Aime, Aimey,** Aimi, Aimia, Aimie, Aimy, Amey, Amie.

ÁINE. *(an-ya) Irish, 'brilliance, wit'.* Name of a fertility goddess said to confer luck on its bearer, though to avoid confusion you may want to use the phonetic spelling Anya or Enya. **Anne, Anya, Enya.**

♂**AINSLEY.** *Scottish, 'one's own meadow'.* While theoretically unisex, this surname name has been edging up the girls' list, perhaps as an Ashley substitute. **Ainslea, Ainslee, Ainsleigh, Ainslie, Ainsly, Ansley, Aynslee, Aynsley, Aynslie.**

♂ **AIR.** *Word name.* Airy hippy dippy nature name, à la River or Sky. **Aer.**

AISHA. *(eye-EE-sha) Arabic, 'woman'; Swahili, 'life'.* Aisha was Muhammad's favourite wife, making this lovely name and its myriad variations increasingly popular. **Aaisha, Aaishah, Aeesha, Aeeshah, Aesha, Aeshah, Aheesha, Aiasha, Aiesha, Aieshah, Aisa, Aischa, Aish, Aishah, Aisheh, Aishia, Aishiah, Aisia, Aisiah, Aixa, Aiyesha, Aiysha, Asha, Ashah,** Ashia, Ashiah, Asia, Asiah, Ayeesa, Ayeesah, Ayeesha, Ayeeshah, Ayeisa, Ayeisah, Ayeisha, Ayeishah, Ayesha, Ayisa, Ayisah, Ayisha, Ayishah, Aysa, Ayse, Aytza, Ieasha, Ieashah, Ieashia, Ieashiah, Iesha, Ieshah, Ieesha, Ieeshah, Ieeshia, Ieeshiah, Yiesha, Yieshah.

AISLINN. *(ash-lin) Irish, 'dream'.* Old Irish name that's taken off in its phonetic forms, mainly Ashlyn or Ashlynn. **Aishellyn, Aishlinn, Aislee, Aisley, Aislin, Aisling, Aislyn, Aislynne, Ashling, Ashlyn, Ashlynn, Isleen.**

AITHNE. *(et-na) Irish, 'fire'.* This soundalike for the famous volcano, Mount Etna, is far more unusual and less attractive than its male equivalent, Aidan. **Aine, Aithnea, Eithne, Ena, Ethnah, Ethnea, Ethnee.**

AJA. *Hindi, 'goat'.* Sounds like and is often confused with Asia, though it has an air of retro cool via the seminal Steely Dan album. **Ahjah, Aija, Aijah, Aijiah, Ajá, Ajada, Ajah, Ajara, Ajaran, Ajare, Ajaree, Ajhia, Aji, Ajia, Ajjia, Azha.**

AKILAH. *Arabic, 'intelligent, logical'.* Rhythmic and exotic. Aikiela, Aikilah, Akeela, Akeelah, Akeila, Akeilah, Akeiyla, Akiela, Akielah, Akila, Akilaih, Akili, Akilia, Akilla, Akillah, Akkila, Akyla, Akylah.

♂ **AKIVA.** *Hebrew, 'to protect, shelter'.* Strong name used in Israel. Akeeva, Akiba, Keeva, Keevah, Kiba, Kibah, Kiva, Kivah, Kivi.

ALABAMA. *Place name.* In the US, hot new southern place name, picking up from Georgia and Savannah.

ALAIA. *(al-EYE-a) Arabic, 'sublime'.* Fashion designer surname could make exotic first.

ALAIR. *Variation of* **HILARY.** Firmer form of Hilary. Alaira, Ali, Allaire.

ALALA. *Greek mythology.* Rhythmic ancient name belonging to the mythological sister of Ares.

ALANA. *Irish, feminine variation of* **ALAN.** Not a bad way to honour Grandpa Alan . . . or Grandma Helen or Elaine. Alaana, Alaina, Alaine, Alanaa, Alanae, Alanah, Alane, Alanea, Alani, Alania, Alanis, Alanna, Alannah, Alawna, Alayna, Alayne, Alene, Aleyna, Aleynah, Aleyne, Aileen, Allana, Allanah, Allena, Ailene, Alleynah, Alleyne, Allina, Allinah, Allyn, Allyna, Alonna, Lana, Lanah, Lanna, Lannah.

♂ **ALANI.** *Hawaiian, 'orange tree'.* More appealing than most other Alan equivalents. Alaini, Alainie, Alania, Alanie, Alaney, Alannie.

ALANIS. *Variation of* **ALANA.** Singer Alanis Morissette made this twist famous.

ALBA. *Latin, 'white'.* Many two-syllable names that start and end in vowels are coming back . . . but not Alba. Albana, Albane, Albani, Albanie, Albany, Albeni, Albina, Albine, Albinia, Albinka, Alva, Elba. **International: Albane** *(French).*

♂ **ALBANY.** *Place name.* The Beckhams have put Brooklyn on the map. Albany – also in New York State – not yet.

ALBERTA. *English, feminine variation of* **ALBERT.** Jazzy old name that could make a comeback, the way Josephine and Ella have. Alberthine, Albertina, Albertine, Albertyna, Albertyne, Auberta, Aubertha, Auberthe, Aubine, Alverta, Berry, Bert, Berta, Berte, Berti, Bertie, Berty, Elberta, Elbertha, Elberthina, Elberthine, Elbertina, Elbertine. **International: Albertine, Auberte** *(French).*

ALBINIA. *Latin, 'white, fair'.* The original male name Alban is a lot sleeker and more usable. Alba, Albina, Alva, Alvina, Aubine.

ALCHEMY. *Latin word name.* One of the most extreme of the new word names, recommended only to the most mystical-minded parents. Metallica hard-rocker Lars Hendrickson spelled his daughter's name Alchamy.

♂ **ALCOTT.** *English, 'dweller at the old cottage'.* Intriguing alternative that goes beyond Louisa and May, for *Little Women* fans.

ALDA. *German, 'old, prosperous'.* Old, indeed. **Aldabella, Aldea, Aldina, Aldine, Aleda, Alida.**

♀ **ALDEN.** *English, 'old, wise friend'.* Tired male surname name that sounds fresh and modern for a girl. **Aldan, Aldon, Aldyn, Alten, Alton.**

ALEAH. *Arabic, 'high, exalted'; Persian, 'God's being'.* Simple and melodic. **Aileah, Ala, Alah, Alea, Aleea, Aleeah, Aleia, Aleiah, Alia, Allea, Alleah, Alleea, Alleeah.**

ALEELA. *Swahili, 'she cries'.* Lilting African name that translates perfectly into other cultures. **Aleelah, Alila, Alile.**

ALEESHA. *Variation of* **ALICIA.** Beginning to be heard more frequently since the birth of the Eastenders baby.

ALEEZA. *Hebrew, 'joy'.* One of the most energetic and exotic of the legion of Alyssa/Alicia/Eliza names. **Aleezah, Aleiza, Alieza, Aliezah, Aliza, Alizah, Alitza, Leeza.**

ALEJANDRA. *(al-eh-HAHN-dra) Spanish, feminine variation of* **ALEJANDRO.** The Spanish form of this popular and multivaried name is attracting good reviews outside the Latino community. **Alandra, Alejandrina, Alexandra.**

ALETHEA. *Greek, 'truth'.* Alicia, with a lisp. **Alathea, Alathia, Aleethia, Aleta, Aletea, Aletha, Aletheia, Alethia, Aletia, Aletta, Alette, Alithea, Alithia, Elethea, Elethia.**

♀ **ALEX.** *Diminutive of* **ALEXANDER, ALEXIS.** One of the most evenly divided unisex names these days; strong and energetic, if overused, for both genders. **Aleix, Aleks, Alexe, Alexx, Alix, Allex, Allexx, Alyx.**

★**ALEXA.** *Diminutive of* **ALEXANDRA.** This simple and most feminine form of the Alexi group retains the greatest freshness, although it's already in with the-in crowd. **Aleixa, Alekia, Aleksa, Aleksha, Aleksi, Alexha, Alexsa, Alexssa, Alexxa, Allexa, Alyxa.**

ALEXANDRA. *Greek, 'man's defender'.* The feminine form of Alexander has been consistent in the bottom half of the Top 100. Why? It's strong, tasteful, and elegant, maintaining a chic aura despite its popularity, has a solid historic pedigree and offers an array of softer nicknames. **Alaxandra, Alecsandra, Aleczandra, Aleksandra, Alesandra, Alessandra, Alex, Alexanda, Alexande, Alexandera, Alexandere, Alexandrea, Alexandreana, Alexandretta, Alexandria, Alexane, Alexea, Alexene, Alexes, Alexi, Alexus, Alexxandra, Alexys, Alexzandra, Alissandre, Alissandrine, Alix, Alixandra, Allessa, Allessandra, Allex, Allexa, Allexandra, Allexandrina, Allexina, Allexine, Alissandre, Alissandrine, Allix, Ally, Alyx, Alyxandra, Cesya, Etena, Lesy, Lesya, Lexandra, Lexi, Lexie, Lexy, Lissandre, Lissandrine, Sandi, Sandie, Sandra, Sandy, Sandye, Sanndra, Sasha, Sohndra, Sondra, Xandra, Xandy, Zandra, Zandy, Zohndra, Zondra.**

ALEXANDRIA. *Variation of* **ALEXANDRA.** Turns Alexandra into a more distinctive place name, in both Egypt and Virginia. **Alaxandria, Alecsandria, Aleczandria, Alexanderine,**

Alexandrea, Alexandrena, Alexandrie, Alexandrina, Alexandrine, Alexandrya, Alexanndria, Alexendria, Alexendrine, Alexia, Alixandrea, Alyxandria.

ALEXIA. *Diminutive of* **ALEXANDRIA.** A pretty name, but it has a slightly pharmaceutical aura. **Aleksia, Aleska, Alexcia, Alexea, Alexsia, Alexsiya, Allexia, Alyxia.**

ALEXINA. *Feminine variation of* **ALEX.** Trying too hard to stand out from the sea of Alexes.

♂ **ALEXIS.** *English variation of* **ALEXIOS.** This one-time Russian boys' name has surpassed sister Alexandra in popularity in the US, where it has made the Top 5. **Aalexis, Ahlexis, Alaxis, Alecsis, Alecxis, Aleexis, Aleksis, Alessa, Alessi, Alexa, Alexcis, Alexi, Alexia, Alexias, Alexiou, Alexiss, Alexiz, Alexsis, Alexxis, Alexys, Alixis, Allexis, Elexis, Lexi, Lexie, Lexis, Lexy. International: Alessia** *(Italian).*

Alexandra's International Variations

Irish	Alastríona
Scottish	Alexina, Kina, Saundra
French	Alexandrie, Alexandrina, Alexandrine, Alexine, Alexius, Sacha, Sandrine
Italian	Alessa, Alessandra, Alessia
Spanish	Alajandra, Alandra, Alandria, Alastrina, Alastriona, Alejandra, Alejandrina, Aleka, Alessanda, Alessandra, Alessandrina, Alessia, Alexa, Alexanderia, Alexandrina, Alexandrita, Alexena, Alexia, Alexina, Ali, Alista, Alla, Alli, Alondra, Anda, Drina, Elena, Lesy, Lexi, Sanda, Sandi, Sandra, Sandrina, Sasha, Sondra, Xandra, Zandra, Zondra
Dutch	Xandra
German	Alexis, Alexius
Polish	Ala, Aleska, Alka, Ola, Olesia
Hungarian	Alexa, Elek, Eli, Lekszi
Czech	Ales, Leska, Lexa, Olexa
Russian	Aleks, Aleksandra, Aleksandrina, Aleksasha, Aleksey, Alesha, Alya, Lelya, Lesya, Oleska, Olesya, Sasa, Sasha, Shura, Shurka
Bulgarian	Alekko, Aleksey, Aleksi, Sander
Ukrainian	Olesya
Greek	Aleka, Alexiou, Ritsa

ALFONSINE. *German, feminine variation of* **ALPHONSE.** Try explaining to your teenager why you named her this. **Alfonsa, Alfonsia, Alonza, Alphonsina.**

ALFREDA. *English, 'elf power', feminine variation of* **ALFRED.** Elf power? We weren't crazy about it even before we knew that. **Alfi, Alfie, Alfre, Alfredah, Alfredda, Alfredia, Alfreeda, Alfreida, Alfri, Alfried, Alfrieda, Alfryda, Alfy, Allfie, Allfreda, Allfredah, Allfredda, Allfrie, Allfrieda, Allfry, Allfryda, Allfy, Elfie, Elfre, Elfrea, Elfredah, Elfredda, Elfreeda, Elfrida, Elfrieda, Elfryda, Elfrydah, Ellfreda, Ellfredah, Ellfredda, Ellfreeda, Ellfrida, Ellfrieda, Ellfryda, Ellfrydah, Elva, Elvah, Freda, Freddi, Freddie, Freddy, Fredi, Fredy, Freeda, Freedah, Frieda, Friedah, Fryda, Frydah.**

♂ **ALI.** *Swahili, 'exalted'.* A sweet, simple short form, balanced enough to stand on its own. **Allea, Alli, Allie, Ally, Aly.**

★**ALICE.** *German, 'noble'.* A classic name that's both strong and sweet, Alice remains popular, though it's slipping down the Top 50. Bonus: it's a darling of literature, from the immortal heroine in *Alice in Wonderland* to fine modern writers like Alices Munro, Walker, Sebold, Hoffman, McDermott, Adams, and Elliott Dark. **Adelice, Aleceea, Alecia, Aleece, Aleetheea, Aleethia, Alessa, Alesia, Ali, Alicah, Alicea, Alicen, Alicia, Alicie, Alidee, Alie, Aliece, Alikah, Aliki, Alis, Alisah, Alisann, Alisanne, Alise, Alisha, Alison, Alissa, Alisz, Alitheea, Alitia, Alix, Alise, Alia, Alla, Allecia, Alleece, Alleeceea, Alles, Alless, Alie, Alli, Allice, Allicea, Allie, Allis, Allise, Allison, Allissa, Allisun, Allisunne, Allix, Allsun, Ally, Allyce, Allyceea, Allys, Allyse, Allysia, Allysiah, Allyson, Allyssa, Allysson, Alyce, Alyceea, Alys, Alysa, Alyse, Alysia, Alyson, Alyss, Alyssa, Alysse, Elissa, Elli, Ellie, Ellissa, Ellsa, Elsa, Elyssa, Ilysa, Ilysah, Ilyssa, Ilysse, Leece, Leese, Lissa, Lyssa, Talicia.** International: **Ailis** *(Irish),* **Aili** *(Scottish),* **Alicia, Licha** *(Spanish),* **Aliz Ala, Alisia** *(Polish),* *(Hungarian),* **Alica.**

(Czech), **Alisa** *(Bulgarian),* **Alisa, Alya** *(Russian),* **Alike, Aliz, Alizka, Lici** *(Greek),* **Aleka, Alika** *(Hawaiian).*

ALICIA. *Variation of* **ALICE.** Almost as popular as its mother name for several years, but it lacks Alice's classic character. **Aelicia, Alaysha, Alaysia, Alecea, Alecia, Aleecia, Ali, Alicea, Alicha, Alichia, Aliciah, Alician, Alicja, Alicya, Aliecia, Alisha, Allicea, Allicia, Alycia, Alyssia, Ilysa.**

ALIKA. *Hawaiian, 'truthful'; Swahili, 'most beautiful'.* Multicultural choice that's far off the beaten track. **Aleeki, Aleka, Alica, Alikah, Alike, Alikee, Aliki, Alliki.**

ALINA. *Variation of* **HELEN.** One of the scores of global variations on the classic Helen. **Aleen, Aleena, Alena, Alenah, Alene, Aliana, Alianna, Alinah, Aline, Alinna, Alleen, Allena, Allene, Alline, Allyna, Allynah, Allyne, Alyna, Alynna, Alynnah, Alyne, Alyona, Leena, Leenah, Lena, Lenah, Lina, Linah, Lyna, Lynah.**

ALISA. *Hebrew, 'great happiness'.* Less popular than more complicated forms like Alyssa or Alicia, perhaps because of its association with the once-overused Lisa. **Alisah, Alissa, Alissah, Alitza, Alitzah, Aliza, Allisa, Allisah, Allissa, Allissah, Allysa, Allysah, Alyssa, Alyssah.**

ALISHA. *Sanskrit, 'protected by God'; also phonetic spelling of* **ALICIA.** Member of the well-populated Alice family with overly literal spelling. **Aaleasha, Aaliesha, Aalisha, Aleasha, Aleesha, Aleisha, Alesha, Ali, Aliesha, Aliscia, Alishah, Alishay, Alishaye, Alishia, Alishya, Alisia, Alissia, Alitsha, Allisha, Allysha, Alysha.**

ALISON. *Scottish, diminutive of* **ALICE.** Widely used since the 1950s, surpassing the original in popularity. **Ali, Alicen, Alicyn, Alisan, Alisann, Alisanne, Alisen, Alisenne, Alisin, Alision, Alisonn, Alisoun, Alisson, Alisun, Allecenne, Alles, Allese, Alleyson, Allice, Allicen, Allicenne, Allie, Allisan, Allisann, Allisanne, Allisen, Allison, Allisoun, Allisson, Allisyn, Allix, Allsun, Ally, Allysann, Allysanne, Allyson, Allysoun, Alysan, Alysann, Alysanne, Alysen, Alyson, Alysoun, Alysun.**

ALIX. *Diminutive of* **ALEXANDRA,** *spelling variation of* **ALEX.** Just like Alex, except you have to spell it every time. **Alex, Alexa, Alexis, Aliki, Aliks, Alixe, Alixia, Allix, Allyx, Alyx.**

ALIZA. *Hebrew, 'joyful'.* The z adds zip. **Aleeza, Aleiza, Aliezа, Aliezah, Alitza, Aliz, Alizah, Alise, Alisee.**

ALIZABETH. *Variation of* **ELIZABETH.** Why make your child's life more complicated than it has to be? **Alyzabeth.**

ALIZÉE. *(al-ee-ZAY) French, 'trade wind'.* This exotic name of a hot young French singer is catching on. **Alise, Aliseh.**

★**ALLEGRA.** *Italian, 'joyous'.* In music, the term allegro means 'quickly, lively tempo,' which makes this still-unusual and quintessential ballet dancer's name all the more appealing. **Ally, Alegra, Alegria, Allegretta, Allegro, Lally, Legra, Leggra.**

ALLENA. *See* **ALANA.** **Alana, Alanicc, Alanis, Alanna, Alena, Alene, Allana, Allene, Alleyne, Allynn, Allynne, Allyn, Alynne.**

ALLURA. *French, 'to entice, attract'.* Sounds like a princess – or an enticingly evil witch – in a fairy tale. **Alloura, Alura.**

ALMA. *Latin, 'soul'.* This somewhat solemn name had a burst of popularity a century ago, then faded into the flowered wallpaper – heard mostly in the term *alma mater.* Always well used in Hispanic families, it could just make a comeback, à la Ella; appreciated for its simplicity and soul. **Almah, Allma.**

ALMOND. *Word name.* Gwyneth Paltrow's Apple has opened the world of botanical names beyond flowers to trees, herbs, fruits, and – why not? – nuts. **Almandina, Almandine, Almondine, Amande, Amandina.**

ALOHA. *Polynesian, 'love'.* This familiar Hawaiian greeting is, à la the Hebrew Shalom, occasionally used for babies.

ALOISIA. *German, 'famous fighter'.* Inventive female form of Aloysius. **Aloisa, Aloysia, Eloisia, Eloysia.**

ALOUETTE. *French, 'lark'.* Gallic twist in the stylish

bird name genre. **Allouette, Alouetta, Alowette.**

ALPHA. *Greek, first letter of the alphabet.* Also the brightest star in every constellation, this would make an interesting choice for a first daughter, though it does give off some spectral sci-fi reverberations. **Alfa, Aphia, Aphra.**

ALTA. *Latin, 'elevated'.* A meaning that might raise a child's self-esteem. **Allta, Altah, Altana, Altanna, Altea, Alto.**

ALTHEA. *Greek, 'with healing power'.* Poetic, almost ethereal name found in Greek myth and pastoral poetry, associated with Althea Gibson, the great black tennis player. **Altha, Althaia, Altheda, Altheya, Althia, Althiaa, Altheda, Althelia, Althia, Eltha, Elthea, Eltheya, Elthia, Thea.**

ALTON. *See* **ALDEN.**

ALURA. *English, 'god-like adviser'.* Stems from a different root than Allura, but has the same feel. **Alurea, Allura, Ellura.**

♂ **ALVA.** *Spanish, 'blond, fair-skinned'; Hebrew, 'foliage'.* Best

known as Thomas Edison's middle name, but sounds distinctly, if frumpily, female. **Alba, Albina, Albine, Albinia, Alvah, Alvana, Alvanna, Alvannah, Alver, Alvit.**

ALVINA. *English, 'noble friend' or 'elf-friend'.* No more stylish than the original Alvin. **Alveanea, Alveen, Alveena, Alveene, Alveenia, Alvenea, Alvie, Alvinae, Alvincia, Alvine, Alvinea, Alvineca, Alvinesha, Alvinia, Alvinna, Alvita, Alvona, Alvyna, Alwin, Alwina, Alwyn, Alwyne, Elveena, Elvena, Elvene, Elvenia, Elvina, Elvine, Elvinia, Vina, Vinni, Vinnie, Vinny.** **International: Alwyne** *(Scottish).*

ALYSSA. *English variation of* **ALICIA.** Hugely popular name in the US, related to the flower alyssum as well as to the classic Alice and variants. **Ahlyssa, Alissa, Allisa, Allissa, Allyssa, Alyesa, Alyessa, Alyissa, Alysa, Alysah, Alysia, Elissa, Ilyssa, Lyssa, Lyssah.**

AMABEL. *French, 'beautiful lover'.* Older than Annabel and a lot more distinctive. Worth consideration, even though your child will have to explain that

no, her name is *not* Annabel. **Ama, Amabelle, Annabelle, Belle, Mab, Mabel.**

AMADEA. *(ah-mah-DAY-a) Latin, 'God's beloved'.* Strong and musical feminine form of Amadeus, as in Mozart. **Amada, Amadee, Amadi, Amadia, Amadita, Amadore, Amadora, Amata, Amedee.**

AMALFI. *Italian place name.* Better as a picturesque town on the Italian Riviera than as a name. **Amalfey, Malfie.**

AMALIA. *(ah-MAH-lee-a or ah-mah-LEE-a) German, 'industrious'.* Italian, German, and Dutch twist on Amelia, recently chosen for the Dutch royal baby. **Ahmalia, Amalberta, Amaleah, Amalee, Amaleta, Amalfried, Amalgunde, Amali, Amalija, Amalina, Amalisa, Amaliya, Amaly, Amalya, Amalyn.** **International: Amalie** *(French),* **Amila, Amalita, Amelida, Amelina, Emala** *(Spanish),* **Amalea, Amelie, Amilia** *(German),* **Amalja, Amelja** *(Polish),* **Mali, Malika** *(Hungarian).*

AMANDA. *Latin, 'much-loved'.*

After a long run as the prettiest name around, this romantic name is losing some of its glossy sheen, though it's still lovely. Possible alternatives: the French Amandine or Shakespearean Miranda. **Amada, Amanada, Amandah, Amandalee, Amandalyn, Amandi, Amandie, Amandine, Amandy, Amata, Manda, Mandaline, Mandee, Mandi, Mandie, Mandy.** International: **Amande, Amandine** *(French)*.

AMANI. *Variation of* **IMANI.** Growing in popularity due to similarity to Armani. **Aamani, Ahmani, Aman, Amane, Amanee, Amaney, Amanie, Ammanu.**

AMARA. *Greek, 'lovely forever'.* Strong, attractive, stylish, with an appealing meaning. **Amar, Amaira, Amairani, Amarah, Amargo, Amargoe, Amargot, Amari, Amaria, Amariah, Amarinda, Amaris, Amarra, Amarrinda, Mara, Marra.**

AMARANTHA. *Greek, 'deathless'.* Botanical name whose mythical equivalent was believed to be immortal. **Amarande, Amaranta, Amarante.** International: **Amaranta** *(Spanish)*.

♂ **AMARI.** *Hebrew, 'eternal'.* Related to names and words in a range of languages – Yoruba, Thai, Hebrew (where it's used primarily for boys) – and with a variety of positive meanings. This inventive, lively choice is gaining notice among American parents.

♂ **AMARIAH.** *Hebrew, 'said of God'.* The name of nine minor male biblical characters, this could make a gender switch as a substitution for the popular Mariah. **Amaria, Amarissa, Amarit, Amarys, Maris.**

AMARYLLIS. *Greek flower name.* Showier name than Lily, but in the same botanical family. **Amarilis, Amarillis, Amarylis.**

AMAYA. *Japanese, 'night rain'.* Growing use relates to the popular name Maya rather than the Japanese root.

AMBER. *Word name.* Still in the Top 50, but Ruby, Jade, or Pearl sound fresher. **Aamber, Ahmber, Ambar, Amberia, Amberise, Amberly, Ambria, Ambur, Ambyr, Ambyre, Ammber, Ember.** International: **Ambrette** *(French)*, **Ambra** *(Italian)*, **Inbar** *(Israeli)*.

Names That Mean Beautiful

Alana
Amara
Anahi
Arabella
Belinda
Bella
Belle
Bonita
Bonnie
Calla
Callista
Hermosa
Ilona
Jamilla
Jolie
Linda
Mei
Mirabella
Naava
Ramana
Rosalind
Shaina
Shakila
Vashti
Venus
Zaina

AMBROSIA. *Greek and Roman mythology name, 'food of the gods'.* Heavenly, if you like your names over the top.

★**AMELIA.** *Variation of* EMILY. Lovely Victorian name, with heroic connection to aviatrix Amelia Earhart, that's on the rise as an alternative to the overused Emily and Amanda. It has made it to the Top 20 in recent years. Warning: we think it could climb even closer to the top. Aemilia, Aimilia, Amaleeda, Amali, Amalia, Amalida, Amalie, Amaliya, Ameila, Ameilia, Amelida, Amelie, Amelina, Ameline, Amelisa, Amelita, Amella, Ami, Amie, Amilia, Amilie, Amilina, Amilisa, Amilita, Amilyn, Amylia, Emelie, Emelina, Emeline, Emelita, Emilia, Emilie, Emily, Emilya, Melia. International: Amilia *(Scottish)*, Amalie, Amelie, Emilie *(French)*, Ama, Amelcia, Melcia *(Polish)*, Amalia, Emilia, Ilma, Malcsi, Mali, Malika *(Hungarian)*, Amalia, Milica *(Czech)*.

AMÉLIE. *French variation of* AMELIA *or* EMILY. French favourite that recently entered the Top 10, perhaps thanks to the film of that name. **Amalie.**

AMENA. *Celtic, 'honest, utterly pure'.* Possible Born Again name – Amen! – in the same class as the rising Neveah (that's Heaven spelled backwards) and Trinity. **Amina, Amine.**

♂ **AMERICA.** *Place name.* Given to children of both sexes as far back as colonial times, this carries a lot of baggage and might be easier to handle as a middle name. **Americana, Americanna, Amerika.** International: **Amérique** *(French)*.

AMETHYST. *Gem name.* This purple birthstone for February could make a comeback, as Ruby and Diamond have.

AMICA. *Latin, 'friend'.* An ancient name with a likeable meaning and well suited to modern style.

AMINA. *Arabic, 'trustworthy, faithful'.* The name of the mother of the prophet Muhammad is well used among Muslims everywhere. **Aamena, Aamina, Aaminah, Ameena, Ameenah, Aminah, Aminata, Aminda, Amindah.**

AMINTA. *Greek, 'defender'.* One of the romantic names favoured by British pastoral poets, more appealing in its longer form, Araminta. **Amintah, Amynta.**

AMIRA. *Hebrew, Arabic, feminine variation of* AMIR. This shimmery name, often given to girls born on the harvest feast of Shavuot, and also used in the Arab community, is increasing in popularity. **Ameera, Ameerah, Amirah.**

AMITA. *Sanskrit, 'infinite'.* Feminine form of Amit that's simple and lyrical and close in spirit to a familiar term for friendship. **Amitah, Amyta, Amytah.**

★**AMITY.** *Latin, 'friendship'.* What nicer gift to give your little girl than a name that signifies friendship and harmony? This virtue name is also more rhythmic and feminine than the single-syllable Hope, Faith, and Grace. **Amitee, Amiti, Amitie.**

♂ **AMORY.** *German, 'industrious leader'.* A prime candidate for feminisation, best known for the hero of Fitzgerald's *This Side of Paradise;* could rise as a stand-in for Emily or Avery. **Amery, Amoree, Amorey, Amori, Amorie.**

AMY. *Latin, 'beloved'; French, 'friend'.* One of the Top 25 for the last few years, Amy remains a short, sweet *Little Women*–style classic. **Aami, Aime, Amatia, Amecia, Amee, Amey, Amia, Amiah, Amice, Amie, Amiee, Amii, Amiiee, Amio, Amiya, Ammee, Ammie, Ammiee, Ammy, Amye, Amylyn. International: Aimeé, Amelie** *(French),* **Amalia, Amadea** *(Italian),* **Amada, Amata** *(Spanish),* **Amata** *(Swedish),* **Ema** *(Romanian),* **Amaliya** *(Russian).*

ANA. *Variation of* **HANNAH.** Pared-down form loses none of the name's grace or power. **Anai, Anaia, Anita, Anna.**

ANAHÍ. *Spanish, 'beautiful like the flower'.* Popular Mexican actress is making this unusual choice better known. **Anahi.**

ANAHITA. *Persian, 'a river and water goddess'.* Stylish choice. **Anahai, Anahi, Anahit, Anahy.**

ANAÏS. *(an-EYE-is* or *an-AY-is) Hebrew, 'gracious'; also French Provençal version of* **ANNE.** An unusual, exotic name forever attached to daring French-born American novelist and diarist Anaïs Nin – and later used for a popular perfume – that would make an attractive, creative choice.

ANALA. *Hindi, 'fire'.* Indian choice in step with American and British styles.

ANALISA. *Combination of* **ANNA** *and* **LISA.** Unlike most combination names, this elegant blend – related to the German Anneliese – is more than the sum of its parts. **Analice, Analicia, Analis, Analise, Analisha, Analisia, Analissa, Annalisa.**

ANAMARIA. *Combination of* **ANA** *and* **MARIA.** More feminine and stylish than Anne-Marie. **Anamarie, Anamary, Annamaria.**

ANANDA. *Hindi, 'bliss'.* Genuine Indian name some parents turn to as an Amanda alternative; also connected to a network of spiritual communities. **Anda.**

★**ANASTASIA.** *Feminine variation of* **ANASTASIOS.** This regal Russian name is now a viable – and increasingly popular – option, elegantly beautiful. An apt choice for an Easter or spring baby. **Ana, Anastacia, Anastascia, Anastase, Anastashia, Anastassya, Anastasya, Anastatia, Anastay, Anastaysia, Anastazia, Anastice, Anasztasia, Anestassia, Annastasia, Annastazia, Anstass, Anstice, Asia, Nastassia, Stace, Stacee, Stacey, Staci, Stacia, Stacie, Stacy, Stasia, Stasiya, Taisie, Tasiya. International: Anastasie** *(French, German),* **Tasia** *(Spanish),* **Anastazja, Anatazja, Nastka, Nastusia** *(Polish),* **Anasztaizia** *(Hungarian),* **Anastászie, Nast'a, Stasa, Staska** *(Czech),* **Anastasiya, Anastassia, Asya, Nastasia, Nastasya, Nastya, Stasya, Taskenka, Tasya** *(Russian),* **Anastacia, Anastasha, Natasa, Tasia, Tasoula** *(Greek).*

ANATOLA. *Greek, 'from the east'.* Attractive place name of a beautiful resort region of Turkey. **Anatolia, Anatolya. International: Anatalya** *(Russian).*

ANDI. *Diminutive of* **ANDREA.** Nickname name that seemed cool in the Ricki/Terri generation. **Ande, Andea, Andee, Andie, Andy.**

ANDORRA. *European place name.* Pretty name of a pocket-sized princedom in the Pyrenees, noted for its skiing. **Andora.**

ANDRA. *Variation of* **ANDREA.** Arty 1970s name usually pronounced *AHN-dra.*

♂ **ANDREA.** *Feminine variation of* **ANDREAS.** Feminine form of Andrew (and a male name in several European cultures) with a choice of pronunciations, whose popularity, while never huge, has remained surprisingly steady. **Aindrea, Andee, Andelis, Andera, Andere, Anderea, Andi, Andis, Andra, Andrae, Andrah, Andraia, Andraya, Andre, Andreah, Andreaka, Andreana, Andreane, Andreanna, Andreas, Andree, Andrée, Andreea, Andreena, Andreia, Andreina, Andreja, Andreka, Andrel, Andrell, Andrelle, Andreo, Andresa, Andressa, Andretta, Andrette, Andrewena, Andrewina, Andreya, Andri, Andria,** Andriana, Andrianna, Andricka, Andrieka, Andrietta, Andrina, Andrine, Andris, Andy, Aundrea, Ohndrea, Ohndreea, Ohndria, Ondrea, Ondreea, Ondria, Onndrea, Onndreea, Onndria.

ANDRÉE. *(AHN-dray) French variation of* **ANDREA.** Gilding the lily.

ANDROMEDA. *Greek mythology name.* Beautiful daughter of Cassiopeia who, like her mother, became a star.

ANEKO. *Japanese, 'older sister'.* If you're planning to have a younger one.

ANEMONE. *(ah-NEM-oh-nee) Greek, 'breath', flower name.* Flower name taken from a mythological nymph who was turned into a flower by the wind; an interesting, if challenging, choice. **Anemona, Ann-Aymone, Anne-Aymone.**

♂ **ANGEL.** *Word name.* Many more sightings of earthly Angels of both sexes have been reported recently, but be aware that a good proportion of them are Latin males. **Angele, Angéle,** Angell, Angelle, Angil, Anjel. International: **Anela** *(Hawaiian).*

ANGELA. *Italian from Greek, feminine variation of* **ANGELO.** Widely used through most of the twentieth century, but now seems terminally dated. **Andzela, Anela, Anelja, Angala, Anganita, Angel, Angelanell, Angelanette, Angele, Angeleigh, Angelene, Angeles, Angeleta, Angeli, Angelic, Angelica, Angelina, Angella, Angelle, Angellina, Angellita, Angi, Angie, Angil, Angiola, Angy, Angyola, Anjali, Anjel, Anjela, Anjele, Anjelica, Anjelina, Anjella, Anji, Anjie, Anjy, Anngela, Anngil, Anngilla, Anngiola, Annjela, Aniujilla, Anyelle, Ohngel, Ohnjella, Onngelle, Onnjelia.** International: **Ange, Angéle, Angelette, Angeline** *(French),* **Angelina** *(Italian, Spanish, Russian, and Greek),* **Ange, Angele, Angeles, Angelia, Angelita** *(Spanish),* **Anhelina** *(Russian),* **Ange, Angele, Angeliki** *(Greek),* **Erela, Erelah** *(Hebrew),* **Fereshteh** *(Persian),* **Anakela** *(Hawaiian).*

★**ANGELICA.** *Latin, 'angelic'.* Lacy and poetic, this is by far the best choice among the many forms of the angelic names – but other kids might relate it to the nasty nursery-schooler Angelica C. Pickles on *Rugrats.* **Angalic, Angelic, Angelici, Angelicia, Angelike, Angeliki, Angelisa, Angelissa, Angellica, Angilica, Angyalka, Anjelica, Anjelika, Anyelika. International: Angélique** *(French),* **Angelika** *(German).*

ANGELINA. *Diminutive of* **ANGELA.** Ms Jolie's star power has changed its image from delicate to intense – unless you think about the ballet-crazy mouse of *Angelina Ballerina.* **Angalena, Angalina, Angeleana, Angeleen, Angelena, Angelene, Angeliana, Angellina, Angelyn, Angelyna, Angelyne, Angelynn, Angelynne, Anhelina, Anjelina.**

ANGÉLIQUE. *French variation of* **ANGELICA.** Proof that a name can be *too* feminine.

ANGELOU. *Literary name.* If you want to move beyond Maya.

ANGIE. *Diminutive of* **ANGELA.** In the pizzeria with Guido. **Ange, Angee, Angey, Angi, Angy.**

ANI. *Hawaiian, 'beautiful'.* Folk singer DiFranco popularised this simple, appealing form. **Aany, Aanye.**

ANICE. *Modern invented name.* Tomorrow's Denise, trendy but destined to be dated. **Anicka, Annice, Annick, Anis, Annis, Annys.**

ANICETA. *Spanish from German, 'unconquerable'.* Delicate name with strong roots. St Anicetus was an ancient pope and martyr. **Anicetta, Anis, Anisa, Anisha, Anissa, Anniceta, Annicetta, Annis, Annissa.**

ANIKA. *(a-NEE-ka) African, Hausa, 'sweetness of face'.* Attractive name with ties to several cultures, both African and Scandinavian.

ANINA. *Aramaic, 'let my prayer be answered'.* Palindrome name rarely heard outside Italy. **Anena, Anhma, Annina.**

ANISA. *Arabic, 'good-natured'.* Phonetic spelling of the Muslim Aanisah, chosen by singer Macy Gray for one of her daughters. **Aanisa, Aanisah, Anisah.**

ANISE. *(ANN-iss) Nature name.* Name of the liquorice plant whose downside, at least in school science classes, is its similarity to an anatomical word. **Aneese, Anis, Anisette.**

ANITA. *Spanish variation of* **ANN.** Mid-century favourite, long in fashion limbo. **Aneeta, Aneetah, Aneethah, Anetha, Anitha, Anithah, Anitia, Anitra, Anitte, Annita, Annitra, Annitta.**

ANIYA, ANIYAH. *Variation of* **ANN.** New hottie, with stylish sound related to the popular Aaliyah.

ANJA. *(AHN-ya) Russian variation of* **ANYA.** A more exotic spelling of a popular ethnic version of Ann.

ANN, ANNE. *Variation of* **HANNAH.** The name of the sainted mother of the Virgin Mary was among the top girls' names for centuries, in both the English Ann spelling and the French Anne. Both have fallen out of favour in recent years and show no signs of returning.

Ann's International Variations

Irish Gaelic	Áine
Scottish	Anice, Annella
French	Anaïs, Anne, Annelle, Annette, Annouche, Anouk
Breton	Annick
Italian	Annetta, Annina
Spanish	Ana, Anica, Anita, Anna, Nana, Nanor, Nina, Nita
Basque	Ane
Portuguese	Ana, Anicuta
Dutch	Anke, Anki, Anneke, Annika, Anouk, Antje
German	Anna, Anitte, Annchen, Anneli, Annelie, Anni, Antje, Hanna, Hanne, Nettchen
Scandinavian	Annika
Danish	Anne, Hanne
Swedish	Anna, Anneka, Annika, Annike
Norwegian	Anette, Anne
Finnish	Annalie, Anneli, Anni, Anniina, Annikki, Annukka, Anu
Polish	Ania, Anieli, Anka, Hania, Hanka
Eastern European	Ayn, Ayna

Anazizi, Anel, Anell, Anissa, Anitra, Anna, Annabel, Annabella, Annabelle, Annaelle, Annalee, Annelore, Anney, Annick, Annimae, Annis, Annise, Annora, Anona, Hanni, Hannie, Hanny, Nan, Nance, Nancee, Nancey, Nancie, Nanete, Nanette, Nanice, Nanine, Nanni, Nannie, Nanny, Nanon, Neti, Nettia, Nettie, Netty, Ninette, Ninon, Ninor, Nona, Nonie.

ANNA. *German, Italian, Czech, and Swedish, 'grace'.* This is the dominant form of the name, in the Top 25 in recent years. It offers a touch of the exotic and more style than the oversimplified Ann. **Ahnna, Ana, Anah, Anica, Anita, Annah, Annina, Annora, Anona, Anyu, Aska. International:** Áine *(Irish Gaelic),* Ana *(Spanish, Portuguese),* Ane *(Danish),* Ania, Anya *(Russian).*

★**ANNABELLE.** *Combination of* **ANNA** *and* **BELLE.** Charming name on the rise along with other-*belle* names, especially in this form. **Amabel, Anabel, Anabela, Anabele, Anabell, Anabella, Annabal, Annabel, Annabelinda, Annabell, Annabella. International: Anabelle** *(French).*

ANNALIE. *Finnish variation of* **HANNAH.** Melodious and unusual form. **Analeah, Analee, Analeigh, Anali, Analie, Annalea, Annaleah, Annalee, Annaleigh, Annaleigha, Annali, Anneli, Annelie.**

ANNALISE. *Combination of* **ANNA** *and* **LISE.** Lovely, but still on the mountain with Heidi. **Analeisa, Analiesa, Analiese, Analisa, Analise, Anelisa, Anelise, Annaleisa, Annalie, Annaliesa, Annaliese, Annalise, Annalissa, Annalisse, Annelie, Annelisa, Annelise, Annelisse, Annelyse, Annissa.** International: **Anneliese** *(German),* **Anneli, Anneliese** *(Scandinavian).*

ANNAMARIA. *Combination of* **ANNA** *and* **MARIA.** Mama Mia! Pretty, if predominantly used by Italian Catholics. **Anna-Maria, Annamarie, Anna-Marie, Annemarie, Annmaria, Annmarie, Anne-Marie.**

ANNETTE. *French, diminutive of* **ANN.** Among the first wave of Frenchified names, but now considered quite passé. **Anet, Aneta, Anetra, Anett, Anetta, Anette, Anneth, Annett, Annetta.**

Ann's International Variations	
Hungarian	Anci, Aniko, Anna, Annus, Annushka, Annuska, Anyu, Nina, Nusi
Romanian	Anicuta
Czech	Andula, Andulka, Anezka, Anicka, Anna, Anca, Anicka, Anuska
Lithuanian	Anikke, Annze, Onele
Russian	Anechka, Anja, Anna, Annik, Annika, Anninka, Annuska, Anushka, Anya, Asenka, Asya, Nyura, Vania, Vanya
Ukranian	Aneta, Nyura
Latvian	Ance, Ansenka, Anya, Anyuta, Asenka, Aska, Asya, Hanna
Greek	Anna, Nani, Noula
Armenian	Anie, Anna
Hebrew	Ana, Ayn, Chana, Channa, Channah, Enye, Hana, Hanna, Ona
Hawaiian	Ana, Ane

ANNIE. *English, diminutive of* **ANN.** Short form perennially fashionable for its casual charm. **Anni, Anny.**

ANNIKA. *Russian variation of* **ANN.** Surprise hit of recent years, inspired by golfer Sorenson.

Aneka, Anekah, Anneka, Anneke, Annica, Annick, Annicka, Annike, Anniki, Annikka, Annikki, Anninka, Anouk.

ANNORA. *Latin, 'honour'.* Noble name but still best in its most essential form: Honor.

Anora, Anorah, Honour, Honora, Onora, Nora, Norah.

ANNUNCIATA. *Latin, 'annunciation'.* Religious name, referring to the announcement to the Virgin Mary that she was with child. **Anunciada, Annunziata, Annunziate, Anunciacíon, Anunciata, Anunziata.**

ANONA. *Latin, 'of the harvest'.* Name of the Roman goddess of harvest, appropriate for an Autumn baby. **Annona, Anonna, Nona.**

ANOUK. *Dutch and French variation of* **ANNA.** Made famous by French actress Anouk Aimée, this singular name is newly popular in the Netherlands.

ANOUSHKA. *Russian, diminutive of* **ANN.** Old-fashioned diminutive wearing a baboushka and embroidered blouse. **Annouska, Annuskha, Anoush, Anushka, Anuska, Anyoushka.**

ANSLEY. *English, 'clearing with a hermitage'.* Ashley alternative climbing up the charts, probably due to the trendy *ley/leigh* ending. **Annesleigh, Annslea,**

Annslee, Annsleigh, Annsley, Annsli, Annsly, Anslea, Anslee, Ansleigh, Ansli, Anslie, Ansly.

ANSONIA. *Feminine variation of* **ANSON.** Sounds like a hotel. **Annesonia, Annsonia, Annsonya, Ansonya.**

ANSWER. *Word name.* Implied spiritual meaning makes this a possible new name.

ANTHEA. *Greek, 'flower-like'.* British upper-class choice used as poetic symbol of spring. **Annthea, Antha, Anthe, Antheemia, Antheia, Anthemia, Anthemya, Antheya, Anthia, Anthymia, Antia, Thia.**

ANTIGONE. *(an-TIG-o-nee) Greek mythology name.* Mythological daughter of Oedipus, never popular in mortal world.

ANTIQUITY. *Word name.* Your daughter will like this better at twenty than she will at fifty.

ANTOINETTE. *French feminine form of* **ANTOINE.** Feminisation of Anthony as out of style as other early French forms, such as Babette and Nanette. **Anta, Antanette,**

Antoinella, Antoinet, Antonetta, Antonette, Antonia, Antonice, Antonie, Antonieta, Antonietta, Antonine, Antonique, Antwahnette, Antwanetta, Antwinett, Antwohnette, Netta, Netti, Nettie, Netty, Toinette, Toni, Tonia, Tonie, Tony, Tonye. International: Antonella *(Italian)*, Antoniná *(Slavic)*.

★**ANTONIA.** *Latin, 'beyond price, invaluable'.* Distinguished female form of Anthony makes a strong, elegant choice, stronger than most feminised boys' names, reflecting the pioneer spirit of Willa Cather's *My Antonia*. **Ansonia, Ansonya, Antania, Antinia, Antona, Antonetta, Antoñía, Antonice, Antonija, Antonine, Antoniya, Antonnea, Antonnia, Antonya, Netta, Netti, Nettie, Nety, Toinetta, Tloinette, Tonechka, Tonette, Toney, Toni, Tonia, Tonie, Tony, Tonya.** International: **Antoinette, Antonie, Toinette, Toinon** *(French)*, **Antonieta, Antonina, Antuca, Tona** *(Spanish)* **Antonetta** *(Swedish)*, **Tonia** *(Polish)*, **Antoniná** *(Slavic)*.

ANWEN. *Welsh, 'very fair'.* One of the simplest and best of the classic Welsh girls' names, more unusual than Bronwen but with the same serene feel. **Anwyn, Anwynne.**

ANYA. *Russian variation of* **ANNA.** Succeeds in making Ann dynamic. **Aaniyah, Aniya, Aniyah, Anja.**

AOBH, AOIBH. *(eev) Irish Gaelic, 'beauty, radiance'.* Irish mythological equivalent of Eve, but prohibitively hard to pronounce. **Aoife.**

AOIFE. *(EE-fa) Irish Gaelic, 'beauty, radiance'.* Very popular in Ireland, but elsewhere in the easier-to-comprehend Anglo forms. **Aife, Ava, Eva.**

APHRA. *Hebrew, 'dust'.* While the Puritans used Dust as a name, Aphra is preferable in the modern world – especially since it's the name of the first published female writer in English, the seventeenth century's Aphra Behn. **Affera, Affery, Afra.**

APHRODITE. *Greek mythology name.* Has never descended to mortal use, though Venus, thanks

to tennis star Williams, seems newly possible. **Afrodita, Afrodite.**

APOLLONIA. *Feminine variation of* **APOLLO.** Name of early Christian martyr with exotic, appealing feel in the modern world. **Abbeline, Abbetina, Apollinia, Apollonia, Apollyne, Appolonia. International: Appoline, Appolinia, Apolline** *(French),* **Apolonia** *(Spanish),* **Abelone** *(Danish).*

APPLE. *Nature name.* Gwyneth Paltrow made international headlines when she chose this wholesome fruit name for her daughter.

APRIL. *Latin, 'to open'.* Still the most popular month name, but we think old-fashioned May is prettier. **Aipril, Aprele, Aprelle, Apriell, Aprielle, Aprila, Aprile, Aprilete, Aprilette, Aprili, Aprill, Aprille, Apryl, Averel, Averell, Averil, Averill, Averyl, Averyll, Averylle, Avrill. International: Avril** *(French),* **Abril** *(Spanish).*

AQUA. *Colour name.* One of the new colour names that is catching on, invoking a calm, blue-green-sea feeling.

AQUILIA. *Latin, 'eagle'.* This and two other female forms – **AQUILA** and **AQUILINA** – of the Roman family name Aquilius might live on in modern times.

AQUINNAH. *Place name.* The Native American name for Martha's Vineyard in New England, this was used by Michael J. Fox and Tracy Pollan for one of their twin daughters.

♂ **ARA.** *Arabic, 'rain-maker'; Armenian, 'handsome'.* Simple and distinctive, also used for boys in the Armenian culture. **Ahraya, Aira, Arae, Arah, Araya, Arayah, Ari, Aria, Arra, Arria.**

★**ARABELLA.** *Latin, 'beautiful altar'.* Well-used in Britain, we think it's as lovely and classy as Isabella, and far more original. Sure to be hotter in the future. **Ara, Arabel, Arabela, Arabele, Arbela, Arbell, Arbella, Arbelle, Bel, Bella, Belle, Orabel, Orabella, Orabelle, Orbel, Orbella, Orbelle. International: Arabelle** *(French).*

ARABESQUE. *Word name, 'ballet position' or 'ornate design'.* Fanciful, edging toward bizarre.

Names with No Nicknames

Ara

Ava

Blair

Bree

Claire

Drew

Faith

Ivy

Jade

Maeve

Nora

Paige

Piper

Ruby

Skye

♂ **ARABIA.** *place name.* Phonetically attractive, politically difficult. **Araby.**

ARACELI. *Spanish, 'altar of the sky'.* Obscure but intriguing Spanish name. Araceli Segarra is a noted mountain climber. **Aracelia, Aracelis, Aracely.**

★**ARAMINTA.** *Hybrid name from* **ARABELLA** *and* **AMINTA.** This is an enchanting eighteenth-century playwright's invention that is more familiar over here than elsewhere. **Arameta, Aramintha, Areminta, Minta, Minty.**

ARANTXA. *(ah-rahn-cha) Basque, 'thornbush'.* Basque names, indeed the entire Basque language, are unrelated to any other. This obscure choice was made known by tennis player Arantxa Sanchez-Vicario.

ARAVA. *Hebrew, 'willow'.* Unknown but eminently usable choice, especially for Jewish parents, with lovely meaning. **Aravah.**

♂ **ARBOR.** *Nature name.* Original unisex tree-related choice we're sure to hear more of.

ARCADIA. *Greek, 'region offering peace and contentment'.* This name for an unspoilt paradise makes a secular alternative to Neveah. **Arcadie, Cadi, Cadia, Cadie, Cady.**

ARCANGELA. *Greek, 'high-ranking angel'.* If Angel or Angela isn't elevated enough for you. **Arcangel, Archangela, Archangella.**

ARCELIA. *Spanish, 'treasure chest'.* Undiscovered Spanish treasure worth considering. **Aricelia, Aricelly.**

♂ **ARCHER.** *Occupational name.* Interesting – if somewhat masculine – choice in the stylish class of occupational names, with the added bonus of being the last name of heroine Isabel in Henry James's *Portrait of a Lady.*

★♂ **ARDEN.** *English, 'valley of the eagle'.* Name of magical forest in Shakespeare's *As You Like It,* poised to move up as stand-in for overused Aidan. **Ardeen, Ardeena, Ardena, Ardene, Ardenia, Ardi, Ardin, Ardina, Ardine, Ardis, Ardon, Ardyn, Ardynn, Ardynne. International: Arddun** *(Welsh).*

ARDITH. *Hebrew, 'flowering field'.* Lispy combination of Arden and Edith. **Ardath, Ardi, Ardice, Ardyth.**

ARELLA. *Hebrew, 'messenger from God, angel'.* Bell-like and original. **Arelle, Orella, Orelle.** International: **Arela** *(English, Hebrew).*

ARETHA. *Greek, 'virtuous'.* There's still only one. **Areatha, Areetha, Areta, Arete, Arethusa, Aretina, Aretta, Arette, Arita, Aritha, Oreta, Oretha, Oretta, Orette, Retha, Ritha.**

ARGENTA. *Latin, 'silvery'.* More modern and exotic than Silver, but sounds a bit medicinal. **Argentia.**

ARGENTINA. *Place name.* South America provides a continent of interesting, undiscovered names – Bolivia, Peru, Brazil and the tango-rhythmed Argentina.

♂ **ARI.** *Hebrew, diminutive variation of* **ARIEL.** Still mostly a boys' name, but works well for girls, too. **Aria, Ariah, Arie, Ariea, Aryia.**

ARIA. *Italian, 'a melody'.* Operatic choice. **Arya.**

ARIADNE. *Greek, 'most holy'.* Name of Cretan goddess of fertility, most popular now as the more melodic Ariana. **Arene, Ariadna, Ariagna, Ariana, Arianie, Aryana, Aryane, Aryanie, Aryanna, Aryanne.** International: **Ariane, Arianne** *(French),* **Arianna** *(Italian).*

★**ARIANA, ARIANNA.** *Italian variation of* **ARIADNE.** Smooth, exotic choice on the rise in both these spellings. **Aeriana, Aerianna, Aerionna, Ahreanna, Ahriana, Ahrianna, Airiana, Ariane, Arieana, Ariona, Arionna, Aryonna.** International: **Aryana, Aryanna** *(Italian).*

ARIANWYN. *Welsh, 'woman of silver'.* A mouthful. Variation Arianell might be slightly more user-friendly. **Arianell, Arianwen, Arianwynn, Arianwynne, Aryanwen.**

♂ **ARIEL.** *Hebrew, 'lion of God'.* Biblical place and name of Shakespearean (male) sprite that enjoyed a burst of popularity with the release of Disney's *The Little Mermaid.* Although its wave has crested, it's still a name any little girl would love. **Aerial, Aeriale, Aeriel, Aeriela, Aeriell, Aeryal, Ahriel, Aire, Aireal, Airial, Airiél, Ari, Aria, Arial,** Ariale, Arieal, Ariela, Ariele, Ariella, Arielle, Ariellel, Arrieal, Arriel, Arriele, Arriell, Arrielle, Aryel, Aryelle, Auriel, Aurielle.**

ARIN. *Hebrew, 'exalted'.* Too close to Erin and Aaron.

ARISSA. *Modern invented name.* If you're torn between Marissa and Alyssa.

ARISTA. *Greek, 'the best'; Latin, 'harvest'.* From the root for aristocrat, an upwardly mobile choice that might put a bit of pressure on a child. **Aris, Arissa, Aristana, Aristella, Aristelle, Aristen.**

ARIZA. *Hebrew, 'cedar panels'.* Breezy modern Israeli choice. **Arza, Arzice, Arzit.**

ARLEIGH. *Modern invented name.* Softer version of hot Harley or Marley. **Arla, Arlea, Arlee, Arley, Arli, Arlie, Arly.**

ARLENE. *Modern invented name.* Busy knitting booties for granddaughter Arleigh. **Airlen, Aria, Arlana, Arlee, Arleen, Arleene, Arlen, Arlena, Arlenis, Arleta, Arletta, Arlette, Arletty,**

Names from Books

Alhambra	Maisie
Antonia	Orleanna
Arwen	Portia
Beloved	Romola
Brett	Sabra
Briony	Scarlett
Daisy	Scout
Denver	Sethe
Emma	Sheba
Esme	Sidda
Faunia	Sula
Jacy	Temple
Juliet	Undine
Kiki	Velvet
Kinsey	Vivi
Lolita	Zora
Lux	

Arleyne, Arlie, Arliene, Arlina, Arlinda, Arline, Arluene, Arly, Arlyn, Arlyne, Arlynn, Lena, Lene, Lina.

ARLETTE. *French, diminutive of* **CHARLETT**, *a variation of* **CHARLOTTE.** In modern times, it can make Arlene seem positively stylish. **Arlet, Arietta.**

ARLISE. *Irish, 'pledge'.* Feminine form of Arliss. But why not just use Arliss? **Arliss, Arlyse, Arlyss.**

ARMANDE. *French, feminine variation of* **ARMAND.** Feminine form of Armand, has an elegant charm. **Armanda, Armonde, Ormonde.**

♂ **ARMANI.** *Persian, 'desire, goal'; Italian surname.* One of the designer baby names – Chanel and Gucci are others – that have appeared in this era of branding everything from your purse to your offspring. **Armahni, Arman, Armanee, Armanii.**

ARMINA. *Italian from German, 'army man'.* Army plus meaner equals an unappealing name. **Armantine, Armeena, Armine, Arminie, Armyne, Erminia, Erminie, Ermyne.**

ARNELLE. *German, 'eagle'.* This is a polyester-like choice. **Arnell, Arnella.**

ARSENIA. *Feminine variation of* **ARSENIO.** Could lead to 'arsenic' teasing. **Arcenia, Arsania, Arsemia.**

ARTEMIS. *Greek mythology name.* Goddess of the moon and the hunt, equivalent to the Roman Diana, but a fresher and more distinctive, if offbeat, choice. **Artemasia, Artemesia, Artemisia.**

ARTIS. *Scottish, 'bear'.* Unusual multicultural choice that may appeal to the artistically inclined. **Arthea, Arthelia, Arthene, Arthette, Arthurette, Arthurina, Arthurine, Artina, Artice.**

ARWEN. *Welsh, 'noble maiden'.* Well-known as princess of the Elves in Tolkien's *Lord of the Rings*: a lovely name with an authentic Welsh ring.

ARZA. *Hebrew, 'panels of cedar'.* Straightforward yet intriguing, a winning combination. **Ariza, Arizit, Arzice, Arzit.**

♂ **ASA.** *Hebrew, 'doctor, healer'; Japanese, 'born in the morning'.* Simple, soft, strong, this usually male biblical choice – he was a king of Judah – may work even better today for girls.

ASENCION. *Spanish, 'ascension'.* Highly religious choice. **Asuncion.**

♂ **ASH.** *Nature name.* The tree, not the charred bit of soot in the fireplace, usually used for boys, but, as a short form of Ashley, works for girls, too.

ASHANTI. *Place name, former kingdom of western Africa.* Authentic African name that rose in popularity a few years ago when US hip-hop singer Ashanti first arrived on the scene. **Achante, Achanti, Asante, Ashanta, Ashantae, Ashantay, Ashante, Ashanté, Ashantee, Ashantie, Ashaunta, Ashauntae, Ashaunte, Ashauntee, Ashaunti, Ashonti, Ashuntae, Ashunti, Shantee, Shanti, Shauntae, Shauntee.**

♂ **ASHBY.** *English, 'ash tree farm'.* Ashley substitute that sacrifices too much of that name's attractiveness for what it gains in originality. **Ashbea, Ashbee, Ashbey, Ashbie.**

ASHIRA. *Hebrew, 'rich' or 'I will sing'.* Unusual name with stylish, silky feel. **Ashirah,**

Ashya, Ashyah, Ashyia, Ashyra, Ashyrah, Ayshia.

♂ **ASHLEY.** *English, 'ash tree meadow'.* Once, this male name hit number 1 on the US girls' list, but nowhere near as popular here. Still pretty but no longer even vaguely stylish. **Ahshlee, Aishlee, Ashala, Ashalee, Ashalei, Ashaley, Ashely, Ashla, Ashlay, Ashlan, Ashlea, Ashleay, Ashlee, Ashleigh, Ashleye, Ashien, Ashli, Ashlie, Ashly, Ashlye.**

ASHLYN, ASHLYNN. *Variation of* **AISLINN.** Though it relates to the Irish original, Ashlyn and its next most popular form, Ashlynn, owe some of their rising popularity to cousin Ashley. **Ashelynn, Ashlan, Ashleann, Ashleen, Ashleene, Ashlen, Ashlene, Ashlin, Ashling, Ashlinne, Ashlyne, Ashlynne.**

♂ **ASHTON.** *English, 'ash tree place'.* In the US, hot star Ashton Kutcher is pushing this unisex choice toward the boys' camp, but its variation Ashtyn is on the rise. **Ashten, Ashtin, Ashtine, Ashtyn, Ashtynne.**

ASIA. *Place name.* This still attractive place name was one of the first to gain popularity, though it now probably owes some of its favour to its similarity to Aisha. **Ahsia, Aisia, Aisian, Aja, Asiah, Asian, Asianae, Asya, Aysia, Aysiah, Aysian, Ayzia, Azha.**

♂ **ASPEN.** *Nature and place name.* Nature name, chic Colorado ski resort name in the US and unisex feel equals red-hot baby name. **Aspin, Aspyn.**

ASSISI. *Italian place name.* This lovely Tuscan hill town became a striking first name for the young daughter of Jade Jagger.

ASTA. *Greek, 'like a star'.* There are many more melodious ways to say star. This was attached to a dog in early Hollywood movies. **Astera, Asteria, Asti, Astra, Estella, Esther, Estrella, Etoile, Hadassah, Hester, Stella.**

ASTRA. *Latin, 'of the stars'.* A kind of Jetsons-like, intergalactic name. **Asta, Astara, Aster, Astera, Asteria, Asterina, Astraea, Astraeia, Astrea, Astri, Astria.**

Poet Names

Angelou

Auden

Blake

Byron

Crane

Dante

Dylan

Eliot

Emerson

Frost

Jarrell

Keats

Millay

Paz

Poe

Poet

Saga

Sonnet

Whitman

Yeats

ASTRID. *Norse, 'divinely beautiful'.* Familiar Scandinavian royal name that never really took off the way Ingrid did. **Assi, Astra, Astri, Astrida, Astride, Astrik, Astrud, Astryr, Atti, Estrid.**

ATALANTA. *Greek mythology name.* Beautiful mythological maiden who refused to marry any man who couldn't beat her in a foot race – some role model! **Atalaya, Atlanta, Atlante, Atlee.**

★**ATARA, ATARAH.** *Hebrew, 'crown'.* Finally, an attractive, undiscovered Old Testament choice for *girls*. **Ataree, Atera, Ateret.**

ATHALIA. *Hebrew, 'the Lord is exalted'.* Old Testament king's wife with a gory history. You don't want to know – and you probably don't want to name your kid after her either. **Atalee, Atalia, Atalie, Atha, Athalee, Athalie, Attalie.**

ATHENA. *Greek mythology name.* The name of the daughter of Zeus who was the goddess of wisdom and fertility could appeal to enlightened parents who particularly prize intelligence. **Athenais, Athene, Athenea, Athie, Athina, Atina, Attie.**

ATLANTA. *Place name.* In the US, Georgia and Savannah are popular, but Atlanta's just entering the baby-name map.

♂ **ATLANTIS.** *Place name.* Mythical wonderland makes strong, evocative first name.

♂ **AUBREY.** *English from French, 'elf ruler'.* This unisex name is moving up the popularity charts, along with the revived Audrey. **Aubary, Auberon, Aubery, Aubray, Aubrea, Aubreah, Aubree, Aubreigh, Aubrette, Aubreyana, Aubreyanna, Aubreyanne, Aubreyena, Aubria, Aubriana, Aubrianna, Aubrianne, Aubrie, Aubry, Aubury, Avery.**

♂ **AUBURN.** *Colour name.* Could be the next Amber, or Scarlett.

★♂ **AUDEN.** *English 'old friend,' literary name.* Softly poetic surname name enjoying quiet but marked fashion status. This will definitely be one to watch during the next few years. **Aud, Auda, Aude, Audine, Audny.**

AUDREY. *English, 'noble strength'.* Saint's name rising again thanks to reverence for the eternally radiant Audrey Hepburn. **Adrey, Audey, Audi, Audie, Audra, Audray, Audre,**

Audrea, Audreanne, Audree, Audreen, Audria, Audriana, Audrianna, Audrianne, Audrie, Audrienna, Audrienne, Audrin, Audrina, Audriya, Audry, Audrye, Audy.

♂ **AUGUST.** *Latin, 'majestic, venerable'; month name.* Though associated traditionally (and fashionably) with boys, it has been used occasionally for girls as well – by Garth Brooks, for one.

AUGUSTA. *Latin, feminine form of* **AUGUSTUS.** Dignified name reminiscent of wealthy great-aunts, but with the fashion for August and Gus for boys, it could get some fresh energy. **Agusta, August, Auguste, Augustia, Augustina, Augustine, Augustus, Augustyna, Augustyne, Austina, Austine, Austyna, Austyne, Gus, Gussie, Gusta, Tina. International: Augusteen** *(Irish).*

AURA. *Latin, 'air'.* This name has an otherworldly glow. **Aure, Aurea, Auria, Oria.**

AURELIA. *Latin, 'gold'.* Richly evocative antique name, very common in the Roman Empire but rarely heard in modern

Britian, has the right stuff to rise again. **Aranka, Aural, Auralee, Auralei, Auralia, Aurea, Aureal, Aurel, Aurele, Aurelea, Aurelee, Aureliana, Aurellana, Aurelle, Aurelina, Aurelle, Auria, Aurie, Aurilia, Aurita, Ora, Oralia, Orel, Orelee, Orelia. International: Aurélie** *(French).*

AURIEL. *Latin, 'gold'.* Roman slave name revived during nineteenth-century craze for unusual names. **Aureola, Aureole, Auriol, Oriel, Oriole.**

AURORA. *Latin, 'dawn'.* Poetic name of the Roman goddess of sunrise and of Sleeping Beauty, sure to make any little girl feel like a princess. **Arora, Ora, Ori, Orie, Rora, Rory, Zora, Zorica. International: Aurore** *(French).*

♂ **AUSTEN.** *Shortened form of* **AUGUSTINE,** *literary surname.* While Austin is a popular boys' name, this version, honouring novelist Jane, is more girlish. **Austin, Austine, Austyn, Austynn.**

AUSTRIA. *Place name.* Interesting, appealing, unexplored geographic destination.

AUTUMN. *Season name.* Crisp and colourful, this is the most popular season name, now rivalled only by the sunnier Summer.

★**AVA.** *Latin, 'like a bird'.* Glamour girl name given big popularity boost – when several high-profile stars such as Reese Witherspoon and Hugh Jackman chose it for their daughters. **Aeva, Aiva, Avada, Avae, Avah, Ave, Aveen, Avis, Eva.**

★**AVALON.** *Celtic, 'island of apples'.* Island paradise of Celtic myth and Arthurian legend makes heavenly first name. **Avallon.**

♂ **AVERILL.** *English.* April with a unisex surname twist. **Averil, Averille, Averyl, Avril, Avrill.**

♂ **AVERY.** *English, 'ruler of the elves'.* Though this unisex name has been around for a few decades, it's just starting to become hot for girls, thanks to its distinctively feminine lilt. **Aivree, Avari, Avary, Averi, Averie, Avori, Avory, Avry.**

Stellar Starbabies Beginning with *A*

Aanisah	Macy Gray
Agnes	Elisabeth Shue, Thom *(Radiohead)* Yorke
Alabama	Travis *(Blink 182)* Barker
Alchamy	Lance Hendrickson
Ali	Ronan & Yvonne Keating
Alice	Tom Cavanaugh, Tina Fey
Aliseh	Geena Davis
Allie Colleen	Garth Brooks
Amandine	John Malkovich
Amba	Jade Jagger
Amelia	Lisa Rinna & Harry Hamlin
Anais	Noel *(Oasis)* Gallagher
Angel Iris	Melanie *(Spice Girls)* Brown
Apple	Gwyneth Paltrow & Chris Martin
Aquinnah	Tracy Pollan & Michael J. Fox
Assisi	Jade Jagger
Astrid	John Hannah
Atherton	Don Johnson
Atlanta	Amanda de Cadenet & John *(Duran Duran)* Taylor
Audrey	Greg Kinnear
August	Garth Brooks
Ava	Kevin Dillon, Hugh Jackman, Heather Locklear & Richie Sambora, Martina McBride, John McEnroe, Aidan Quinn, Reese Witherspoon & Ryan Phillippe

AVIS. *Latin, 'bird'.* This is one bird name that's sitting in the rental car park. **Avais, Avi, Avia, Aviana, Avianca, Aviance, Avianna, Avice, Avys.**

AVIVA. *Hebrew, 'spring-like, fresh, dewy'.* Vivacious and memorable. **Auvit, Avi, Aviv, Avivah, Avivi, Avivice, Avivit, Avni, Avnit, Avri, Avrit, Avy, Viva.**

AVRIL. *French variation of* APRIL. French-Canadian pop star Avril Lavigne has put the spotlight on her name. **Averel, Averell, Averil, Averill, Averyl, Avra, Avri, Avrilia, Avrill, Avrille, Avrillia, Avy.**

AYA. *Hebrew, 'bird'.* Similar and prettier: Maya or Anya. **Ayala, Ayla.**

AYANNA. *Modern invented name.* Trendy blend of Ayesha and Bryanna. **Ahyana, Aiyana, Aiyanna, Ayan, Ayana, Ayania, Ayannia, Iana, Ianna.**

AYELET. *(eye-uh-LET) Hebrew, 'deer, gazelle'.* Unusual – and somewhat challenging – Israeli name familiar thanks to writer Ayelet Waldman.

AYESHA. *Variation of* **AISHA.** This phonetic form may ease pronunciation but it undercuts the name's inherent grace. **Ayasha, Ayeshah, Ayessa, Ayisha, Ayishah, Aysha, Ayshah, Ayshe, Ayshea, Aysia.**

AYN. *(rhymes with mine) Finnish variation of* **ANN.** Nonconformist name associated with controversial Russian-born writer and philosopher Ayn Rand, (born Alisa) author of *The Fountainhead.*

♂ **AZA.** *Arabic, 'comfort'.* Great Arabic choice: elegant and simple. **Aiza, Aizha, Aizia, Azia.**

AZALEA. *Flower name.* If Lily and Rose are too tame for you, consider this brilliant pink springtime blossom with a touch of the exotic. **Azaleia, Azalia.**

AZAMI. *Japanese, 'thistle flower'.* Prickly image and feel.

AZIZA. *Hebrew, 'mighty'; Arabic and Swahili, 'precious'.* Zippy palindromic choice. **Azise.**

AZURE. *Colour name.* Good choice for a blue-eyed child. **Azor, Azora, Azura, Azzura, Azzurra.**

B *girls*

BABE. *Diminutive of* **BARBARA.** You can call your baby 'babe,' but don't name her that. **Bebe, Babby, Baby.**

BABETTE. *French, diminutive of* **ELIZABETH** *or* **BARBARA.** A less common relic of the Claudette-Paulette-Annette era. **Barbette.**

BAEZ. *Spanish surname.* Plausible music hero choice with undertones of Joan Baez's social activist folkie persona.

BAHAAR. *Hindi, 'springtime'.* Invokes images of colourful bazaars.

BAHIA. *Spanish, 'bay'.* Cool tropical Latin word name.

BAHIRA. *Arabic, 'dazzling, brilliant'.* Sultry.

BAI. *Chinese, 'outgoing'.* Attractive middle name option.

BAILA. *Spanish, 'dance'.* An offbeat approach to Bella. **Bailee, Bayla, Beyla.**

♂ **BAILEY.** *Occupational name, 'law enforcer, bailiff'.* This jaunty unisex surname was chosen for her daughter by Stella McCartney. **Bailee, Baileigh, Bailie, Baillie, Baily, Bayleah, Baylee, Bayleigh, Bayley, Baylie, Bayly.**

BAISE. *French, 'dark brown'.* This fabric word name would be a one-of-a-kind. **Bayze, Baze.**

BAJA. *Spanish place name, 'lower'.* Pronounced Bah-hah, this name of the Mexican peninsula attached to California makes for an out-of-the ordinary, exotic possibility. **Baha.**

BALA. *Sanskrit, 'a young girl'.* Exotic alternative to Bella.

BALI. *Sanskrit, 'strength'; also place name.* Evokes picture-postcard image of colourful Indonesia.

♂ **BALDWIN.** *German, 'brave friend'.* Writer James Baldwin could make this an inspirational choice for a child of either sex. **Baldwen, Baldwinne, Baldwyn, Baldwynne.**

BALLENCIA. *Variation of* **VALENCIA,** *Spanish place name.* Might sound as if your child had the sniffles every time she said her name.

♂ **BALLOU.** *French, 'from Bellou'.* Unusual surname name with rowdy quality. **Bailou, Balou.**

BAMBALINA. *Italian, 'little girl'.* Better saved for a doll.

BAMBI. *Italian, 'child,' diminutive for* **BAMBINA,** *'baby girl'.* Although Disney's cute deer was a male, Bambi's always been used for girls, but it sounds far too flimsy to face the modern world. **Bambee, Bambie.**

♂ **BAO.** *Chinese, 'adorable' or 'creative'.* Name introduced via Chinese cinema, it has middle-place potential.

BAPTISTA. *Latin, 'the baptised one'.* Probably too evangelical for mass importation. **International:** Baptiste *(French),* Batista *(Italian),* Bautista *(Spanish).*

BARA. *Hebrew, 'to select'.* Gently appealing. **Barah, Bari, Barra, Barrie.**

♂ **BARAKA.** *Kiswahili, 'blessings'.* Its resonant rhythm and positive connotations have led to some popularity with parents of African heritage, though it tends to have a masculine feel.

BARBARA. *Latin, 'foreign woman'.* Fashionable from the 1920s through to the 50s, it's very much a grey-haired name now. **Bab, Baba, Babba, Babbie, Babs, Bar, Barb, Barbe, Barbee, Barbi, Barbie, Barby, Barra, Bobbee, Bobbi, Bobbie, Bobby. International:** Barbary *(English, earlier form),* **Baírbre, Baibín** *(Irish Gaelic),* Barabal *(Scottish Gaelic),* Babette *(French),* Barbarella *(Italian),* Barbro *(Swedish),* **Barbica, Barbika** *(Nordic),* **Basha, Basia** *(Polish),* Borbála, *(Hungarian),* **Varvara, Varenka, Varinka, Vary, Varyusha** *(Russian),* Babara *(Hawaiian).*

BARBIE. *Diminutive of* **BARBARA.** Despite the voluptuous doll's various career choices, from astronaut to doctor, her name still remains a euphemism for 'bimbo'.

BARBRO. *Scandinavian variation of* **BARBARA.** A more upbeat, modern-sounding version of a gereatric name.

♂ **BARCELONA.** *Place name.* This is an attractive but somewhat unwieldy place-name name. **Lona.**

BARIAH. *Arabic, 'does well'.* A name to consider when seeking an offbeat substitute for the more familiar Mariah.

♂ **BARRETT.** *German, ' bear strength'.* Masculine sounding surname. **Baret, Barett, Barit, Baritt, Barret, Barrit, Barritt, Barryt, Baryt, Barytt.**

♂ **BARRY, BARRIE.** *Irish 'spear'.* Out of date for a boy, innovative for a girl. **Bari, Barree, Barrey, Barri, Barry.**

BASHA. *Polish, 'stranger'.* Sounds a bit like other newly popular Slavic names Sasha and Mischa, but also a bit like 'basher'. **Basia, Basja, Bashya, Batia, Batya.**

BASILIA. *Greek, feminine variation of* **BASIL**. Rare but attractive female form of Basil. **Basilie, Bassilly.**

BATHSHEBA. *Hebrew, 'daughter of the oath' or 'seventh daughter'.* Popular with the Puritans, this name of the shrewd and beautiful wife of King David would be a heavy load for a modern girl to carry. **Bat-Sheba, Bat-Sheva, Bathseva, Bathshua, Bathsua, Batsheba, Batsheva, Batshua, Batya, Bethsabee, Bethsheba, Sheba, Sheva.**

BATHSHIRA. *Arabian, 'seventh daughter'.* The short form Shira is more manageable. **Shira.**

BATYA. *Hebrew, 'daughter of God'.* With Katya catching on, this sound-related name could too, though there is the Batgirl association. **Basha, Basya, Batyah, Bitya, Peshe, Pessel** *(Yiddish).*

★ ♂ **BAY.** *Vietnamese, 'seventh child,' nature name.* One of the most usable of the pleasant, newly adopted nature/water names (like Lake and Ocean), especially in middle position. **Bae, Baye. International: Baie,** Baye *(French),* **Bahia, Estera** *(Spanish),* **Selka** *(Finnish),* **Zaliv** *(Russian),* **Bandar** *(Persian),* **Floi** *(Icelandic).*

BAYA. *Spanish, 'berry'.* Maya is exotic, Baya is singular.

BAYLEE. *See* **BAILEY.**

♂ **BAYLOR.** *English, 'horse trainer'.* Possible alternative to the tired Taylor. **Bailer, Bailor, Bayler.**

★**BAYO.** *African, Nigerian, Yoruba, 'joy has found us'.* Conjures up a Harry Belafonte-ish calypso beat.

BEA. *Diminutive of* **BEATRICE**. Former old lady name gets cute again as a short form – but too brief to stand on its own.

BEAH. *Short form of* **BEATRICE**. A rarely seen member of the Beatrice clan.

BEATA. *Swedish, Italian, 'blessed'; Italian version pronounced* bay-AH-tah. Playground alert: apt to be mispronounced Beeta – or 'beat her'. **Bea, Beatta.**

BEATHA. *(BEH-tha) Irish, 'life, livelihood'.* Another candidate for mispronunciation. **Betha.**

Water Names	
Aqua	Lake
Aquarius	Loire
Arno	Lucerne
Bay	Marina
Bayou	Marsh
Brook	Misty
Cascade	Neptune
Caspian	Nile
Como	Oceane
Danube	Po
Delta	Rain
Evian	Rainey
Firth	Rio
Fjord	River
Ford	Tahoe
Harbor	Thames
Hudson	Wade
Jordan	Zambezi
Laguna	Zarya

★**BEATRICE.** *Latin, 'blessed' or 'she who brings happiness'.* Beatrice is back. Stored in the attic for almost a century, this lovely name with a long literary (Shakespeare, Dante) and royal history is being looked at with fresh eyes by parents (such as Paul McCartney) seeking a classic name with character and lots of upbeat nicknames. **Bea, Beah, Beat, Beata, Beatie, Bee, Beatris, Beatriss, Bice, Trix, Trixi, Trixie, Trixy.** International: **Beatha** (*Irish*), **Beitris** (*Scottish Gaelic*), **Betrys** (*Welsh,*) **Béatrice** (*French*), **Beatrice** (*Italian*), **Beatriz** (*Spanish*), **Beatrix** (*Dutch*), **Beatrisa** (*German*), **Beate** (*Norwegian*).

★**BEATRIX.** *Latin, 'blessed' or 'she who brings happiness'.* Beatrix has a solid history of its own (think Beatrix Potter), and that final *x* adds a playful, animated note.

BEATRIZ. *Spanish variation of* **BEATRICE.** Another attractive translation of Beatrice, popular with Hispanic parents.

BEBE. *Diminutive of* **BEATRICE, BEATRIX.** High-kicking cohort of Coco, Gigi, Fifi, Kiki, et al. **Beebee, Bibi.**

BECCA. *Diminutive of* **REBECCA.** The currently preferred replacement for Becky, sometimes used on its own. **Beccah, Becka, Beckah, Bekka, Bekkah.**

♂**BECHET.** *French surname.* Naming babies for personal heroes is the cool contemporary trend followed by Woody Allen when he honoured New Orleans jazz musician Sidney Bechet in his daughter's name. Has a nice, catchy Gallic feel.

BECHETTE. *French, 'little spade'.* Pronounced *Beshette,* this unfamiliar French appellation sounds fresh and feminine.

♂**BECK.** *English, 'one living beside a small stream', short form of* **REBECCA.** Although the single-named singer is male, this remains a girl's nickname name.

BECKY. *Diminutive of* **REBECCA.** One of those casual down-home names last popular in the 1960s. **Beckey, Becki, Beckie.**

BEDELIA. *Irish, 'strength, power'.* This fanciful Irish extension of Bridget is known here through the wacky Amelia Bedelia books for kids – an association your child may or may not like. **Bedeelia, Biddy, Bidelia, Bridget, Delia.**

BEE. *Diminutive of* **BEATRICE.** This buzzy form is for middle name consideration only.

BEEJA. *Hindi, 'the beginning' or 'happy'.* Rhythmic and exotic. **Beej.**

BEGONIA. *Flower name.* One flower name that doesn't smell or sound sweet enough for baby name use.

BEIGE. *Colour name.* Nice sound, colourless image.

♂**BELA.** *Czech, 'white'.* Since this is strictly a male name in Slavic cultures, better to stick with the 'Bella' spelling here. **Belah, Belalia, Biela.**

BELÉN. *Spanish, 'at Bethlehem'; Hebrew, 'house of bread'.* Popular throughout the Spanish-speaking world.

★BELIA. *Spanish variation of* **BELLA.** This is a pretty and unusual translation of Bella. **Belicia, Belita.**

BELINDA. *Spanish, 'pretty one'; German, 'serpent'.* Belinda sits on the 'Not in Current Usage' shelf alongside cousins Linda and Melinda. **Bel, Bellinda, Bellynda, Linda, Lindie, Lindy.**

BELINE. *French, 'goddess'.* Possible Gallic import in the Celine mode.

★BELLA. *Diminutive of* **ISABELLA.** Ciao, Bella. Everything *ella,* from Ella to Bella to Gabriella, is red hot right now, and this is one of the less overused examples, with the hint of a nice old-fashioned grandmotherly veneer. **Bela, Belia, Bell, Bellette.**

BELLE. *French, 'beautiful'.* Nothing but positive associations come with this name, from 'belle of the ball' to 'Southern belle' to the heroine of Disney's *Beauty and the Beast.* **Bel, Bela, Belia, Belinda, Belisse, Bell, Bellina.**

BELLEZZA. *Italian, 'beauty'.* Beauty con brio italiano.

BELOVED. *Literary word name.* Toni Morrison, the modern master of literary names, made this one famous as the title character of a novel. But things didn't work out so well for that Beloved.

BELVA. *Latin, 'beautiful view'.* Has a decidedly middle-aged image. **Belvah, Belvia.**

BENEDETTA. *Latin, 'blessed'.* Saintly. **Benita.**

BENEDICTA. *Latin, 'blessed'.* Saintly, and a Mother Superior to boot. **Benna, Benni, Bennie. International: Bénédicte** *(French),* **Benicia** *(Spanish),* **Benedikta** *(German),* **Benedeka, Benedika, Benke** *(Eastern European),* **Benci** *(Hungarian),* **Venedicta** *(Greek).*

♂ BENILDE. *(ben-NIL-dee) French variation of Latin, 'good'.* Strong and unusual name of a medieval (male) saint and a contemporary (female) novelist, Benilde Little.

BENITA. *Latin, 'blessed'.* In fashion limbo with Anita and Juanita. **Bena, Beneta, Benetta, Benni, Bennie, Benny, Binnie, Binny, Nita.**

BENJAMINA. *Hebrew, 'daughter of the right hand'.* The kind of feminised male name that never caught on. **Benay, Jamina. International: Bannerjee** *(Gaelic),* **Vernamina** *(Greek).*

BERENICE. *See* **BERNICE.**

BERIT. *Scandinavian variation of* **BIRGIT.** Well used in northern Europe. **Beret, Berette, Beri, Berry, Berta, Beryt.**

BERMUDA. *Place name.* Maybe if you spent your honeymoon there. We did say maybe.

BERNADETTE. *German, 'brave as a bear'.* Pleasant, feminine, but strong name associated with the saint who saw visions of the Virgin Mary, now no longer strictly inhabiting the Catholic diocese. **Bern, Berna, Bernadene, Bernadina, Bernadine, Bernarda, Bernardette, Bernetta, Bernette, Berni, Bernie, Bernita, Berny, Berrie, Berry. International: Berneen** *(Irish),* **Bernardetta**

(Italian), **Bernardita** *(Spanish),* **Bernadett** *(Hungarian).*

BERNADINE, BERNARDINE. *German, 'brave as a bear'.* This is as dated as an old Pat Boone song. **Berna, Bernadeene, Bernadina, Bernadyne, Bernardin, Bernardine, Berni, Bernideene, Bernidine, Bernie, Bernydeene, Bernydine.**

BERNARDA. *German, 'brave as a bear'.* Too close in sound to the so-far-out-it-will-always-be-out Bernard. **Bennie, Benny, Berna, Bernadeena, Bernadett, Bernadetta, Bernata, Bernette, Bernie, Bernina, Bernita.** International: **Benadette, Bernadette, Bernardine, Bernardene** *(French),* **Bernadina** *(Spanish),* **Bernharda** *(German and Austrian),* **Bernarda** *(Eastern European),* **Vernada** *(Greek).*

BERNICE, BERENICE. *Greek, 'she who brings victory'.* Since most Bernices were called Binnie, Benny or Bunny anyway, few will notice that this old Greek name has faded away. **Beranyce, Bereniece, Berenyce, Bern, Bernee, Berni, Bernie, Berry, Bunny.**

International: **Bernise, Bearnas** *(Scottish Gaelic),* **Bérénice, Berenicia, Bernelle** *(French),* **Beronia** *(Italian),* **Bernessa, Bernise** *(German),* **Beranice, Beraniece, Berenice, Berenike** *(Greek).*

♂ **BERRY.** *Nature name.* With the recent arrival of fruit names like Apple, Peaches and Plum, this older example might also rise in popularity. **Berree, Berri, Berrie.**

BERTHA. *German, 'bright, glorious'.* Ever since the enormous German cannon was dubbed 'Big Bertha' in World War I, this name hasn't worked for a sweet little baby girl. Not true of the Polish version, Berta. International: **Berthe, Bertille** *(French),* **Berrta, Berrti, Berrty, Berti, Bertilde, Bertina, Bettina** *(German),* **Berit, Bertie, Bird, Birdie, Birta** *(Swedish),* **Berte** *(Norwegian),* **Berta** *(Polish).*

BERTILLE. *French, 'heroine, bright maiden'.* Name of medieval French saint and still often found preceded by the word 'Sister'. **Bertilla.**

BERTRICE. *Combination of* **BERTHA** *and* **BERNICE.** One not-very-attractive name combined with another not-very-attractive name will usually equal a third not-very-attractive name. **Bert, Bertee, Berti, Bertie, Berty.**

BERYL. *Greek, 'sea-green jewel'.* World War II-period favourite. Why not try Jade as a more popular green gem choice. **Barry, Beril, Berri, Berrie, Berrill, Berry, Beryle, Berylla, Beryn.**

BESS. *Diminutive of* **ELIZABETH.** Declared its independence as far back as the reign of Elizabeth I, yet now sounds less passé than Beth or Betsy. **Bessa, Besse.**

BESSIE. *Diminutive of* **ELIZABETH.** After a century of association with names for horses and cows, Bessie could be ready for revival by a fearless baby namer – after all, it did happen to Jessie and Becky. **Bessee, Bessey, Bessi, Bessie, Bessy.**

BETA. *Greek, second letter of the Greek alphabet.* If you can't have an Alpha male, how about a Beta girl?

BETH. *Diminutive of* **ELIZABETH.** The sweetest and most sensitive of the pet names for Elizabeth, now also one of the most dated. **Betha, Bethah, Bethia.**

BETHAN. *Welsh, diminutive of* **ELIZABETH.** Very popular in Wales, this perfectly nice name's only problem is its similarity to the dated Beth Ann.

BETHANY. *Hebrew, 'house of figs'; also New Testament place name.* Though beginning to slip on the popularity lists, this lyrical name still strikes many parents as a fresher, more substantial substitute for the overused Brittany/Brittney. **Beth, Bethanee, Bethaney, Bethani, Bethanie, Bethanne, Bethannie, Bethanny, Bethenee, Betheney, Betheny.**

BETHEL. *Hebrew, 'house of God'.* A rarely used Biblical place name with a soft and pleasant sound. **Bethell.**

BETHESDA. *Hebrew, 'house of mercy'.* Beware if you plan to move to the US – this might be too closely associated with a Maryland suburb of D.C.

BETHIA. *Hebrew, 'daughter of Jehovah'.* Long forgotten Old Testament name with modern potential. **Betia, Bithia.**

BETSY. *Diminutive of* **ELIZABETH.** From Betsy Ross to the Betsy Wetsy doll, this was seen as a perkier, younger-sounding alternative to Betty. No longer. **Bets, Betsey, Betsi, Betsie, Betts.**

BETTE. *Diminutive of* **ELIZABETH.** Pronounced à la Bette (Betty) Davis or Bette (Bet) Midler, a twentieth-century relic.

BETTINA. *Diminutive of* **ELIZABETH.** Ballerina version of Betty. **Battina, Betiana, Betina, Bettine.**

BETTY. *Diminutive of* **ELIZABETH.** Popular during World War II, when it blanketed the English-speaking world. **Bett, Betta, Betti, Bettie, Bettye.**

BEULAH. *Hebrew, 'married'; another name for Palestine.* Fatally stereotyped as a black

Nicknames for Elizabeth

Bess

Bessie

Beth

Betsy

Bette

Bettina

Betty

Eliza

Libby

Lisa

Liz

Liza

Lizbeth

Lizzie

Tibby

maid's name in movies and TV, the biblical Beulah would challenge the most audacious baby namer. **Beula, Bewlah, Byulah.**

BEVERLY. *English, 'dweller near the beaver stream'.* More visible in reference to a posh California community than as a girls' name. **Bev, Bevalee,**

Beverle, Beverlee, Beverley, Beverlie, Beverlye, Bevverly, Bevvy, Buffy.

♀ **BEVIN**. *Scottish, 'sweet, melodious woman'*. Possible alternative to Devin. **Bev, Bevan, Bevann**. International: **Bébhinn** *(Irish Gaelic)*.

BEYONCÉ. *Modern invented name*. The unique name of the hot young singer will not remain unique for long.

BIANCA. *Italian, 'white'*. Livelier Shakespearean version of Blanche; Blanca is a favourite in the Spanish-speaking community. **Beanka, Beonca, Beyonca, Beyonka, Biancha, Bianka, Blancha**. International: **Blanche** *(French)*, **Blanca** *(Spanish)*, **Blanka** *(Czech)*.

BIBI. *French, 'toy' or 'delight'; Persian, 'lady of the house'; diminutive of* **BIBIANA**. A spunky nickname name for parents with showbiz aspirations for their daughter. **Bebe, Beebee**.

BIBIANA. *Latin, 'animated'*. Melodic and unusual, and she *will* outgrow any bib jokes. **Bibi, Bibianna, Biviane**. International: **Bibiane** *(French)*.

BICE. *Italian, diminutive of* **BEATRICE**. Though Beatrice has the lovely Italian pronunciation bay-uh-TREE-chay, Bice has the problematic BEE-chay – a bit too close to 'bitchy'.

BICHETTE. *French, 'little doe'*. Charming Gallic possibility but with some obvious playground problems.

BIDDY. *Diminutive of* **BRIDGET**. In this country, it usually follows the word *old*. **Biddie, Bidou**.

BIDU. *Diminutive of* **BRIDGET**. Uncommon choice too reminiscent of 'bidet'.

BIENVENIDA. *Spanish, 'welcome'*. Somewhat unwieldy, but would certainly make your little girl feel wanted.

★**BIJOU**. *French, 'jewel', from Old English 'bizou'*. A name that lives up to its definition – a real jewel. Warning: not unheard of on poodles' dog collars. **Bijoux, Bizou**.

BILLIE. *English, diminutive of* **WILHELMINA, WILMA**. Tomboyish nickname name and a possible retro choice for fans of jazz great Billie Holiday. **Billa, Billee, Billi, Billina, Billy, Willa**.

BINA. *Hebrew, 'understanding'; Yiddish, 'bee'; also diminutive of* **SABINA** *and other -ina names*. Tends to sound incomplete. **Binah, Bine**.

BINNIE. *Celtic, 'crib, wicker basket'*. Like Minnie and Winnie, eccentric enough to appeal to the iconoclastic parent. **Binne, Binni, Binny**.

BIONDA. *Italian, 'blond'*. As with the pop singer Blondie, more a description than a name.

♀ **BIRD**. *Nature name*. Too flighty. **Birdella, Birdena, Birdey, Birdie, Byrd, Byrdie**.

BIRDIE. *English, 'bird'.* A middle-aged Ladies' Club member wearing a bird-decorated hat.

BIRGIT. *Scandinavian variation of* **BRIGHID.** Pronounced with a hard *g* and sure to be misunderstood in more ways than that. **Bergette, Berit, Birget, Birgetta, Birgite Birgitt, Birgitta, Birgitte, Britta.**

BJÖRK. *Icelandic, 'birch tree'.* Destined to remain a one-person name – in this country anyway.

♂ **BLAINE.** *Irish, 'slender, angular'.* Best friend of Blair, Blake, and Brooke. **Blain, Blane, Blayn, Blayne.**

♂ **BLAIR.** *Scottish, 'dweller on the plain'.* One of the first upwardly mobile unisex names to hit the charts, Blair retains its air of slightly snobby sophistication. **Blaire, Blare, Blayr, Blayre.**

♂ **BLAISE.** *Latin, 'one who stutters'.* Blaze with a French accent. **Blaise, Blasé, Blasia, Blaza, Blaze.**

♂ **BLAKE.** *English, means both 'fair-haired' and 'dark'.* The unisex Blake has a briskly efficient image when used for a girl. **Blaike, Blaque, Blayke.**

BLANCA. *Spanish, 'white'.* More colourful than Blanche, but blanker than Bianca. **Bellanca, Blanka, Blankah.**

BLANCHE. *French, 'white'.* Originally a nickname for a blonde, Blanche was in style a century ago, then became a faded Southern belle, now might be preparing for revival. **Blanchette.**

♂ **BLAZE.** *English, 'one who stutters'.* This is a hot name, but more in the stripper sense. **Blais, Blaise, Blaiz, Blaise, Blase.**

BLEU. *French, 'blue'.* The middle name of the Travoltas' Ella, this French colour alternative hasn't caught on with many other parents.

BLISS. *English word name.* Only for parents positive their daughter won't ever have a tantrum. **Blisse, Blyss, Blysse.**

Names for Blond Babies

Alben
Alva
Aubrey
Banning
Blake
Blanca/Blanche
Bionda
Bowie
Boyd
Dory
Elvira
Fairfax
Finn
Finnian
Flavian
Gaynor
Gwynn
Kyle
Linus
Xanthus

BLODWEN. *Welsh, 'white flower'.* One of the less-appealing Welsh *wen* names. **Blodwyn.**

BLOSSOM. *English, 'to bloom'.* Few parents today would pick this dated generic flower name that had a showgirl aura in the Floradora days. **International: Bluma** *(German),* **Blume** *(Yiddish).*

♂ **BLUE.** *Colour name.* Blue is the starbaby middle name du jour, occasionally used as a first. **Bleu, Blu.**

BLUEBELL. *Flower name.* Geri 'Ginger Spice' Halliwell joined her former Spice Sisters in creative baby-naming with this adventurous – some might say outlandish – choice. Distinctive and charming? Or better suited to a farmyard animal? Your call. **Bluebelle.**

BLUMA. *Hebrew, 'flower'.* See **BLOSSOM.**

BLYTHE. *English, 'free spirit, happy, carefree'.* Embodies a cheerful, carefree spirit and could be the next Brooke. **Blithe, Blyth.**

BOBBIE. *English, diminutive of* **ROBERTA, BARBARA.** Dated nickname of the 1930s and 40s; Barbie without the wasp waist. **Bobbe, Bobbee, Bobbi, Bobby.**

BOHEMIA. *Place or word name.* More a concept than a place – or a name.

♂ **BOLIVIA.** *Place name.* If you're tired of Olivia, you could be the first on your road to introduce this unique sound-related place name with Latin flair.

BONITA. *Spanish, 'pretty'.* Like Benita, had some popularity in the 1950s. **Boni, Bonie, Bonni, Bonnie, Bonny, Bunita, Bunnie, Bunny, Nita.**

BONNIE. *Scottish, 'beautiful and cheerful'.* Despite its appealing meaning and amiable air, Bonnie's been out of the fashion loop since *Bonnie and Clyde*'s 1967 Oscar nomination. **Boni, Bonne, Bonnee, Bonni, Bonnibel, Bonny, Bunni, Bunnie, Bunny.**

BORA. *Czech, diminutive of* **BARBARA.** 'Bore' and 'boring' are teasing possibilities; Thora, Nora and Flora are alternatives.

♂ **BRADLEY.** *English 'broad clearing'.* Fading boys' name making fresh start for girls, aided by *-ley* ending. **Brad, Bradlee, Bradleigh, Bradli, Bradlie, Bradly.**

♂ **BRADY.** *Irish, 'broad meadow,' 'one with broad eyes'.* Has the energetic-Irish-slightly-boyish image that many modern parents love. **Bradee, Bradey, Braedi.**

BRAE. *Modern invented name.* A newly hatched cousin of Bree and Brea.

♂ **BRAEDEN.** *English, 'broad hill'.* One of several trendy boys' names now being adopted for girls with feminised spellings. **Bradyn, Bradynn, Braedan, Braedyn, Braedynn, Braedynne, Braiden, Braidin, Braidyn, Braidynn, Braidynne, Braydon, Braydyn, Braydynn, Braydynne.**

BRAELYN. *Modern invented name.* One of the most girlish offshoots of Braeden. **Braelan, Braelen, Braelin, Braelinn, Braelon, Braelynn, Braelynne, Braylan, Braylen,**

Braylin, Braylinn, Braylon, Braylyn, Braylynn, Braylynne.

BRANDY. *Dutch, 'burnt wine'.* The alcohol-laced member of the Randy-Candy-Mandy sorority of 1970s to 80s nickname names; now pretty much on the wagon. **Bran, Brande, Brandea, Brandee, Brandey, Brandi, Brandie, Brandye, Branndea, Branndi, Branndie.**

BRANWEN. *Celtic, 'blessed raven'.* Attractive Celtic mythological name, possibly a variant of Bronwyn. **Branwyn.**

♂ **BRAYDEN.** *English, 'broad hill'.* One in the currently modish *aden* family of boys' names beginning to be used for girls.

♂ **BRAZIL.** *Place name.* Place name with character. **Brasilia.**

BREA. *Short form of* **BREANA.** See **BRIA.**

BREANA. *See* **BRIANA.** This spelling is running a close second in pereference to Briana. **Breann, Breanna, Breanne, Breawna, Bryanna, Bryanne.**

★**BREE.** *Variation of* **BRIGHID** *or* **BRIANA.** Sophisticated yet upbeat image, preferable to the cheese-related Brie; featured on *Desperate Housewives* and in several films. **Brae, Bray, Bre, Brei, Breigh, Bri, Brie, Brielle.**

BREEZE. *Word name.* Refreshing middle name possibility.

BRENDA. *Celtic, 'blade of a sword'.* First a glamorous 1940s debutante, now fading in favour of more modern Brenna, Briana, and Bryn. **Bren, Brenn, Brenna, Brennda, Brenndah.**

BRENNA. *Irish, 'raven'.* As Jennifer begat Jenna, so did Brenda lead to the steady use of this female form of Brendan. **Branna, Bren, Brenn, Brennah, Brenne, Brinna, Brynna, Brynne.**

♂ **BRENNAN.** *Irish, 'descendent of the sad one'.* Poised for popularity, an Irish last name soft enough to borrow from the boys.

♂ **BRETT.** *Celtic, 'from Brittany'.* First spotted as a female name in Hemingway's *The Sun Also Rises,* Brett retains its pleasingly brisk, executive air. **Bret, Brette, Britt.**

BRIA. *Short form of* **BRIANA.** Sweet but spirited shortening of Briana, becoming increasingly popular. **Brea.**

BRIALLEN. *Welsh, 'a primrose'.* Unusual combination choice.

BRIANNA, BRIANA. *Feminine variation of* **BRIAN.** There are nine different popular versions of this name in the US – a sure sign that, though pretty, it's getting more and more difficult to make it distinctive. **Brana, Breana, Breann, Breanne, Breeanna, Breeanne, Bria, Brianna, Brianne, Brielle, Brienna, Brinn, Brinna, Briny, Bryana, Bryann, Bryanna, Bryannah, Bryanne, Bryn, Bryna, Brynne.**

BRIAR. *English, 'a thorny patch'.* Fairy-tale memories of 'Sleeping Beauty' inspire some parents to call their daughters Briar Rose. **Brier, Bryar.**

♂ **BRICE.** *Celtic, 'bright strength'; Welsh, 'speckled, freckled'.* Among the more masculine of the short unisex *B* names. **Bryce.**

BRIDE. *(BREE-da) Irish, 'strength'.* Pronunciation problems complicate this choice. **Breeda, Bridie, Brídín.**

BRIDGET. *Anglicised variation of* **BRIGHID.** This most familiar form of the name of the Celtic goddess of wisdom is still used by traditionalists. **Biddy, Bidu, Bree, Bridey, Bridgette, Bridgie, Bridgit, Bridgitte, Bridie, Brie, Brigid, Brigit, Brigita, Brigitte. International: Breda, Bríd, Bride, Brigid, Brighid** *(Irish),* **Ffraid** *(Welsh),* **Brigitte** *(French),* **Brigida** *(Italian),* **Brigitta, Gitta** *(German),* **Birgit, Birgitta, Bridgette, Brigitta** *(Scandinavian),* **Berget, Brigitta, Brita, Britt, Britta, Gittan** *(Swedish),* **Berit, Birgit, Birgitte, Birte** *(Norwegian),* **Piritta, Pirjo, Pirkko, Riitta** *(Finnish),* **Brygid, Brygida** *(Polish).*

BRIE. *French, place name of cheese-producing region.* Place name and homonym of Bree, less popular than its enlargement, Brielle. **Bree, Briella, Brielle, Briette.**

BRIELLE, BRIELLA. *Long form of* **BRIE.** Feminine, breezy name but lacks heft.

BRIGHID. *Irish, 'strength, power'.* This is the original Gaelic form of the name of the mythological goddess of fire, poetry, and wisdom.

BRIGIDINE. *Irish variation of* **BRIGHID.** Unique take on Bridget used by singer Sinead O'Connor.

BRIGITTE. *French variation of* **BRIGHID.** French version long associated with 1950s sex symbol Brigitte Bardot.

BRILIE. *Modern invented name.* Combines elements of the megapopular Briana and Riley to form a pleasant merger. **Brilee, Brileigh, Briley, Brily, Brylee, Bryleigh, Bryley, Bryli, Brylie, Bryly.**

♂ **BRIO.** *Italian, 'vivacity, zest'.* Musical term with great verve and energy.

BRIONA, BRIONNA. *Variation of* **BRIANA.** Another increasingly popular *Bri* pick. **Breona, Breonna, Brione, Brionne.**

BRIONY. *See* **BRYONY.**

BRISA. *Spanish, 'beloved'.* Commonly used in Latino families, all but unheard of in others. **Breza, Brisha, Brishia, Brissa, Bryssa.**

BRITANNIA. *Latin, 'Britain'.* Hail Britannia? We think not. **Britania, Britanja, Britanya, Brittannia, Brittanja, Brittanya.**

BRITNEY. *Variation of* **BRITTANY.** This abbreviated spelling, which also relates to Whitney, quickly took on a life of its own, thanks to the megafame of Ms Spears, but it's already beginning to burn out. **Britini, Britnee, Britni, Britny, Britnye.**

BRITT. *Swedish, contracted form of* **BIRGIT.** Brisk but rather brittle. **Brita, Brite, Britta.**

BRITTANY. *Celtic, 'from Brittany, a Breton'.* One of the sensations of the last two decades, it started as an upscale name, quickly became overused to the point of cliché, now almost overtaken by little sister Britney. **Brett, Brit, Briteney,**

Briteny, Britni, Britny, Britt, Britta, Brittan, Brittanee, Brittaney, Brittani, Britteny, Brittin, Brittnee, Brittni, Brittny, Britton.

BRONNEN. *Cornish, 'a rush'.* Similar to so many others, sure to provoke a lot of 'What was that again?' queries.

★**BRONTË.** *Greek, 'thunder'.* Lovely surname of the three novel-writing sisters, now used as a baby name; a fitting tribute for lovers of *Jane Eyre* and *Wuthering Heights*.

★**BRONWEN.** *Welsh, 'fair-bosomed'.* Widespread in Wales, but not as common in the rest of Britain, we think it's a real winner. (Note: the Bronwyn spelling is strictly for males in its native land.) **Branwen, Bronnie, Bronny, Browin, Bronwyn, Bronwynn, Bronwynne, Bronya.**

BRONYA. *Polish, 'protection'.* Evokes an image of peasant blouses, dirndl skirts and babushkas. **Bronia, Bronja.**

BROOKE. *English, 'small stream'.* Brooke still retains a large measure of freshness and sophistication. **Brook, Brooks. International:** Bahr *(Arabic).*

♂ **BROOKLYN.** *Place name.* Although known more for the borough in New York City, it has become a popular feminine girl's name. **Brookelyn, Brookelynn, Brooklen, Brooklin, Brooklinn, Brooklyne, Brooklynn, Brooklynne.**

BRUNA. *Italian, 'brown'.* Possibility for a dark-haired babe. **International: Brunette** *(French),* **Brona, Brune, Brunetta** *(Italian).*

BRUNHILD, BRUNHILDA. *Norse, 'armour-wearing fighting maid'.* One of the Valkyries, still clad in heavy armour. **Brinhild, Brinhilda, Brinhilde, Brunhilde, Brynhild, Hilda, Hilde, Hildi, Hildie, Hildy.**

BRYANA, BRYANNA. *Variations of* **BRIANA.** More of the seemingly infinite variations of this name. **Bryann, Bryanne, Bryanni.**

♂ **BRYCE.** *See* **BRICE.**

★↑♂ **BRYN, BRYNN.** *Welsh, 'hill'.* An up-and-coming gentle, yet substantial, Welsh name, would also be effective in the middle spot. **Brin, Brinn, Brinne, Brynne.**

Stellar Starbabies Beginning with *B*

Bailey	Stella McCartney & Alasdhair Willis
Beatrice	Heather Mills & Paul McCartney
Bechet	Soon-Yi & Woody Allen
Bella	Eddie Murphy, Keenen Ivory Wayans
Billie	Carrie Fisher
Blossom	Kacey *(Little Mo, Eastenders)* Ainsworth
Blue Angel	Dave *(The Edge)* Evans
Bluebell	Geri *(Ginger Spice)* Halliwell
Bobbi Kristina	Bobby Brown & Whitney Houston
Bria	Eddie Murphy
Brielle	Blair Underwood
Brighton	Jon Favreau
Brigidine	Sinead O'Connor

BRYNNA. *Welsh, 'hill'.* You say Bryn, he says Bryana – here's a name you might agree on. **Brena, Breena, Brinah, Brinna, Brinnah, Bryna, Brynah, Brynnah.**

★**BRYONY.** *Latin, 'to sprout'; botanical name, vine with green flowers.* Unusually strong plant name with the popular *Bry* beginning. **Brihoney, Brioney, Briony, Bryonie. International: Bryonia** *(Greek).*

BUENA. *Spanish, 'good, excellent'.* Affirmative adjective that is occasionally used as a name. **Buona.**

BUFFY. *Diminutive of* **ELIZABETH.** One-time sorority girl with a roommate named Muffy, then a fearless vampire slayer, though still basically fluffy. **Buffee, Buffey, Buffi, Buffie.**

BUNNY. *Nickname deriving from a variety of* B *names.*

If Buffy is fluffy, what would that make this? **Bunnee, Bunni, Bunnie.**

BUONA. *Italian, 'good'.* Naming your child the word for *good* comes with no guarantees.

♂ **BURGUNDY.** *French place name; also colour name.* It's a place! It's a wine! And a colour! – no wonder trend-heavy Burgundy's been discovered as a name. **Burgandi, Burgandie, Burgandy, Burgundee, Burgundey, Burgundi, Burgundie.**

♂ **BURMA.** *Place name.* Less-travelled member of this fashionable group, with less than attractive sound.

BUTTERFLY. *English word name.* Fluttery and flighty. **International: Papillon** *(French),* **Fella** *(Italian),* **Borboleta** *(Portuguese),* **Babochka** *(Russian),* **Farasha** *(Arabic).*

C *girls*

CACHET. *(ka-SHAY) French, 'prestigious, desirable'.* One of those word names – Cliché is the most egregious example – that sounds lovely but seems slightly ridiculous when taken literally. **Cachae, Cache, Cachea, Cachee, Cachée.**

CADEAU. *(kad-DOH) French, 'gift'.* A decidedly exotic twist on the word name trend, but don't be surprised if you encounter ponies and poodles with the same moniker.

CADENCE. *Latin, 'rhythm, beat'.* Musical word name zooming up the American charts. **Cadencia, Cady, Kadena, Kadence. International: Cadenza** *(Italian).*

CADY. *English, diminutive of* **CADENCE** *and surname.* Stylish name that might relate to nickname names like Katie or Kaylee or may honor women's rights leader Elizabeth Cady Stanton. **Cade, Cadee, Cadey, Cadi, Cadie, Cadye, Caidie, Kade, Kadee, Kadi, Kadie, Kady, Kadye.**

CAI. *Vietnamese, 'feminine'.* Unusual, exotic, simple. **Cae, Cay, Caye.**

CAILIN. *American variation of* **CAITLIN** *or* **KAYLIN.** While this spelling doesn't appear on popularity charts, other forms do, along with several similar names, from Caitlin to Jalen to Kayla. The result: a name that feels more common than it actually is. **Caelin, Caelyn, Caileen, Cailen, Cailene, Cailine, Cailyn, Cailynn, Cailynne, Calen, Calin, Cayleen, Caylen, Caylene, Caylin, Cayline, Caylyn, Caylyne, Caylynn, Caylynne.**

♀ **CAIRO.** *Place name.* American model Beverly Peele put this exotic name on the map when she chose it for her daughter; it's much less faddish sounding than more typical US place names like Dallas and Dakota.

CAITLIN. *Irish variation of* **CATHERINE.** Most forms of this megapopular name, which is in the Top 50, including this most-authentic one, are starting to dip, though there have been thousands of girls named Caitlin – and Katelyn and Kaitlyn ad infinitum – every year for the past two decades. **Caetlin, Cailin, Caithlin, Caitlan,** **Caitland, Caitlandt, Caitlann, Caitleen, Caitlen, Caitlene, Caitlenn, Caitline, Caitlinn, Caitlon, Caitlyn, Caitlyne, Caitlynn, Caitlynne, Catelin, Cateline, Catelinn, Catelyn, Catelyne, Catelynn, Catlee, Catleen, Catleene, Catlin, Catlinn, Catlyn, Catlynn, Catlynne, Cayetin, Caylin, Haitian, Kaitlann, Kaitlin, Kaitlinn, Kaitlyn, Kaitlynn, Katelan, Katelin, Katelynn, Kayelin, Kayelyn.**

CAITRIONA. *Scottish variation of* **CATHERINE.** Considerably less exotic – and less appealing – when you know it's pronounced like Katrina. **Catriona.**

CALA. *Arabic, 'castle, fortress'.* Extremely simple and extremely distinctive – a winning combination, though more often spelled Calla. **Calah, Calan, Calla, Callah.**

CALAIS. *(kal-LAY) French place name.* Undiscovered name of the picturesque northern French port.

CALANDRA. *Greek, 'lark'.* Calista Flockhart opened the door to a whole flock of graceful

Music Names

Allegra

Alto

Amadea

Banjo

Brio

Cadence

Calliope

Calypso

Clarion

Corisande

Danae

Drum

Fife

Guitar

Harmony

Harper

Haydn

Jaz/Jazz

Lyric

Music

Octavia

Piano

Piper

Viola

and unusual Greek names like this. **Cal, Calan, Calandre, Calandrea, Calandria, Caleida, Calendra, Calendre, Calee, Calley, Calli, Callie, Cally, Kalandra, Kalandria.**

CALANTHA. *Greek, 'lovely flower'.* Another of the new Greek-accented *Cal-* names. **Cal, Calanthe, Callee, Calley, Calli, Callie, Cally, Kalantha.**

CALEDONIA. *Latin, 'poetic appelation for Scotland'.* This is a rhythmic place name appropriate for a child with Scottish roots.

CALI. *Diminutive of any CAL-name.* A short form that can stand on its own, though not all that steadily.

CALICO. *English word name.* Word name with fashionable *o* ending that has associations with both the homespun fabric and the mottled cat.

CALIDA. *Spanish, 'heated'.* Unusual but accessible Hispanic choice with stylish sound. **Calina, Calinda, Calla, Calli, Callida, Callinda, Kalida.**

♂ **CALIFORNIA.** *Place name.* Has not caught on as much as other place names linked to the American state– Sierra, Marin, West, or even Francisco – probably because of its length.

★**CALISTA.** *Greek, 'most beautiful'. Ally McBeal* actress Calista Flockhart didn't just introduce a name (or a body type or a skirt length), she introduced a whole sensibility. Pretty and delicate, it's definitely worthy of consideration, especially for parents with Greek roots. **Cala, Calesta, Calixta, Calla, Callesta, Calli, Callie, Callista, Callixta, Cally, Callysta, Calysta, Kala, Kalesta, Kalista, Kalla, Kallesta, Kalfi, Kallie, Kallista, Kally, Kallysta.**

CALLA. *Greek, 'beautiful'.* Flower name more distinctive and delicate than Lily.

CALLIE. *Greek diminutive, 'beautiful'.* This Hallie-esque nickname name is starting to dip, while the sleeker, more nouveau Cali is rising. **Cal, Calee, Caleigh, Cali, Calie, Callee, Calley, Calli, Cally, Caly, Kallee, Kaleigh, Kalley, Kalli, Kallie, Kally.**

CALLIOPE. *(ka-LYE-oh-pee)*
Greek mythology name. Calliope
is the name of the muse of epic
poetry – and also the musical
instrument on the merry-go-
round. Bold and creative, it
would not be the easiest name
for a girl lacking such qualities.
Callia, Callyope, Kalliope.

CALVINA. *Latin, feminine form
of* CALVIN. There are several
better *Cal-* names that don't
simply echo a male form.
Calvine, Calvinetta, Calvinette.

♂ **CALYPSO.** *Greek, 'she who
hides'.* Name of a mythological
nymph and West Indian music
makes a dramatic, rhythmic
choice. **Calipso, Callypso, Caly,
Kallypso, Kalypso, Lypsie, Lypsy.**

CAMBRIA. *Place name.* Most
names that start with *Cam-* are
on the up, so why not this obscure
term for Wales as well as for a
prehistoric time period? **Cambaria,
Camberry, Cambie, Cambrea,
Cambreah, Cambreia, Cambrie,
Cambrina, Cambrya, Cami.**

CAMBRIE. *Modern invented
name.* Cute but slight mix of
stylish sounds Cam and Bree.

**Cambree, Cambreigh, Cambrey,
Cambri, Cambry.**

♂ **CAMDEN.** *Scottish,
'winding valley'; American
and British place name.* Newly
popular boys' name could cross
over in much the way the
related Cameron has. **Camdan,
Camdin, Camdon, Camdyn,
Camdynne, Kamden.**

CAMELLIA. *Flower name.*
Exotic flower name with distinct
roots related to the Camille/
Camila group. Could be a floral
replacement for Amelia. **Camala,
Camalia, Camallia, Camela,
Camelia, Camelita, Camella,
Camellita, Cami, Canunelia,
Kamelia, Kamellia.**

CAMEO. *Word name.* This
evocative term for a stone or
shell carved in relief could make
a striking first name for a girl,
though she would have a starring
role in her story, rather than a
cameo. **Cami, Cammeo, Kameo.**

CAMERA. *Word name.* Late
tennis great Arthur Ashe (whose
wife was a photographer)
pioneered word names when
he used this for his daughter.
Camara, Kamara, Kamera.

♂ **CAMERON.** *Scottish,
'crooked nose'.* Cameron Diaz
almost single-handedly
transported this sophisticated
Scottish male surname into the
girls' camp, where it is proving
increasingly popular – though it
hasn't caught up with the boys.
The phonetic, more feminine
spelling of Camryn is also a
possibility. **Cam, Camaran,
Cameran, Cameren, Cameri,
Cameria, Camerin, Camie,
Camira, Camiran, Camiron,
Camran, Camren, Camrin,
Camron, Camry, Camryn,
Kameran, Kameren, Kamerin,
Kameron, Kamran, Kamren,
Kamrin, Kamron, Kamryn.**

CAMILA, CAMILLA. *Latin,
'young ceremonial attendant'.*
The Spanish Camila, pronounced
ka-MEE-la, is the fastest rising
version of this ancient Roman
name, but recent royal Camilla
may have helped promote the
brand. In Roman myth, Camilla
was a swift-footed huntress so
fast she could run over a field
without bending a blade of
grass. **Cam, Cami, Camia,
Camilia, Camilya, Cammi,
Cammie, Cammilla, Cammille,
Cammy, Cammylle, Camyla,
Camylla, Camylle, Chamelea,**

Chamelia, Chamika, Chamila, Chamilia, Kamille, Kamyla, Mille, Millee, Milley, Milli, Millie, Milly. **International: Cama, Camala, Camile** (*Spanish*), **Kamilka, Milla** (*Polish*), **Kamila, Kamilla** (*Hungarian*), **Camelia** (*Romanian*).

★**CAMILLE.** *French variation of* **CAMILLA.** Once connected to Greta Garbo's tragic 'Lady of the Camellias,' but that image has faded, replaced by a sleek, chic, highly attractive one. **Cam, Cami, Camia, Camiel, Camielle, Camil, Camila, Camile, Camilia, Camill, Camilla, Camillia, Camilya, Camylle, Camyle, Camyll, Cammilla, Cammille, Cammillie, Cammilyn, Cammyl, Cammyll, Camylle, Chamelea, Chamelia, Chamelle, Chamika, Chamila, Chamilia, Chamille, Kamille.**

♂ **CAMPBELL.** *Scottish 'crooked mouth'.* This unisex name, which is also a family surname, can make a more unusual Cameron alternative.

CAMRYN. *See* **CAMERON.**

♂ **CANADA.** *Iroquois place name, 'where the heavens*

touch the earth'. Undiscovered but attractive place name possibility, up till now a masculine territory.

CANDACE. *Latin, 'white, pure, sincere'.* This ancient title of a dynasty of Ethiopian queens, associated both with actress Candice Bergen and *Sex and the City* writer Candace Bushnell, is rarely used for babies today, perhaps due to the sticky sweetness of nickname Candy. **Cace, Canace, Canda, Candaice, Candas, Candase, Candayce, Candece, Candee, Candelle, Candes, Candi, Candiace, Candias, Candice, Candie, Candies, Candis, Candise, Candiss, Candus, Candy, Candyce, Candys, Candyse, Cyndyss, Dace, Dacee, Dacey, Dacie, Dacy, Kandace, Kandice, Kandiss, Kandy.**

CANDIDA. *Latin, 'white'.* Attractive ancient name borne by several saints but sullied by association with the yeast infection. **Candeea, Candi, Candia, Candie, Candita, Candy. International: Candide** (*French*).

CANDY. *Diminutive of* **CANDACE.** Too sugary sweet and inconsequential for a modern girl.

CANTARA. *Arabic, 'little bridge'.* Lovely and unusual choice, with a choral feel. **Cantarah.**

CANTRELLE. *French, 'song'.* Vocal name seldom heard, with most *elle*-ending names these days dropped in favour of the more straightforward Elle and Ella. **Cantrella.**

♂ **CANYON.** *Spanish word name.* Rugged nature name with possibilities . . . but more for boys.

CAPRICE. *French from Italian, 'impulsive change of mind'.* This word name has an appealing sound, however it's spoilt by its trivialising meaning. **Cappi, Caprece, Caprecia, Capreece, Capresha, Capri, Capria, Capricia, Caprie, Capriese, Caprina, Capris, Caprise, Caprisha, Capritta, Capry.**

CAPUCINE. *French, 'cowled monk'.* Capucine was a sexy French actress half a century ago, but today, the name is more likely to be mistaken for a cup of coffee – or a long-tailed monkey. **Cappucine.**

CARA. *Latin, 'dear'.* Simple, sweet, Italian endearment that enjoyed some popularity from the 1970s through the 1990s. It's faded now . . . though that may be a good reason to use it. Caira, Carabel, Carabell, Carabelle, Caragh, Carah, Caralea, Caralee, Caraleigh, Caralia, Caralie, Caranda, Carely, Caretta, Carey, Carina, Carine, Carrah, Carrie, Carry, Kara, Karina, Karine, Karra, Karrie, Karry. International: Carra *(Irish)*.

♂ **CARBRY.** *Irish, 'charioteer'.* Male name from Irish mythology makes stylish-sounding choice for girls. Cáirbre, Carbery, Carbury.

♂ **CARDEN.** *English occupational name, 'wool carder'.* Unusual, serious, no-nonsense occupational surname that could be borrowed from the boys. Cardin, Cardon, Cardyn.

CAREY. *Irish, 'dark, black'.* Variously spelt trendy name in the 1970s, but it hasn't been used much in the last decade. Caree, Cari, Carie, Carrey, Cary, Kari.

CARINA. *Italian, 'dear little one'.* Pretty feminissima name whose fall from popularity may be speeded by similarity to (hurricane name) Katrina. Careena, Caren, Carena, Caridad, Carin, Carinah, Carine, Carinn, Carinne, Carinna, Kareena, Karena, Karina, Karine.

CARISSA. *Greek, 'grace'.* Trending down, along with others of both the *Car* and the *issa* groups. Caresa, Carese, Caressa, Caresse, Carisa, Carise, Carisha, Carisia, Carrisa, Charessa, Charesse, Charisa, Charissa, Karessa, Karisa, Karissa, Kharissa.

CARITA. *Latin, 'beloved'.* Sweet as a nickname – but it's like naming your child 'Dearie'. Caritta, Karita, Karitta.

CARLA. *Feminine variation of* CARL. While the *K* version is still rising, Carla-with-a-*C*, the somewhat severe feminisation of the Germanic Carl, gets more unfashionable every year. Carila, Carilla, Carlah, Carlana, Carleta, Carletta, Carlette, Carlia, Carliqua, Carliyle, Carlla, Carlonda, Carlyjo, Carlyle, Carlysle, Karla, Karlla.

CARLEIGH. *See* **CARLY.**

♂ **CARLIN.** *Irish, 'little champion'.* Stronger and more contemporary twist on Carla or Carly. Carlan, Carlana, Carlandra, Carlina, Carlinda, Carline, Carling, Carllan, Carlyn, Carlyna, Carlynn, Carlynne, Carllen, Carrlin.

CARLOTTA. *Italian variation of* CHARLOTTE. Familiar name that retains its Latin rhythm. Carletta, Carlita, Carlota.

CARLY. *Feminine diminutive of* CARL. Though a couple of its more 'creative' spellings – Carli and Karlee, for example – are still on the rise, this feminine form of Carl, popularised by singer Carly Simon in the 1970s, could by no stretch be considered fashionable. Carle, Carlea, Carleah, Carlee, Carleen, Carleh, Carleigh, Carlene, Carley, Carli, Carlie, Carline, Carlita, Carlye, Carlyne, Carlyta, Karlee, Karleigh, Karlene,

Karli, Karlie, Karline, Karlita, Karly, Kavlyta.

CARMEL. *Hebrew, 'garden'.* Biblical place name with sweet association, commonly heard in Ireland. Carma, Carmaletta, Carmalit, Carmalita, Carmalla, Carman, Carmania, Carmanya, Carmarit, Carmeli, Carmelia, Carmelina, Carmelit, Carmelita, Carmelitha, Carmelitia, Carmella, Carmelle, Carmellia, Carmellina, Carmellit, Carmellita, Carmellitha, Carmellitia, Carmesa, Carmesha, Carmi, Carmia, Carmie, Carmiel, Carmiela, Carmil, Carmila, Carmile, Carmilla, Carmille, Carmina, Carmine, Carmisha, Carmit, Carmiya, Carmy, Karmel, Karmela, Karmelit, Karmen, Leeta, Lina, Lita, Melina, Melita, Mina.

CARMELA. *Italian and Spanish variation of* **CARMEL.** It will be a long time before Carmela shakes the image of TV's *Sopranos* wife. Carmela.

♂ **CARMEN.** *Spanish variation of* **CARMEL.** Carmel's sexier, more operatic sister, also used for boys in Hispanic culture. Carma, Carmaine, Carman,

Carmelia, Carmelina, Carmelita, Carmencita, Carmene, Carmi, Carmia, Carmie, Carmin, Carmina, Carmine, Carmita, Carmon, Carmyna, Carmynn, Carmyta, Charmaine, Karmen, Karmia, Karmina, Karmita, Lita, Mina.

♂ **CARO.** *Italian, 'dear', Short form of* **CAROL** or **CAROLINE.** Upper-crusty nickname occasionally used in Britain; in the US it's been eclipsed by Carrie et al.

CAROL. *English, feminine variation of* **CHARLES.** Caroline abbreviation wildly popular with Mum's generation . . . or Grandma's. Caral, Carel, Carey, Cari, Cariel, Carla, Carleen, Carlene, Carley, Carlin, Carlina, Carline, Carlita, Carlota, Carlotta, Carly, Carlyn, Carlynn, Carlynne, Carola, Carole, Carolee, Carolena, Carolenia, Carolin, Carolina, Carolinda, Caroline, Caroll, Caroly, Carolyn, Carolynn, Carolynne, Carri, Carrie, Carrol, Carroll, Carrolyn, Carry, Cary, Caryl, Caryle, Caryll, Carylle, Charla, Charleen, Charlena, Charlene, Charlotta, Charmain, Charmaine, Charmian,

Charmion, Charyl, Cheryl, Cherlyn, Karel, Kari, Karla, Karleen, Karli, Karlie, Karlina, Karinka, Karlote, Karlotta, Karole, Karolina, Karyl, Karyll, Karrole, Karryl, Karryll, Kerril, Kerryl, Keryl, Lola, Loleta, Lolita, Lotta, Lotte, Lotti, Lottie, Sharleen, Sharlene, Sharline, Sharmain, Sharmian.

★**CAROLINA.** *Variation of* **CAROLINE;** *also place name in US.* Languid, romantic and classy, this variation heats up Caroline and modernises Carol.

↑**CAROLINE, CAROLYN.** *French, feminine variation of* **CHARLES.** Royal name with a well-earned patina. Caroline's only downside: it's quite straightlaced. Carolyn, while less formal, brings the name distinctly down-market. Caraleen, Caraleena, Caralin, Caraline, Caralyn, Caralyne, Caralynn, Caralynna, Caralynne, Cari, Carileen, Carilena, Carilene, Carilin, Cariline, Carilyn, Carilynn, Carilynne, Carleen, Carleena, Carlen, Carlena, Carlene, Carley, Carli, Carlie, Carlin, Carline, Carly, Carlyn, Carlyna, Carlyne,

Carlynn, Carlynne, Carlyne, Caro, Carol, Carola, Carolann, Carole, Caroleen, Caroleena, Caroleina, Carolena, Carolin, Carolina, Carolyn, Carolyne, Carolynn, Carolynne, Carollyn, Carri, Carrie, Carroleen, Carrolena, Carrolene, Carrolin, Carroline, Carroll, Carrolyn, Carrolynn, Carrolynne, Cary, Caryl, Carylin, Carylyn, Carylynn, Charla, Charleen, Charleena, Charlena, Charlene, Charlyne, Ina, Karaleen, Karaleena, Karalina, Karaline, Karalyn, Karalynna, Karalynne, Kari, Karie, Karla, Karleen, Karlen, Karlena, Karli, Karlie, Karlina, Karoline, Karolyn, Karolyna, Karolyne, Karolynn, Karolynne, Leena, Sharla, Sharleen, Sharlene, Sharline, Sharlyne. International: Karoline, Lina, Linchen, Line *(German),* Carolinda, Karila *(Swedish),* Karoliina *(Finnish),* Karolina, Karolinka *(Polish),* Karola, Karolina *(Czech).*

CARON. *Welsh, 'loving, kind-hearted, charitable', or variation of* **KAREN.** Though it sounds like Karen, this spelling makes the name more distinctive. **Caren, Carin,**

Caronne, Carren, Carron, Carrone, Caryn.

CARRIE. *Diminutive of* **CAROL** *or* **CAROLINE.** Retains some charm, thanks to *Sex and the City* heroine Carrie Bradshaw, but was last stylish in the disco era. **Carey, Carree, Carrey, Carri, Carria, Carry, Cary, Kari, Karri.**

♂ **CARSON.** *Scottish and Irish, 'son of the marsh dwellers'.* Very popular surname choice – at least as a boy's name – beginning to catch on for girls. **Carsen, Carsin, Carsyn, Karsen, Karsin, Karson, Karsyn.**

♂ **CARTER.** *English occupational name, 'cart maker or driver'.* One of the megapopular Wasp-ish surname names for boys just dipping its toe into the girls' pool.

CARYN. *Danish variation of* **KAREN.** Modernised spelling not enough to revive Karen. **Caren, Carren, Carrin, Carryn, Caryna, Caryne, Carynn.**

CARYS. *(KAR-is) Welsh, 'love'.* Common in Wales, this name was introduced elsewhere when

Welsh-born Catherine Zeta-Jones and husband Michael Douglas chose it for their daughter. **Caris, Caryse, Ceris, Cerys.**

CASCADE. *Word name.* It's a nature name evocative of waterfalls. But in the US it's also a washing-up detergent.

♂ **CASEY.** *Irish, 'brave in battle'.* One of the original unisex Irish surname names, energetic Casey bounced onto the scene in the 1960s, then peaked in the 1980s for both boys and girls. **Cacey, Caci, Cacie, Cacy, Caesi, Caisee, Caisie, Caisey, Caisi, Caisie, Casce, Casci, Cascy, Casi, Casie, Casse, Cassee, Cassey, Cassye, Casy, Cayce, Caycee, Caycey, Cayci, Caycie, Cayse, Caysee, Caysey, Caysi, Caysie, Caysy, Cazzi, Kacey, Kacie, Kacy, Kacyee, Kasey, Kaycee, Kaycey, Kayci, Kaycie, Kaysee, Kaysey, Kaysi, Kaysie, Kaysy, Kaysyee.**

CASHMERE. *Word name.* Soft, luxurious – and out of the ordinary.

♂ **CASS.** *Diminutive of* **CASSANDRA.** Once tied to

the unfortunate Mama Cass, still feels a bit flimsy to stand on its own. **Cassee, Cassey, Cassi, Cassii, Cassy, Casy, Kass, Kassi, Kassie, Kassy.**

CASSANDRA. *Greek, 'prophetess'.* The name of the mythological sibyl condemned never to be believed has been used for exotic characters in movies and soap operas. Ethereal and delicate, it was well used in the 1990s, but is now descending in popularity. **Casandera, Casandra, Casandre, Casandrea, Casandrey, Casandri, Casandria, Casanndra, Casaundra, Casaundre, Casaundri, Casaundria, Casondra, Casondre, Casondri, Casondria, Cass, Cassandre, Cassandry, Cassatindra, Cassaundra, Cassaundre, Cassaundri, Cassi, Cassie, Cassondra, Cassondre, Cassondri, Cassondria, Cassundra, Cassundre, Cassundri, Cassundrai, Kasandera, Kassandra, Kassi, Kassie, Kassy, Sande, Sandee, Sandera, Sandi, Sandie, Sandy, Saundra, Sohndra, Sondra, Zandra.**

★**CASSIA.** *Greek, 'cinnamon'.* It's rare to find a name that's truly unusual yet has a stylish feel. This one has the added attraction of the sweet smell of cinnamon. **Casia, Casiah, Cass, Cassa, Casya.**

CASSIDY. *Irish 'curly-haired'.* This one has fallen off its peak. **Casadee, Casadi, Casadie, Casidee, Casidi, Casidy, Cass, Cassaday, Cassadee, Cassadey, Cassadi, Cassadie, Cassadina, Cassady, Cassandre, Cassandri, Cassandry, Cassaundra, Casseday, Cassi, Cassiddy, Cassidee, Cassidey, Cassidi, Cassidie, Cassie, Cassity, Cassondra, Kassadey, Kassidy, Kassodey. International: Caiside** *(Irish).*

CASSIE. *Diminutive of* **CASSANDRA.** Though not much in use, still retains a cozy *Little House on the Prairie-type* pioneer feel.

CASSIOPEIA. *(kass-ee-OH-pee-uh) Greek mythology name.* This name of a mythological mother who became a stellar constellation is challenging but intriguing, and has all those softening Cass nicknames

available. **Cassio, Cassiopia, Kassiopeia, Kassiopia.**

★**CATALINA.** *Spanish variation of* **CATHERINE,** *place name.* This name of an island in sight of Los Angeles makes an attractive and newly stylish variation on the overused Catherine or Caitlin. **Cataleen, Catalena, Catalene, Catalia, Catalin, Catalyn, Catalyna, Cateline.**

CATERINA. *Italian variation of* **KATHERINE.** If your ancestry is Italian, you may want to consider this elegant twist on a classic.

CATHERINE. *Greek, 'pure'.* One of the oldest and most consistently well-used female names, with endless variations and nicknames. The *C* form feels more gently old-fashioned and feminine than the more popular *K* versions. Most stylish nickname right now: Kate . . . or Cate, à la Blanchett. **Caitlinn, Caity, Caren, Carri, Carrin, Caryn, Carynn, Cass, Cassey, Cassi, Cassie, Cataina, Cataleena, Catarena, Cate, Caterin, Caterine, Catey, Catha, Cathaleen, Cathaline, Catharen,**

Catharin, Catharyn, Catharyna, Catharyne, Cathe, Cathee, Cathelin, Cathenne, Catheren, Catherene, Catheria, Catherin, Catherina, Catherinn, Catheryn, Cathey, Cathi, Cathie, Cathirin, Cathiryn, Cathleen, Cathlene, Cathline, Cathrinn, Cathryn, Catina, Catlaina, Catreeka, Catreena, Catrelle, Catrice, Catricia, Catrika, Catrine, Kait, Kaitey, Kaitie, Kaitlin, Kaitlinne, Kaitrin, Kaitrine, Kaitrinna, Kaitriona, Kaitrionagh, Kaity, Kat, Kataleen, Katalina, Katchen, Kate, Katee, Katelle, Katey, Katha, Katharyn, Katherin, Katherina, Katherine, Katheryn, Katherynn, Kathi, Kathie, Kathileen, Kathiryn, Kathleen, Kathlene, Kathleyn, Kathline, Kathrine, Kathrinna, Kathryn, Kathryne, Kathy, Kathyleen, Kathyrine, Katica, Katie, Katina, Katinka, Trina, Trinette.

CATHLEEN. *Spelling variation of* **KATHLEEN.** Way more unusual, and distinctive, than the now-cliched *K* version. Caithlyn, Cathaleen, Cathelin, Cathelina, Cathelyn, Cathi, Cathleana, Cathleene, Cathlene, Cathleyn, Cathlin, Cathline, Cathlyn, Cathlyne, Cathlynn, Cathy, Catleen, Catlin, Catline.

Catherine/Katherine's International Variations

Irish	Cáit, Caitlín, Caitria, Caitríona, Cathleen, Catrina, Kathleen
Scottish	Caitrìona, Catriona, Catrona
Welsh	Catrin
French	Carine, Trinette
Breton	Katarin, Katell
Italian	Catarina, Caterina
Spanish	Catalina
Basque	Katalin
Portuguese	Catarina
Dutch	Katelijne, Kaatje, Katrien, Katrijn, Katrine
German	Katarine, Katharina, Kathe, Kathrin, Katja, Katrin, Katrine
Scandinavian	Cathrine, Kaja
Danish	Caja, Katrine, Trine
Swedish	Cajsa, Kai, Kaj, Kajsa
Norwegian	Kaia
Finnish	Kaarina, Kaija, Kaisa, Kata, Katariina, Kati, Katri, Katriina
Polish	Kasia, Katarzyna
Hungarian	Kata, Katalin, Kato

(continued)

Catherine/Katherine's International Variations

Romanian	Ecaterina
Czech	Kata, Katarina, Kateřina, Katica
Russian	Ekaterina, Katenka, Katerina, Katerinka, Kati, Katia, Katinka, Katka, Katushka, Katya, Yekaterina
Greek	Aikaterine
Yiddish	Reina
Hawaiian	Kakalina, Kalena

CAYENNE. *Word name.* Spicy.

CAYLEE. *Spelling variation of* **KAYLEE.** Softer spelling of the wildly trendy Kaylee. **Caela, Caelee, Caeleigh, Caeley, Caeli, Caelie, Caelly, Cailee, Caileigh, Cailey, Caili, Cailie, Cailley, Caillie, Caleah, Caleigh, Caley, Cayle, Cayleah, Cayleigh, Cayley, Cayli, Caylie, Cayly, Kaileigh, Kailey, Kailie, Kaleigh, Kaylee, Kayleigh, Kayley.**

CEARA. *(KEER-ah) Spelling variation of Italian* **CIARA.** Would tend to be mispronounced as Sierra.

CECILIA. *Latin, 'blind one'.* Delicate feminine form of Cecil, from a Roman clan name, beginning to be rediscovered. Saint Cecilia is the patron of music. **Caceli, Cacelia, Cece, Ceceilia, Ceceley, Cecely, Ceceli, Cecil, Cecila, Cecilea, Ceciley, Ceciliane, Cecilija, Cecilla, Cecille, Cecillia, Cecilya, Cecilyann, Ceclia, Cecyl, Cecyle, Cee, Ceil, Ceila, Ceilagh, Ceileh, Ceileigh, Ceilena, Cela, Cele, Celia, Celie, Celli, Cellie, Cesia, Cesilia, Cesya, Cicelia, Cicely, Cicily, Cile, Cilia, Cilly, Cissey, Cissi, Cissie, Cissy, Kikelia, Kikylia, Sacilia, Sasilia, Sasilie,** Seelia, Seelie, Seely, Sesilia, Sessaley, Sesseelya, Sessile, Sessilly, Sessily, Sheila, Sile, Siseel, Sisely, Siselya, Sisile, Sisifiya, Sissela, Sissie, Sissy. International: **Síle** *(Irish),* **Sìleas** *(Scottish),* **Cécile** *(French),* **Caecilia** *(German),* **Silje** *(Norwegian, Danish),* **Silja** *(Finnish),* **Cecylia** *(Polish),* **Cecilija, Cilka** *(Slovene),* **Sisel, Zisel** *(Yiddish).*

CECILY. *Feminine variation of* **CECIL.** As dainty as a lace handkerchief.

♂ **CEDAR.** *Word name.* Fresh and fragrant nature name more apt to be used for a boy.

CEIL. *Short form of* **CECILIA.** Vintage canasta-playing name that could be due for a comeback.

★**CELESTE.** *Latin, 'heavenly'.* Softly pretty and somewhat quaint name with heavenly overtones, which kids might associate with Queen Celeste of Babar's elephant kingdom: a light and lovely choice that's finally getting noticed. If you want a more unusual variation, consider Celestia – or even Celestial. **Cela, Cele, Celeeste,**

Celense, Celes, Celesia, Celesley, Celest, Celesta, Celestena, Celestene, Celestia, Celestial, Celestijna, Celestin, Celestine, Celestyn, Celestyna, Celestyne, Celia, Celie, Celina, Celinda, Celine, Celinka, Celka, Cellest, Celleste, Celueste, Celyna, Saleste, Salestia, Seleste, Selestia, Selestina, Selestine, Selestyna, Selestyne, Silesta, Silestena, Silestia, Silestijna, Silestina, Silestyna, Silestyne, Tina, Tinka. International: Celestina *(Italian, Spanish).*

★CELIA. *Diminutive of* CECILIA. Underused today, but splendidly sleek and feminine, Celia was scattered throughout Shakespeare and other Elizabethan literature, but still manages to feel totally modern. **Ceilia, Celie, Celya.**

CELIE. *(seel-ee) French variation of* CECELIA. Attractive, underused name made famous by the heroine of *The Color Purple.* Author Toni Morrison is widely acknowledged as a master of character names.

CELINDA. *Variation of* CELESTE. Feels like a hybrid of Celine and Melinda – either of which would be preferable. **Celinde, Salinda, Salinde, Selinda, Selinde.**

CÉLINE. *French variation of* CELESTE. French Canadian singer Dion made us notice this variation, but most parents would prefer the Selene spelling. **Celina, Selene.**

CERELIA. *Latin, 'relating to springtime'.* Melodic and unusual choice, perfect for a child born in April or May. **Cerelia, Cerelisa, Cerella, Ceres, Sarelia, Sarilia.**

CERES, CERYS. *(SEER-eez) Roman mythology name.* Little known name of the goddess of the harvest, a possibility for the parent seeking something original, but with the aura of classical myth. Cerys made a brief appearance in the Top 100 in recent years.

CERIDWEN. *(keh-RID-wen) Welsh, 'beautiful as a poem'.* Celtic goddess of poetry, though less-than-poetic name. **Ceri.**

CERISE. *(se-rees) French, 'cherry'.* Preferable to the English version. **Cera, Cerea, Cerese, Ceri, Ceria, Cerice, Cericia, Cerissa, Cerisse, Cerra, Cerria, Cerrice, Cerrina, Cerrita, Cerryce, Ceryce, Cherise, Sarese, Sherise.**

♂ CERULEAN. *Colour name.* Vivid new sky-blue colour name, at present used mostly for boys.

CESSAIR. *(KAH-seer) Irish, 'sorrow, affliction'.* Mythological widow whose tears rained on Ireland, and whose name is lovely but, if pronounced phonetically, might be taken for a charter airline.

★CEYLON. *(say-lon) place name.* Lovely, exotic, tea-scented possibility undiscovered by baby namers.

CÉZANNE. *Artist name.* The last syllable being a female name makes the surname of the great French Post-Impressionist a creative natural for a girl.

CHABLIS. *(sha-BLEE) French place and wine name.* Chardonnay's twin sister. **Chabeli, Chabelly, Chabely, Chablee, Chabley, Chabli.**

CHAKA. *Hebrew, 'life'.* We all know that Chaka really means disco.

♀ **CHAKRA.** *Sanskrit, 'wheel, circle'.* For devoted New Agers only: yoga practitioners know this as the centre of spiritual energy in the body. **Chaka, Chakara, Chakaria, Chakena, Chakina, Chakira, Chakrah, Chakria, Chakriya, Chakyra.**

CHAMBRAY. *French word name.* Another one of those word names, like Cachet, with a pretty sound and a silly meaning: chambray is a fabric. **Chambrae, Chambre, Chambree, Chambrée, Chambrey, Chambria, Chambrie.**

♀ **CHAN.** *Cambodian, 'sweet-smelling tree'.* Common Asian surname also works as a first.

CHANAH. *Hebrew variation of* HANNAH. Begs for the guttural pronunciation that's a problem in this culture. **Chaanach, Chaanah, Chana, Chanae, Chanach, Chanai, Chanay, Chanea, Chanie.**

CHANDELLE. *French, 'candle'.* Sounds classy . . . but isn't. **Chandal, Chandel, Chantelle, Shandal, Shandel, Shandelle, Shantelle.**

CHANDRA. *Hindi, 'goddess of the moon'.* Name last groovy when incense and meditation were hot new concepts. **Candra, Chanda, Chandee, Chandi, Chandie, Chandin, Chandrae, Chandrah, Chandray, Chandre, Chandrea, Chandrelle, Chandria, Shandra.**

CHANEL. *French, 'dweller near the canal'.* Fans of the classic French designer would now more fashionably choose Coco. **Chanal, Chaneel, Chaneil, Chanele, Chanell, Chanelle, Channal, Channel, Channell, Channelle, Chenel, Chenell, Chenelle, Shanel, Shanell, Shanelle, Shannel, Shannelle, Shenelle, Shynelle.**

CHANTAL. *French, 'stone, boulder'.* Better to look to one of the more modern names popular for little girls in France today: Océane, Léa, Manon. **Chandal, Chanta, Chantaal, Chantae, Chantael, Chantai, Chantala,** Chantale, Chantall, Chantalle, Chantara, Chantarai, Chantasia, Chantay, Chantaye, Chante, Chanté, Chantéa, Chanteau, Chantee, Chanteese, Chantel, Chantela, Chantele, Chantell, Chantella, Chantelle, Chanter, Chantey, Chantez, Chanti, Chantia, Chantle, Chantoya, Chantrel, Chantrell, Chantrelle, Chantrill, Chatell, Chaunte, Chauntea, Chauntéa, Chauntee, Chauntel, Shantal, Shantalle, Shantel, Shantell, Shantelle, Shontel, Shontelle.

CHANTILLY. *French place name noted for lace.* Look for it in the credits of a soft-porn film. **Chantiel, Chantielle, Chantil, Chantila, Chantilée, Chantill, Chantille.**

CHARDONNAY. *French, a dry white wine.* If you're actually considering this as a name for your child, you must have had a glass too many. Save it for your poodle. **Char, Chardae, Chardnay, Chardney, Chardon, Chardonae, Chardonai, Chardonay, Chardonaye, Chardonee, Chardonna, Chardonnae, Chardonnai, Chardonnee, Chardonnée,**

Chardonney, Shardonay, Shardonnay.

CHARIS. *(KAR-is) Greek, 'grace'.* Reference to the mythological Three Graces of womanly charm, this one representing charity. **Charece, Chareece, Chareesse, Chareeze, Charese, Chari, Charice, Charie, Charish, Charissa, Charisse, Charysse, Karas, Karis, Karisse.**

CHARISMA. *Word name.* Trying to imbue your child with charisma at birth involves a certain degree of chutzpah. It was brought into the mix by ex–*Buffy the Vampire Slayer* actress Charisma Carpenter, who was named after an Avon perfume.

CHARITY. *Virtue name.* Faith and Hope are on the rise, while the arguably more melodic Charity is fading. **Carissa, Carita, Chareese, Charesa, Charese, Charessa, Charesse, Chariety, Charis, Charisa, Charise, Charisha, Charissa, Charisse, Charissee, Charista, Charita, Charitee, Chariti, Charitey, Charitye, Chariza, Charyssa, Cherri, Cherry, Sharitee, Sharitey, Shanty, Sharity, Sharitye.**

CHARLENE. *Variation of* **CAROLINE** *or* **CHARLOTTE.** Charlene wears a beehive hairdo and a too-tight turquoise tube top. **Char, Charla, Charlaina, Charlaine, Charlane, Charlanna, Charlayna, Charlayne, Charlea, Charlean, Charleen, Charleene, Charleesa, Charlena, Charlenae, Charlesena, Charline, Charlyn, Charlyne, Charlynn, Charlynne, Charlzina, Charoline.**

♂♀ CHARLIE. *Diminutive of* **CHARLES** *or* **CHARLOTTE.** One of the original oh-so-cute boys' names for girls, now a bit last decade, recently falling out of the Top 100. **Charle, Charlee, Charleigh, Charley, Charli, Charly, Chatty, Sharli, Sharlie.**

CHARLISE. *Variation of* **CHARLOTTE.** A name that owes its very life to a star: elegant blond South African actress Theron. **Charlise.**

★CHARLOTTE. *French, 'little and womanly'.* An elegant royal name now at Number 12 with such varied role models as Charlotte Bronte and Charlotte of E. B. White's *Web* – not to mention Charlotte Church.

Carleen, Carline, Carlyne, Char, Chara, Charil, Charill, Charl, Charla, Charlaine, Charlet, Charlett, Charletta, Charlette, Chariot, Charlisa, Charlita, Charlott, Charlottie,

If You Like Charlotte, *You Might Love . . .*

Arabella

Caroline

Celia

Clementine

Colette

Georgina

Jane

Juliet

Lucy

Madeline

Margaret

Nora

Rosa

Sophia

Susannah

Charlotty, Charolet, Charolette, Charolot, Charolotte, Charly, Charlyne, Charmain, Charmion, Charo, Charty, Cheryn, Cheryll, Karleen, Karlene, Karlika, Karlotte, Karlyne, Lotta, Lottey, Lotty, Sharel, Sharil, Sharla, Sharlaine, Sharlet, Sharlette, Sharlot, Sharmain, Sharmayne, Sharmian, Sharmion, Sharyl, Sherie, Sherye, Sheryl. International: Séarlait *(Irish Gaelic)*, Carlotta *(Italian)*, Carlota *(Spanish)*, Karlotta *(German and Greek)*, Charlotta *(Swedish)*, Sarolta *(Hungarian)*, Sharlotta *(Russian)*.

CHARMAINE. *Latin, 'a singer'.* An ancient name soiled by toilet paper association. **Charamy, Charma, Charmae, Charmagne, Charmaigne, Charmain, Charmalique, Charman, Charmane, Charmar, Charmara, Charmayane, Charmayne, Charmeen, Charmeine, Charmene, Charmese, Charmian, Charmin, Charmine, Charmion, Charmisa, Charmon, Charmyan, Charmyn, Charmyne, Charmynne, Sharmain, Sharman, Sharmane,**

Sharmayne, Sharmian, Sharmion, Sharmyn.

CHARMIAN. *Greek, 'joy'.* Shakespearean name less charming than the sound might imply. **Charmiane, Charmin, Charmyan, Sharmian, Sharmiane, Sharmyan.**

CHARNA. *Jewish/Yiddish, 'dark, black'.* Popular name in Israel, worth considering for a dark-haired daughter with a bit of a bohemian cast. **Charnke, Charnele.**

CHARO. *Spanish variation of* **ROSA.** Arriba!

CHASTITY. *Virtue name.* One of the original so-weird-it's-cruel starbaby names. **Chasa Dee, Chasadie, Chasady, Chasaty, Chasidee, Chasidey, Chasidie, Chasidy, Chasiti, Chasitie, Chasitti, Chasity, Chassedi, Chassidi, Chassidy, Chassiti, Chassity, Chassy, Chasta, Chastady, Chastidy, Chastin, Chastitee, Chastitie, Chastitey, Chastney, Chasty, Chasydi.**

CHAVA. *Hebrew, 'life'.* Ava or Eva are more appealing. **Chabah,**

Chavae, Chavah, Chavalah, Chavarra, Chavarria, Chave, Chavé, Chavette, Chaviva, Chavvis, Chaya, Chayka, Eva, Hava, Haya, Kaija, Kaÿa.

CHAYA. *Hebrew, 'life'.* For parents who want the kosher version of Eve. **Chaike, Chaye, Chayka, Chayla, Chaylah, Chaylea, Chaylee, Chaylene, Chayra.**

CHELSEA. *London and New York place name.* Once swinging but it recently dropped out of the Top 100. **Chelce, Chelcee, Chelcey, Chelci, Chelcie, Chelcy, Chelese, Chelesia, Chelli, Chellie, Chellise, Chellsie, Chelsa, Chelsae, Chelsah, Chelsay, Chelse, Chelseah, Chelsee, Chelsei, Chelseigh, Chelsey, Chelsi, Chelsia, Chelsie, Chelssie, Chelssey, Chelssy, Chelsy, Chelsye, Cheslea, Cheslee, Chesley, Cheslie, Chessea, Chessie.**

CHER. *French, 'beloved'.* There's only one – and that's plenty. **Chere, Cheree, Cherey, Cheri, Cherice, Cherie, Cheriee, Cherise, Cherish, Cherri, Cherrie, Cherry, Chery, Cherye,**

Cherylee, Cheryiie, Sher, Sherelle, Sherey, Sheri, Sherice, Sherie, Sherry, Sheryll.

CHERILYN. *Variation of* **CHERYL.** Cher's pre-icon birth name. **Charalin, Charalyn, Charalynne, Charelin, Charelyn, Charelynn, Charilyn, Charilynn, Cheralin, Cheralyn, Cherilin, Cherilynn, Cherilynne, Cherralyn, Cherrilin, Cherrilyn, Cherrylene, Cherrylin, Cherryline, Cherrylyn, Cherylin, Cheryline, Cheryllyn, Cherylyn, Sharalin, Sharalyn, Sharelyn, Sharelynne, Sharilynn, Sheralin, Shera-Lynne, Sheritin, Sherralin, Sherrilyn, Sherrylene, Sherryline, Sherrylyn, Sherylin, Sherylyn.**

CHERISH. *English word name.* So sweet it makes our teeth hurt. **Charisa, Charise, Charish, Charisha, Cheerish, Cherece, Chereese, Cheresa, Cherese, Cheresse, Cherice, Cherise, Cherishe, Cheriss, Cherissa, Cherisse, Cherrise, Cherrish, Sherish.**

CHERRY. *Fruit name.* Why give your future teenager even more reason to hate you? **Chere,** Cheree, Cherey, Cherida, Cherise, Cherita, Cherrey, Cherri, Cherrie, Cherrita, Cherry-Ann, Cherry-Anne, Cherrye, Chery, Cherye.

CHERYL. *Modern invented name.* As frozen in the pre-Beatles era as short white gloves. **Charel, Charell, Charelle, Charil, Charyl, Cherell, Cherelle, Cheriann, Cherianne, Cherell, Cherrelle, Cherryl, Cheryl-Ann, Cheryl-Anne, Cheryle, Charylee, Cheryll, Cherylle, Cheryl-Lee, Cherilynn, Chyril, Chyrill, Sharel, Sharil, Sharyl, Sharyll, Sheral, Sherianne, Sheril, Sherill, Sheryl, Shyril, Shyrill.**

CHESLEIGH. *English, 'camp on the meadow'.* Chelsea with dyslexia. **Cheslea, Chesley, Chesli, Cheslie, Chesly, Chesslea, Chesslee, Chessley, Chessli, Chesslie, Chessly.**

CHESNEY. *English from French, 'oak grove'.* We don't care how much you love Kenny: this is going too far. **Chesnea, Chesneigh, Chesnie, Chesni, Chesny, Chessnea, Chessney, Chessni, Chessnie, Chessny.**

♂ **CHEYENNE.** *Sioux, 'people of a different language'.* The name of a courageous tribe, Cheyenne became popular in the US in the 1990s, inspiring a wide range of spelling variations – ShyAnne is one example that's still on the rise. **Chayan, Chayanne, Chey, Cheyan, Cheyana, Cheyane, Cheyann, Cheyanna, Cheyanne, Cheye, Cheyeana, Cheyeanna, Cheyeanne, Cheyeene, Cheyena, Cheyene, Cheyenna, Cheyna, Cheyne, Cheynee, Cheyney, Cheynna, Chi, Chi-Anna, Chie, Chyan, Chyana, Chyane, Chyann, Chyanna, Chyanne, Chyeana, Chyenn, Chyenna, Chyenne, Chyennee, Shayan, Shayanne, Shianne, Shyann, Shyanne.**

★**CHIARA.** *(kee-AHR-a) Italian, 'light' or 'clear'.* Romantic Italian name that's familiar but not widely used: a winner. **Cheara, Chiarra, Kiara, Kiarra.**

CHINA. *Place name.* One of the first and still most striking place names; preferably used in its original spelling. **Chinaetta, Chinah, Chinasa, Chinda, Chinea, Chinesia, Chinita,**

Chinna, Chinwa, Chyna, Chynna.

CHIQUITA. *Spanish, 'little one'.* Banana. **Chaqueta, Chaquita, Chica, Chickie, Chicky, Chikata, Chikita, Chiqueeta, Chiqueta, Chiquila, Chiquin, Chiquite, Chiquitha, Chiquithe, Chiquitia, Chiquitta.**

CHLOE. *Greek, 'young green shoot'.* Pretty Greek name found in romantic poetry is in the Top 10, and for several years has been one of the most popular names in England. **Chlöe, Chloee, Chloie, Clo, Cloe, Cloei, Cloey, Cloie, Khloe, Khloey, Kloe.** International: **Chloé** *(French).*

CHLORIS. *Greek, 'pale'.* Antiseptic sounding. **Caloress, Cloris, Clorissa, Khloris, Kloris.**

CHRISTA. *German, short form of* **CHRISTINA.** Fading since the 1970s – but still a lovely name.

CHRISTABEL. *Latin/French, 'fair Christian'.* Though Isabel is a smash hit, Christabel still sounds slightly like what you'd name a cow. **Charystobel, Christabell, Christabella, Christabelle, Christable, Christobel, Chrystabel, Chrystabelle, Cristabel, Cristabella, Cristabelle, Crystabel, Crystabella, Kristabel.**

♂ **CHRISTIAN.** *Greek, 'anointed one,' English, from Latin, 'follower of Christ'.* While Christian is still on the rise for boys, for girls it's heading down along with the rest of the *Chris* names. But we like it and think it sounds more original than the girlier versions. International: **Carsten** *(Low German),* **Kristen** *(Danish).*

CHRISTIANA. *Feminine variation of* **CHRISTIAN.** Not cutting edge, but still graceful and feminine. **Christiane, Christianna.**

CHRISTINA. *Greek, 'anointed, Christian'.* This pretty and feminine classic may be trending downwards, but it's never out of style. A royal name best used in its full glory. **Chris, Chrisa, Chrisie, Chrissa, Chrissee, Chrissta, Chrisstan, Chrissten, Chrissti, Chrisstie, Chrissty,**

Christa, Christain, Christal, Christalene, Christalin, Christaline, Christall, Christalle, Christalyn, Christan, Christana, Christann, Christanna, Christeen, Christeena, Christella, Christen, Christena, Christene, Christi, Christian, Christiana, Christiann, Christi-Ann, Christianna, Christianne, Christi-Anne, Christianni, Christiaun, Christie, Christiean, Christien, Christiena, Christienne, Christin, Christinaa, Christinan, Christinea, Christini, Christinia, Christinna, Christinnah, Christiona, Christmar, Christum, Christy, Christy-Ann, Christy-Anne, Christyn, Christyna, Christynna, Chrys, Chrysa, Chryssa, Chrysta, Chrystalle, Chrystee, Chrystelle, Chrysten, Chrystena, Chrysti, Chrystie, Chrystina, Chrystine, Chrystle, Chrysty, Chrystyan, Chrystyna, Cris, Crissa, Crissey, Crissie, Crissy, Cristal, Cristeena, Cristelle, Cristi, Cristiann, Cristie, Cryssa, Crysta, Crystene, Crystian, Crystie, Crystin, Crystine, Crystyn, Crystyna, Crystyne, Khrissy, Khristeen, Khristena, Khristine, Kit, Kris, Kristeen, Kristeena, Kristena, Kristi, Kristie, Kristy, Kristyna, Krystina, Krystyna, Teena, Teyna.

♂ CHRISTMAS. *English word name.* Day name long and quietly used. Prettier and more modern than Noel or Noelle.

CIA. *Short form.* What's it short for? Cynthia or most any other C name. But too close to the Central Intelligence Agency.

CIARA. *(KEER-a) Irish, 'black-haired'.* Very popular in Ireland, more familiar here as the more easily pronounced Keira or Kyra. **Ceaira, Ceairah, Ceairra, Cearaa, Cearie, Cearah, Cearra, Ceira, Ceirah, Ceire, Ceiria, Ceirra, Cera, Chiarah, Ciaara, Ciaera, Ciaira, Ciarah, Ciaria, Ciarra, Ciarrah, Cieara, Ciearra, Ciearria, Ciera, Cierra, Cierrah, Cierre, Cierria, Cierro, Cioria, Cyarra, Cyera, Cyerra, Cyerria, Keera, Kira, Searra, Siara.** International: **Ceara, Ciar** *(Irish).*

CICELY. *English variation of* **CECILIA.** Prissy but pretty Victorian name, a surprise choice for comedienne Sandra Bernhard. **Cecilie, Cecily, Chilla, Chilli, Cicelia, Cicelie, Ciciley, Cicilia, Cicilie, Cicily, Cile, Cillie, Cilly, Cilka.**

Christina's International Variations

Irish	**Cristin, Cristiona**
Scottish	**Cairistìona, Kirsteen, Kirstie, Kirstin, Kirsty**
French	**Christele, Christine, Crestienne**
Italian	**Cristiana, Cristina**
Spanish	**Crista, Cristiana, Cristina, Cristy**
German	**Christa, Christel, Christiane, Chrystel, Crista, Kerstin, Krista, Kristen, Kristin, Stina, Stine, Tine**
Danish	**Kirsten, Stinne**
Swedish	**Kerstin, Kia, Kolina, Kristina**
Norwegian	**Kjersti, Kjerstin, Kristin, Stina**
Finnish	**Kirsi, Kirsikka, Kristia, Kristiina, Stiina, Tiina**
Polish	**Krysia, Krysta, Krystka, Krystyn, Krystyna, Krystynka**
Hungarian	**Kriska, Kriszta, Krisztina**
Czech	**Crystina, Krista, Kristina, Kristinka, Tyna**
Bulgarian	**Khrustina**
Russian	**Khristina, Khristya, Khrysta, Tina**
Latvian	**Krista, Kristine**
Estonian	**Krista**
Greek	**Christina, Tina**
Hawaiian	**Kilikina**

CIEL. *(see-EL) French, 'sky'.* Simple yet evocative, though many will misunderstand it as 'seal'.

CILLA. *Diminutive of* **PRISCILLA.** Takes the priss out of Priscilla.

CIMMARON. *Place name.* A name that conjures up rugged images of the American wild west. **Cimeron, Simarron, Simeron.**

CINDERELLA. *French, 'little ash-girl'.* One familiar name never used for real people, for obvious reasons. **Cendrillon, Cenerentola, Cindella, Cindie, Cindy, Ella.**

CINDY. *Diminutive of* **CYNTHIA** *or* **LUCINDA.** Cindy's gone from cute teenager to peppy mum, but it's not for her daughter. **Cindee, Cindi, Cindie, Cynda, Cyndal, Cyndale, Cyndall, Cyndee, Cyndel, Cyndi, Cyndia, Cyndie, Cyndle, Cyndy, Sindi, Sindie, Sindy, Syndi, Syndie, Syndy.**

CINNABAR. *Word name.* Associated with a vivid red-orange-coloured lacquer, would make a more than distinctive colour-related choice.

CINNAMON. *Word name.* The only spice name we have a taste for is Saffron. **Cynnamon, Sinemmon, Sinnamon.**

CIPRIANA. *Greek, 'from the Island of Cyprus'.* Offbeat and exotic place name.

CIRCE. *(SUR-see) Greek mythology name.* In *The Odyssey,* she's the nymph who can turn men into swine.

CITRON. *French, 'lemon'.* Gallic twist on word or nature name, has a nice lemony feel.

★**CLAIRE.** *French variation of* **CLARE.** Luminous, simple and strong, Claire is one of those special names that is familiar yet distinctive, feminine but not frilly, combining historical depth with a modern edge. And though it's enjoying revived popularity, it will never be seen as trendy. Great middle name choice as well. **Ceara, Cearra, Cheeara, Ciara, Ciarra, Clair, Claireen, Claireta, Clairey, Clairice, Clairinda, Clairine, Clairissa, Clairita, Clairy,**

Clarabel, Clarabelle, Clare, Clarene, Claresta, Clareta, Clarey, Clari, Claribel, Claribella, Claribelle, Clarice, Clarie, Clarinda, Clarine, Clarisse, Clarita, Clarrie, Clarry, Clary, Claryce, Clayre, Clayrette, Clayrice, Clayrinda, Clayrissa, Cliara, Clorinda, Klaire, Klare, Klaretta, Klaryce, Klayre, Kliara, Klyara, Sinclair, Sinclaire. International: **Clairette, Clarette** *(French),* **Chiara, Chiarina, Claretta, Clarina, Clarissa** *(Italian),* **Clareta, Clarisa, Clarita** *(Spanish),* **Clarissa, Klarissa** *(German),* **Klarika** *(Hungarian),* **Klara** *(Slavic),* **Kalea** *(Hawaiian).*

♂ **CLANCY.** *Irish 'red-haired warrior'.* Irish surnames are hot, and this one can cross the line to work for girls, replacing the outdated Casey.

CLARA. *Latin, 'bright, clear'.* European-sounding Claire variation that was hugely popular a century ago, and is just starting to revive today, picked up on by parents like Ewan McGregor. **Claira, Claire, Clarabelle, Claramae, Claramay, Clare, Claresta, Claretha, Clarey, Clari, Claribel, Clarie, Clarina, Clarinda,**

Clarine, Claris, Clarisse, Claritza, Clarry, Clary, Claryce, Cleriese, Klara, Klarice, Klarise, Klarra. International: Clarice, Clarissa *(Italian)*, **Clarita** *(Spanish)*.

CLARABELLE. *Latin, 'bright and beautiful'.* This is a clown and cow name. **Clarabella, Claribel, Claribell.**

CLARE. *Latin, 'bright'.* This is the original, more prosaic spelling, but the airier Claire now dominates.

CLARET. *Colour name, also Bordeaux wine.* Rich purplish-red colour choice that may gain favour along with Claire, though the wine connection can't be ignored.

CLARICE. *Variation of* **CLARE.** Murdered by Hannibal Lecter. **Claris, Clarise, Clarisse, Claryce, Cleriese, Clerissa, Clerisse, Clerysse, Klarice, Klarise, Klarissa, Klaryce.**

CLARION. *Music name.* Tuneful variation on the Claire names.

CLARISSA. *Italian, variation of* **CLARA.** Although it had

its day in the 1990s, it still could make a pretty and dainty alternative to the overused Melissa and Vanessa. **Clairisa, Clairissa, Clairisse, Claraissa, Clarecia, Claressa, Claresta, Clarisa, Clarissia, Claritza, Clarizza, Clarrisa, Clarrissa, Clerissa.**

CLARITY. *Virtue name.* One of the newly rediscovered virtue names, like Peace and Justice, with old-fashioned charm and a clear vision for the future.

♂ **CLAUDE.** *Latin, 'lame'.* Ancient clan name used in France for girls as well as boys, which makes a distinctive choice here, too.

CLAUDETTE. *French, feminine variation of* **CLAUDE.** Leave this dated feminisation back with Annette and Paulette.

★**CLAUDIA.** *Latin, feminine variation of* **CLAUDE.** A classic name with a hint of ancient Roman splendour that has never been truly in or truly out, Claudia still feels like a strong, modern choice – though Claude or Claudie may be more special. **Claudee, Claudeen,**

Claudel, Claudella, Claudelle, Claudetta, Claudex, Claudey, Claudi, Claudiana, Claudiane, Claudie, Claudie-Anne, Claudy, Claudya, Clodia, Klaudia, Klod. International: Claude, Claudette, Claudine *(French)*, **Claudeta, Claudina, Claudita** *(Spanish)*.

CLAUDIE. *French, feminine variation of* **CLAUDE.**

Attractive form still très Parisienne.

CLAUDINE. *French, feminine variation of* **CLAUD.** There are much chicer versions of this name today.

★**CLEA.** *(CLAY-uh) Literary name.* Attractive and unusual name that may be a variation of Cleo, possibly invented by Lawrence Durrell for a character in his *Alexandria Quartet.* **Claea, Klea.**

CLELIA. *Latin, 'glorious'.* Obscure yet not unappealing name of a legendary heroine of Rome.

CLEMATIS. *Greek flower name.* Flower name that sounds a bit too much like a disease. **Clematia, Clematice, Clematiss.**

CLEMENCE. *(CLAY-mahnz) French feminine variation of* **CLEMENT.** Calm, composed and chic. **Clemency.**

CLEMENCIA. *Latin, 'mercy'.* This ancient feminine form is the kind of name your child will grow into . . . at least by her fiftieth birthday.

CLEMENCY. *Virtue name.* May come back along with the more familiar Puritan virtue names, like Hope and Faith; has a nice three-syllable sound, and funky nickname. Clem. **Clem, Clemmie.**

★**CLEMENTINE.** *Latin, 'mercy'.* Fashionable name, but if 'Oh, My Darlin' ' still rings too loudly in your ears, consider pronouncing it Clement*een* – or even using Clementina, which rhymes with Christina. Stylish supermodel Claudia Schiffer chose it for her daughter. **Clem, Clemencia, Clemencie, Clemency, Clementya, Clementyna, Clementyn, Clemenza, Clemette, Clemmie, Clemmy, Klementina.** **International: Clémence** *(French),* **Clementia, Clementina** *(Spanish),* **Clemenza, Klementyna** *(Polish).*

CLEO. *English, short form of* **CLEOPATRA.** One of the few girls' names to boast the cool-yet-lively *o* ending, but we prefer Clio's history. **Clio.**

CLEOPATRA. *Greek, 'her father's renown'.* A royal name in ancient Egypt that's never quite made it to the modern world. **Chleo, Clea, Cleo, Cleona, Cleone, Cleonie, Cleta, Clio.**

CLIANTHA. *Greek, 'glory-flower'.* Another flower name that sounds uncomfortably disease-like. **Cleantha, Cleanthe, Clianthe, Kliantha, Klianthe.**

★**CLIO.** *(CLEE-o) Greek mythology name.* The name of the ancient Greek mythological muse of history is rich with modern charm and would make an intriguing choice. **Clea, Klio.**

CLODAGH. *(CLO-dah) Irish river name.* Extremely popular in Ireland, but here, we're afraid, a bit cloddy.

CLORINDA. *Latin literary name.* Romantic name invented by a sixteenth-century poet, but has a synthetic sound today. **Chlorinda, Clarinda.**

CLOTILDA. *German, 'renowned battle'.* Old and aristocratic European name that would be tough for a kid to pull off today. **Clothilda, Clothilde, Clotilde, Klothilda, Klothilde.**

♂ CLOUD. *Nature name.*
This kind of plainspoken
nature name (think River and
Sunshine) still carries a whiff
of the hippy. **Cloudy.**

♂ CLOVE. *Nature name.* Spice
name a tad more piquant than
Saffron or Cinnamon.

★CLOVER. *Flower name.*
Charming, perky choice if you
want to move beyond hothouse
blooms like Rose and Lily.

♂ COBALT. *Colour and nature
name.* Even among the range of
blue names on the current baby
naming palette – Blue itself,
Azure, Cerulean, Teal, Aqua,
Cyan, Indigo – Cobalt remains
the most unusual.

★COCO. *Spanish nickname.* A
new starbaby favourite, inspired
by legendary designer Chanel
and chosen by Courteney Cox,
that the press loves to ridicule –
but we predict it's heading for
more widespread acceptance and
even popularity.

♂ COLBY. *English, 'from a coal
town'.* One of the first reality
show-inspired names in the US;
hugely trendy for
boys but just starting for
girls. **Colbee, Colbey, Colbi,
Colbie, Kolbee, Kolbey,
Kolbi, Kolbie, Kolby.**

COLETTE. *French, diminutive
of* **NICOLE.** Modern parents
might be attracted to this name
because of the French novelist –
though pen name Colette was
actually her last name, Sidonie
her first. **Coe, Coetta, Coleta,
Coletta, Collet, Collete, Collett,
Colletta, Collette, Kolette,
Kollette, Nicolette.**

COLINE. *Feminine variation
of* **COLIN.** Wishy-washy, and
too similar to Colleen. **Colena,
Colene, Coletta, Collina, Colline,
Niceleen, Nicolene, Nicoline,
Nicolyne. International:
Colina** *(Spanish).*

COLLEEN. *Irish, 'girl'.* Mid-
century Irish-American
favourite, never used in Ireland
itself, being the generic word
for 'girl'; rarely given today.
**Coe, Coel, Cole, Coleen,
Colena, Colene, Coley,
Colina, Colinda, Coline,
Colleene, Collen, Collene,
Collie, Collina, Colline,
Colly, Kolleen, Kolline.**

COLOMBIA. *Latin, 'dove,'
place name.* South American
country name, with peaceful
connotations.

COLOMBINE. *English from
Latin, 'dove'.* Flower name
too redolent of disaster.
Columbine.

♂ COLORADO. *Place name.*
Inspired by the American
western state.

★COLUMBA. *Latin, 'dove'.*
Early saint's name that rhumbas
to a modern beat. **Collie, Colly,
Colombe, Columbana, Columbia,
Columbine. International:
Colombe** *(French),* **Colomba,
Colombina, Colombita,
Columbias, Columbita** *(Spanish).*

♂ COMET. *Nature name.*
Soaring astral name with two
strikes against it: a masculine
feel, and the fact that it's also a
well-known cleanser in the US.

COMFORT. *Word name.* This
Puritan virtue name is unstylish,
but sympathetic and appealing, in
these largely uncomfortable times.

CONCEPCIÒN. *Latin,
'conception'.* Enshrined in the

Latin and Catholic culture. **Chiquin, Chita, Concetta, Concha, Concheta, Conchissa, Conchita.**

CONCETTA. *Italian, 'pure'.* A name that relates to Concepcion and the Virgin Mary, but feels a good deal more secular. **Concettina, Conchetta.**

CONCHITA. *Spanish, diminutive of* **CONCEPCIÒN.** Concepciòn dressed in red satin. **Chita, Conceptia, Concha, Conchata, Conchissa, Conciana.**

CONCORDIA. *Latin, 'peace, harmony'.* The name of the goddess of peace. **Con, Concord, Concorde, Cordae, Cordaye.**

CONDOLEEZZA. *Modern invented name.* Made famous by US Secretary of State Condoleezza Rice, whose parents fashioned her name from a musical term meaning 'with sweetness'. **Conde, Condi, Condie, Condy.**

♂ **CONNELLY.** *Irish, 'love, friendship'.* Rollicking and rare example of this popular genre that may work even better for girls. **Con, Conn, Connally,** **Connaly, Connelli, Connely, Connolly, Connoly.**

CONNEMARA. *(kahn-ah-MAHR-ah) place name.* Wild, lovely place in western Ireland makes wild, lovely name.

♂ **CONNOR.** *Irish, 'lover of hounds'.* Popular boys' name that might – but that's a big might – work for girls. **Con, Conn, Connar, Conner, Connery, Conor.**

CONSTANCE. *Latin, 'steadfastness'.* With its icy and forbidding image, this is the kind of name given to the strong matriarch in American TV dynasties, while nickname Connie brings it downscale – all of which gives it little appeal for modern parents. **Con, Conetta, Connee, Conney, Conni, Connie, Conny, Constancy, Constanta, Constantine, Constantya, Constanze, Constynse, Konnie, Konny, Konstance.** International: **Concettina, Constantia, Constanza** *(Italian),* **Constancia, Constanza** *(Spanish),* **Constanz, Konstanze** *(German),* **Konstancji, Konstanty** *(Polish),* **Konstantin, Kostenka, Kostya, Kostyusha, Kotik** *(Russian),* **Dina, Kosta,** **Kostantina, Tina** *(Greek),* **Kani** *(Hawaiian).*

CONSUELO. *Spanish, 'consolation, comfort'.* Sophisticated Spanish name works well with Anglo surnames. **Chela, Chelo, Consolata, Consuela, Consuella, Consula, Conzuelo.**

★**CORA.** *Greek, 'maiden'.* A lovely, old-fashioned name – she was a daughter of Zeus and the heroine of *The Last of the Mohicans* – recently rejuvenated and strengthened by its contemporary-feeling simplicity. **Corabel, Corabella, Corabelle, Corabellia, Corah, Coralee, Coree, Corella, Corena, Corene, Coresa, Coressa, Coretta, Corey, Cori, Corie, Corilla, Corine, Corinna, Corinne, Corisa, Corissa, Corita, Corra, Correen, Corrella, Correlle, Correna, Correnda, Correne, Correy, Correye, Corri, Corrie, Cortina, Corrine, Corrissa, Corry, Corynna, Corynne, Coryssa, Kora, Korabell, Kore, Koreen, Korella, Koretta, Korey, Korilla, Korina, Korinne, Korissa, Korry, Koryne, Korynna, Koryssa.**

CORAL. *Nature name.* First used during the Victorian craze for jewel names; it could rise again, along with Ruby and Pearl, although it doesn't have as much lustre. **Coraal, Coralee, Coralena, Coralie, Coralina, Coraline, Corallina, Coraly, Coralyn, Coralyne, Corral, Koral, Korall, Koralig, Koralline.**

CORALIE. *French extension of* **CORA** *or* **CORAL.** Unusual name, afforded some appeal by Neil Gaiman's spooky and lovely children's book. **Coralea, Cora-Lee, Coralee, Coralena, Coralene, Coraley, Corali, Coralia, Coralina, Coraline, Coraly, Coralyn, Coralynn, Coralynne, Corella, Corilee, Koralee, Koraley, Korali, Koralie, Koraly.**

CORAZÒN. *Spanish, 'heart'.* Well-used Spanish name expressing heart-filled emotion, with religious relevance to the Sacred Heart of Jesus.

♂ **CORBIN.** *Latin, 'raven'.* Rising boys' name could cross the gender line. **Corban, Corbe, Corben, Corbi, Corbinne, Corby, Corbyn, Corbynn, Corbynne, Korban, Korben, Korbin, Korbinn, Korbyn, Korbynn.**

★**CORDELIA.** *Latin, 'heart'; Celtic, 'daughter of the sea'.* The name of King Lear's one sympathetic daughter has style and substance, and is exactly the kind of old-fashioned, grown-up name that many parents are seeking today. **Cordae, Cordelie, Cordelle, Cordett, Cordette, Cordey, Cordia, Cordie, Cordilia, Cordilla, Cordula, Cordy, Delia, Delie, Kordella, Kordella, Kordelie, Kordelia, Kordula.** International: **Cordi** *(Welsh).*

♂ **CORDIS.** *Latin, 'of the heart'.* Unusual and substantial unisex choice. **Cordiss.**

CORETTA. *English, elaborated form of* **CORA.** Famous in the US as the name of the widow of Dr Martin Luther King Jr.

♂ **COREY.** *Irish, 'from the hollow'.* Cool a few decades ago, along with Lori and Tori – but no more. **Coree, Cori,**

Antiques Ready for Restoration

Adeline
Amabel
Amity
Beatrice
Celia/Cecilia
Cecily
Clarissa
Clementine
Cora
Cordelia
Edith
Eliza
Emmeline
Evangeline
Flora
Genevieve
Lavinia
Letitia
Matilda
Maude
May, Mae
Millicent
Mirabel
Nell
Violet

Corie, Correy, Correye, Corrie, Corry, Cory, Korie, Korrey, Korri, Korry.

CORINNA. *Greek, 'maiden'.* Delicate and gentle old-fashioned name, the kind found in early English poetry.

CORINNE. *French variation of* **CORINNA.** 1930s era name, much prettier when the second syllable is pronounced *in,* rather than *een.* Carinna, Carinne, Carine, Carynna, Carynne, Coreen, Coreena, Coren, Corenne, Coriana, Corianna, Corin, Corina, Corinda, Corine, Corinee, Corinn, Correen, Corren, Correna, Corrianne, Corrienne, Corrin, Corrina, Corrinda, Corrine, Corrinn, Corrinna, Corrinne, Corryn, Coryn, Coryna, Corynn, Corynne, Karinne, Karynna, Koreen, Korina, Korinne.

CORISANDE. *Greek, 'chorus-singer'.* Very unusual choice, musical in every way. Corissanda, Corissande, Corrisande.

CORLISS. *English, 'carefree person'.* Eccentric yet well-established, has an independent and artistic air. Corlee, Corless, Corley, Corlie, Corlisa, Corlise, Corlissa, Corly, Korliss.

★CORNELIA. *Latin, feminine variation of* **CORNELIUS.** In ancient Rome, Cornelia was considered the paragon of womanly virtue, making it a handsome name with an excellent pedigree. Rare today, so if you want a name no one else is using, this should be on your list. Carna, Carniella, Cornalia, Corneelia, Corneelija, Corneilla, Cornela, Cornelija, Cornella, Cornelle, Cornelya, Cornie, Cornilear, Cornisha, Corny, Korneelia, Korneelya, Kornelija, Neely, Nell, Nelli, Nellie, Nelly. International: Cornelie *(French),* Melia, Nelia *(Spanish),* Kornelia, Nele *(German),* Kornelis *(Swedish),* Kornelia *(Czech).*

CORONA. *Spanish, 'crown'.* Let's face it – most modern British men will think of the beer. Coronetta, Coronette, Coronna.

CORSICA. *Place name.* The picturesque Mediterrean island birthplace of Napoleon makes an easy switch from atlas to baby name book, with its delicate, feminine ending. Just don't consider neighbouring island Sardinia.

CORVINA. *Latin, 'like a raven'.* Sounds too much like a car model. Corva, Corveena, Corvetta.

COSETTE. *French, 'victorious people'.* This female version of Nicholas is best known as the heroine of *Les Misérables.* Cossetta, Cossette, Cozette. International: Cosetta *(Italian).*

★COSIMA. *(KO-see-mah) Greek, feminine variation of* **COSMO.** The kind of exotic name the British upper classes once used for their daughters; most often heard in the classical music world. Cosma, Cosme, Kosma.

♂ **COURTNEY.** *French, courteous, from the court, also Old French nickname, 'short nose'.* Although still in the Top 100, today's Courtney is more apt to be the babysitter than the baby. Cordney, Cordni, Cortenay, Corteney, Cortland, Cortne, Cortnea, Cortnee, Cortneia, Cortneigh, Cortney,

Cortni, Cortnie, Cortny,
Corttney, Courtaney, Courtany,
Courtena, Courtenay, Courtene,
Courteneigh, Courteney,
Courteny, Courtland, Courtnae,
Courtnay, Courtne, Courtnee,
Courtnée, Courtnei, Courtneigh,
Courtni, Courtnie, Courtnii,
Courtny, Courtonie, Kordney,
Kortney, Kortni, Kortnie,
Kortny, Kourtenay, Kourtneigh,
Kourtney, Kourtnee, Kourtnie.

CRESCENT. *French, 'increasing,
growing'.* Intriguing word name
with a pretty sound. **Crescence,
Crescenta, Crescentia, Cressant,
Cressent, Cressentia, Cressentya.**

★**CRESSIDA.** *(KRESS-i-da)
Greek, 'gold'.* Mythological and
Shakespearean heroine name
much better known among
theatre-goers. It is worth
considering by the more
adventurous baby namer. **Cressa.**

CRIMSON. *Colour name.* A
possible competitor for Scarlett's
success, though lacking that
Gone With the Wind charm.

CRISANTA. *Spanish from
Greek, 'golden flower,
chrysanthemum'.* Pretty and
highly unusual Christine

alternative. **Chrisanta,
Chrisantha, Chrissanta,
Chrissantha, Chryssantha.**

CRISPINA. *Latin, 'curly-
haired'.* Unfortunately,
everyone will hear this
feminine form of Crispin
as Christina.

CRISTINA. *Italian, Spanish,
Portuguese, and Romanian
variation of* **CHRISTINA.** One
case where the streamlined
version feels more exotic.

♂**CRUZ.** *Spanish, 'cross'.*
A sister for Concepciòn and
Corazòn, although its masculine
side was emphasised when

Stellar Starbabies Beginning with C

Caledonia	Shawn Colvin
Carys	Catherine Zeta-Jones & Michael Douglas
Cecilia	Vera Wang
Celeste	Catherine Oxenberg & Casper van Dien
Chanel	Nelly
Charlotte	Amy Brenneman, Harry Connick Jr, Sigourney Weaver, Dylan McDermott
Chloe	Rupert Murdoch
Cicely	Sandra Bernhard
Clara	Ewan McGregor
Clementine	Claudia Schiffer
Coco	Courteney Cox & David Arquette
Cosima	Nigella Lawson
Cosma	Nina Hagen

the high profile David Beckhams chose it for their son. **Crucita, Cruise.**

CRYSTAL. *Gem name.* Originally a male name, Crystal was hot in the 1980s along with shoulder pads and big hair, but retains none of the sparkle it once had. **Christal, Christalle, Chrystalle, Chrystal-Lynn, Chrystel, Chrystle, Cristal, Cristalie, Cristalina, Cristalle, Cristel, Cristela, Cristelia, Cristella, Cristelle, Cristhie, Cristle, Crysta, Crystala, Crystale, Crystalee, Crystalin, Crystall, Crystalle, Crystaly, Crystel, Crystela, Crystelia, Crystelle, Crysthelle, Crystl, Crystle, Crystol, Crystole, Crystyl, Khristalle, Khrystle, Kristle, Krystal, Krystle.** **International: Criostal** *(Irish Gaelic),* **Chrystal** *(Irish),* **Christel, Christelle** *(French),* **Krystalle** *(German).*

♂ **CUBA.** *Place name.* Cuba Gooding Jr notwithstanding, this sounds better for girls.

♂ **CURRAN.** *Irish, 'hero, champion'.* Curry-flavoured Irish surname-y name that could work as well for girls as boys.

Cura, Curin, Curina, Curinna, Curren, Currin, Curryn.

♂ **CURRY.** *Word name.* Peppy choice. **Currey, Curri, Currie, Kurri, Kurry.**

♂ **CURTIS.** *French, 'courteous, polite'.* This familiar boys' name could be considered as a fresh girls' choice.

CYANE. *(SY-an) Greek, 'bright blue enamel'.* Mythological Sicilian nymph who lived in a pool and whose name is an intriguing twist on the colour name trend. **Cyan.**

CYBELE. *(si-BELL) Greek, 'the mother of all gods'.* This name of a Greek goddess of fertility, health and nature would undoubtedly be confused with Sybil. **Cybel, Cybela, Cybil, Cybill, Cybille, Cyebele, Sibyl, Sybil.**

CYDNEY. *Spelling variation of* **SYDNEY.** *Unnecessary complication.* **Cydne, Cydnee, Cydnei, Cydni, Cydnie, Cydny.**

CYMBELINE. *Greek, 'hollow'; Celtic, 'sun lord'.* Musical name

that is the title of a Shakespeare play. **Cymbaline.**

CYNARA. *Greek, 'thistly plant'.* Poetic though thorny. **Cinara, Zinara.**

CYNTHIA. *Greek, 'of the moon'.* Attractive name – in classical mythology an alternate for Artemis or Diana – that was so overexposed in the middle of the twentieth century that few style-conscious parents would choose it today. **Cia, Cinda, Cindee, Cindi, Cindra, Cindy, Cinnie, Cinny, Cinthia, Cyn, Cynda, Cyndee, Cyndi, Cyndia, Cyndie, Cyndra, Cyndy, Cyneria, Cynethia, Cynithia, Cynnie, Cynthy, Cynthea, Cynthiana, Cynthiann, Cynthie, Cynthria, Cynthy, Cynthya, Cyntia, Cyntria, Cythia, Cytia, Kynthija, Sindee, Sindi, Sindy, Sindya, Sinnie, Sinny, Synda, Syndee, Syndi, Syndy, Syntha, Synthee, Syntheea, Synthia, Synthie, Synthya.** **International: Cinzia** *(Italian),* **Cinta** *(Spanish),* **Cintia** *(Spanish, Portuguese),* **Kynthia** *(Greek).*

CYRA. *(SEER-a) Persian, 'sun' or 'throne'.* Twist on all those Keiras, but not as attractive.

CYRILLA. *Latin, 'lordly'.* If you want something even more tightly laced than Priscilla. **Cerelia, Cerella, Ciri, Cirilla, Cyrella, Cyrille, Siri, Sirilla, Syrilla.** International: **Cira** *(Spanish)*.

CYTHEREA. *Greek, 'from the island of Cythera'.* Home of Aphrodite, this name seems stuck in ancient Greece.

D *girls*

♂ **DACEY.** *Irish, 'from the south'.* Delicate and lacy Irish name with real possibilities. **Dacee, Dacei, Daci, Dacia, Dacie, Dacy, Daicee, Daici, Daicie, Daicy, Daycee, Daycie, Daycy.**

DACIA. *Latin place name.* Ancient place name – it was in Eastern Europe – as lacy as Dacey, but more substantial.

DAEL. *Dutch variation of* **DALE.** Vowel switch gives an old nature name a hipper look.

DAFFODIL. *Flower name.* Yes, girls were actually sometimes given this name a century ago;

now so uncommon it would make a strong springtime statement. Biggest obstacle: the nickname Daffy.

♀ **DAGAN.** *(dah-ghan) Hebrew, 'corn, grain'.* Popular in Israel for girls and boys born on Shavout, a harvest festival.

DAGMAR. *Norse, 'Dane's joy'.* Royal Danish name, unlikely choice for British commoners. **Dagna, Dagomar.**

DAGNY. *Scandinavian, 'new day'.* If you're looking for a name with Scandinavian roots, this would make a stronger and more appealing import than Dagmar. **Dagna, Dagnanna, Dagne, Dagney, Dagnie.**

DAHLIA. *Flower name.* One of the rarer flower names, used occasionally in Britain (where it's pronounced *DAY-lee-a*); can have a slightly affected la-di-dah air. **Dahiana, Dahliah, Dahlya, Dahlye, Dalia, Dalla, Dalya.**

♂ **DAI.** *(dah-ee) Japanese, ' great,' also Welsh, 'to shine'.* Pronunciation is not obvious to English speakers. **Dae.**

DAIJA, DAIJAH. *French variations of* **DÉJA.** *See* **DEJA.**

★**DAISY.** *Flower name, diminutive of* **MARGARET.** Fresh, wholesome and energetic, Daisy is one of the flower names bursting back into bloom after a century's hibernation. Has a colourful literary history

(Henry James, F. Scott Fitzgerald), and is currently in the Top 25. **Daisee, Daisey, Daisi, Daisie, Daizy, Dasey, Dasi, Dasie, Daysee, Daysey, Daysi, Daysie, Daysy, Deisy, Deysi.**

DAKIRA. *Modern invented name.* Like cousin Shakira, exotic and evocative. **Dakara, Dakaria, Dakarra, Dakirah, Dakyra.**

♂ **DAKOTA.** *Native American, Sioux, 'friendly one'.* One of the first trendy 1990s American place names, now galloping into the sunset. **Dakkota, Dakoda, Dakodah, Dakotah, Dekota, Dekotah.**

♂ **DALE.** *English, 'valley'.* An early unisex name, now outmoded but still simple and serene. **Daelyn, Dalena, Dalene, Dalenna, Dayle, Deal.** International: **Dael** *(Dutch),* **Dair** *(Norse).*

DALIA, DALYA. *Hebrew, 'branch'; Swahili, 'gentle'.* Similar in sound to the flower name Dahlia, this gentle but distinctive name, heard in many cultures, shows signs of being on the rise. **Daleah, Daleia, Daliah, Dalit, Dalya, Dalyah.**

DALILA. *Swahili, 'gentle'.* Rhythmic name that sounds similar to Delilah and is heard in several different languages: Hebrew, Spanish, Tanzanian and Swahili. **Dalilah, Dalilia.**

DALILI. *Swahili, 'a sign from the gods'.* Lovely, melodic Dalila/Delilah cousin. **Leeli, Lilie.**

♂ **DALLAS.** *Irish, 'skilled'; place name in Scotland and Texas.* This was a trendy name a decade ago. **Dalis, Dalise, Dalisha, Dalisse, Dalles, Dallis.**

DAMARA. *Greek, 'gentle girl'.* This name of an ancient fertility goddess is associated with the month of May and could make a pretty, unusual choice for a springtime baby. **Damaris, Mara, Mari.**

DAMARIS. *Greek, 'sweet heifer'.* New Testament Puritan favourite that's still attractive and accessible. **Damara, Damarys, Damiris, Dammaris.**

DAMIA. *Greek mythology name.* Greek nature goddess name that, though lacking a specific image, has a pleasing femininity. **Damiane, Damienne.**

DAMIANA. *Greek, 'tame, domesticated'.* This feminine form of **DAMIAN** projects a positive and lilting image, a distinct contrast to its male counterpart. **Damiane, Damianna, Damienne, Damiona, Damya, Damyan, Damyana, Damyenne.**

DAMICA. *French, 'open-spirited, friendly'.* Rarely heard but pleasing feminissima name for a baby girl. **Dameeka, Dameka, Damekah, Damicah, Damie, Damika, Damikah, Demeeka, Demeka, Demekah, Demica, Demicah, Damicia, Damicka.**

DAMITA. *Spanish, 'little noblewoman'.* Has a petite, dainty charm. **Dametia, Dametra.**

♂ **DANA.** *English, 'from Denmark'; also feminine variation of **DANIEL**.* This name found in both Celtic and Scandinavian mythology has gone from all-boy to almost all-girl, retaining a strong, slightly boyish quality; the birth name of Queen Latifah. **Daina, Dainna, Danacia, Danae, Danah, Danalee, Danette, Danka, Danna, Danula, Dayna.** International: *Danuta (Polish),* **Danka,** *Danulka (Czech).*

DANAË. *(dah-NAY) Greek mythology name.* A Greek goddess of music and poetry, Danae has a novel yet familiar sound. **Danai, Danay, Danaye, Danayla, Danea, Danee, Dani, Danie, Dannae, Denae, Denee, Dinae, Donnay.**

DANCER. *Word name.* Appealing when applied to a person boogying or doing ballet; a different story in the context of Santa's reindeer.

DANE. *English, 'from Denmark'.* This rarely heard name pares down all the ultrafeminine *Dan* names to one that's much more powerful, for both boys and girls.

DANI. *Hebrew and Italian, diminutive of* **DANIELLA, DANIELLE, DANITA.** Short form occasionally used on its own, with an open and friendly androgynous quality. **Danee, Daney, Danie, Dany.**

DANIA. *Hebrew, diminutive of* **DANIELLE,** *'God is my judge'.* Offbeat name with a multi-ethnic flavour. **Daniah, Danya, Danyah.**

DANICA. *Norse, 'morning star,' the planet Venus.* Unique and accessible European spin on the no longer fresh Danielle and Daniela. **Danaca, Daneca, Daneeka, Danicah, Danicka, Danika, Danikah, Danikka, Danneeka, Dannica, Dannika.**

DANIELLA. *Italian, Polish, Czech, feminine variation of* **DANIEL.** Daniela (and Danielle) were among the hottest names for twenty years, but now, though still popular, they can no longer be considered stylish options, lagging behind the newer Ella, Stella, Bella, Gabriella, and Isabella. **Dalella, Dani, Dania, Daniellah, Danijela, Danila, Danna, Danni, Danniella, Dannilla, Danny, Dany, Danya, Danyela, Danyella.** International: **Daniéle, Danelle, Danette, Danice** *(French),* **Danele** *(Basque),* **Daneila, Daniela** *(Eastern European),* **Daniyelle** *(Israeli).*

DANIELLE. *Hebrew, feminine variation of* **DANIEL.** Well used for decades, now not even in the Top 100. **Danelle, Dani, Danialle, Daniele, Daniell, Daniyelle, Danny.**

DANIKA. *Eastern European, 'morning star'. See* **DANICA.** **Danica, Danicka, Danyca, Danycka, Danyka.**

DANIQUE. *French variation of* **DANICA.** This Danielle/Monique hybrid offers a new twist on an old favourite.

DANIT. *Hebrew, 'God is my judge'.* Israeli spin on Danielle is rarely heard here. **Danita.**

DANNA. *Modern invented name.* This Dana-Donna variation has started to gain in popularity; an interesting alternative to Daniella as a namesake for a relative named Daniel.

DANU. *(DAH-noo) Celtic, goddess of fruitfulness.* This sprightly Irish mythology name would make an attention-grabbing choice.

High-Energy Names

Barnaby

Clancy

Dart

Dash

Dasha

Finian

Ivo

Juniper

Keagan

Keenan

Lulu

March

Mateo

Mitzi

Murphy

Piper

Pippa

Poppy

Rory

Rosie

Tatum

Ving

Viva

♀ **DANUBE.** *River name.* Unique and fluid river name with the lilt of a Viennese waltz.

DANY. *French, diminutive of* **DANIÈLLE.** Sometimes used on its own. *See* **DANI.**

DANYA. *Hebrew, 'judgment of God', Russian, diminutive of Daniel.* Ethnic, embroidered feel. **Dania, Daniah, Daniya.**

DAPHNE. *Greek, 'laurel tree'.* Its origins may be Greek, but it's seen as quintessentially British. **Daffy, Dafnee, Dafneigh, Dafny, Daphnee, Daphney, Daphni, Daphnie, Daphny.**

DARA. *Hebrew, 'pearl of wisdom'; Irish, 'son of the oak tree'.* Though Dara was an (extremely wise) male figure in the Bible, this name couldn't be more feminine sounding. **Dahra, Dahrah, Darah, Daralis, Darda, Darelle, Dareth, Daria, Darice, Darissa, Darra, Darrah, Darya.** International: **Darach** *(Irish Gaelic).*

♂ **DARBY.** *Irish, 'free one,' or 'free from envy'; Norse, 'from the deer estate'.* Once a common boys' name in Ireland (e.g., *Darby*

O'Gill and the Little People), the dynamic Darby now has a definite unisex feel. **Darbee, Darbey, Darbi, Darbie, Derby.**

DARCY, DARCI. *Irish, 'dark one,' originally d'Arcy; French, 'from Arcy' or 'from the fortress'.* Delicate ballerina name with grace, charm, and heft courtesy of Jane Austen's Mr Darcy. **D'Arcy, Darce, Darcee, Darcel, Darcelle, Darcey, Darcia, Darsey, Darsi, Darsie.**

DARI. *Variation of* **DARA** *or* **DARIUS.** Breezy and flyaway.

DARIA. *Persian, 'having many possessions'; feminine variation of* **DARIUS.** An early Christian martyr, and now a Canadian supermodel: Daria Werbowy. **Dariah, Darie, Darina, Darinka, Darissa, Dariya, Darria, Darriah, Darrya, Darryah, Darya, Daryah, Daryia.** International: **Daruška** *(Czech),* **Dariya, Darya, Dasha** *(Russian).*

♂ **DARIAN.** *Variation of* **DARIUS.** A rarely heard member of the Darren-Darius clan. **Darien, Daryan, Daryen.**

DARLA. *English, 'darling'.*
Dimpled *Our Gang* comedy
name. **Darlah, Darlie, Darly.**

DARLENE. *English, 'darling'.*
Attending crochet classes for the
seniors at the community centre
with her friends Arlene and
Marlene. **Darleen, Darleena,
Darleene, Darlina, Darline,
Darlonna, Darlyn, Darlyne.**

♂ **DARREN.** *Irish, 'little great
one'.* Once-popular boys' name
works better now for girls, as a
kind of Dara/Karen blend. **Daran,
Daren, Darin, Daron, Darran,
Darrin, Darron, Darryn, Daryn.**

DARSHA. *Hindi, 'to see, to
perceive, to have vision'.* This
is an Indian name similar
in feeling to some of the
increasingly popular Russian
names. **Darshika, Darshina,
Darshini, Darshna.**

DARU. *Hindi, 'pine or cedar'.*
Exotic, aromatic Indian name.

DARVA. *Slavic, 'honeybee'.*
Reality TV show-type name.

DARYA. *Russian variation of*
DARIA. *See* **DARIA. Dariya,
Dasha.**

♂ **DARYL.** *Variation of*
DARRELL. Actress Daryl
Hannah made this a girls'
name. **Darel, Darelle, Daril,
Darille, Darrel, Darrell,
Darrellem, Darrill, Darryl,
Darryll, Daryll, Derel.**

DASHA. *Russian, diminutive
of* **DARIYA** *or* **DARYA.** Nice,
energetic – dare we say dashing?
– quality. **Dasia.**

DASHAWNA. *American
variation of* **SHAWNA.** One
of many now-downscale names
that begin with *Da-* or *De-*, a
prefix that originally indicated
patrimony. **Daseana, Dashauna,
Dashona, Deseana, Deshauna,
Deshawna, Deshona, Seshawna.**

DATYAH. *(dah-TI-ah) Hebrew,
'belief in God'.* Heard more in
Israel than the UK. **Datia,
Datiah, Datiya, Datya.**

DAVIDA. *Feminine variation of*
DAVID. As passé as Bernarda
and Benjamina. **Daveeda,
Daveen, Daveisha, Davene,
Davesia, Daveta. International:
Daibhidha** *(Scottish Gaelic),* **Taffy**
(Welsh), **Dabida** *(Basque),* **Daven**
(Scandinavian), **Davita** *(Israeli).*

DAVINA. *Hebrew, 'beloved';
Scottish, 'little deer'.* A Scottish
favourite occasionally heard in
the UK. **Dava, Davannah,
Daveen, Daveena, Davene,
Davenia, Davi, Davia, Davida,
Davinah, Davita, Devina,
Devinah, Devinia, Divina,
Divinah.**

DAWN. *Word name.* There are
more substantial names with
the same golden meaning:
Aurora (Latin), Zora (Arabic),
and Roxana (Persian). **Daun,
Daune, Dawna, Dawne,
Dawnelle, Duwad, Dwan.**

♂ **DAY.** *Word name.* This is a
bright and optimistic middle
name choice.

DAYA. *Hebrew, 'bird of prey'.*
Possible alternative to the trendy
Maya. **Dayah.**

DAYAA. *(dah-YAH) Hindi,
'compassion'.* The double vowel
changes this name's pronunciation
and gives it a novel twist.

DAYANA. *Latin variation
of* **DIANA.** This creative
spelling of Diana has taken
on a life of its own. **Dayani,
Dayanita, Dayanna.**

DAYANARA. *Modern invented name.* Too close to 'sayanara'. **Dayanarah.**

♀ **DAYO.** *Nigerian, 'joy arrives'.* This has an evocative African beat.

♀ **DAYTON.** *English variation of* **DEIGHTON,** *'place with a dike'.* A city name in the US that is more successful as a girl's name than some others due to similarity in sound to Peyton et al. **Deyton.**

♀ **DEAN.** *English, 'valley,' or 'church official'.* Like many passé boys' names, this one sounds fresh again for girls. **Deani, Deanie, Deen, Deeni, Deenie, Deeny, Dene, Deni, Denie, Deny.**

DEANA. *Variation of* **DIANA** *or feminine variation of* **DEAN.** Depending on how you say it, either a streamlined version of Deanna, or the namesake of a male Dean. But today, why not name her Dean? **Deanah, Deanna, Deeana, Deeanna, Dena.**

DEANNA. *English spelling variation of* **DIANA.** Though still being used, Deanna hit its peak in the 1940s. **Deana, Deandra, Deanne, Dee, Deeana, Deona, Deonna.**

★**DEBORAH.** *Hebrew, 'bee'.* In the mid-twentieth century, there were so many Debbies on the block that the beauty and meaning of the original name got lost. Now this lovely name of an Old Testament prophetess and the only female judge of Israel suddenly sounds fresher than overused Sarah, Rachel and Rebecca. **Deb, Debara, Debbi, Debbie, Debbora, Debborah, Debbra, Debbrah, Debby, Debera, Deberah, Debi, Debora, Deboreh, Deborrah, Debra, Debrah, Debs, Devora, Devorah.**

DEBRA. *Spelling variation of* **DEBORAH.** When Deborah seemed too formal in the laid-back 1960s, Debra stepped in as a pared-down alternative, but the pendulum is about to swing back. **Deb, Debbie, Debbra, Debbrah, Debrah, Debry.**

♀ **DECEMBER.** *Word name.* Cooler than April, May or June, but also a tad icy. **Decembra.** **International: Dicembre** *(Italian).*

DECIMA. *Latin, 'tenth'.* In the days of huge families, this Roman goddess of childbirth's name would be saved for bambina number ten. Now might be used for a girl born in October, the tenth month. **Decia.**

DECLA. *Irish, feminine variation of* **DECLAN.** Has an incomplete feeling . . .

DEIRDRE. *Irish, 'sorrowful'.* Sadly, this strong Celtic name often has 'of the sorrows' attached to it because of the tragic character in Irish legend. Also a bit drab when compared with newer Irish imports. **Dedre, Deedra, Deedrah, Deedre, Deerdra, Deerdre, Deidre, Deirdra, Deirdrah, Deirdre, Dierdra, Dierdre, Dierdree, Dierdrie.**

DÉJA. *French, 'already'.* Déja was a name sensation of the 1990s in the US, reaching the Top 15 in African-Caribbean popularity lists, but it has déja fallen far from those lofty heights. **D'Ja, Daeja, Daija, Déjah, Dejai, DeJana, Dejana.**

★♂ **DELANCEY.** *French, 'from Lancey'.* Energetic dance of an Irish surname, great for both genders. **Delancie, Delancy.**

♀ **DELANEY.** *Irish, 'dark challenger'.* A top Irish surname name for a decade, projecting buoyant enthusiasm plus a feminine feel. **Dalaney, Dalayne, Daleney, Del, Delaina, Delaine, Delainey, Delanee, Delani, Delanie, Delany, Delayna, Delaynie, Dellaney.**

DELFINA. *Italian and Spanish variation of* **DELPHINE.** *See* **DELPHINE.**

DELIA. *Greek, 'born on the island of Delos'.* Seductive charmer associated with cookery writer Delia Smith. **Dehlia, Deilyuh, Delea, Deliah, Dellya, Delya.**

DÉLICE. *French, 'delight'.* French delicacy.

DELICIA. *Latin, 'delight'.* Tastier than Alicia or Felicia. **Daleesha, Dalicia, Dalisha, Dalisia, Deleesha, Delesha, Delica, Delight, Delisa, Delisha, Delishia, Delisia, Delisiah, Delite.**

DELIGHT. *Word name.* The mythical daughter of Eros and Psyche becomes a modern-sounding word name. Danger: could be seen as X-rated.

★**DELILAH.** *Hebrew, 'desirable, seductive', Arabic, 'guide'.* Has shed the stigma of its biblical beguiling-temptress image, and is now appreciated for its haunting, melodic, feminine qualities. **Dalialah, Dalila, Dalilah, Delila, Delilia.**

DELISE. *Latin, 'delight'.* Variation on the Delight-Delicia theme. **Delesha, Delisa, Delisha, Delisiah, Delissa.**

DELJA. *(DEHL-yah) Polish, diminutive of* **KORDELJA**, *'daughter of the sea'.* Pretty in a polka-dancing way.

DELLA. *Diminutive of* **ADELA.** One of the few *ella* names that's not on every other new mother's lips – a definite plus. **Dell, Dellah, Delle, Dellia, Dellya, Delya, Delyah.**

♂ **DELLEN.** *Cornish, 'petal'.* Intriguing combo of elements. **Dellan, Dellin, Dellon.**

DELORES. *Variation of* **DOLORES.** *See* **DOLORES.** **Deloris.**

★**DELPHINE.** *French from Greek, 'woman from Delphi'.* Sleek, chic French name with two nature associations – the dolphin and the delphinium – definitely fresher than over-the-hill Danielle. **Adephine, Dauphin, Delfa, Delfine, Delpha, Delphene, Delphi, Delphia, Delphina, Delphinea, Delphinia, Delphy, Delphyne, Delpina. International: Delfina** *(Italian and Spanish).*

DELTA. *Greek, fourth letter of Greek alphabet.* This name has a lazy-day-down-by-the-river feel.

DELYTH. *Welsh, 'pretty and blessed'.* If you like soft, lispy Welsh names like Gwyneth, consider this out-of-the-ordinary one.

DEMELZA. *Cornish, 'fort on the hill'.* Complex and challenging – but aren't childhood and parenthood challenging enough?

Da & De Names

Dajuana

Dameesha

Danacia

Da'nell

Darenda

D'arline

Dashawn

Dashay

Dejana

Deleanna

Delinda

Delisa

Delondra

Demika

Denisha

Denita

Deondray

Deshandra

Dewanda

D'shay

DEMETRIA. *Greek, goddess of fertility.* Dramatic earth goddess possibility with film-star nickname. **Demeta, Demeter, Demeteria, Demetra, Demetras, Demetris, Demi, Demita, Demitra, Detria, Dimetra, Dimitra.**

DEMI. *(de-MEE) Greek, 'half'; diminutive of* **DEMETRIA.** Tied to a single celeb in Hollywood, megapopular in Holland and just appearing in the Top 100 here. **Deme, Demee, Demeter, Demetra, Demetria, Demia, Demie, Demitra, Demmi, Demy, Dimitira, Dimitra.**

DENA. *English, 'valley'.* Dated namesake of dated Dean. **Deana, Deanna, Deena, Dina.**

DENI. *English, diminutive of* **DENISE.** Cute nickname name used by Woody Harrelson for his daughter. **Denee, Deney, Denie, Denni, Dennie, Denny, Deny.**

DENISE. *French, feminine variation of* **DENIS.** A French favourite of the 1950s and 1960s, not exactly chic now. **Danica, Danice, Daniece,** Danise, Denese, Deni, Denice, Deniece, Deniese, Denisse, Denni, Dennise, Denny, Denyce, Denyse. International: **Dinisia** *(Portuguese),* **Deniska** *(Russian).*

DENISHA. *American variation of* **DENISE.** Typical of formula that takes a traditional name syllable and adds *-isha* ending. **Daneesha, Danisha, Danysha, Deneesha, Denishe, Denita, Denysha.**

DERVLA. *Anglicised form of Irish* **DEARBHÁIL,** *'daughter of Fál'.* Tongue twister of a name common in Ireland in both its Gaelic and its Anglicised forms. **Deirbhile, Derbáil, Derval, Dervila, Dervilia.**

DERYN. *Welsh, 'bird'.* This 1950s Welsh bird name sounds less dated than Robin, popular at the same time. **Deron, Derren, Derrin, Derrine, Derron.**

DESDEMONA. *Greek, 'ill-starred'.* Shakespearean as a name can be, but because the beautiful and innocent wife of Othello came to such a tragic end, her name's been avoided for centuries.

DESIRÉE. *French, 'desired'.* Desired and chosen by many, despite (or because of) its blatantly sensual image. **Desairee, Desarae, Desaray, Desaraye, Desaree, Desarhea, Desary, Deseri, Desi, Desirae, Desirai, Desiray, Desree, Des'ree, Des-ree, Desyrae, Desyray, Desyree, Dezarae, Dezaray, Dezeret, Dezirae, Deziree, Dezray, Dez'ree.**

DESTINY. *Word name.* This is a popular girl's name in the US, and there are three alternate spellings in hot pursuit. **Destanee, Destanie, Destany, Destenee, Desteney, Desteny, Destinay, Destinee, Destinei, Destiney, Destini, Destinie, Destinni, Destinny, Destinyi, Destnay, Destney, Destonie, Destony, Destunee, Destynee, Destyni.**

★♂ **DESTRY.** *English variation of French, 'warhorse'.* It was the hero's last name in the classic film *Destry Rides Again,* but in today's anything-goes naming climate, nobody blinked when the Steven Spielbergs picked it for their daughter. A real winner. **Destrey, Destri, Destrie.**

DEVA. *Hindi, 'divine, shining one'.* If you don't want your daughter to be a Diva, try this Hindu moon goddess name instead. **Deeva, Devi.**

DEVI. *Sanskrit, 'divine'.* This Hindu goddess name has a powerful heritage plus lively sound with a devilish edge. **Devaki, Devee.**

♂ **DEVIN.** *Irish, 'poet'.* Used far more for boys with this spelling, but still has a nice impish Irish feel for a girl. **Davin, Devan, Deven, Devena, Devini, Devinn, Devinne, Devyn, Devynne.**

♂ **DEVON.** *English place name.* This spelling makes it a pretty and popular British place name, evoking dramatic seascapes and moors. **Davon, Deaven, Devan, Devann, Devaughn, Deven, Devin, Devinne, Devona, Devonne, Devvon, Devyn.**

DEVORA, DEVORAH. *Variation of* **DEBORAH.** Both a biblical and an Israeli place name, this can be used as an offbeat substitute for

Deborah. **Deva, Devra, Devrah, Devoria, Dvora, Dvorit.**

DEVYN. *Spelling variation of* **DEVIN.** A more feminine version of Devin.

♂ **DEXTER.** *Latin, 'right-handed, skillful'.* Perfect example of a name that's nerdy for a boy, but turns ultracool for a girl; Diane Keaton named her daughter Dexter Dean. **Dex, Dexee, Dexey, Dexie, Dextra, Dexy.**

DHARA. *Hindi, 'the earth'.* An exotic take on Dara.

DHARMA. *Buddhist and Hindu basic principle of cosmic existence.* Rarely used in real life; the name of the hippyish character on the sitcom *Dharma & Greg* and part of the title of a Kerouac novel. **Dharana.**

DIA. *Spanish, 'day'.* One fine day.

DIAHANN. *Alternate spelling of* **DIANE.** *See* **DIANE.**

DIAMANTA. *Greek, 'unconquerable'.* Softens the

Names Kids Love Having

Angelica

Ariel

Belle

Britney

Daisy

Diamond

Jade

Jasmine

Miranda

Princess

Rosie

Silver

Skye

Starr

Willow

Zoe

hardness of the stone. **Diamante, Diamantina.**

DIAMOND. *Gem name.* Sparkled all through the 1990s, now its shine is slightly diminished. **Diamin, Diamon, Diamonda, Diamonde,** Diamonte, Diamund, Diamunde, Diamyn, Dyamond.

DIANA. *Latin, 'divine'.* The tragic British princess inspired many fashions, but strangely, not one for her classic and lovely moon-goddess name, which is infrequently used today. **Daiana, Daianna, Dayana, Dayanna, Deana, Deanna, Dede, Dee, DeeDee, Di, Dia, Dianah, Dianca, Diandra, Diane, Diania, Dyana, Dyanna.**

DIANDRA. *Greek, 'twice a man'.* One of many variations on Diana, but lacking its classic class. **Deandra, Deandre, Diandrea, Dyandra.**

DIANE. *French variation of* **DIANA.** Like Joanne and Christine, middle-aged Diane has been overshadowed by the a- ending version of her name. **Deanne, Dede, Dee, DeeDee, Di, Diahann, Dian, Dianne, Dione, Dionne, Dyan, Dyane, Dyann, Dyanne.**

DIANTHA. *Greek, 'divine flower'.* Mythological flower of Zeus, melodious and more unusual Diana cousin. **Dianthe, Dianthia.**

DIARRA. *African, 'gift'.* Could lead to teasing *re* association with certain digestive problem. **Diara, Diera, Dierra, Dyara, Dyarra, Dyera.**

♂ **DIAZ.** *Spanish from Latin, 'days'.* If Cameron's first name could start a girl's name craze, why not her second?

DIDI. *Pet name for* Di-starting names. Not as lively or independent as Gigi, Kiki or Coco. **Dee, DeeDee.**

DIDO. *Greek, meaning obscure.* Heroine of Virgil's *Aeneid;* could have some awkward associations down the line.

DIGNA. *Latin, 'worthy'.* Seems to cry out for another syllable.

DIJA. *(DEE-jah) Diminutive of* **KHADIJA.** Uncommon and cool.

DILLIAN. *Latin, 'image of worship'.* Real name that sounds like a made-up combination of Dillon and Lillian. **Diliana, Dilla, Dillianna, Dillanne, Dilly.**

♂ **DILLON.** *Irish, 'loyal'.* Turns trendy boy's name into trendy surname name. **Dilen, Dillan, Dillen, Dillin, Dillyn, Dillynn, Dillynne, Dilynn, Dilynne.**

DILLY. *Diminutive of* **DILYS, DILWEN** *and* **DAFFODIL.** Silly.

DILYS. *(DILL-is) Welsh, 'genuine, steadfast, true'.* Common in Wales, but would really stand out here.

DIMANCHE. *(dee-MAHNZH) French, 'Sunday'.* Pleasant-sounding word that could morph into a unique Sunday-picnic-type name.

DINA. *English, feminine variation of* **DINO.** OK, as long as it's not pronounced *diner*.

★**DINAH.** *Hebrew, 'God will judge'.* As the song says, 'Dinah, is there anyone finer?' Charming, underused Old Testament name, long shunned for old slave-name stereotype, but has a rich literary and musical résumé and would make a vivid name for a contemporary girl. **Deena, Dina, Dinna, Dyna, Dynah. International: Dine** *(Yiddish).*

DIONE. *(dy-OH-nee) Greek, 'divine queen'.* In Greek mythology the mother of Aphrodite by Zeus, and also one of Saturn's moons; this is an astral name quite distinct from the better known Dionne. **Dion, Dionne.**

DIONNE. *(dee-ahn) Greek, feminine variation of* **DION.** Americanised version of the Greek Dione, with many sub-versions of its own. **Deona, Deonne, Dion, Diona, Diondra, Dione, Dionis, Dionna, Dyon, Dyone, Dyonne.**

DIOR. *French surname.* Could join Chanel and Armani on the fashionista hit parade of names.

♂ **DISCOVERY.** *Word name.* A lot to handle, but it does give a sense of openness, joy and awe.

DIVA. *Latin, 'goddess'.* Once unique to the Zappa family, now you can have your own little prima donna. **Deeva, Dyva.**

♂ **DIVERSITY.** *Word name.* As a name, it's a bit too politically correct.

DIVINA. *Variation of* **DAVINA.** A choice of two pronunciations, making this little girl divine or diveen.

DIVINITY. *Word name.* A sister to Trinity, Genesis or Heaven.

DIXIE. *Latin, 'I have spoken'; French, 'tenth'.* Saucy American showgirl, wise-cracking waitress. **Dixee, Dixey, Dixi, Dixy.**

DJUNA. *(JOON-a) Meaning unknown.* Novelist Djuna (born Djalma) Barnes introduced this interesting name to the mix.

DODIE. *English, diminutive of* **DOROTHY.** Good only up to the age of 2½ years old.

DOE. *English, 'a female deer'.* Soft and gentle-eyed middle name possibility.

DOLLY. *English, diminutive of* **DOROTHY** *and* **DOLORES.** Goodbye, Dolly. **Dolley.**

DOLORES. *Spanish, 'lady of sorrows'.* Though it's related to the Virgin Mary, this name was once perceived as the height of exotic sensuality, a role since taken over by nickname Lola.

Dalora, Dalores, Daloris, Dalorita, Delora, Delores, Deloris, Dolly, Dolora, Dolorcita, Doloriana, Doloris, Dolorita, Doloritta, Dolours, Lola, Loli, Lolica, Lolicia, Lolita. International: Dores *(Portuguese)*.

DOMINI. *Latin variation of* **DOMINIC.** Most distinctive of the Dominic-related girls' names. **Dominee, Dominey, Dominie, Dominy.**

DOMINGA. *Spanish, feminine variation of* **DOMINGO.** Nice for a little girl born on Sunday.

♂ **DOMINIC.** *Latin, 'lord'.* Instead of trying to feminise it, actor Andy Garcia gave this historically male name to his daughter, making it instantly and appealingly unisex.

DOMINICA. *Italian, feminine variation of* **DOMINIC.** Fashionably continental, much fresher than Dominique. **Domenica, Domenika, Domineca, Domineka, Domini, Dominicka, Dominika, Domynica, Domynicka, Domynika.**

DOMINIQUE. *French, feminine variation of* **DOMINIC.** Had a surge of popularity in the *Dynasty* days, now has subsided in the wake of fresher French choices like Destry and Delphine. **Domaneke, Domanique, Domeneque, Domenique, Domineek, Domineke, Domineque, Dominika, Dominiqua, Meeka, Mika.**

♂ **DOMINO.** *Latin, 'lord, master'.* One of those ultimate cool-girl names, played by Keira Knightley in a film about a supermodel-turned-bounty hunter, but kids might associate it with the game.

DONATA. *Latin, 'given'.* Evokes a sympathetic feeling of generosity and charity. **Donada, Donatila, Donatilia, Donatta.**

DONATELLA. *Italian, feminine diminutive of* **DONATO.** Stylish and dramatic, à la Donatella Versace.

DONNA. *Italian, 'lady'.* The perfect housewife of the 1950s.

♂ **DONNELLY.** *Celtic, 'dark brave one'.* Makes Donna into a cool twenty-first-century unisex Irish surname.

♂ **DOON, DOONE.** *Scottish surname.* Photographer Diane Arbus named her daughter Doon, inspired by the sand dunes she walked among when pregnant.

DORA. *Greek, 'gift'; diminutive of* **THEODORA.** Poised for a comeback, right behind Laura, Nora, Cora, and Flora. **Dorah, Doro, Dory.**

DORCAS. *Greek, 'doe, gazelle'.* Classic name used by the Romans, the Puritans, and the Bard, but pretty much taboo today due to the objectionable connotations of both its front and back ends. **Dorcia, Dorkas.**

DORÉ. *(dor-AY) French, 'gilded'.* Glitzy and pretentious.

DOREEN. *Variation of* **DORA;** *also Anglicised variation of Irish* **DOIREANN,** *'sullen'.* Much fresher Irish imports available for colleens now. **Dairinn, Dorean, Doreena, Dorena, Dorene, Dorienne, Dorina, Dorine.**

DORETTA. *Variation of* **DOROTHY.** Frilly, feminissima, unstylish *Dor* name.

DORIA. *Variation of* **DOROTHY.** Not quite Dora or Daria, this name suffers from an identity crisis. **Dorria, Dorrya, Dorya.**

♂ **DORIAN.** *Greek, 'from Doris'.* Strictly male in the Oscar Wilde days, the attractive Dorian crossed the lake into the girls' camp several years ago. **Dorea, Dorean, Doreane, Doria, Doriana, Doriane, Doriann, Dorianna, Dorianne.**

DORINDA. *Greek, 'bountiful gift'; also extension of* **DORA.** Cinderella stepsister-type Victorian-valentine name. **Derinda, Dori, Dorin, Dorrinda, Dory, Drinda, Dyrinda.**

DORIS. *Greek, 'gift of the ocean'.* Has long been on our so-far-out-it-will-always-be-out-for-babies list, and seems written there in indelible ink. **Doria, Dorice, Dorika, Dorise, Doriss, Dorita, Dorrise, Dorrit, Dorrys, Dorys.**

DORIT. *(do-REET) Hebrew, ' of this generation'.* Popular in Israel, sounds a lot more current than Doris. **Dorith, Doritt, Dorritt, Dorli.**

DORKAS. *See* **DORCAS.** **Dorca, Dorcas, Dorcea, Dorcia.**

DORO. *Diminutive of* **DOROTHY.** Improvement on Dotty, but still not quite a name.

★**DOROTHEA.** *Greek, 'gift of God'.* Flowing and romantic Victorian-sounding name with a literary heritage and choice of two appealing nicknames. **Dorete, Dorethea, Doretta, Dorine, Dorita, Doro, Dorota, Dortha, Dorthea, Thea.** International: **Díorbhail** *(Scottish Gaelic),* **Dorothée** *(French),* **Dorotea** *(Italian),* **Doortje** *(Dutch),* **Dorotea** *(Swedish and Italian),* **Dorete, Dorte, Dorthe** *(Danish),* **Dortea, Tea** *(Norwegian),* **Dorota, Dosia** *(Polish, Czech),* **Dorika, Dorottya** *(Hungarian),* **Doroteya, Dosya** *(Russian).*

DOROTHY. *English variation of* **DOROTHEA.** In the 1930s Dorothy left Kansas for Oz, but by the 1980s she was ready for retirement. **Do, Doa, Doe, Dodo, Dodie, Dollie, Dolly, Dorettam, Dori, Dorothea, Dorothee, Dorothey, Dorothi, Dorothie, Dorthee, Dorthy, Dorrit, Dot, Dotti, Dottie, Dotty, Totie.**

♂ **DORSEY.** English from *French, 'from Orsay'.* Big Band-ish name could easily be confused with Darcy. **Dorsee, Dorsi, Dorsie, Dorsy.**

DORY. *French, 'golden', or diminutive of* **DOROTHY.** Dorothy nickname name with a measure of modern charm. **Doree, Dorey, Dori, Dorie, Dorree, Dorrey, Dorri, Dorrie, Dorry.**

DOT. *English, diminutive of* **DOROTHY.** Old-fangled nickname could make dot.com era short form or middle name.

DOTTIE. *English, diminutive of* **DOROTHY.** Synonym of screwy – but London tastemakers are restoring it to style. **Dottey, Dotti, Dotty.**

Ancient Roman Names

Aeliana	Laurentia
Albia	Livia
Aquilia	Marilla
Argentia	Martia
Aurelia	Maxima
Avita	Mila
Cassia	Nerilla
Clemensia	Prima
Decima	Quintia
Dulcia	Rufina
Fabia	Septima
Faustina	Sergia
Florentina	Tanaquil
Fortunata	Tauria
Galla	Tertia
Horatia	Tullia
Junia	Urbana
Laelia	Varinia

DOUCE. *(doos) French, ' gentle, sweet'.* A sweet French word name possibility, but with unsavoury teasing potential. **Docina, Douceline, Doucette, Duce.**

♂ **DOVE.** *Nature name.* One of the new bird names, like Lark and Wren, this one's associated with the billing and cooing sounds of love.

DOVEVA. *Hebrew, 'graceful'.* Feminine but strong name heard in Israel. **Dova, Dovevet, Dovit.**

DREA. *(DRAY-a) Diminutive of* **ALEXANDRIA** *or* **ANDREA.** Introduced via *Sopranos* star Drea (born Andrea) de Matteo, and catching on with a wider audience.

DREAM. *Word name.* Singular and serene noun name.

DREE. *Diminutive of* **ALEXANDRIA** *or* **ANDREA.** Unique one-syllable name added to the mix by Mariel Hemingway for her daughter; could make a distinctive middle name or Bree substitute.

♂ **DREW.** *Diminutive of* **ANDREW.** Elegant formerly male alternative to Andy, now in the stylishly upscale Paige-Brooke-Blair sorority, thanks largely to Drew Barrymore. **Dru, Drue.**

DRU. *Diminutive of* **DRUCILLA.** Flimsier than *Drew* spelling. **Drew, Drue.**

DRUCILLA, DRUSILLA. *Latin, 'strong'.* Pleasingly quaint and dainty New Testament possibility; the nickname Dru modernises it. **Dru, Drucella, Drucila, Druesila, Druscila, Druscilla, Drusila.**

DRUELLA. *German, 'elfin vision'.* A little too close to Cruella.

DUANA. *Irish, 'song'.* Name her after a Duane relative if you like, but please pronounce it *doo-ahn-a* and not *doo-wain-a*.

♂ **DUANE.** *Irish, 'swarthy'.* On second thought, why not just call her Duane, putting her in synch with her girlfriends Dylan, Dustin and Daryl?

♂ **DUFFY.** *Irish, 'dark'.* This Irish surname packs a lot of attitude, projecting an image of spunk and sass. **Duff.**

DULCE. *(DOOL-chay) Latin, 'sweet'.* Popular Spanish name that refers to *'dulce nombre de*

Maria' – the sweet name of the Virgin Mary. **Douce, Doucie, Dulcea, Dulcee, Dulcey, Dulci, Dulcia, Dulcie, Dulcina, Dulcinea, Dulcinia, Dulcy.**

DULCIE, DULCY. *Latin, 'sweet'.* Dating back to the Roman Empire, Dulcy may be too lightweight to merit a revival. **Dulciana, Dulcine, Dulcita. International: Dulcet, Dulcette** *(French),* **Dulce, Dulcea, Dulcia, Dulcinea** *(Spanish and Italian).*

★♂ **DUNE.** *Nature name.* Haunting and evocative sandy-beach name, also with sci-fi connections. **Doon, Doone.**

DUNYA. *Russian, 'well-regarded'.* Courageous sister of Raskolnikov in Dostoyevsky's *Crime and Punishment.*

DUŠANA. *(doo-sha-nah) Slavic, 'spirit or soul'.* Pretty Slavic name, with some obvious pronunciation challenges. **Dušanka, Dušička, Duška.**

DUSCHA. *(DYOO-sha) Russian, 'happy'.* Possible alternative to the more

popular Sascha. **Dusa, Duschinka, Dusica.**

♂ **DUSTIN.** *German, 'brave warrior'.* Just a few years ago, Dustin, Dylan and Daryl seemed like radical, edgy names for girls; now even Great-aunt Alberta wouldn't raise an eyebrow. **Dustan, Dusten, Duston, Dusty, Dustyn.**

DWYN. *Diminutive of* **DWYNWEN.** Short, but still

kind of a mouthful. **Dwynwen.**

DWYNWEN. *Welsh, 'wave'.* Far from a win-win.

DYAN. *Variation of* **DIANE.** Creative spelling can't revive uncreative name. **Dian, Dyana, Dyane, Dyani, Dyann, Dyanna, Dyanne.**

DYANI. *Native American, 'deer'.* Could sound like a babyish nickname for Diane.

Stellar Starbabies Beginning with *D*

Daisy	Lucy Lawless, Jamie Oliver, Meg Ryan
Dakota Rain	Dolores O' Riordan
Deanna	James Brown
Delilah	Lisa Rinna & Harry Hamlin
Deni	Woody Harrelson
Destry	Kate Capshaw & Steven Spielberg
Dexter	Diane Keaton
D'Lila Star	Sean 'Diddy' Combs
Dixie Dot	Anna Ryder Richardson
Dominik	Andy Garcia
Dree	Mariel Hemingway
Dylan	Robin Wright & Sean Penn

♂ **DYLAN.** *Welsh, 'son of the sea'.* A favourite boy's name that retains more of its poetic, windswept quality when used for a girl, as Robin Wright and Sean Penn did. **Dylann, Dylen, Dylin, Dyllan, Dyllen, Dyllon, Dylon, Dylynn.**

DYLANA. *Feminine variation of* **DYLAN.** Feminises Dylan – but why bother?

E girls

EACHNA. *(EEK-na) Irish, 'horse'.* Irish goddess renowned for her beauty and fashion sense – though her name has neither.

♂ **EARHART.** *German surname, 'honor, bravery'.* Conceivable middle name choice for admirers of flyer Amelia.

EARLA. *English, feminine variation* of **EARL.** If there's an ancestral Earl you want to honour, consider Early instead. **Earldena, Earldene, Earldina, Earlean, Earlecia, Earleen, Earlena, Earlene, Earletta, Earley, Earlie, Earlina, Earlinda, Earline,**

Erla, Erlana, Erlene, Erlenne, Erletta, Erlette, Erlina, Erlinda, Erline, Erlinia, Erlisha, Ireleen, Irelene, Irelina, Irelene.

♂ **EARLY.** *Word name.* A word that's been used, very infrequently, as a name for hundreds of years. Interesting sound and meaning.

EARTHA. *English, 'earth'.* Used by the Puritans, and, three hundred years later, by Eartha Kitt's parents, it sounds dated and dry. **Earth, Erda, Ertha, Herta, Hertha.**

EAST. *Word name.* North and West are easier on the ear, but this works fine if it has some significance for your family.

★**EASTER.** *Word name.* Used as a name for several hundred years, as part of the day-naming tradition, this rarely heard holiday celebration would make a novel choice for a springtime baby. **Eastan, Eastlyn, Easton.**

EAVAN. *(EE-vahn) Irish, 'beautiful, radiant'.* Anglicised spelling of the unpronounceable Aoibheann, the name of several

Irish princesses, this has pronunciation problems of its own, as most people would think it rhymed with 'heaven'.

EBBA. *English, 'fortress of riches'; German, 'strength of a boar'.* Soft yet strong name heard in Germany and Scandinavia could be readily assimilated. **Ebbe.**

EBONY. *English, 'deeply black wood'.* Word name that came into favour because of its connotations of blackness and beauty, trending down since the 1980s. **Abonee, Abony, Eban, Ebanee, Ebanie, Ebany, Ebboney, Ebbony, Ebone, Eboné, Ebonea, Ebonee, Eboney, Eboni, Ebonie, Ebonique, Ebonisha, Ebonne, Ebonnee, Ebonney, Ebonni, Ebonny, Eboni, Ebonie, Ebonye, Ebonyi.**

ECCENTRICITY. *Word name.* The definition of quirky.

ECHO. *Greek mythology name.* Pretty choice, though the legendary nymph Echo became *only* a voice. **Echoe, Ecko, Ekko, Ekkoe.**

ECRU. *Colour name.* Neutral colour, but as a name, too much of an oddity.

EDA. *German, 'wealthy, happy'.* Sounds too much like 'eater'.

EDANA. *Irish, 'fire'.* Feminine of Aidan, but now girls would prefer to use the original. **Aydana, Eda, Edan, Edanna.**

EDDA. *Italian variation of* HEDDA. If her dad's name is Ed, then name her . . . Emily, Margot, Susannah, but not Edda. **Etta.**

★EDEN. *Hebrew, 'place of pleasure, delight'.* Attractive paradise-equivalent of the more-popular Nevaeh (yes, that's heaven spelled backwards). The two long *e*'s make it sound especially serene. **Eaden, Eadin, Ede, Edena, Edene, Edenia, Edin, Edyn.**

EDINA. *English, 'wealthy'.* Infectious-sounding Minnesota place name, featured in the British cult hit TV show *Absolutely Fabulous.* **Adena, Adina, Edeena, Edyna.**

EDIE. *English, diminutive of* EDITH. Cute short form that sometimes stands on its own, due for rediscovery along with Warhol 'It Girl' Edie Sedgwick. **Edea, Edee, Edeigh, Edi, Edy.**

EDITH. *English, 'prosperous in war'.* Hugely popular name a hundred years ago that's being revived among stylish parents in London. Definitely worth considering for those with a taste for forgotten, old-fashioned names. **Eadie, Eadith, Ede, Edie, Edit, Edithe, Ediva, Edy, Edyth, Edythe, Eidith, Eidyth, Eyde, Eydie, Eydith, Edyte.** International: **Edetta, Edita, Editta** *(Italian),* **Edita, Dita** *(Spanish),* **Editha** *(German),* **Eda, Edda, Edka, Edyta, Ita** *(Polish),* **Dita, Ditka, Edita** *(Czech),* **Edi, Ekika** *(Hawaiian).*

EDLYN. *English, 'small, noble one'.* Feels like a hybrid. It would be better to go for Edith or Evelyn. **Edelynn, Edlin, Edlinn, Edlinna, Edlynn.**

EDNA. *Hebrew, 'rejuvenation, delight'.* Though Emma and Ella have had successful return engagements, we don't see much hope for Edna. **Adna, Adnisha, Eddi, Eddie, Eddna, Eddnah, Eddy, Ednah, Edneisha, Edneshia, Ednisha, Ednita, Edona.**

EDWIGE. *(ed-WEEG) French from German* HEDWIG. Haitian writer Edwidge Danticat highlighted this sophisticated, chignon-wearing choice for literate parents. **Edvig, Edwidge, Edwig.** International: **Edvige** *(Italian),* **Hedwig** *(German).*

Clunky but Cool Names

Agatha	Iris
Agnes	Isadora
Augusta	Josephine
Edith	Mabel
Eleonora	Margaret
Eudora	Matilda
Florence	Myrtle
Frances	Olive
Frederica	Pearl
Harriet	Phoebe
Helen	Prudence
Henrietta	Rosamund
Ida	Theodora
Imogen	

EDWINA. *Feminine variation of* **EDWIN.** Edwina's still a little old-fashioned, but we can see her joining friends like Matilda and Josephine for a comeback. Better pronounced like Edwin than Edween. **Eady, Eddi, Eddie, Eddy, Edina, Edweena, Edweina, Edwena, Edwine, Edwinna, Edwyna, Edwynn, Edy, Win, Winnie.** International: **Edwynna, Edwynne** *(Welsh),* **Eduina** *(Spanish),* **Edvina** *(Eastern European).*

EFFIE. *Greek, 'pleasant speech'.* Old-fashioned short form for Euphemia, a little too barefoot and tattered to be worth reviving. **Effemie, Effemy, Effi, Effia, Effy, Efthemia, Ephie, Eppie, Euphemia, Euphemie, Euphie.**

EGLANTINE. *French botanical name.* This name is for the sweetbriar shrub – where is should remain, not the best choice your daughter. **Eglantyne.**

EGYPT. *place name.* Ever since Little Egypt practically invented the belly dance in the 1890s, this name has had a suggestive aura. Try Cairo instead.

EIBHLIN. *(ev-lin) Irish, 'shining, brilliant'.* Gaelic spelling complicates what is, phonetically, Evelyn. **Aibhlin.**

EILA. *Hebrew, 'oak tree'.* Hebrew name heard in Israel, without much spark. **Ayla, Eilah, Eilona, Ela, Elah, Eyla, Ila.**

EILEEN. *Irish variation of* **HELEN.** Plain-Jane Irish name that's so far out it's . . . still out. **Aileen, Ailene, Alene, Aline, Ayleen, Eila, Eilah, Eilean, Eileena, Eileene, Eilena, Eilene, Eiley, Eilie, Eilieh, Eilina, Eiline, Eilleen, Eillen, Eiley, Eily, Eilyn, Eleen, Elene, Ilene Ilianna, Leana, Lena, Lianna, Lina.**

EILIDH. *(ay-lee) Scottish, 'sun'.* A pretty name obscured outside of Scotland by difficult spelling and impossible pronunciation.

EILIS. *(eh-LEESH) Irish variation of* **ELIZABETH.** Interesting, but far too susceptible to confusion with the Alicia family of names. **Ailis, Ailish, Eilish, Elis, Elish.**

EIR. *(air) Norse, 'peacefulness, mercy'.* So airy, it's almost not there.

EIRA. *(I-ra or AY-ra) Welsh, 'snow'.* Or, to avoid confusion with the outmoded male Ira, you could just name her Snow.

ÉIRE. *(air-ih), Irish place name.* Eire was a mythological goddess who named Ireland after herself. Rarely used today, even in Eire.

EIRIAN. *Welsh, 'silver'.* A modern Welsh name that will be misunderstood as Irene.

EITHNE. *(ETH-na, EN-ya) Irish, 'fire'.* Name of a goddess who survived only on milk. Pretty and soulful, but the phonetic spelling may save everyone a lot of trouble. **Aine, Aithnea, Eithne, Ena, Enya, Ethnah, Ethnea, Ethnee.**

EKATERINA. *Slavic variation of* **CATHERINE.** This exotic variation was publicised by Olympic skater Ekaterina Gordeeva. **Ekaterine, Ekaterini, Yekaterina.**

ELAINA. *Variation of* **ELAINE** *or* **ELENA.** Sounds exotic, feels familiar.

ELAINE. *French variation of* **HELEN.** Form of Helen first popularised in Arthurian legend, it is now unfashionable, except in its *a*-ending forms. **Alaina, Alayna, Alayne, Allaine, Eilane, Elaene, Elain, Elainea, Elaini, Elainia, Elainna, Elan, Elana, Elane, Elania, Elanie, Elanit, Elanna, Elauna, Elayna, Elayne, Ellaina, Ellaine, Ellane, Ellayne, Lainey, Layney.** International: **Elaina** *(French)*, **Elena** *(Spanish and Italian)*, **Eline** *(Scandinavian)*.

★**ELARA.** *Greek mythology name.* Elara, a lover of Zeus who gave birth to a giant son (ouch!); it's also the lovely name of one of the moons of Jupiter.

ELBA. *Place name.* The site of Napoleon's exile became the great-great-aunt in the purple hat. **Elbe, Ellba.**

ELBERTA. *English, 'highborn, shining'.* The great-great-aunt in the purple hat, singing jazz. **Elbertha, Elberthe, Elberthina, Elberthine, Elbertina, Elbertine.**

ELDORA. *Spanish, 'covered with gold'.* Elderly. **Eldorada, Eldoree, Eldorey, Eldori, Eldoria, Eldorie, Eldoris, Eldory.**

ELEANOR. *French variation of* **HELEN.** In and out of fashion since Queen Eleanor of Aquitaine brought it from France to England in the twelfth century, this stately name is hot again and in the Top 50. Big plus: it's a serious name, with a nickname – Ellie – that's endearing. **Aleanor, Alenor, Aleonore, Aline, Allinor, Eileen, El, Elaine, Elan, Elana, Elanee, Elaney, Elani, Elania, Elanie, Elanna, Elanni, Elanor, Elanore, Ele, Elea, Eleanora, Elen, Elena, Eleni, Elenie, Elenor, Elenorah, Elenore, Eleny, Elianora, Elianore, Elie, Elienora, Elienore, Ell, Ella, Elladine, Elle, Elleanor, Ellee, Elleigh, Ellen, Ellene, Ellenor, Ellenora, Ellenorah, Ellenore, Elleonor, Elli, Ellie, Ellin, Elliner, Ellinor, Ellinore, Elly, Ellyn, Elna, Elnora, Elnore, Elyn, Elynor, Elynora, Elynore, Enora, Heleanor, Helen, Helena, Helene, Helenora, Heleonor, Leanora, Lena, Lenora, Lenore, Leonora, Leonore, Leora, Lina, Nelda, Nell, Nelle, Nelley, Nelli, Nellie, Nelly, Nonnie, Nora, Norah, Norina.** International: **Eileanóra** *(Irish)*, **Ealanor, Eilonóra** *(Gaelic)*, **Eleanore, Eléonore, Elinor, Élénora, Elinore** *(French)*, **Eleonora** *(Spanish, Italian, and Swedish)*, **Eleonore** *(German)*.

★**ELECTRA.** *Greek, 'shining, bright'.* Though the tragedies, of the Greeks and Eugene O'Neill, that used this name are filled with incest and murder, Electra is still a brilliant choice. **Alectra, Elektra, Elettra, Ellectra, Ellektra, Oectra.** International: **Elettra** *(Italian)*.

ELENA. *(ee-LAY-na) Spanish variation of* **HELEN.** The rising popularity of this name is undoubtedly due to its being 'exotic lite'. **Elaina, Elana, Eleana, Eleen, Eleena, Elen, Elene, Elenitsa, Elenka, Elenna, Elenoa, Elenola, Elina, Ellena, Lena.**

ELENI. *(ee-LAY-nee) Greek variation of* **HELEN.** Much more old-fashioned than Elena, very common in Greece.

ELERI. *(el-AYR-ee) Welsh, 'greatly bitter'.* Striking name of a legendary princess and a Welsh river that feels both moody and modern.

⚲ **ELEVEN.** *Word name.* If Erykah Badu can name her son Seven, why can't you name your daughter (or son) this? Though it could lead to some confusing wordplay.

ELEXIS. *Greek variation of* **ALEXIS.** We'd stick with the original *A* version. **Elexas, Elexes, Elexess, Elexeya, Elexia, Elexiah, Elexius, Elexsus, Elexus, Elexxus, Elexys.**

ELFRIDA. *English, 'elf power'.* Unappealing on every level. **Alfrida, Alfrieda, Elfie, Elfre, Elfrea, Elfreda, Elfredah, Elfredda, Elfreeda, Elfreyda, Elfrieda, Elfryda, Elfrydah, Ellfreda, Elva, Elvah, Freda, Freddi, Freddy, Freeda, Frieda, Friedah, Fryda.**

ELGA. *Slavic, 'sacred'.* Olga variant without the Russian spirit. **Elgiva, Ellga, Helga.**

⚲ **ELIA.** *Diminutive of* **ELIJAH.** Though the most famous Elia, screenwriter Kazan, was male, this name sounds purely female.

★**ELIANA.** *Hebrew, 'my God has answered me'; Greek, 'sun'.* Lilting, rhythmic choice, more distinctive than Elena, heard in Israel, Italy, Spain and Portugal, but rarely used here. One celebrity who chose it is Christian Slater. **Eilane, Elia, Eliah, Elianna, Elliana, Ellianna, Liana, Liane, Lianne.**

ÉLIANE. *(ae-lee-AHN) French variation of* **ELIANA.** The soignée French member of this family of names. **Elia, Eliana, Elianna, Elianne, Eliette, Elice, Eline, Elliane, Ellianne, Elyette.** International: **Eline** *(Dutch).*

ELIDI. *Greek, 'gift of the sun'.* Try Elodie instead. **Elida, Elide, Elidee, Elidia, Elidy.**

ELIN. *Swedish variation of* **ELLEN.** Makes an old favourite sleeker and more modern.

ELIORA. *Hebrew, 'the Lord is my light'.* Melodic name ripe with vowel sounds. **Eleora, Eliorah, Elira, Elleora, Elliora, Elora.**

ELISA. *Spanish and Italian, diminutive of* **ELIZABETH.** The variations that start with

A are heading up, the *E* versions down. **Alisa, Elecea, Eleesa, Elesa, Elesia, Elise, Elisia, Elisya, Ellisa, Ellisia, Ellissa, Ellissia, Ellissya, Ellisya, Elysa, Elysia, Elyssia, Elyssya, Elysya, Ilisa, Lisa.**

ELISABETH. *Spelling variation of* **ELIZABETH.** Found in France, Germany, Greece and other cultures, and represented by such notables as Swiss-born psychiatrist and author Elisabeth Kubler-Ross.

ELISE. *French variation of* **ELIZABETH.** This form maintains a steady popularity, due to its dash of French flair. **Eilis, Eilise, Elese, Eliese, Elisa, Elisee, Elisie, Elisse, Elise, Elizé, Ellecia, Ellice, Ellise, Ellyce, Ellyse, Ellyze, Elsey, Elsie, Elsy, Elyce, Elyci, Elyse, Elyze, Ilise, Liese, Liesel, Lieselotte, Liesl, Lise, Lisel, Lisl, Lisette, Lison, Lissie, Lise.**

⚲ **ELISHA.** *Hebrew, 'God is my salvation'.* An Old Testament male name, sometimes borrowed for girls. **Eleacia, Eleasha, Elecia, Eleesha, Eleisha, Elesha, Eleshia, Eleticia, Elicia, Elishah, Elisheva, Elica, Elicea, Elicet, Elichia,**

Elishia, Elishua, Elisia, Eliska, Elissia, Ellecia, Ellesha, Ellexia, Ellicia, Ellisha, Elsha, Elysha, Elyshia.

ELISHEVA. *Hebrew, 'the Lord is my pledge'.* The name of Aaron's wife in the Book of Exodus, it gains strength and distinction via the *v* sound. **Eliseva, Elisheba.**

ELISSA. *Variation of* **ALICE** *or* **ELIZABETH.** This version of a long-popular name is fading in favour of Alyssa and other variants. **Alissa, Allissa, Allyssa, Alyssa, Elissah, Ellisa, Ellissa, Ellyssa, Elys, Elyssa, Elyssia, Ilissa, Ilysa, Ilyssa, Lissa, Lissie, Lissy Lyssa.**

ELIXYVETT. *Hybrid name.* Few people go to such lengths to make a name different. Aren't you glad? **Alixevette, Alixyvetha, Elixevetta, Elixyvetha, Elixyvette.**

★**ELIZA.** *Diminutive of* **ELIZABETH.** Okay, we admit it, this one of our favourite names; we love its combination of streamlined modernity and

Elizabeth's International Variations

Irish Gaelic	Eilís
Scottish Gaelic	Ealasaid
Scottish	Elsbeth, Elspeth
French	Babette, Elisabeth, Elise, Lise, Lisette, Lisette
Italian	Betta, Bettina, Elisa, Elisabetta
Spanish	Belita, Bella, Chabica, Chavelle, Chela, Elisa, Isa, Isabel, Isabelita, Isabella, Issa, Iza, Izabel, Izabela, Izabella, Liseta, Sabela, Ysabel, Yza, Yzabel, Yzabela
Basque	Elizabete
Portuguese	Elzira, Isabela, Izabel
Dutch	Els, Liesje, Liesbeth
German	Betti, Bettina, Elis, Elisabet, Elsbeth, Elschen, Else, Isle, Lieschen, Liese, Liesel
Danish	Ailsa, Elisabet, Lisbet
Swedish	Elisabet, Elsa, Lisa
Norwegian	Elise, Ellisif, Lise
Finnish	Elisa, Elli, Liisa, Lusa
Polish	Ela, Eliza, Elizaveta, Elka, Elżbieta, Elzunia
Hungarian	Boski, Bozsi, Erzsébet, Orzsebet

Elizabeth's International Variations *(continued)*

Romanian	Elisabeta
Czech	Alzbet, Alžběta, Beta, Betka, Betuska, Bozena
Lithuanian	Elzbieta, Elzbute
Bulgarian	Elisveta
Russian	Elisaveta, Elsavetta, Liza, Yelizaveta
Ukrainian	Yelysaveta, Lisaveta
Latvian	Elizabete, Lizina
Estonian	Elts, Etti, Etty, Liisa, Liisi
Greek	Elisavet
Armenian	Yeghisapet
Hawaiian	Elikapeka

Eliza Doolittle charm and spunk, and offer it as one of our top recommendations. **Aliza, Alizah, Eliz, Elizah, Elizaida, Elizalina, Elise, Elisea, Elyza, Elyzza, Liza.**

ELIZABELLA. *Combination of* **ELIZA** *and* **BELLA.** The megapopularity of Isabella may give this awkward hybrid a boost. **Elizabel, Elizabell, Elizabelle.**

★**ELIZABETH.** *Hebrew, 'pledged to God'.* While Elizabeth, one of the premiere classic girls' names, is still in the Top 50, there are actually fewer babies getting the name these days. It has so much going for it – rich history, broad appeal and timeless style – that no matter how many little Lizzies, Elizas and Beths are out there, you can still make it your own. **Alizabeth, Bess, Bessi, Bessie,** Bessy, Bet, Beth, Betsey, Betsi, Betsie, Betsy, Bett, Bette, Bettey, Bettie, Betty, Buffy, Elisabeth, Elisabith, Elisheba, Elisheva, Elizabee, Ellie, Ellisa, Ellsi, Ellspet, Ellyse, Ellyssa, Ellyza, Elsee, Elsy, Elysabeth, Elyse, Elyssa, Elyza, Elyzza, Leesa, Leeza, Libbi, Libby, Lilabet, Lilibet, Lilibeth, Lisabet, Lisabeth, Lisanne, Lisbeth, Liz, Lizabeth, Lizanne, Lizbet, Lizbeth, Lizzi, Lizzie, Lizzy, Lysa, Lyssie, Lyza, Lyzanne, Lyzbet, Lyzbeth, Lyzbette, Lyzette.

ELKE. *(el-kee) Dutch, diminutive of* **ADELHEID.** Creates a seemingly contradictory image: a German sex kitten – though there was one, Elke Sommer, in the 1960s. **Elka, Elki, Ellke, Ilka, Ilki.**

ELLA. *German, 'all, completely'; English, 'fairy maiden'.* Staying strong in the Top 20 and one of the fastest rising names among the glitterati – including the John Travoltas, the Warren Beattys, and Eric Clapton – riding on the coat-tails of both the Isabella and Emma bandwagons. Ella Fitzgerald adds jazzy edge. **Alia, Ela, Elladine, Ellah, Ellamae,**

Elletta, Ellette, Elley, Elli, Ellia, Ellie, Ellina, Elly.

ELLAMAE. *Combination of* ELLA *and* MAE. Proof that one plus one sometimes equals zero. **Ellamay.**

★**ELLE.** *French, 'she'.* Add the charming heroine of the film *Clueless* to a supermodel (Elle Macpherson) and to another charming movie heroine in the *Legally Blonde* films, and you have one hit name.

↓**ELLEN.** *English variation of* HELEN. Fading fast, in favour of Ella, Eleanor, Ellie – a Top 10 favourite – Elle and even Elena. **Elan, Elea, Elen, Elena, Elene, Elenee, Eleni, Elenita, Eleny, Elenyi, Elin, Elina, Elinda, Ellan, Ellena, Ellene, Ellie, Ellin, Ellon, Elly, Ellyn, Ellynn, Ellynne, Elon, Elyn.**

♂**ELLERY.** *English, 'island with elder trees'.* In the past few years this formerly male-only name has become a hot girls' name. **Eleree, Eleri, Elerie, Elery, Elleree, Elleri, Ellerie, Ellerie.**

♂**ELLIOT.** *Anglicisation of* ELIJAH *or* ELIAS. This is

another boy's name that has been lured into the girls' camp. Variously spelled Eliot, Elliot and Elliott, its star is definitely on the rise for girls, as it wanes for boys. Bonus is cute and feminine nickname, Ellie. **Eliot, Eliott, Elliott, Ellyot, Ellyott, Elyot, Elyott.**

♂**ELLIS.** *Welsh, 'benevolent'.* Surname name that was used as first in the Wallace/Morris period, but it sounds new now for girls. **Elice, Ellice.**

♂**ELLISON.** *English, 'son of Ellis'.* Updates Allison – which everyone will misunderstand it as. **Elisan, Elisen, Elison, Elisyn, Ellisan, Ellisen, Ellisin, Ellisyn, Ellyson, Ellysyn.**

♂**ELM.** *Nature name.* This is for tree huggers.

ELMA. *Diminutive of names like* WILHELMINA. Elma's rocking on the porch, with Thelma and Velma (and Wilhelmina, too). **Ellma.**

ELMIRA. *English, 'noblewoman'; also New York State place name.* Has hardly been heard of since Mark Twain was buried there

in 1910. **Allmera, Almyra, Elmeera, Elmera, Elmeria, Elmyra, Mera, Meera, Mira, Mirah, Myra, Myrah.** International: **Almeria, Almira** *(Spanish).*

★**ELODIE.** *French, from Greek, 'marsh flower'.* Overlooked medieval saint's name that could be a more sophisticated tribute to an Aunt Melody. Recommended to parents with exotic tastes and a short and simple last name. **Elodea, Elodee, Elodia, Elody, Helodea, Helodia, Helodie.** International: **Elodia** *(Spanish).*

ELOISE. *French variation of* LOUISE. Brought to England by the Normans, Eloise is still in common use. **Aloysia, Elois, Eloisa, Eloisia, Elouisa, Elouise, Heloise.** International: **Eloisa, Elsita, Ilsa** *(Spanish).*

ELOQUENT. *Word name.* If you want to give your child the gift of . . . gab.

ELSA. *Diminutive of* ELIZABETH. Operatic and leonine name not enjoying the resurgence of Ella and her sisters. **Ellsa, Ellse, Ellsie, Ellsy, Else, Elsi, Elsia, Elsie, Elsje, Elssa, Elsy, Elza, Lisa.** International: **Elsje, Ilsa** *(Dutch)*, **Else** *(Scandinavian)*.

ELSIE. *Diminutive of* **ELIZABETH** *via its Scottish variation,* **ELSPETH.** Popular name at the end of the nineteenth century; it's faded during the twentieth century – however it could conceivably rise again on the heels of Ella and Ellie. **Ellsey, Ellsi, Ellsie, Elsea, Elsee, Elsey, Elsi.**

ELSPETH, ELSBETH. *Scottish variation of* **ELIZABETH.** This Scottish contraction of Elizabeth does have a certain childlike charm. **Elsbeth, Elsbet, Elsepet, Elspet, Elspie.**

ELUNED. *(el-LOOND)* *Welsh, 'idol, image'.* Exotic and mysterious, like the heroine of a medieval Welsh fairy tale, but another of those Celtic names that would not be easy for a girl living elsewhere to carry. **Elined, Eiluned, Lanet, Lanette, Linet, Linette, Luned, Lunette, Lynnette.**

ELVA. *Irish, 'leader of the elves'.* Anglicised version of Ailbhe, growing more popular in Ireland. **Ailbhe, Elfie, Elvia, Elvie.**

ELVINA. *English, 'noble friend'* *or 'elf friend'.* Sounds elven in every sense of the word. **Alveena, Alvina, Alvine, Alvinia, Ehrena, Elveena, Elvenea, Elvenia, Elvine, Elvinea, Elvinia, Elvinna, Vina, Vinni, Vinnie, Vinny.**

ELVIRA. *Spanish, 'white, fair'.* Elvira was the long-suffering wife of Don Juan, and unfortunately this negative image still clings to it. **Ellvira, Elva, Elveera, Elvina, Elvyra, Vira.** International: **Elvéra, Elvire** *(French)*, **Elvera** *(Italian)*, **Albira, Alvira** *(Spanish)*, **Alviria** *(German)*, **Elwira** *(Polish)*.

ELYSE. *Variation of* **ELISE** *or* **ELYSIA.** Yet another variation on a familiar theme.

ELYSIA. *Latin, from 'Elysium'.* This version stands out from the pack, as it relates to Elysian Fields, the mythological home of dead heroes. **Aleesyia, Eleese, Eliese, Elise, Elishia, Elisia, Ellicia, Ellysa, Ellyse, Ellyssa,** **Elyce, Elycia, Elys, Elyse, Elysee, Elyssa, Elysse, Ileesia, Ilise, Ilysa, Ilyse, Ilysha, Ilysia.**

ELZA. *Hebrew, 'God is my joy'; Russian from German, 'noble'.* Intriguing twist on several familiar names, though many people will mistake this for Elsa, Eliza and so on.

EMANI. *Arabic variation of* **IMAN.** While this spelling is unusual, the *I*-beginning version is quite popular. **Eman, Emane, Emaneé, Emanie, Emann.**

EMBER. *French variation of* **AMBER.** Unlike Amber, still has a bit of a glow left – though confusions between the two will inevitably arise. **Emberlee, Emberly.**

EMBETH. *Combination of* **EMMA** *and* **BETH.** South African–raised actress Embeth Davidtz added this unique name to the mix.

EMELINE. *German, 'industrious'.* An old name, with a history separate from Emily and Emma and a different kind of vintage feel, that's a possible alternative to top-of-the-pops names. **Em, Emaleen, Emalene, Emaline, Emalyn, Embline, Emblyn, Emelen, Emelyn, Emiline, Emlyn, Emmalee, Emmalene, Emmaline, Emmalyn, Emmalynne, Emmeline, Emmiline, Emmy, Emylin, Emylynn.**

EMENY. *English, uncertain origin.* Emily substitute, though it sounds like a child's mispronunciation of 'enemy'. **Emonie, Imanie, Ismene.**

ÉMER. *(EE-mer) Irish mythology name.* The wife of legendary Irish hero Cú Chulainn, blessed with the gifts of beauty, sweet speech, wisdom, needlework and chastity – a mixed bag. **Ema, Eamhair, Eimear, Eimer.** International: **Éimhear** *(Scottish Gaelic).*

EMERALD. *Gem name; Persian, 'green'.* Colour and jewel name of the deep green stone treasured as far back as ancient Egypt, could make for an interesting, unusual name. International: **Emeraude** *(French),* **Emelda, Emeralda, Emeraldina, Esmeralda** *(Spanish).*

♂ **EMERSON.** *German, 'son of the chief'.* The combination of Emily and Emma's popularity have put this choice in the limelight. *Desperate Housewives'* star Teri Hatcher's daughter is named Emerson.

♂ **EMERY.** *German, 'industrious'.* The popularity of Emily and Emma could boost the unisex Emery. **Emeri, Emerie.**

EMILIA. *Feminine variation of* EMIL. This lovely feminine form of the Roman clan name Aemilius is rising as an Emily/Amelia alternative.

EMILY. *Latin, 'industrious'; Teutonic, 'energetic'.* Reaching Number 1 in recent years, this popular name appeals on many levels: it's feminine, classic, simple, pretty, and strong. But, at this point, waaaaaaay overused. **Aemiley, Aemilie, Amalea, Ameldy, Amelia, Ameline, Amelita, Amella, Em, Ema, Emaili, Emaily, Emalee, Emaleigh, Emali, Emalie, Emalina, Emaly, Emelea, Emelina, Emeline, Emellie, Emelly, Emely, Emelyn, Emelyne, Emera, Emi, Emie, Emilee, Emileigh, Emiley,**

If You Like Emily, You Might Love . . .

Amalia

Amelia

Amelie

Ellery

Emery

Emilia

Emiliana

Emlyn

Emmeline

Emmi

Emmy

Mallory

Millie

Emilie, Emilienne, Emilis, Emilla, Emillea, Emillee, Emilley, Emillie, Emilly, Emillyn, Emillynn, Emlin, Emlyn, Emlynn, Emlynne, Emma, Emmalee, Emmalene, Emmalie, Emmalina, Emmaline, Emmaly, Emmalyn, Emmalynn, Emmalynne, Emmelee, Emmelie, Emmeline, Emmely, Emmey, Emmi, Emmie, Emmilee,

Emmilie, Emmy, Emmye, Emyle, Emylee, Melia, Mila, Milia. International: Aimiliona, Eimile *(Irish)*, Aimil *(Scottish)*, Amalie, Émilie *(French)*, Emilia, Emiliana *(Italian)*, Amalia, Ema, Emelia, Emilia, Emilita *(Spanish)*, Amilie, Amma, Emelie, Emmi *(German)*, Amalia, Emelia, Emilka *(Eastern European)*, Alalija *(Russian)*, Aimilios *(Greek)*, Emele, Emalia *(Hawaiian)*.

↑**EMMA.** *German, 'healer of the universe'.* This is a long-time favourite that has consistently been in the Top 30 list in recent years, thanks to a legion of Emma heroines, from Bovary to Jane Austen's protagonist to *The Avengers'* Mrs Peel. So parents who have turned from Emily to Emma seeking something more distinctive will have to keep looking. Em, Ema, Emelina, Emeline, Emelyne, Emmah, Emmaline, Emmalyn, Emmalynn, Emmalynne, Emme, Emmeleia, Emmeline, Emmelyn, Emmelyne, Emmet, Emmett, Emmette, Emmi, Emmie, Emmy, Emmye.

EMMALEE. *Combination of* EMMA *and* LEE. Parents trying to personalise Emily have hit on this a combo of Emma and Lee, but it still sounds just like the popular Emily. Emalea, Emalee, Emi, Emie, Emilee, Emily, Emmalea, Emmalei, Emmaleigh, Emmaley, Emmali, Emmalia, Emmalie, Emmaliese, Emmalyse, Emmi, Emmie, Emmye, Emy, Emylee.

EMMALYNN. *Combination of* EMMA *and* LYNN. Not the classiest variation. Emelyn, Emelyne, Emelynne, Emilyn, Emilynn, Emilynne, Emlyn, Emlynn, Emlynne, Emmalin, Emmalinn, Emmalyn, Emmalynne.

EMMANUELLE. *French, feminine variation of* EMANUEL. The female version of Emanuel could become more prominent, but for some it still carries a steamy image dating back to an erotic French film. Emanual, Emanuel, Emanuela, Emanuella, Emanuelle, Emmanuel, Emmanuella, Emonualle, Manuella, Manuelle. International: Emmanuela, Manuela *(Spanish)*.

EMMY. *Diminutive of* EMILY. Long a nickname for all the Em-names, as well as an annual award in the US, Emmy is now being given on its own, as are soundalikes Emme and Emmi. Emme, Emmee, Emmi, Emmie.

EMMYLOU. *Combination of* EMMY *and* LOU. There's only one: Emmylou Harris, the US country singer who gives dignity to an old-style combo name. Emlou, Emmalou, Emmelou, Emmilou, Emylou.

ENA. *Diminutive of several names.* Names that started off as diminutives – Ena, Ita, Etta – seem too insubstantial for a modern female. Eena, Enna, Ina.

♂ **ENDEAVOUR.** *Word name.* Neo–word name that maybe tries too hard.

♂ **ENERGY.** *Word name.* Better than Synergy.

♂ **ENGLAND.** *Place name.* Most parents would prefer London for their daughters.

ENGRACIA. *Spanish from Latin, 'endowed with God's grace'.* Exotic and charming alternative to the overused Grace. Agraciana, Agracianna.

ENID. *Welsh, 'life, spirit'.* Celtic goddess and Arthurian name that sounds terminally old-ladyish. **Eanid, Ened, Enedd, Enidd, Enyd, Enydd.**

ENJOLI. *Modern invented name.* This perfume name, undoubtedly a takeoff on the French word for pretty, has somehow wafted into the girls' lexicon. It's a bit too commercial for our tastes. **Enjolie.**

♂ **ENNIS.** *Irish, 'from the island'.* Irish town names are now fair game – as are most other places with connections to Ireland – but are much better suited to boys.

ENORA. *Breton, 'honour'.* Unusual Honor or Nora alternative, but we prefer the originals.

ENRICA. *Italian, feminine form of* **ENRICO.** Novel way to honour Grandpa Henry. **Enricketta, Enrieta, Enrietta, Enrika, Enriqua, Enriqueta, Enriquetta, Enriquette, Rica, Rika. International: Enriqua (Spanish).**

ENTERPRISE. *Word name.* The virtue? Or the Starship?

ENYA. *Irish, 'fire'.* New Agey name that's an Anglicisation of Eithne, brought to attention here by the popular Irish singer. **Aenya, Ennya.**

ÉPIPHANIE. *French word name, 'realisation'.* You could just spell it epiphany, but that's so much more pedestrian. It's also a holiday name, à la Christmas and Easter: the Epiphany marked the visitation of the Three Wise Men to Baby Jesus. **Epiphany.**

ERGA. *Hebrew, 'yearning, craving'.* Urgh.

ERICA. *Norse 'eternal ruler'.* Cool name . . . over thirty years ago, but its use is still widespread in some countries. **Aerica, Aericka, Africa, Airicka, Airika, Enrica, Enrika, Eraca, Ereka, Ericca, Ericha, Ericka, Erickah, Erika, Erikaa, Erikah, Erikka, Errica, Erricka, Errika, Eryca, Erycka, Eryka, Erykah, Erykka, Eyrica, Eyrika, Rickee, Ricki, Rickie, Ricky, Rikki, Rikky.**

ERIN. *Irish, 'from the island to the west'.* First-wave Irish name and place name – the poetical name for Ireland – now supplanted by newer alternatives. **Aeran, Aerenne, Aerin, Airin, Earin, Earrin, Eire, Eirin, Eirinn, Eiryn, Eiryne, Eirynn, Eran, Eren, Erena, Erene, Ereni, Eri, Erian, Erina, Erine, Erinetta, Erinn, Erinna, Erinne, Errin, Eryn, Eryne, Erynn, Erynne.**

ERMA. *Variation of* **IRMA.** Once, believe it or not, this name seemed more stylish than Irma. **Ermelinda, Ermina, Erminia, Erminie, Hermia, Hermine, Herminie, Hermione, Irma, Irminia, Irminie.**

ERMINE. *French, 'weasel'; English variation of* **HERMINE.** Fur names? We don't think so. **Erma, Ermin, Ermina, Erminda, Erminia, Erminie, Erminne.**

ERNA. *Irish, 'to know'.* That *er* sound – as in Myrna, Myrtle and Bernice – sounds terminally dated. **Ernaline, Ernalynn, Irna.**

ERNESTINE. *Feminine variation of* **ERNEST.** Joke name in the US, that of a character created by comedienne Lily Tomlin. **Erna, Ernaline, Ernesia, Ernestina, Ernestyna.** International: **Ernesta** *(Spanish and Italian)*, **Ernesztina** *(Hungarian)*.

EROICA. *Latin, 'heroic'.* The name of Beethoven's third symphony, and too close to the word erotica. **Eroiqua, Eroique, Heroica.**

★**ESMÉ.** *French, 'esteemed'; Persian, 'emerald'.* This is a sophisticated, distinctive and charming name used by the author J. D. Salinger and also a current favourite among celebs, including Michael J. Fox. **Esma, Esmae, Esmay, Esmée, Esmëe, Isme.**

ESMERALDA. *Spanish, 'emerald'.* Emerald equivalent long popular with Hispanic parents, given increased visibility via the Disney version of *The Hunchback of Notre Dame.* **Em, Emelda, Emerald, Emerant, Emeraude, Emmie, Esma, Esmarada, Esmaralda, Esmarelda, Esmaria, Esmé, Esmeralda, Esmeraldina, Esmeranda, Esmerelda, Esmerilda, Esmie, Esmiralda,**

Esmiralde, Esmirelda, Ezmirilda, Ismaerelda, Ismaralda. International: **Ismeralda** *(Spanish).*

ESPERANZA. *Spanish, 'hope, expectation'.* Another Spanish classic finding its way onto the popularity list in the US. **Esparanza, Espe, Esperance, Esperans, Esperansa, Esperanta, Esperantia, Esperanz, Esperenza.**

ESSENCE. *Word name.* Heavily perfumed word name that peaked a few years ago. **Essa, Essenc, Essencee, Essences, Essenes, Essense, Essynce.**

ESTEFANIA. *Spanish variation of* **STEPHANIE.** Attractively exotic Stephanie alternative. **Estafania, Estefana, Estefane, Estefani, Estefanie, Estefany, Estephani, Estephania, Estephanie, Estephany.**

ESTELLA. *See* **ESTELLE.**

ESTELLE. *French, 'star'.* Estelle is a muumuu-wearing canasta player of a certain age; Estella, introduced in *Great Expectations,* has more energy and charm, while Estrella is the most stylish of the trio. **Essa, Essey, Essie,**

Essy, Esta, Estee, Estée, Estel, Estela, Estele, Esteley, Estelina, Estelita, Estell, Estella, Estellina, Estellita, Esthella, Esti, Estrella, Estrellita, Stelle.

ESTHER. *Persian, 'star'.* One of the major female figures in the Old Testament, quiet, studious Esther was popular a hundred years ago, but is rarely used today; it could appeal to parents – Ewan McGregor is one – seeking an underused biblical name with a history and serious image. **Essa, Essey, Essie, Essy, Esta, Estee, Esti, Esthur, Ettey, Etti, Ettie, Etty, Hesther, Hettie, Hetty, Hittie.** International: **Eistir** *(Irish)*, **Estée** *(French)*, **Ester** *(Scandinavian)*, **Ester, Estzer, Eszter, Eszti** *(Slavic).*

ESTRELLA. *(es-STRAY-a) Spanish, 'star'.* Rising star among Hispanic families, would make a good cross-cultural choice. **Estrela, Estrelinda, Estrell, Estrelle, Estrellita.**

ETANA. *Hebrew, 'strength of purpose'.* Girlish for Ethan: attractive and unusual.

ÉTAOIN. *(AY-deen) Irish, 'jealousy'.* This name of a

mythical beauty transformed into a scarlet fly by a jealous wife is popular in its native land; elsewhere, while pleasant to the ear, it's bewildering on paper.

♂ ETERNITY. *Word name.* Might have a shot as a name, à la Genesis and Destiny, if it weren't for yet another perfume connection. **Eternal.**

ETHEL. *English, 'noble maiden'.* Sounds as dated today as the old Anglo-Saxon names that hatched it – Ethelreda and Elthelburga – though it was the Ashley of a hundred years ago. **Ethelda, Ethelin, Ethelinda, Etheline, Ethelle, Ethelyn, Ethelynn, Ethelynne, Ethill, Ethille, Ethlin, Ethlyn, Ethlynn, Ethyl, Ethyll.**

ETHEREAL. *Word name.* Otherworldly.

♂ ETHICAL. *Word name.* Upstanding to a fault.

ÉTOILE. *(ay-TWAHL) French, 'star'.* Novel French twist on Starr or Stella.

ETTA. *English and Scottish, feminine diminutive suffix.* Once a short form of Henrietta, it has long been used on its own, and we wonder if it could follow the progression of Emma to Ella to . . . Etta? **Etka, Etke, Etti, Ettie, Etty, Itke, Itta.**

EUDORA. *Greek, 'generous gift'.* The name of five minor goddesses of Greek mythology and a major goddess (in the person of Eudora Welty) of modern literature, Eudora is pleasant and euphoneous. **Dora, Dorey, Doric, Eudore.**

EUGENIA, EUGENIE. *Feminine variations of* EUGENE. The elegant Eugenie enjoyed a major dusting off when Fergie and Prince Andrew chose it for their daughter, restoring some its tarnished royal sheen. **Eugenee, Eugenina, Eugina, Geena, Gena, Gene, Genia, Genie, Janie, Jeena, Jenna, Jennie. International: Eugénie, Génie** *(French),* **Evgenia, Yevgenia, Zenechka, Zenya** *(Russian).*

EULALIA. *Greek, 'sweet-speaking'.* Melodious name with a lilt. **Eula, Eulala,** Eulalee, Eulalya, Eulaylie, Eulia, Lallie, Lally, Ulalia. **International: Eulalie** *(French),* **Eulaylia, Olalla** *(Spanish).*

EUNICE. *Greek, 'victorious'.* New Testament name that sounds terminally gawky. **Euna, Eunices, Eunike, Eunique, Eunise, Euniss, Eunisse, Unice, Uniss.**

EUPHEMIA. *(yu-FEM-ee-a) Greek, 'well spoken'.* Ancient martyr's name that, though not especially appealing, might still be mildly possible. **Effam, Effie, Effy, Ephan, Ephie, Eppie, Eppy, Euphan, Euphemie, Euphenia, Euphie, Fanny, Mia, Phemie. International: Eadaoine** *(Irish),* **Euphème** *(French),* **Eufemia** *(Italian and Spanish).*

EURYDICE. *(yu-RID-ih-see) Greek mythology name.* Poisoned by a snake and condemned to the underworld, where her husband, musician Orpheus, tried and failed to bring her back: this is a name too tragic for real life. **Euridice, Euridiss, Euridyce, Eurydyce.**

Cool Biblical Names

Deborah

Delilah

Dinah

Eve

Jemima

Keturah

Keziah

Leah

Lydia

Sela

Susannah

Tabitha

Tamar

EUSTACIA. *Greek, 'fruitful'.* Ancestor of Stacy, both now have disappeared in limbo. **Eustacie, Eustasia, Stacey, Stacia, Stacie, Stacy.**

EVA. *Variation of* **EVE.** Simple, classic name, with a recent appearance in the Top 100, but be warned: There are suddenly a lot of little Evas (and Avas and Eves) around. **Eba, Ebba, Eeva, Éva, Evah, Evalea, Evalee, Eve, Evelin, Evelina, Evelyn, Evita, Evlyn.**

EVADNE. *(ee-VOD-neh) Greek, 'pleasing one'.* This is a difficult to pronounce name, à la Ariadne. **Evadney, Evadnie, Evanne.**

♂ **EVAN.** *Welsh variation of* **JOHN.** Boys' favourite recently brought to the girls' side.

★♂ **EVANGELINE.** *Greek, 'bearer of good news'.* Old name on the brink of a major comeback, via religious overtones, Eva popularity and hot star of TV megahit *Lost*, Evangeline Lilly. Evangelica and Evangelina are sure to tag along for the ride. **Eva, Evangel, Evangelene, Evangelia, Evangelica, Evangelina, Evangelique, Evangelista, Evangelyn, Evangelynn, Eve, Vangie, Vangy.**

EVANTHE. *(ee-VAHN-thuh) Greek, 'fair flower'.* Leave it at Eva or Evan. **Evanthey, Evanthie.**

★↑ **EVE.** *Hebrew, 'life'.* The oldest name in the Book, and consistently in the Top 100, it has the virtues of simplicity and purity, yet has more strength and resonance than other single-syllable names like Ann. Clive

Owen chose it for his daughter. **Eba, Ebba, Eva, Evaleen, Evelina, Eveline, Evelyn, Evetta, Evette, Evey, Evicka, Evie, Evike, Evka, Evlyn, Evonne, Evuska, Evvie, Evvy, Evy, Evyn, Ewa, Ewie, Ewy, Yeva. International: Aioffe Aobh, Aoibh, Aoife, Eeve, Éahba Eibhlin** *(Irish Gaelic),* **Efa** *(Welsh),* **Evaine** *(French),* **Evelia, Evetta, Evia, Eviana, Evita** *(Spanish),* **Evchen, Evi** *(German),* **Eeva** *(Finnish),* **Ewa** *(Polish),* **Evicka, Evka, Evuska** *(Czech),* **Evva, Yeva, Yevka** *(Russian),* **Evathia** *(Greek),* **Chava, Chaya, Hava** *(Yiddish),* **Ewalina** *(Hawaiian).*

EVELINA. *Latin variation of* **EVELYN.** Eclipsed by Evelyn in the last century, but has a chance at a well-deserved comeback now. **Eveleen, Evelene, Eveline, Evelyne.**

EVELYN. *English, 'dear youth'.* Soft and feminine, and hugely popular a hundred years ago (especially in the 1910s), Evelyn is just beginning to return to favour now. **Avalyn, Evalin, Evalina, Evaline, Evalyn, Evalynn, Evalynne, Eveleen, Evelene, Evelin, Evelina, Eveline,**

Evelyna, Evelyne, Evelynn, Evelynne, Evilyn, Evleen, Evlene, Evlin, Evlina, Evline, Evlyn, Evlynn, Evlynne, Ewalina. *International:* Aveline, Evaleen *(Irish).*

★♂ **EVER.** *Word name.* Truly unusual and simple name with evocative meaning.

♂ **EVEREST.** *Place name, world's tallest mountain.* Attractive enough sound and lofty enough meaning to come into style, à la Sierra.

♂ **EVERETT.** *German, 'brave boar'.* Male name that's a prime crossover candidate, much like Eliot and Ellery.

♂ **EVERLY.** *English, 'wild boar in woodland clearing'.* Part Eva, part Emily and a large part Everly Brothers.

♂ **EVERY.** *Word name.* All-inclusive word name.

♂ **EVIAN.** *Variation of* **EVAN.** Might sound elegant, if you could forget the water. But no one will. **Evyan.**

EVIE. *Diminutive of* **EVE** *or* **EVA.** Evie has zoomed in popularity, making into the Top 25 in recent years, with nickname names such as Ellie, Rosie, Billy, and Archie all the rage. **Evi, Evy.**

EVITA. *Spanish, diminutive of* **EVA.** There's only one Evita.

EVONNE. *French variation of* **YVONNE.** *See* **YVONNE.** Evanne, Eve, Evenie, Evenne, Eveny, Evette, Evin, Evon, Evona,

Evone, Evoni, Evonna, Evonnie, Evony, Evyn, Evynn, Evyonne, Eyona, Eyvone.

♀ **EXPERIENCE.** *Word name.* Used by the Puritans but probably too joke-worthy for a modern child . . . or teenager.

♀ **EXPLORER.** *Word name.* One occupational name destined to seek and find greater things.

♀ **EZRI.** *Hebrew, 'helper, strong'.* Boys' name that sounds quirky and cute for a girl. **Ezra, Ezria.**

F girls

FABIA. *(FAH-bia) Latin female variation of* **FABIAN.** One of several pleasant international-accented female versions of Fabian. **Fabiane, Fabianna, Fabianne, Fabiola, Fabra, Favianna, Faviola. International: Fabienne** *(French),* **Fabiana** *(Italian, Spanish).*

★**FABIENNE.** *French variation of* **FABIA.** Instead of the usual French suspects – Danielle, Isabelle, Gabrielle – why not consider Fabienne, which is less common and just as pretty?

FABIOLA. *French, Italian, and German variation of* **FABIA.** Romantically elaborate name of a saint who organised the first hospice. **Fabiana, Fabiane, Fabianna, Fabienne, Fabra, Fania, Fanianne, Favianna, Favilola.**

♀ **FABLE.** *Word name.* Like Story, a word name with real potential, combining enchanted tale-telling with a moral edge.

FABRIZIA. *Italian, 'works with the hands'.* An Italian name sizzling with electricity. **Fabrice, Fabricia, Fabrienne, Fabriqua, Fabritzia.**

♀ **FAINE.** *English, 'joyful'.* A very unusual one-syllable option. **Faina, Fayna, Fayne.**

FAIRUZA. *Turkish, 'turquoise'.* Instead of the more obvious Aqua or Blue, why not consider this offbeat Turkish name.

FAITH. *Virtue name.* Several of the Puritan virtue names have recently come back into fashion, with Faith, Grace and Hope in the vanguard. At the moment Faith is rising quickly in the Top 100. Many parents still choose Faith as an indicator of their religious conviction. **Fa, Fae, Faithe, Fay, Fayanna, Faye, Fayette, Fayth, Faythe. International: Fe** *(Spanish).*

FAIZAH. *(FAH-ee-zah) Arabic, 'victorious'.* Hauntingly exotic. **Faiza, Fayza.**

FALALA. *African, 'born in abundance'.* Add a few more *la*'s and you have a jolly Christmas refrain. **Fala.**

FALINE. *Latin, 'catlike'.* A Disneyfied name: Faline was the sweet doe Bambi fell in love with. **Faeleen, Faleen, Falene, Fallyne, Fayline, Felina, Feyline.**

♀ **FALLON.** *Irish, 'leader'.* One of several boyish surname names introduced in the over-the-top 1980s American TV programme *Dynasty:* they sounded cutting-edge at the time, but no longer. **Falan,**

Fallan, Fallen, Fallyn, Falon, Falyn, Falynn.

FAMKE. *Dutch, 'little girl'.* Introduced elsewhere via Dutch-born actress Famke Janssen, but not likely to appeal to many non-Dutch parents.

FANA. *African, 'light'; also West African word for 'jungle'.* Simple, delicate and unusual.

FANCHON. *(fahn-shon) French variation of* **FRANÇOISE.** Sweet and affectionate Gallic choice.

FANIA. *Anglicisation of Irish* **FAINNE,** *'ring'.* Would make an interesting choice for a child of Irish-Russian heritage, being a Celtic name with a Russian Tania-like feel. **Fanya.**

FANNY. *Diminutive of* **FRANCES.** A staple of Brit Lit, appearing in novels by Fielding, Dickens, Trollope, Eliot and Hardy, this nickname could make a comeback. **Fan, Fania, Fannee, Fanney, Fanni, Fannia, Fannie.**

FANTASIA. *Greek, 'imagination'.* One of the more prominent by-products of reality TV, via Disney. **Faintasi, Fantasy, Fantasya, Fantaysia, Fantazia.**

FANTINE. *Latin, 'infant'.* Rarely heard French name, a character in the Victor Hugo novel *Les Misérables.*

FARAH. *Arabic, 'happiness'. See* **FARRAH.** **Fara, Fariha, Farra, Farrah.**

FARIDA. *Arabic, 'unique, precious pearl'.* A Muslim name more distinctive than the Americanised Farah/Farrah. **Fareeda, Fareedah, Farideh.** **International: Faridah** *(Persian).*

FARRAH. *English, 'lovely, pleasant'; Arabic, 'happiness'.* For a few seconds there in the late 1970s, Farrah Fawcett's name was as frequently copied as her hairstyle: both are now equally unfashionable. **Fara, Farah, Farra, Fayre, Ferra, Ferrah.**

♂ **FARRELL.** *Irish, 'courageous'.* Though usually considered a boy's name, the soft sound of this Irish surname makes it perfectly appropriate for a girl. **Farrelly.**

FATIMA. *Arabic, 'captivating, a woman who abstains'.* Thousands of Muslim girls are annually given this name of the daughter of Muhammad and one of the four perfect women according to the Koran – unlikely to cross cultures. **Fateema, Fateemah, Fatia, Fatimah, Fatina, Fatma, Fatmah. International: Fatemeh** *(Persian).*

FAUNA. *Latin, 'the animals of a specific area'; Roman goddess of nature and animals.* Fauna was one of the fairies who protected Disney's Sleeping Beauty, but it's still a bit too generic to be recommended as a baby name. **Faune, Fauniel, Fauniella, Fawna.**

FAUSTINE. *Latin, feminine variation of* **FAUST.** Although it means good luck, the association with the character who sold his soul to the devil is off-putting. Consider one of the other 'lucky' names, like Felicity, instead. **Fauste, Faustena, Faustia, Faustiana, Faustyna. International: Fausta** *(Italian),* **Faustina** *(Spanish).*

♂ **FAVOR.** *Word name.* This word has too many conflicting associations to make a satisfying name.

FAWN. *Nature name, 'a young deer'.* The doe-eyed Fawn, like other retrograde names such as Tawny and Taffy, does not, in our opinion, give a girl enough to live up to. **Faan, Faandelia, Fahn, Fahndelia, Faina, Faun, Fauna, Faunia, Fawna, Fawndelia, Fawne, Fawnia, Fawniah, Fawne, Fawnya.**

FAY, FAYE. *French, 'fairy'; shortened form of* **FAITH.** Napping quietly since the 1930s,

Fay/Faye, like cousins May/Mae and Ray/Rae, has sat up and started rubbing her eyes, ready for a minicomeback, especially as a middle name. **Fae, Fay, Fee, Fey, Fayette.**

FEATHER. *Word name.* Though it was used for a character in a novel, Feather seems too light and fluttery for a real-life girl.

FEDERICA. *Italian, feminine variation of* **FREDERICK.** Latin version of one of those formerly stuffy female names – think Josephine and Eleanor – that feels fresh and elegant again.

FEDORA. *Greek variation of* **THEODORA.** Occasionally heard among the Mayfair and Belgravia set, but we're afraid that in some places there would be too strong an association with the man's felt hat. **Fadora, Feodora, Fyodora.**

FEE. *Diminutive of* **FIONA.** Too fiscal.

FELICE. *Italian, 'lucky'.* The Italians pronounce it *fa-LEECH-ay;* the Americanised

version, *feh-LEESE,* now sounds dated and not very appealing.

FELICIA. *Latin, 'lucky'; feminine variation of* **FELIX.** A lacy, lucky name very popular in the Hispanic community a decade ago, less so now. **Falecia, Faleece, Faleshia, Falicia, Falisha, Felecia, Felica, Felice, Feliciana, Felicidad, Felicie, Felicity, Felis, Felisa, Felise, Felisha, Feliss, Felita, Fellysse, Felyssia, Filicia, Filisha, Phalisha, Phelicia, Phylicia, Phyllicia, Phyllisha. International: Felicita, Felicitas, Felisa, Felixa, Feliz** *(Spanish).*

FELICIDAD. *Spanish, 'happiness'.* Used exclusively in Latino families.

★**FELICITY.** *Latin, 'happy'.* As accessible as Hope and Faith, but more feminine – and dare we say happier? **Felecia, Felice, Feliciona, Felicitee, Felicitie, Felise, Felisha, Felita, Feliza, Filicia, Flick. International: Felicienne, Félicité** *(French),* **Felicita** *(Italian),* **Felice, Felicia, Felicidad, Felicita, Felisa, Felixa, Feliz** *(Spanish),* **Felicidade** *(Portuguese),* **Felicie** *(German),* **Fela, Felka** *(Polish).*

FELIXA. *(fay-LEEK-sah) Spanish, 'happy, lucky'.* The futuristic consonant *x* sets this apart – for better and worse – from all the other Felices, Felicias and Felicitys. **Felecia, Felia, Felica, Felicanna, Feliciania, Felicianna, Felicina, Felisa, Felixia, Felizia.**

★**FENELLA.** *Celtic, 'white-shouldered one'.* This engaging Scottish name, the heroine of a Sir Walter Scott novel, is, though scarcely heard elsewhere, much more user-friendly than some of the Irish versions. **Fennella, Finella, Finola, Fionnuala, Fionola, Fynella.**

♂ **FENNEL.** *Vegetable and herb name.* Word name possibility carrying the scent of liquorice-like anise.

FEODORA. *(fay-oh-DOR-a) Slavic variation of* **THEODORA.** An interesting choice for the intrepid name giver, especially with its dynamic nickname, Feo *(pronounced FAY-oh)*. **Feo.**

FERGIE. *Diminutive of* **FERGUS.** One Fergie was an aberration. But two women with that nickname – the duchess and the Black Eyed Pea – might make a trend.

FERN. *Nature name.* Of all the botanicals, Fern has never really moved from the conservatory into the nursery, despite the appealing girl character in the children's classic *Charlotte's Web.* **Fearne, Ferna, Ferne.**

FERNANDA. *Spanish and Portuguese, feminine variation of* **FERDINAND.** Very popular in the Latino community, with a lot more charm than its male counterpart. **Anda, Annda, Ferdinanda, Ferdinande, Fern, Fernande, Fernandina, Fernandine, Nan, Nanda.**

FERNANDE. *French, feminine variation of* **FERDINAND.** A dark-haired femme fatale choice.

FEY. *Word name.* For middle name purposes, could be thought of as a fey spelling of Fay. **International: Feya** *(Hebrew).*

FFLUR. *(Fleer) Welsh, 'flower'.* Why bother to invent a new name or spelling when there are intriguing oddities like this in existence? Also in the Welsh encyclopedia of names: Ffion, Ffiona and Ffraid, the Welsh form of Brigid.

FIA. *Irish, diminutive of* **FIACHNA,** *'raven'.* A pleasantly light and distinctive possible alternative to Mia.

FIAMMETTA. *Italian, 'little fiery one'.* Derived from the Italian word for flame, this name has both femininity and fire. **Fiamma.**

FIANNA. *Irish, 'fair' or 'white'.* This virtually unknown Irish name combines the best elements of Fiona and Brianna.

FIDELITY. *Word name.* An admirable virtue, yes, but as a name it tends to sound like a financial institution. **Fedelia, Fedila, Fideila, Fidela, Fidele, Fidelia, Fidelina, Fidelita, Fidella, Fidylia.**

FIFI. *French, diminutive of* **JOSEPHINE.** A perfect name – for a French poodle. **Fifine.**

FILIPA. *Slavic variation of* **PHILIPPA.** *See* **PHILIPPA.**

FILOMENA. *Greek, 'lover of singing'; Spanish variation of* **PHILOMENA.** *See* **PHILOMENA. Filomela.**

FINELLA. *Irish variation of* **FINOLA.** *See* **FINOLA.**

♂ **FINLEY.** *Irish, 'fair-haired hero'.* This was a 100 per cent male name until recently. Can Finleigh be far behind? **Finlay, Finlea, Finleah, Finlee, Finleigh, Finli, Finlie, Finly, Fynley, Fynlie, Fynly.**

♂ **FINN.** *Irish, 'bright, fair'.* The most enduringly popular hero of Irish myth was Finn McCool, whose name is one of the coolest ever. When used for the female protagonist of *How to Make an American Quilt*, it established its hipness for girls as well.

FINOLA. *Irish, 'white shoulders'.* This readily accessible version of some of the more problematic Gaelic versions would make a welcome addition to the stockpot of Irish girls' names. **Fennela, Finella, Finnguala, Finoula, Fionnala, Nola.**

FIONA. *Scottish, 'the fair one'.* This late nineteenth-century Scottish invention is still being given to baby girls today. Also popular in the US since the 1954 musical *Brigadoon* had a character with the name. **Fee, Ffion, Ffiona, Ffyona, Fina, Fione, Fionn, Fionna, Fiora, Fyona.**

FIONNUALA. *(fin-OO-lah) Irish Gaelic, 'white shoulders'.* This lovely Gaelic name, very popular in the Emerald Isle, would pose obvious pronunciation problems elsewhere. Simplify to Finola or Fenella. **Fenella, Finella, Finola, Fionnuala, Fionnualagh, Nola, Nuala.**

FIORELLA. *Italian, 'little flower'.* Feminine, floral and rarely enough heard here to be exotic.

FLAIR. *Word name.* Beware: extremely high pressure, high-expectation name.

♂ **FLAME.** *Word name.* Beware again: the kind of name used by women named Fran when engaging in endeavours they'd just as soon their parents weren't aware of.

FLANNA. *Irish, 'red-haired'.* An uncommon name for a red-haired girl, not as familiar as its nickname, Flannery. **Flana, Flanagh, Flannerey, Flannery.**

★**FLANNERY.** *Irish, diminutive of* **FLANNA.** Long before the vogue of using Irish surnames for girls names, writer Flannery O'Connor gave this one some visibility. It has a warm (flannelly) feel and the currently popular three-syllable *ee*-ending sound.

FLAVIA. *Latin, 'golden, blond'; from ancient Roman family name* **FLAVIUS.** An ancient Roman clan name, Flavia is one choice that's unusual but historic. **International: Flaviana, Flavie, Flaviere, Flavyere** *(French).*

FLEUR. *French, 'flower'.* This generic, delicate flower name risks sounding a bit precious. **Fleurette, Fleurine.**

FLOR. *Spanish, 'flower'.* Attractive Spanish name heard in the film *Spanglish*. Roll that final *r*.

★**FLORA.** *Latin, 'flower'.* The name of the Roman goddess of flowers and spring, who enjoyed eternal youth, is one of the gently old-fashioned flowery classics we think is due for a comeback. **Fiora, Fiordenni, Fiore, Fiorella, Fiori, Flo, Floralia, Florella, Florelle, Florentia, Florentina, Florenza, Floressa, Floretta, Florette, Flori, Floria, Florianna, Florinda, Florrie.** International: **Floraigh** *(Gaelic),* **Fleur, Flore, Fleurette** *(French),* **Flor, Florida, Florinda, Florita, Floridita** *(Spanish),* **Florka** *(Hungarian).*

FLORENCE. *Latin, 'blooming, flowering,' place name.* Connection to the lovely Italian city got lost in Florence's last flowering as a name – but the association to the place seems to be helping it stir back to style life. **Flo, Florance, Florella, Florentina, Florentine, Florentyna, Florian, Florice,**

Stellar Starbabies Beginning with *F*

Faith	Rick Schroder
Fifi Trixiebelle	Bob Geldof
Fiona	Jenni Garth
Florence	Rupert Penry-Jones & Dervla Kirwan
Frances Bean	Courtney Love & Kurt Cobain. Amanda Peet, Kate Spade
Francesca	Erik Estrada, Frances Fisher & Clint Eastwood, Martin Scorsese
Fuchsia	Trudi Styler & Sting

Florie, Florina, Florinda, Florine, Floris, Florrance, Florrie, Florry, Florynce, Floss, Flossey, Flossie, Flossy. International: **Blathnaid** *(Irish),* **Fiorentina, Fiorenza** *(Italian),* **Florencia, Florinia, Floriana, Florencita** *(Spanish),* **Florentia** *(German).*

FLORIDA. *Latin, 'flowery'; Spanish, variation of* **FLORA**; *also place name.* It lacks the cachet found in some newer place names.

FLOWER. *Word name.* It may sound sweet smelling, but remember, it *was* the name of the little skunk in *Bambi*. Better

to pick a single bloom from the bouquet, like Violet or Lily or Daisy.

★♂ **FLYNN.** *Irish 'son of the red-haired one'.* A winning last-name-first Celtic choice. **Flinn, Flyn.**

FOLAMI. *African, 'honour and respect me'.* Nigerian name with some teasing potential: 'follow me'? 'salami'?

♂ **FOREVER.** *Word name.* Timeless.

FORSYTHIA. *Flower name.* This yellow spring bloom is not as sweet as such other exotic species as Acacia and Azalea.

♀ **FORTUNE.** *Latin 'luck, fate, wealth'.* Contemporary sounding word name with an ancient history, widely used in the Roman Empire, and based on the mythic goddess of good luck and fertility. **International: Fortuna, Fortunata** *(Spanish)*.

FRANCA. *Latin, 'free'.* One of the most attractive and exotic spins on the 'Fran' franchise. **International: Franka** *(German)*.

FRANCE. *Place name.* Geographic name with lots of Gallic élan. **Fran, Franci, Francie.**

♀ **FRANCES.** *Latin, 'from France'.* This soft and gentle classic, last popular a hundred years ago, was as faded as old wallpaper until such hip parents as Courtney Love, Sean Penn, Michael J. Fox and Brooke Shields picked it as a first or middle name for their daughters. **Fan, Fancey, Fanchette, Fancie, Fancy, Fanechka, Fani, Fania, Fanni, Fannia, Fannie, Fanny, Fran, France, Franceen, Franci, Francie, Francille, Francina,** Francique, Francis, Francys, Franki, Frankie, Franky, Franni, Frannie, Franny, Fransabelle, Franze, Franzetta, Franzi, Fronia. **International: Proinséas** *(Irish Gaelic)*, **Fanchon, Francine, Franette, Françoise** *(French)*, **Franca, Francesca** *(Italian)*, **Francisca, Paquita** *(Spanish)*, **Franziska, Ziska** *(German)*, **Franka** *(Russian)*, **Fanya** *(Slavic)*.

★**FRANCESCA.** *Italian variation of* **FRANCES.** Lighter and more feminine than the English classic, Francesca is popular with upscale parents, such as movie directors Martin Scorsese and Clint Eastwood.

FRANCINE. *French variation of* **FRANCES.** Dated and déclassé. **Franceen, Francene, Franci.**

FRANÇOISE. *(frahn-SWAHZ) French variation of* **FRANCES.** In France it's sometimes bestowed as a patriotic gesture; elsewhere it has an air of genteel sophistication. **Fanchon, Fanchone, France, Franchon, Francine.**

♀ **FRANKIE.** *Diminutive of* **FRANCES.** *Really* retro name, part of the nickname revolution. **Frankee, Frankey, Franki, Franky.**

FRAYDA. *Yiddish, 'joy'.* An old favourite in traditional Jewish families. **Frayde, Fraydel, Freyda, Freyde, Freydel.**

FREDA. *German, 'peaceful,' diminutive of* **FREDERICA, ALFREDA,** *and* **WINIFRED.** Pronounced as Fred with an *a*, it has been surpassed by Freya. **Freada, Freeda, Freida, Frida, Frieda, Frydda.**

FREDERICA. *Feminine variation of* **FREDERICK.** An interesting possibility for the parent unintimidated by its old-fashioned formality, Frederica has some vintage charm and verve lurking inside its stuffiness. **Farica, Farika, Federica, Fred, Freda, Fredalena, Fredda, Freddee, Freddi, Freddie, Freddey, Fredericha, Fredericka, Frederickina, Frederine, Fredi, Fredia, Fredie, Fredricia, Fredrika, Frerika, Frida, Frieda, Friedegard, Friederike, Frika, Frikka, Fritzi, Fritzie, Fryda, Rica, Ricki, Rickie, Ricky, Rikki, Rikky. International: Frédérique** *(French)*, **Federica**

(*Italian*), **Friederika, Frerika**
(*German*), **Frederika, Frideborg**
(*Swedish*), **Frydryka** (*Polish*),
Frici (*Hungarian*).

FREE. *Word name.* The 1960s
are back! **Freedom.**

FREESIA. *Flower name.* A really
exotic flower name for the parent
who wants to move beyond Rose
and Daisy. **Freezia, Fresia.**

FREYA. (*FRAY-a*) *Norse, 'a noble
woman'.* The name of the Norse
goddess of love and fertility is
very popular, making a recent
appearance in the Top 25.
International: Freja (*Swedish*),
Freyde (*Yiddish*).

FRIDA. *German, 'peaceful'.*
The dynamic personality and
paintings of Mexican artist Frida
Kahlo have inspired growing
numbers of parents to resurrect
this form of the name.

FRIEDA. *German, 'peaceful
ruler'.* The traditional Germanic
Frieda holds little appeal for the
modern baby namer. **Frayda,
Freda, Fredia, Freeda, Freeha,
Freia, Freida, Frida.**

FRITZI. *German, diminutive of*

FREDERICA. Like Mitzi, the
bubbly Fritzi shows signs of
rising again.

FUCHSIA. *Plant and colour
name.* A plausible colour name,
it was chosen by the singer
Sting as a middle name for his
daughter, after a character in the
Gormenghast fantasy trilogy.

FULVIA. *Latin, 'blond one'.*
This name of the wife of Mark
Antony in ancient Rome sounds
a tad too anatomical for a
modern girl.

♂ **FUTURE.** *Word name.*
Gives the message that you
want your daughter to keep
her eye on the prize.

G *girls*

★**GABRIELA, GABRIELLA.**
*Italian and Spanish, feminine
variation of* **GABRIEL.** This
strong yet graceful feminine
form of Gabriel is on the rise,
given to many baby girls each
year, with the double *L* spelling
more popular. **Gabbe, Gabbey,
Gabbi, Gabbie, Gabbriel,**

Gabbrielle, Gabbryel, Gabby,
Gabey, Gabie, Gabielle, Gabreal,
Gabreale, Gabrealle, Gabreil,
Gabrial, Gabriala, Gabrialla,
Gabriana, Gabrielia, Gabriell,
Gabriellen, Gabriellia, Gabrila,
Gabrilla, Gabrille, Gabrina,
Gabriyelle, Gabryel, Gabryell,
Gabryella, Gabryelle.
International: Gabriel, Gabrielle,

**Stylish Girly-Girl
Names**

Angelina

Arabella

Carolina

Cassandra

Cecily

Clarissa

Gabriella

Georgiana

Isabella

Juliana

Larissa

Mirabelle

Savannah

Scarlett

Tatiana

Valentina

Gaby, Gigi *(French)*, Gabriela, Gabriella *(Italian)*, Gabella, Gabrela, Gabriela, Gebriela, Graviella *(Spanish)*, Gába, Gabi, Gabina, Gabinka, Gabra *(Czech)*, Gavi, Gavriela, Gavriella, Gavrielle, Gavrilla *(Hebrew)*.

GABRIELLE. *French, feminine variation of* **GABRIEL.** Just beginning its descent after years on the rise, the quintessentially elegant and worldly Gabrielle – designer Coco Chanel's real name – has recently fallen from the Top 100. For variations, see above.

GAETANA. *(gy-TAH-nah) Italian place name.* Gaeta is a southern Italian region; this makes a sunny first name. **Gaetan, Gaetanne. International: Gaetane** *(French)*.

GAIA, GAEA. *(GAY-ah or GUY-ah) Greek, 'earth mother'.* The name of the Greek mythological earth goddess and universal mother; actress Emma Thompson stated that she was attracted by its ecological element. **Gaea, Gaiea, Gaya, Kaia.**

GAIL. *Hebrew, 'my father rejoices'.* Mid-twentieth century

favourite, now far surpassed by its original form, Abigail. **Gael, Gaela, Gahl, Gaila, Gaile, Gaill, Gal, Gale, Gayel, Gayelle, Gayla, Gayle, Gayleen, Gaylene, Gayline, Gayll, Gaylla. International: Gaelle** *(French)*.

GALA. *Russian, diminutive of* **GALINA**; *English word name.* Festive name of the wife of Salvador Dalí. **Gaila, Galla.**

GALATEA. *(gal-ah-TEH-ah) Greek, 'white as milk'.* Mythical statue sculpted by Pygmalion and brought to life by Aphrodite, the inspiration for *My Fair Lady.* **Galatee, Galathea.**

GALAXY. *Word name.* Otherworldly. **Galaxia.**

GALE. *See* **GAIL.**

♂ **GALEN.** *Greek, 'healer, calm'.* The final *n* makes this choice infinitely more modern than Gail. **Gaelen, Gaelin, Gaellen, Gailen, Gailin, Gailyn, Galin, Galyn, Gaylaine, Gayleen, Gaylen, Gaylene, Gaylyn.**

GALI. *Hebrew, 'wave, billow'.* Sprightly. **Gal, Galice, Galie, Galila, Galiya, Galya.**

GALILA. *Hebrew, 'rolling hills'.* Interesting alternative to Dalila, relates to the Biblical Galilee. **Galilah, Galilea, Galilee, Galya, Gelila, Gelilah, Gelifia, Getilya, Glila, Glilah.**

GALINA. *Latin, 'hen'; Russian variation of* **HELEN.** Commonly used in Russia, has an old-fashioned Slavic feel. **Gailya, Gala, Galayna, Galena, Galenka, Galia, Galiana, Galiena, Galinka, Gallina, Galochka, Galya, Galyna, Lina.**

♂ **GALWAY.** *place name.* The familiar Irish city and bay is one place name that seems distinctly masculine.

GALYA. *Hebrew, 'God has redeemed, hill of God'.* Well used in Israel and in Russia, either on its own or as an endearment for Galila or Galina. **Galenka, Galia, Galina, Gallia, Gallya, Galochka.**

GANESHA. *(gay-NAY-sha) Hindi, 'fortunate'.* The name of the Hindu elephant-headed goddess of success and wisdom. **Ganesa.**

GANYA. *Hebrew, 'garden of the Lord'; Zulu, 'clever'.* Tanya with a *G*. **Gana, Gani, Gania, Ganice, Ganit.**

GARBO. *Italian nickname, 'polite, kind'.* Patricia Arquette named her daughter Harlow, so why not consider this other great early screen icon?

GARCELLE. *Modern invented name.* Although it sounds like it could be a genuine French name, it's an invention.

♂ **GARCIA.** *Spanish and Portuguese, 'fox'.* Evocative ethnic surname choice for a girl.

GARDENIA. *Flower name.* More exotic and powerful than garden varieties like Rose and Lily. **Deeni, Denia, Gardeenia, Gardena, Gardinia.**

♂ **GARDNER.** *English, 'keeper of the garden'.* One of the best of this fashionable occupational group, strong and particularly well suited to a girl, also with alluring connection to glamour girl Ava Gardner. **Gardener, Gardie, Gardiner.**

GARLAND. *Word name.* Fragrant and celebratory, and also has a celebrity-tribute tie to the star of *The Wizard of Oz*. **Garlan, Garlande, Garlandina, Garlen, Garlin, Garlind, Garlinde, Garlyn, Garlynd, Garlynde.**

GARNET. *Jewel name, from the French, 'pomegranate'.* One of the jewel names in use a hundred years ago, due for revival along with sisters Ruby and Pearl. **Garnetta, Garnette, Granata, Grenata, Grenatta.**

♂ **GARY.** *English, 'spear man'.* While not generally thought of as unisex, this is a male name that, like Perry and Barry, has occasionally been used for girls over the years. **Gari, Garri, Garry.**

GAURI. *(GAU-ree) Hindi, 'fair, pale'.* Gauri the Brilliant is one of the many names for the Hindu goddess Shakti, but it's not very euphonious to the Western ear. **Gawri, Gori, Gowri.**

♂ **GAY.** *Word name.* Out of the question these days. **Gae, Gai, Gaye.**

♂ **GAYNOR.** *Welsh, 'white and smooth, soft'.* Early androgynous name with a positive association, related to the Cornish megastar Jennifer. **Gaenor, Gayna, Gayner.**

GAZELLA. *Latin, 'gazelle'.* Graceful. **Gazelle.**

GEENA. *Variation of* **GINA.** Actress Geena Davis (born Virginia) put her own distinctive stamp on the spelling of Gina. **Geania, Geeana, Geeanna, Gena.**

GEELA. *(GEE-lah) Hebrew, 'joy'.* Gay, nearly giddy, gee-whiz feel; also too reminscent of a gila monster. **Geela, Geelah, Geelan, Geila, Geiliya, Geiliyah, Gila, Gilah, Gilalah, Gilana.**

GELSEY. *Persian, 'flower'.* Given a lithe and graceful image by ballerina Gelsey Kirkland, but since surpassed by Kelsey and Chelsea. **Gelsomina, Jelsomina.**

GEMINI. *Latin, 'twins'.* Astrological sign with enough rhythm to make a plausible astral name. **Gemella, Gemelle, Gemima, Gemina, Geminine, Gemmina.**

GEMMA. *(JEM-mah) Italian, 'precious stone'.* Very popular in 1980s England, but it hasn't been seen in the Top 100 since 2002. **Gem, Gema, Gèmma, Gemmey, Gemmie, Gemmy, Jemma, Jemsa.**

GEN. *Japanese, 'spring,' or diminutive of names beginning with 'Gen'.* Commonly used in Japan, and so much more distinguished than Jen.

GENA. *Variation of* **GINA.** Actress Gena Rowlands publicised this name, which she pronounces with a soft *e*.

♂ **GENE.** *Diminutive of* **EUGENIA** *or variation of* **JEAN.** This is still usually the boy's spelling. **Genie.**

GENEEN. *Scottish variation of* **JEANINE.** Somewhat flat-footed spelling variation. **Geanine, Geannine, Gen, Genene, Genine, Gineen, Ginene.**

GENEROSITY. *Word name.* Full-hearted new virtue choice, though five syllables is a lot to handle. **Generous.**

GENESIS. *Word name.* The name of the first book of the Bible, not nearly as original for babies as you'd think, since it has recently been used for thousands of baby girls in the US. **Genes, Genese, Genesha, Genesia, Genesies, Genesiss, Genessa, Genesse, Genessie, Genessis, Genicis, Genises, Genisis, Gennesis, Gennesiss, Genysis, Jenesis, Jenesyss, Jennasis, Yenesis.**

★**GENEVA.** *French, 'juniper tree'; Swiss place name.* Unlike its somewhat formal Swiss city namesake, this is a lively and appealing place name that also has a real history as a female name. **Geena, Gen, Gena, Geneieve, Geneiva, Geneive, Genever, Genevia, Genevre, Genovela, Genovella, Genovova, Ginebra, Ginevre, Ginneva, Janeva, Janevra, Jeaneva, Jeneva, Jenovefa, Jineeva, Jineva, Joneva, Jonevah. International: Genève** *(French),* **Genevra, Genoveffa, Ginevra** *(Italian).*

GENEVIEVE. *(zhahn-vee-EV or GEN-uh-veev) French 'woman of the people'; Celtic, 'white wave'.* Perfect choice for anyone who wants to retain the *gen* sound but is tired of all the overused Jen names. The medieval saint Genevieve, patroness of Paris, defended the city against Attila the Hun. **Gen, Gena, Genaveeve, Genaveve, Genavie, Genavieve, Genavive, Geneva, Geneveeve, Genever, Genevera, Geneveve, Genevie, Genevievre, Genevive, Genivieve, Gennie, Genny, Genoveve, Genovieve, Genovive, Genvieve, Gin, Gina, Ginata, Ginett, Ginetta, Ginette, Gineveve, Ginevieve, Ginevive, Ginnetta, Ginnette, Guinevieve, Guinivive, Gwenevieve, Gwenivive, Janeva, Jenevieve, Jennavieve, Jennie, Jenny. International: Geneviève, Yevette** *(French),* **Genoveffa, Genovova, Genoviva, Ginevra** *(Italian),* **Genobeba** *(Spanish),* **Januveva** *(Slavic),* **Zenevieva** *(Hungarian and Polish).*

GENNIFER. *English variation of* **JENNIFER.** Does not improve on the pretty but overused favourite. **Gen, Genifer, Ginnifer.**

★**GENOA.** *Italian place name.* One of the newer geographical site names, it has the advantage of sounding like a real girl's name because of its *jen* beginning and feminine *a* ending.

♂ **GEORGE.** *Greek, 'farmer'.* One frankly boys' name that can work in an offbeat way for girls; a few celebrities have used it as their daughters' middle names.

GEORGEANNA. *English, combination of* **GEORGIA** *and* **ANNA.** With the first two syllables pronounced Georgie, it has a stylish air. Georgana, Georganna, Georgeana, Georgi, Georgiana, Georgiann, Georgianna, Georgianne, Georgie, Georgieann, Georgianna, Georgy, Georgyanna, Giorgi, Giorgianna, Giorgina.

GEORGEANNE. *English, combination of* **GEORGIA** *and* **ANNE.** Has none of the élan of the *a*-ending version. Georgann, Georganne, Georgean, Georgeann, Georgie, Georgyann, Georgyanne.

GEORGETTE. *French, feminine variation of* **GEORGE.** Has a musty 1940s feel. Georgeta, Georgett, Georgetta, Georjetta, Jorjetta, Jorjette.

★**GEORGIA.** *English, feminine variation of* **GEORGE.** A name so rich, so lush and luscious, it's almost irresistible. With a strong place in the Top 50, it's now a rising star among the feminisations of George, helped by associations with the painter O'Keeffe and the Ray Charles song playing in the background. George, Georgeann, Georgeanne, Georgeena, Georgeina, Georgena, Georgene, Georgenia, Georgetta, Georgi, Georgiana, Georgianna, Georgianne, Georgie, Georgiena, Georgine, Georgy, Georgyana, Georgyann, Georgyanne, Giorgi, Giorgina, Giorgyna, Jorja. International: Georgette, Georgienne, Gigi *(French)*, Giorgia *(Italian)*, Georgina, Georginita, Gina, Jorgina *(Spanish)*, Gyorgi, Gyorgyi, Gyuri *(Hungarian)*, Jirca, Jirina, Jirka *(Czech)*, Gerda *(Latvian)*.

GEORGIANA. *English, feminine variation of* **GEORGE.** This has been a long-time favourite among the upper-class, where it's pronounced *George-ayna.*

GEORGINA. *English, feminine variation of* **GEORGE.** Now more popular than Georgiana,

If You Like Georgia,
You Might Love . . .

Ava
Bella
Cara
Carolina
Eudora
Eva
Francesca
Geneva
Georgiana
Gianna
Louisiana
Miranda
Savannah
Stella

this elegant Dickens–Jane Austen name deserves more attention. Georgeina, Georgena, Georgene, Georgejean, Georgiana, Georgianna, Georgianne, Georgienne, Georgine, Georgyana, Giorgina, Jorgina.

GERALDINE. *German and French, feminine variation of* **GERALD.** Almost, but not quite as tired as her male name-mate. **Deena, Dina, Dyna, Geraldeen, Geraldene, Geraldyna, Geraldyne, Geralyn, Geralynne, Gerdene, Gerdine, Geri, Gerianna, Gerianne, Gerilynn, Gerri, Gerrie, Gerrilee, Gerrilyn, Gerroldine, Gerry, Jeraldeen, Jeraldene, Jeraldine, Jeralee, Jere, Jeri, Jerilene, Jerrie, Jerrileen, Jerroldeen, Jerry.** International: **Gearóidin** *(Irish Gaelic)*, **Giralda** *(Italian)*, **Geralda, Geraldina** *(Spanish)*, **Gerhardine** *(German)*.

GERANIUM. *Flower name.* Offbeat flower name, sure to raise some eyebrows.

GERARDINE. *French, feminine variation of* **GERARD.** Makes Geraldine seem positively groovy. **Gerarda, Gerardina, Gerardyne, Gererdina, Gerrardene.**

GERDA. *Scandinavian, 'enclosure, stronghold'.* Mythological goddess of fertility whose name seems, ironically, among the least attractive.

Garda, Geerda, Gerd, Gerta. International: **Gerde** *(German)*.

GERMAINE. *French, feminine variation of* **GERMAIN.** Name linked to the early days of feminism via Germaine Greer, this saint's name feels neither French nor German enough. **Germain, Germana, Germane, Germanee, Germani, Germanie, Germaya, Germayn, Germayne, Germine, Jarmaine, Jermain, Jermaine, Jermane, Jermayn, Jermayne.**

♂ **GERRY.** *English, diminutive of* **GERALDINE.** Gerry was hep along with poodle skirts and banana splits. **Geri, Gerri, Gerrie, Jeri, Jerri, Jerrie, Jerry.**

GERTRUDE. *German, 'strength of a spear'.* Enormously popular a hundred years ago but feels as heavy as lead today. Though we must admit, nickname Gertie sounded kind of cute on the young Drew Barrymore in *E.T.* **Gehtruda, Gehtrudis, Gerda, Gert, Gerta, Gerte, Gertey, Gerti, Gertie, Gertina, Gertraud, Gertrudis, Gerty, Traudl, Trude, Trudi, Trudie, Trudy.** International: **Geerta** *(Dutch)*,

Gertraud, Gertrud, Gertruda *(German)*.

♂ **GERVAISE.** *French, 'skilled with a spear'.* Predominantly male choice that nevertheless has a pretty sound and fashionable unisex feel. **Gervase, Jervaise, Jervase.** International: **Gervasia** *(Spanish)*.

GHISLAINE. *(gees-LANE) French from German, 'pledge'.* Still sounds exotic to us, even though in France this name – which can be pronounced with a hard or soft initial *G* – is dated. **Gislan, Gislaine.**

GIACINTA. *(jee-ah-SEEN-tah) Italian, from Greek, 'hyacinth'.* As pretty in its way as Jacinta, the Spanish name for the same flower. **Giacintha, Jacinta, Jacintha, Jacynth, Jiacintha, Yacinta, Yacintha.**

GIADA. *(jee-AH-dah) Italian, 'jade'.* More unusual Italian possibility to consider.

GIANNA. *(jee-AH-nah) Italian, feminine variation of* **JOHN.** Feminisation of John gaining favour outside

the confines of Italian culture.
**Gian, Giann, Giannetta,
Giannina.**

GIGI. *French diminutive.*
Like high-kicking *amies* Coco
and Fifi, it has a lot of Gallic
spunk but lacks substance.
GeeGee, G.G., Giggi.

GILA, GILIA. *Hebrew, 'joy of
the Lord'.* Gila and its variants
have joyous meanings in
Hebrew, but other children in
the playground might connect
them to the monster. **Geela,
Gil, Gilah, Giliah, Gilana,
Gilat, Gilada, Gilit, Giliya,
Giliyah, Gill.**

GILBERTE. *French, feminine
variation of* **GILBERT.** You
might be able to make this
work if you pronounce it the
sophisticated French way:
zhil-bare. **Berta, Bertie,
Berty, Gigi, Gilbert, Gilberta,
Gilbertha, Gilbertina,
Gilbertine, Gili, Gill,
Gilli, Gillie, Gilly.**

GILDA. *English, 'covered with
gold'.* Sexy 1940s film heroine,
once shimmering gold, now
tarnished. **Gilde, Gildi,
Gildie, Gildy.**

GILLIAN. *(JILL-ee-an)
Feminine variation of* **JULIAN.**
Very British, with a soft *G,*
but also spelled phonetically as
Jillian – it's a very attractive
choice either way. **Gila, Gilana,
Gilenia, Gili, Gilian, Gill, Gilli,
Gilliana, Gilliane, Gilliann,
Gillianna, Gillianne, Gillie,
Gilly, Gillyan, Gillyane,
Gillyann, Gillyanne, Gyllian,
Jillian, Jilly, Jillyan, Lian.**

GIN. *(jin) 'silver'.* Although
it's a common name in Japan,
it would definitely have alcoholic
allusions here.

GINA. *Diminutive of* **REGINA,
ANGELINA,** *etc.* Has been
used on its own since the 1920s,
but still seems like only part
of a name. **Geanna, Geena,
Geenah, Geina, Gen, Gena,
Genae, Genah, Genai,
Genea, Geneja, Geni, Genia,
Genie, Gin, Ginah, Ginai,
Ginette, Ginna, Jena, J
eena, Jenna.**

★**GINEVRA.** *Italian variation
of* **GUINEVERE.** A lovely
alternative for the Jennifer-
lover.

GINGER. *English diminutive.*
Originally a unisex nickname
for a redhead – since 'ginger'
is a nickname for red hair –
or for the name Virginia,
Ginger perennially wears pink
gingham and spike heels. **Gin,
Gingee, Gingie, Ginja, Ginjer,
Ginny, Jinger.**

GINNY. *English, diminutive of*
VIRGINIA. More common
before Jenny and its myriad
variants came along. **Gin, Gini,
Ginia, Ginnee, Ginney, Ginni,
Ginnie, Giny, Gionni, Gionny,
Jinnee, Jinnie, Jinny.**

GIOCONDA. Italian,
'lighthearted woman'. Another
name for the Mona Lisa, who
was married to a Florentine
businessman surnamed
Giocondo; others say the title
referred to her mysterious smile.
Geoconda, Jeoconda.

GIOIA. *(JOY-a) Italian, 'joy'.*
Prettier than Joy and just being
used elsewhere. **Gioya, Joya.**

GIORDANA. *Italian variation
of* **JORDANA.** Spelling twist
makes it exotic.

★GIOVANNA. *(joh-VAH-nah) Italian, feminine variation of* GIOVANNI. Like Leonardo, one of the Italian names that fashionable American parents – with or without Italian roots – have started to choose for their daughters. **Anna, Geona, Geonna, Geovana, Geovanna, Geovonna, Gian, Giana, Gianella, Gianetta, Gianina, Gianinna, Giann, Gianna, Gianne, Giannee, Giannella, Giannetta, Gianni, Giannie, Giannina, Gianny, Gianoula, Giavanna, Giavonna, Giovana, Giovanetta, Giovanne, Giovanni, Giovannia, Giovonna, Givonnie, Jeveny, Jovana, Jovanna, Jovanne.**

GISELLE, GISELE. *(GEE-zah-lah) German, 'pledge/hostage'.* Brazilian supermodel Gisele Bundchen undoubtedly gave this name a boost. The French pronunciation *(jiz-ELLE)* gives it a more graceful, balletic, gazellelike feel. **Gella, Ghisele, Ghisella, Gigi, Gisel, Giseli, Gisell, Gissela, Gissell, Gissella, Gisel, Gisella, Giselle, Gysell.** International: **Ghislaine, Gisele, Gisella** *(French),* **Gisela** *(Italian and Spanish),* **Gisela, Gisella,** **Giselda** *(German),* **Gizi, Gizike, Gizus** *(Hungarian),* **Giza, Gisela** *(Slavic).*

GISH. *Chinese, meaning unknown.* This name was brought to the fore by acclaimed Chinese-American novelist and short story writer Gish Jen, whose birth name was Lillian.

GITA. *Sanskrit, 'song'; Yiddish, 'good'; Polish, diminutive of* MARGARITA. Harsh and slight – an unfortunate combination. **Geeta, Gitika, Gitka, Gitta, Gituska.**

GITANA. *Spanish, 'gypsy, wanderer'.* Too close to jeans brand. **Gitane, Jeetanna.**

GIUDITTA. *(jyoo-dit-tah) Italian variation of* JUDITH. Italian accent glamorises even Judith.

GIULIA. *(jyoo-lee-ah) Italian variation of* JULIA. Another Italian spelling beginning to be adopted. **Giula, Giulana, Giuliana, Giulianna, Giulliana, Giulietta, Giullia, Guila, Guiliana, Guilietta, Jiulia,** **Jiuliana, Jiulla, Jiullya, Julia, Juliana, Julie, Juliet, Julietta, Juliette, Jullia, Julliana, Julliane.**

GIUSEPPINA. *(jyoo-sep-PEE-nah) Italian, feminine variation of* GIUSEPPE. One case where the English version – Josephine – is far preferable. **Giuseppa, Josefina.**

♂ GLADE. *Nature name, 'forest'.* One of the evocative new nature names with a simple, stylish feel.

GLADYS. *Welsh variation of* CLAUDIA. The cat's miaow a century ago, featured in many romantic novels, and now anything but. Hard to imagine it ever coming back. **Glad, Gladdis, Gladdys, Gladi, Gladis, Gladiz, Gladness, Gladwyse, Glady, Gladyss, Gwladys, Gwyladyss.**

♀ GLASGOW. *Scottish place name.* Prettier: Paisley, a suburb of Glasgow, or even Scotland itself.

GLENDA. *Welsh, 'fair and good'.* There aren't many Glendas under forty. **Glennda.**

♀ GLENN. *Scottish, 'a narrow valley'.* While actress Glenn Close didn't inspire many parents to give their daughters her name in particular, she did help launch a general trend towards boys' names for girls. **Glen.**

GLENNA. *Irish, 'glen'.* Honouring a male relative? Be bold and go with Glenn. **Glanda, Gleana, Glenda, Gleneen, Glenene, Glenesha, Glenetta, Glenice, Glenina, Glenine, Glenis, Glenise, Glenisha, Glen, Glenn, Glennda, Glenne, Glennene, Glennesha, Glennette, Glennia, Glennie, Glennis, Glennisha, Glennishia, Glennys, Glenora, Glenwys, Gleny, Glenys, Glenyse, Glenyss, Glinnis, Glinys, Glyn, Glynda, Glynesha, Glynice, Glynis, Glynisha, Glyniss, Glynitra, Glynnis, Glynys, Glynyss.**

GLENYS. *Welsh, 'riverbank, shore'.* Any elaboration of Glen (or Glenn) feels like frippery. **Glenice, Glenis, Glennice, Glennis, Glennys, Glynis.**

GLIMMER. *Word name.* Shimmery but a little too showy, as is Glitter.

GLORIA. *Latin, 'glory'.* Once-sultry name now relegated to grandmas. **Glaura, Glaurea, Glora, Glorea, Gloree, Gloresha, Glori, Gloriah, Gloriana, Gloriane, Gloribel, Glorie, Gloriela, Gloriella, Glorielle, Gloris, Glorisha, Glorra, Glorri, Glorvina, Glory, Glorya, Gloryan, Gloryanna, Gloryanne.**

GLYNIS. *Welsh, 'small glen, valley'.* The feminine version of the common Welsh name Glyn, rarely heard elsewhere. **Glinnis, Glinyce, Glinys, Glinyss, Glyn, Glynnis.**

GOD'ISS LOVE. *Modern invented name.* R & B singer Lil' Mo decided to move beyond Trinity and Genesis and turn her daughter's name into a statement. Her sister is called Heaven.

GODIVA. *English, 'God's gift'.* Whether you think of the chocolates or the naked long-haired lady on the horse, this is a name with baggage no child should have to carry.

GOLDA. *English, 'gold'.* As grandmotherly as Golda Meir. **Goldarina, Goldarine, Goldee, Golden, Goldi, Goldia, Goldie, Goldina, Goldy.**

GOLDIE. *Anglicised form of Yiddish* **GOLDE** *or* **GOLDA.** Goldie Hawn made it work, but don't try this at home – most other Goldies are doing sit-down exercises.

GOYA. *Artist name.* Passion for the Spanish painter may transcend the difficulty of this name – just don't say it in a Jewish community.

★GRACE. *Virtue name.* Who'd have thought a simple and pure virtue name like Grace, which originally referred to divine grace, could ever become trendy? But that's what it is, chosen by many celebrities. If it's too overused for you (it's now at Number 2 on the list), try an exotic variation like Engracia or Graziella – or the earthier Gracie. **Gracey, Graci, Gracia, Graciana, Graciane, Gracie, Graciela, Graciella, Gracina, Gracinia, Gracious, Gracy, Graecie, Graice, Gratia, Gratiana, Gratiela, Gratiella, Gray, Grayce, Graysie. International: Grainne, Grania**

Names That Are Trendier Than You'd Guess

Ava

Chloe

Claire

Destiny

Eleanor

Ella

Eva

Faith

Grace

Julia

Laura

Lily

Lucy

Madeline

Olivia

Ruby

Sadie

Sophia

Sophie

Stella

Trinity

Zoe

(Irish), **Grazielle** *(French),* **Grazia, Graziella, Graziosa** *(Italian),* **Engracia, Gracia, Graciana, Graciela** *(Spanish),* **Graca, Gracinha** *(Portuguese),* **Gratia** *(German),* **Grazyna** *(Polish),* **Arete** *(Greek),* **Kalake** *(Hawaiian).*

GRACIE. *English, diminutive of* **GRACE.** An increasing number of parents are opting to put the pet form on the birth certificate.

♂ **GRADY.** *Irish 'noble'.* A name that's on the rise for boys but rarely used – though possible – for girls. **Gradee, Gradey, Gradi, Gradie.**

GRÁINNE. *(grahn-ya) Irish, 'the loved one' or 'grain of corn'.* Name of both a goddess and a heroine in Irish mythology, it's popular in Ireland and possible here, especially in its Anglicised spelling, Grania. **Grainnia, Grania.**

GRANADA. *Spanish place name.* Moorish region and city in Spain that makes a melodic and unusual first name. **Granadda, Grenada, Grenadda.**

♂ **GRAVITY.** *Word name.* Spacey.

GRAZIANA. *Italian variation of* **GRAZIA,** *'grace'.* An appealingly exotic spin on Grace.

GRAZIELLA. *Italian, diminutive variation of* **GRAZIA.** Another Italian version that adds spice. **Chelita, Cheya, Chita, Graciela, Gracella, Gracensia, Graciella, Graziana.** International: **Graziela, Graziella** *(Spanish).*

♂ **GREEN.** *Colour name.* Best in the middle.

★**GREER.** *Scottish, contraction of surname Gregor; Latin, 'alert, watchful'.* Early and still attractive surname choice, popularised by 1940s Academy Award winner Greer Garson (born Eileen; Greer was her mother's maiden name), and chosen much more recently by Kelsey Grammer for his daughter and by Brooke Shields in the Grier form. **Grear, Grier.**

GREGORIA. *Latin, 'alert, watchful'.* Sounds like a child in a Gothic novel. **Gregoriana, Gregorijana, Gregorina, Gregorine, Gregorya, Gregoryna.**

GREIGE. *Colour name.* Better on your living-room walls.

GRETA. *German, diminutive of* MARGARETHE. This old-fashioned name once tied to Garbo seems to be showing slight signs of a comeback; chosen by Kevin Kline. **Greatal, Greatel, Greet, Greeta, Gretal, Gretchen, Grete, Gretel, Gretha, Grethal, Grethel, Gretna, Grieta, Grytta.** International: **Ghita** *(Italian),* **Grietje** *(Dutch),* **Gretta, Grette** *(German),* **Grethe** *(Scandinavian),* **Gryta** *(Slavic),* **Gretl** *(Eastern European).*

GRETCHEN. *German, diminutive of* MARGARETHE. With Heidi, still wearing its dirndl skirt. **Greta, Gretchin, Gretchyn.**

♂ **GREY.** *Colour name.* Works for a boy, but a bit drab for a girl. **Gray.**

GRISELDA. *German, 'grey fighting maid'.* Wicked stepsister name. **Chriselda, Gricelda, Gricelle, Gricely, Grisel, Griseldis,** Grisell, Griselle, Griselly, Grishelda, Grishilde, Grissele, Grissell, Grisel, Griselda, Gryselde, Gryzelde, Selda, Zelda.

♂ **GROVE.** *Nature name.* Fresh, evocative choice.

GUADALUPE. *Spanish place name; Arabic, 'river of black stones'.* Popular Spanish name that relates to the patron saint of Mexico; could conceivably, like Soledad and Consuelo, cross the border into multicultural territory. **Guadalup, Guadelupe, Guadlupe, Guadulupe, Gudalupe, Lupita.**

GUCCI. *(GOO-chee) Designer name.* Makeup artist to the stars Gucci Westman has made this Italian fashion name a first.

GUDRUN. *(goo-drun) Scandinavian, 'battle'.* Difficult name familiar mainly via D. H. Lawrence's *Women in Love.* **Gudren, Gudrid, Gudrin, Gudrinn, Gudritin, Gudruna, Gudrunn, Gudrunne, Guthrun, Guthrunn, Guthrunne.**

♂ **GUERNSEY.** *place name.* The name of an island in the English Channel that might make an attractive first name . . . until you remember it's also a kind of cow. Works better for a boy.

♂ **GUEVARA.** *Basque place and surname.* Revolutionary choice.

GUINEVERE. *Welsh, 'white shadow, white wave'.* The name of the ill-fated queen of Camelot, for so many years eclipsed by its modern Cornish form Jennifer, could be a possibility for adventurous parents intrigued by this richly evocative and romantic choice. **Gaenna, Gayna, Gaynah, Gayner, Generva, Genever, Genevieve, Genevra, Geniffer, Geniver, Genivra, Genn, Genna, Gennie, Gennifer, Genny, Ginette, Ginevra, Guenever, Guenevere, Gueniveer, Guenna, Guenola, Guinever, Guinivere, Guinna, Gwen, Gwenevere, Gwenivere, Gwenn, Gwenrie, Gwennola, Gwennora, Gwennore, Gwenny, Gwenora, Gwenore, Gwyn, Gwynn, Gwynna, Gwynne, Gwynnevere, Jen, Jeni, Jenifer, Jennee, Jenni, Jennie, Jennifer, Jenny, Wendee, Wendie, Wendy, Win, Winne, Winny.** International: **Gaenor, Gaynor, Guenevere** *(Welsh),* **Gweniver** *(Cornish).*

Stellar Starbabies Beginning with *G*

Gaia	Emma Thompson
Galen	Dennis Hopper
Georgia	Harry Connick Jr., Hope Davis, Jerry Hall & Mick Jagger
Georgina	Caroline Corr
God'iss Love	Lil' Mo
Grace	Lance Armstrong, Elisabeth & Tim Hasselback, Wynonna Judd, Christy Turlington & Ed Burns
Gracie	Anna Friel & David Thewlis
Greer	Kelsey Grammer
Grier	Brooke Shields
Greta	Phoebe Cates & Kevin Kline

GUNDRUNA. *Swedish, 'divine wisdom'.* Baby-naming rule No. 487: it's probably best to avoid names whose only possible nickname is Gun. **Gundrun.**

GUNHILDA. *Norse, 'battle maid'.* Rule No. 488: Or Hilda. **Gunhilde, Gunilda, Gunilla, Gunna, Gunnel, Gunnhilda.**

GUNILLA. *Swedish, 'battle maiden'.* This popular old Swedish name is not one that would appeal to many modern parents elsewhere. **Nilla.**

GUSTA. *Diminutive of* **AUGUSTA.** Stick with the long form. **Gus, Gussi, Gussie, Gussy, Gusti, Gustie, Gusty.**

GUSTAVA. *Swedish, 'staff of the gods'.* Imposing. **Gusta, Gustha.**

♂ **GUTHRIE.** *Scottish, 'windy spot'.* Folk singer Woody's last name makes a fine first choice for a girl.

GWEN. *Diminutive of* **GWENDOLYN, GUINEVERE.** These days, usually stands on its own. Rocker Gwen Stefani has given it a shot of cool. **Gwenesha, Gweness, Gweneta, Gwenetta, Gwenette, Gweni, Gwenisha, Gwenita, Gwenn, Gwenna, Gwennie, Gwenny, Gwyn, Gwynn.**

GWENDA. *Welsh, 'fair and good'.* The Good Witch's first cousin. **Gwennda, Gwinda, Gwynda, Gwynedd.**

GWENDOLEN, GWENDOLYN. *Welsh, 'white circle'.* Retired years ago in favour of the short form Gwen, but now, like many other old-fashioned names, this ancient Welsh favourite is up for reappraisal. **Guendolen, Guendolin, Guendolinn, Guendolynn, Guenna, Gwen, Gwendalee, Gwendalin,**

Gwendaline, Gwendalyn, Gwendalynn, Gwendela, Gwendelyn, Gwendelynn, Gwendilyn, Gwendolen, Gwendolene, Gwendolyne, Gwendolynn, Gwendolynne, Gwendylan, Gwenna, Gwenette, Gwenndolen, Gwenni, Gwennie, Gwenny, Gwenyth, Gwyn, Gwyndolyn, Gwynn, Gwynna, Gwynndolen, Wendi, Wendie, Wendy, Win, Winne, Winnie, Wynne. International: Gwenda, Gwendolin, Gwendoline, Gwyneth, Gwynne, Wendolen, Wendolyn (Welsh).

GWYNETH. *Welsh, 'blessed, happy'.* Gwyneth Paltrow made this name famous, but even her star power hasn't made it popular. However we think its mellifluous sound and wonderful meaning make it a candidate for more widespread use. **Gweneth, Gwenith, Gwenneth, Gwennyth, Gwenyth, Gwineth, Gwinn, Gwinne, Gwinneth, Gwinyth, Gwyn, Gwynith, Gwynn, Gwynna, Gwynne, Gwynneth, Winnie, Winny, Wynne, Wynnie.**

★♂ GWYNN. *Welsh, 'fair, blessed'.* The most modern choice in this group, and the most distinctive; the Gwyn form is a common male name in Wales. **Gwin, Gwinn, Gwinna, Gwinne, Gwyn, Gwynna, Gwynne.**

GYPSY. *English, 'wanderer'.* Even though it has a certain exotic charm, Gypsy is the ultimate stripper name. **Gipsee, Gipsey, Gipsy, Gypsie, Jipsi.**

H *girls*

HABIBAH. *Arabic, 'beloved'.* Strong and memorable. **Habiba, Habibi, Haviva, Havivah, Hebiba.**

♂ HADAR *(had-DAHR) Hebrew, 'ornament, glory, respect'.* Also a city near Tel Aviv, this is a name found primarily in Israel. **Hadara, Hadarit, Hadura.**

HADASSAH. *Hebrew, 'myrtle tree'.* This Hebrew name of Queen Esther is well used in Israel (especially for girls born around the holiday of Purim) but has been shunned elsewhere as hyperreligious, being the name of a Zionist women's philanthropic organisation. **Dassa, Hada, Hadas, Hadasa, Hadasah, Hadaseh, Hadassa, Haddasah, Hodel.**

HADIYA. *(hah-DEE-yah) Arabic, 'guide to righteousness'.* A pleasant, welcoming Middle Eastern choice. **Hadi, Hadiyh, Hadya.**

★♂ HADLEY. *English, 'heathery field'.* Hadley, most famous as the name of Ernest Hemingway's first wife, is more sophisticated, professional and modern than cousins Heather, Haley or Hayden. This one's heading up. **Hadlea, Hadlee, Hadleigh, Hadli, Hadlie, Hadly, Hedlea, Hedleigh, Hedley.**

HAGAR. *Hebrew, 'flight' or 'forsaken'.* Old Testament name as horrible as the eponymous comic strip character. **Hager, Haggar, Hagir, Hagur, Hajar.**

HAIDEE. *English, 'modest'.* Sounds like a variant of Heidi or Hailey, but actually a separate name with a literary history, used in Byron's epic poem *Don Juan*.

If You Like Hailey,
You Might Love . . .

Ali

Bailey

Haidee

Halsey

Harley

Harper

Haven

Hazel

Holly

Layla

Leigh

Marley

Sadie

Sailor

Tally

Wylie

HAILEY. *English, 'hay field'.* There are no less than ten different variations of this name that are currently competing for a popularity contest, with this spelling the most popular one.

So, although the name has a shiny, unpretentious charm, its mass popularity makes it very much of the moment. **Haeley, Haelie, Haely, Haile, Hailea, Hailee, Hailie, Haily, Halea, Halee, Haleigh, Haley, Halie, Halle, Halleigh, Hallie, Hally, Haylea, Haylee, Heyleigh, Hayley, Haylie.**

HALA. *Arab, 'halo'.* Joyous quality. **Halah.**

♂ **HALCYON.** *(HAL-see-on) Greek, 'kingfisher bird'.* This highly unusual name – the Halycyone was a mythic bird who could calm the seas – conjures up images of utter peace and tranquility because of the phrase 'Halycon days' . . . and the sleeping pill. **Alcione, Alcyonne, Halcione, Halcyone, Halcyonne.**

HALDIS. *German, 'purposeful'.* A German name with little chance of adoption elsewhere. **Halda, Haldi, Haldie, Haldisse.**

HALEIGH. *See* **HAILEY.**

HALEY. *English, 'hay field'.* The second most popular spelling of

this name is also the most straightforward.

HALI. *Greek, 'the sea'.* Another culture's take on the Hailey/Halle phenomenon. **Halle, Halli, Hallie, Hally.**

HALIA. *Hawaiian, 'remembrance of a loved one'.* Adds the element of Pacific island rhythm.

HALIMAH. *Arabic, 'gentle and patient'.* The name of the Prophet Muhammad's childhood nurse carries special resonance for Muslim parents. **Haleema, Halima.**

♂ **HALLE.** *Norse, male diminutive of* **HARALD.** Until the beautiful actress Halle Berry inspired hundreds of parents to emulate her name, it was the diminutive Swedish families used for their sons christened Harald. Now, in a complete turnaround, it couldn't be more feminine.

HALLIE. *Norse, 'heroic'; English, 'the meadow by the manor'.* Hallie – it rhymes with alley and is not to be confused with Hailey or Holly – is one of those comfy nicknamish names that are in style in these complicated times. **Hali, Halie, Halle, Hallea, Hallee, Halleigh, Halli, Hallie, Hally, Hallye.**

HALONA. *Native American, 'happy fortune'.* Resonant and unusual. **Lona.**

HANA. *(hah-NAH) Japanese, 'flower, blossom'.* Many things to many peoples: a flower, name, also spelled Hanae, to the Japanese; a Czech and Polish short form of Johana; and an alternate form of the biblical name Hannah in the US. **Hanae, Hanako.**

HANAKO. *Japanese, 'flower child'.* Delicate. **Hana, Hanae.**

HANI. *Hawaiian, 'light-footed, to move softly, to touch'; Arabic, 'joyful'.* This is a sweet multicultural name.

HANIFA. *Arabic, 'true believer'.* Could serve as an alternative to the more common Latifah. **Haneefa, Hanifah.**

HANITA. *Hindi, 'divine grace'.* The added *h* turns Anita exotic and breathy.

HANNAH. *Hebrew, 'the Lord has favoured me'.* Hannah is one of the top biblical girl's name, due to its many sources of appeal: Old Testament roots, soft and gentle sound, and a homey yet aristocratic image. All in all, a wonderful if very widely used name. **Chana, Chanah, Chanha, Channach, Channah, Hanae, Hanah, Hanan, Hanna, Hannaa, Hanne, Hanni, Hannie, Hanny, Honna, Nan, Nanney.** International: **Anne, Ann** *(English)*, **Anna** *(Italian)*, **Ana** *(Spanish)*, **Hannele** *(German)*, **Anneka** *(Swedish)*, **Hanne** *(Nordic)*, **Annalie** *(Finnish)*, **Ania, Anka, Hania** *(Polish)*, **Hajina, Analee, Anci, Nusi** *(Hungarian)*, **Anezka** *(Czech)*, **Anya** *(Russian)*, **Hana** *(Slavic)*, **Haniyah** *(Moroccan)*, **Haniyyah** *(Tunisian)*.

HAPPY. *English word name.* As dated as Merry and Gay.

HAQIKAH. *Arabic, 'truthful'.* North African name with a distinctive beat.

HARA. *(HAH-rah) Hindi, 'to seise'.* One of the 1,008 names for the god Siva; parents of

other ethnicities might prefer the Irish O'Hara.

♀ **HARBOR.** *Word name.* We've seen Haven take off as a nouveau girls' name; Harbor could follow in its wake.

HARIATA. *Hawaiian variation of* **HARRIET.** A feminissima version of a super-serious name. **Haliaka, Hariala.**

HARIKA. *Turkish, 'a miracle, beautiful'.* Pretty and exotic.

♀ **HARLEY.** *English, 'the long field'.* Might be considered just another commonplace unisex surname name if it weren't for the motorcycle connection, which gives it some extra voltage. **Arlea, Arlee, Arleigh, Arley, Harlea, Harlee, Harleen, Harleey, Harleigh, Harli, Harlie, Harly.**

HARLOW. *English, 'army'.* Jean Harlow, the original platinum blonde, was a symbol of 1930s glamour, a factor Patricia Arquette probably had in mind when she gave her daughter this distinctive name.

HARMONIA. *Greek, 'agreement, concord'.* One Greek mythological name – she was the goddess of order – not likely to be embraced by modern parents elsewhere.

HARMONY. *Word name.* If Melody and Lyric are on your style sheet, the peaceful Harmony, popularised by *Buffy the Vampire Slayer,* should be too. Harmonee, Harmoney, Harmoni, Harmonia, Harmonie.

★♂ **HARPER.** *English, 'harp player'.* To Kill a Mockingbird author Harper Lee brought this family name into the public consciousness as a female first name with offbeat, boyish charm.

HARRIET. *English, feminine variation of* **HARRY.** Long considered a stylish, upscale name, it's related to the French Henriette. Etta, Etti, Ettie, Etty, Harietta, Hariette, Harri, Harrie, Harrieta, Harrietta, Harriette, Harriot, Harriott, Hat, Hatsy, Hatti, Hattie, Hatty, Hetta, Hetti, Hetty, Yetta, Yettie, Yetty.

♂ **HARTLEY.** *English, 'stag meadow'.* Brisk and business-like, with a can-do image . . . and a little heart too. Hartlee, Hartleigh, Hartli, Hartlie, Hartly.

HARUKO. *Japanese, 'tranquil' or 'born in spring'.* A traditional possibility for a child born in April or May. Hayu.

HATTIE. *English, diminutive of* **HARRIET.** Could be one of the next wave of vintage grandma nicknames, supplanting Annie and Jenny, and joining the spunkier Mamie and Mitzies. Hatti, Hatty, Hettie, Hetty.

HAVA. *Modern variation of* **EVE.** Caution: might be too close to phrases beginning with 'Have a', as in 'Have a burger'. Havva.

♂ **HAVANA.** *Cuban place name.* Politics aside, the Cuban capital is one of the most rhythmic and exotic of place names. The question is: can politics be put aside? Havanah, Havane, Havanna, Havvanah, Havanuh.

♂ **HAVEN.** *Word name.* Recently invented safe-harbour name that appeals to an increasing number of parents who don't want to voyage quite as far as Heaven. Havin, Havun, Hayven, Hayvin.

HAVIVA. *Hebrew, 'well loved'.* An alternative to the more familiar Aviva. Havivah, Havviva, Havvivah.

HAYA. *Hebrew, 'life'.* Too close to 'Hi ya'.

♂ **HAYDEN.** *English, 'heather-grown hill'.* A newly successful surname for girls, which, like Brayden and Caden, used to be strictly for the boys.

HAYLEY. *English, 'hay field'.* It all started in 1946, when Hayley Mills was given her mother's maiden name. Now that spelling has been joined by Hailey and Haley, with all three adding up to a lot of babies with a similar name. Haeley, Haelie, Haely, Haile, Hailea, Hailee, Haileigh, Hailey, Hailie, Halea, Haleigh, Halle, Halleigh, Hallie, Hally, Hailee, Haily, Halee, Haleigh, Haley, Halie, Haylea, Haylee, Hayleigh, Hayli, Haylie.

★HAZEL. *English, 'the hazelnut tree'.* When Julia Roberts first named one of her twins Hazel, there was a great public outcry in the US against 'another one of those nutty celebrity names!' However we don't see why the fuss. After all, what's wrong with the pleasantly hazy, brownish-green-eyed, old-fashioned image created by this name. We predict more and more parents will want to share. **Hayzel, Hazell, Hazelle, Hazie, Hazyl, Hazzell. International: Aveline** *(French).*

HEA. *Korean, 'grace'.* For English speakers, a little too he for a she.

HEATHER. *Scottish botanical name.* This flower name was one of the most popular in her class in the 1970s and 1980s, but now, though still pretty and evocative of the Scottish moors, it's beginning to feel as dusty as a bouquet of dried flowers. **Hether.**

HEAVEN. *Word name.* Last year hundreds of little Heavens came down to earth in the US. Rap singer Lil' Mo has two daughters, Heaven and God'iss Love. Some parents have taken to using Neveah instead – Heaven spelled backwards. **Heavyn, Hevin.**

HEAVENLY. *Word name.* Turns the noun into an adoring adjective. **Heaven, Heavenlee, Heavenley, Heavynlie.**

HEDDA. *Scandinavian, diminutive of* HEDVIG. A card-carrying member of the league of older, slightly bohemian urban names like Nedda, Andra and Petra; also linked to Ibsen heroine *Hedda Gabler,* as well as being the basis of cruel joke names like Hedda Hare. **Heda, Hedde, Heddi, Heddie, Heddy, Hedi, Hedie, Hedy. International: Edda** *(Italian).*

HEDWIG. *German, 'war'.* Insurmountable teasing opportunities. **Hadwig, Hedda. Hedva, Hedvika, Hedy. International: Edwige** *(French),* **Edvige** *(Italian),* **Hedvig** *(Scandinavian),* **Jadwiga** *(Polish),* **Hedvika** *(Czech).*

HEDY. *Diminutive of* HEDWIG. Linked to one of the great screen beauties, but has never appealed much to the British. **Hedi.**

HEIDI. *Diminutive of* ADELHEID; *German, 'of noble birth'.* Despite decades of international Heidis of all sizes, shapes and personalities, the name seems permanently tethered to that spunky little girl on the Alpine mountaintop in the 1891 children's book and Shirley Temple film. **Heida, Heide, Heidey, Heidy, Hydee.**

HELAINE. *French variation of* HELEN. Like twins Helene and Elaine, a relic of the 1930s to 40s French Renaissance of names. **Helainne, Helayne.**

HELEN. *Greek, 'bright, shining one'.* A name that has connoted beauty since ancient times (the mythological 'face that launched a thousand ships'), Helen has moved in and out of favour over the centuries, often alternating with Ellen. Now, after being unfashionable for decades, we see signs of a comeback (it's the kind of serious, unadorned classic many parents are returning to).

Helen's International Variations

Irish	Ena, Ileene, Ilene, Léana
Scottish	Aileen, Eilidh
Welsh	Elen, Elin, Ellin
French	Héléne
Italian	Elena, Lina
Spanish	Alena, Elaina, Elena, Elina, Ilene, Ileana, Leonora
Basque	Nora
Portuguese	Elena, Eliana
Dutch	Leonora, Nel
German	Helena, Helene, Lele, Leni
Danish	Ellen, Elna
Swedish	Eleonora, Helena
Norwegian	Eli, Lene
Finnish	Aili, Helli, Ilona, Laina
Polish	Haliana, Halina
Hungarian	Helenka, Ilka, Ilona, Ilonka, Iluska
Romanian	Elena, Ileana
Czech	Elenka, Helena
Bulgarian	Elena
Russian	Alena, Alyena, Alyiona, Elena, Elina, Elya, Galina, Gayla, Halina, Jelena, Lelya, Lena, Leonora, Nelli, Nelya, Olenka, Yalena, Yelena
Ukrainian	Galena, Olena
Greek	Elena, Eleni, Helena, Hellae, Hellais, Lena
Estonian	Leena
Israeli	Eliora

HELENA. *(HELL-en-a) Greek, 'bright, shining one'.* This Shakespearean favourite, a more delicate and dainty version of Helen, is the preferred choice for those who find the classic version a bit bland.

HELENE. *French variation of* **HELEN.** Pronounced with an *een* – or an *aine* – sound at the end, a dated variation.

HELGA. *Scandinavian, 'prosperous, successful'.* Flat-footed and broad-bottomed. **Hella.** International: Helje *(Danish)* **Helge** *(Norwegian).*

HELIA. *Greek, 'sun'.* Most parents would prefer Delia, Lelia, or Amelia. **Heleah, Helya, Helyah.**

HÉLOÏSE. *French, 'famous warrior'.* This rather pretentious sounding French version of Eloise was borne by one of the most learned women of the Middle Ages. **Aloysia, Eloisa, Eloise, Heloisa.**

HELSA. *Danish, diminutive of* **ELIZABETH.** One of the least appealing of the Elizabeth nicknames.

HENRIETTA. *Feminine variation of* **HENRY.** Despite a return to such feminisations of male names as Josephine, Clementine and Theodora, starchy Henrietta has not made it into that group. Still, if you look hard enough, you'll see that Henrietta has the same vintage charm. **Etta, Ettie, Etty, Hanrietta, Hanriette, Harriet, Harrietta, Hatsie, Hatsy, Hattie, Hatty, Hen, Henia, Henie, Hennie, Henny, Hettie.** International: **Harriette, Henriette** *(French),* **Enrica** *(Italian and Spanish),* **Hendrika, Jetje, Rika** *(Dutch),* **Enrika, Heinricka, Henrika, Rike** *(German),* **Henrika** *(Swedish),* **Rikka** *(Finnish),* **Henka, Henrieta** *(Polish).*

HEPHZIBAH. *Hebrew, 'my delight is in her'.* A 'you can't do this to your daughter' name. **Hephziba, Hepzi, Hepzia, Hepziba, Hepzibah, Hesba.**

HERA. *(HEH-rah) Greek, 'protectress'.* She may have been queen of the Greek gods, but her name is wispy and wan.

HERMIONE. *(hehr-MY-o-nee) Greek, 'messenger, earthly'; feminine variation of* **HERMES.** Her costarring role in *Harry Potter* has made this previously ignored, stodgy name of the daughter of Venus and Mars suddenly viable, and it could really take off once today's children start having kids of their own. **Hermia, Hermina, Hermine, Herminia.**

♂ **HERO.** *Greek mythology name, English word name.* Gender confusion: the Hero in Greek myth was a woman.

HESTER. *Medieval variation of* **ESTHER.** Disgraced heroine of *The Scarlet Letter*'s name is so far out it might come back but only among those with the most adventurous (some would say reckless) tastes. **Hetti, Hettie, Hetty, Hestia.**

HETTIE. *English, diminutive of* **HENRIETTA.** It may take another generation or so, but this category of Hettie-Lettie-Lottie names could make a comeback.

HIALEAH. *Native American, Seminole, 'pretty prairie'.* It has

a pleasant sound but unlikely to find many takers.

♂ **HILARY, HILLARY.** *Latin, 'cheerful, happy'.* Hilary is strongly linked to Mrs Clinton in the US, making it difficult for Americans to see it as a baby name, which is not a problem in the UK. It has a rhythmic three-syllable structure, it's strong but light, proper but jaunty, with an irresistible meaning – having the same root as *hilarious.* **Hallarie, Hallary, Hilaree, Hilari, Hilarie, Hilery, Hillaree, Hillari, Hillarie, Hilleree, Hilleri, Hillerie, Hillery, Hillory.** International: **Hilaire** *(French),* **Ilaria** *(Italian).*

HILDA. *German, 'battle woman'.* Short for Brunhilda, the operatic Valkyrie of Teutonic legend, Hilda still retains that image. **Hildie, Hildy, Hylda.** International: **Hilde** *(German),* **Hilde** *(Scandinavian),* **Ildikó** *(Hungarian).*

HILDEGARDE. *German, 'comrade in arms'.* Unfortunate name that evokes a caricature of heavy, plodding, Teutonic stodginess. **Heidi, Hilda, Hildagard, Hilde, Hildegard, Hildie, Hildy.**

Stellar Starbabies Beginning with *H*

Hailie	Eminem
Hannah	Clive Owen, Vendela
Happy	Macy Gray
Harlow	Patricia Arquette
Hazel	Julia Roberts
Honey	Gail Porter
Honey Kinney	Jane Goldman & Jonathan Ross
Honor	Tilda Swinton

⚥ **HIMALAYA.** *Place name.* place name that suggests the highest heights and carries a hippyish aura.

HIROKO. *Japanese, 'generous, fair'.* Commonly used in Japanese families.

HJÖRDIS. *(HYOR-dis) Scandinavian, 'sword goddess'.* Pronunciation problems overwhelm this name.

♂ **HOLIDAY.** *Word name.* Free and fun name if you don't want to be pinned down to Noelle, Pasqua or Valentine. **Holidae, Holidaye, Holladay, Holliday, Holly.**

★♂ **HOLLAND.** *Dutch, place name.* One of the coolest geographical names, unadorned and elegant, evocative of fine Rembrandt portraits and fields of pink and yellow tulips.

HOLLIE. *A variation of* **HOLLY**. This spelling has been sliding down the Top 100 in recent years.

♂ **HOLLIS.** *English, 'dweller at the holly trees'.* Puts Holly into a 'dress-for-success' suit.

HOLLY. *Nature name.* Jolly, retains it's long-running popularity. **Hollee, Holleigh, Holley, Holli, Hollie, Hollye.**

⚥ **HONESTY.** *Word name.* Probably not the best (naming) policy. **Honestee, Honesti.**

HONEY. *Word name.* A new celebrity favourite.

★**HONOR.** *Virtue name.* A more pressured virtue name than Hope or Grace, placing a high standard on any girl carrying it, but it's a goal worth setting. **Honora, Honorata, Honorea, Honoria, Honorine, Honour, Nora, Norah, Noreen, Norine, Norrie, Nureen. International: Onóra** *(Irish Gaelic),* **Honore, Honoria Honorine** *(French),* **Honora, Honorata** *(Italian),* **Honorina** *(Filipino).*

HONORA. *Latin, 'woman of honor'.* Honora and Honoria are two ways of softening the severity of Honor, while retaining its righteous meaning. **Annora, Anora, Honour, Honorah, Honorata, Honoratas, Honoratia, Honoria, Honorina, Honorine, Honour, Onora, Nora, Norah, Norina.**

★**HOPE.** *Virtue name.* Can a name as virtuous as Hope be cool and trendy? Strangely enough – yes. But though this optimistic Puritan favourite is experiencing increasing popularity, it is too pure to be corrupted, a lovely classic that deserves all the attention it's getting.

HORATIA. *Latin feminine variation of* **HORATIO.** Has the fusty charm of recently excavated ancient Roman male names like Augustus and Magnus, which might just appeal to the fearless baby namer. **Horacia.**

HORTENSE. *Latin, 'of the garden'.* See **HEPHZIBAH.** **Hartinsia, Hortencia, Hortensia, Ortense.** International: **Ortensia** *(Italian).*

HOSHI. *Japanese, 'star'.* Short and catchy form of traditional Asian name.

HUALI. *Hawaiian, 'bright, polished, gleaming, unsullied'.* Evocative of hulas, leis and luaus.

HULDA. *Hebrew, 'mole'; Swedish, 'sweet, lovable'.* Hilda with a stuffed nose. **Huldah, Huldie.**

♂ **HUNTER.** *English, 'one who hunts'.* One of the trendy formerly male surname names, like Taylor and Carson, that sounded cool in the 1990s, but soon lost their edge.

HUYANA. *Native American, 'rain falling'.* A Miwok tribe name with a pleasant meaning.

HYACINTH. *Flower name.* Not as lovely as Lily or as gentle as Jasmine, Hyacinth still might hold some appeal for the parent seeking a truly exotic flower name. **Cintha, Cinthia, Cinthie, Cinthy, Hyacintha, Hyacinthe, Hyacinthia, Hyacinthie, Hyacintia.** International: **Giacinta** *(Italian),* **Jacinda, Jacinta** *(Spanish),* **Jakinda** *(Basque),* **Hyacinthe, Hyacynthe** *(Greek).*

♀ **IAN.** *Scottish variation of* **JOHN.** A boys' name with every possibility of crossing over. **Iaian, Iain, Iana, Iann, Ianna, Iannel, Iyana.**

IANTHE. *Greek, 'purple flower'.* An unusual, romantic, almost ethereal Greek name of the mythological daughter of Oceanus, supreme ruler of the seas, chosen by the poet Shelley for his daughter. **Iantha, Ianthina, Janthia.**

IBERIA. *Place name.* Spanish-Portuguese peninsula makes an exotic, unusual name. **Ibeeria.**

IDA. *German, 'industrious one'; English, 'prosperous, happy'; Norse, 'womanly'.* Many vowel names stylish a century ago are coming back, though Ida still sounds more old ladyish than Ada or Eva. **Eida, Eidah, Idah, Idaia, Idaleen, Idalene, Idalia, Idalina, Idaline, Idalis, Idaly, Idalya, Idalyne, Idamae, Idania, Idarina, Idarine, Idaya, Ideleen, Idelfa, Idelfia, Idell, Idella, Idelle, Idetta, Idette, Idys.**

International: **Ide** *(French)*, **Aida**, **Idalia** *(Italian)*, **Itka** *(Polish)*, **Iduska** *(Czech)*, **Ita** *(Yiddish)*.

IDALINA. *English elaboration of* **IDA**. Makes Ida more feminine but no more fashionable. **Idaleena, Idaleene, Idalena, Idalene, Idaline.**

IDINA. *English variation of* **EDINA**, *'from Edinburgh, Scotland'*. Has little to recommend it.

IDONY. *Norse, 'renewal'.* Idony was the Norse goddess of spring and eternal youth, and variants of her obscure name could come under consideration with the rest of the fashionable *I* pack. **Idona, Idonah, Idone, Idonea, Idonia, Idonie, Idonna, Idun, Iduna, Idunna.** International: **Idonea** *(Scottish)*, **Idonia** *(Spanish)*, **Idony** *(Slavic)*.

IDRA. *(ih-dra) Aramaic, 'fig tree'.* In ancient times, a fig tree was a symbol of learning, peace and prosperity.

IEESHA. *Variation of* **AISHA**. One of a legion of Americanised spellings of Aisha,

the name of the Prophet Muhammad's favourite wife. **Eyeesha, Ieachia, Ieaisha, Ieasha, Ieashe, Ieashia, Ieashiah, Ieeshah, Ieeshia, Ieisha, Ieishia, Iescha, Iesha, Ieshah, Ieshea, Iesheia, Ieshia, Iesha, Iisha, Iyisha, Iyishah, Yeesha.**

IGNACIA. *Latin, 'ardent, burning'.* No more attractive as a girls' name than in the male version, Ignatius. **Ignacie, Ignasha, Ignashia, Ignatia, Ignatzia, Ignazia, Iniga.**

IKEA. *(eye-KEE-uh* or *eye-KAY-uh) Word name.* Down-market version of the Chanel/Tiffany/Porsche brand-name-as-first idea. **Ikaisha, Ikeea, Ikeia, Ikeisha, Ikeishi, Ikeishia, Ikesha, Ikeshia, Ikeya, Ikeyia, Ikia, Ikiea, Ikiia.**

ILA. *French, 'from the island'.* A simple name occasionally heard a couple of generations back. **Eila, Ilanis, Ilanys, Isla.**

ILANA. *Hebrew, 'oak tree'.* A name with seemingly endless variations, well used in Israel, sometimes chosen for little girls born on the holiday of TuB'Shevat, the New Year of the Trees. **Elana, Elanit, Eleana,**

Eleanna, Ilaina, Ilainie, Ilane, Ilani, Ilania, Ilanit, Ileana, Ileanna, Iliana, Ilianna, Illana, Illane, Illani, Illania, Illanie, Illanit.

ILARIA. *Italian variation of* **HILARY**. This version offers a fresh and interesting alternative to Hilary.

ILENA. *(ill-AY-nuh) Greek variation of* **HELEN**. Ilena-style variants have all been considered more stylish than Helen for many years. **Ileana, Ileena, Ileina, Ilina, Ilyna.**

ILENE. *(eye-leen) Greek variation of* **HELEN**. Phonetic way to spell Aileen or Eileen. **Ilean, Ileen, Ileene, Iline, Ilyne.**

ILESHA. *Hindi, 'earth lord'.* Unusual choice that will undoubtedly be confused with similar and far more common names such as Alicia and Elissa.

ILIANA. *Greek, 'from Ilium or Troy'; Spanish variation of* **HELEN**. Ilium was the poetic name of the city of Troy, and variations of this name – especially Ileana and Ileanna –

have been widely used, projecting a rather bohemian image. **Ileana, Ileane, Ileanna, Ileanne, Ili, Ilia, Iliani, Illeanna, Illia, Illiana, Illiani, Illianna, Illyana, Illyanna.**

ILISA. *Scottish and English variation of* **ALISA** *and* **ELISA.** A spelling variant that's less appealing than the original. **Ilicia, Ilissa, Iliza, Illisa, Illissa, Illysa, Illyssa, Ilycia, Ilysa, Ilysia, Ilyssa, Ilyza.**

ILISE. *German variation of* **ELISE.** The *E* version is more attractive. **Ilese, Illyse, Ilyce, Ilyse.**

ILISHA. *Hebrew variation of* **ALISHA, ELISHA.** The relationship to *'ill'* makes this and similar names less pleasing than the versions that start with *A* or *E*. **Ileshia, Ilishia, Ilysha, Ilyshia.**

ILKA. *Hungarian, diminutive of* **ILONA**; *variation of* **HELEN.** To some, may have the same warm feeling of Russian nicknames like Sasha and Misha. **Ilke, Ilonka.**

♂ **ILLUMINATION.** *Word name.* Many-syllabled entrant in the new-fashioned virtue name group, doesn't stand much chance of rivaling shorter choices.

ILLUMINÉE. *French word name, 'illuminated'.* Illumination with a French accent.

ILONA. *Hungarian variation of* **HELEN.** Never used much elsewhere, not a likely candidate for success. **Elona, Ellona, Elonna, Ilka, Illona, Illone, Illonia, Illonya, Ilonka, Ilonna, Ilyona, Yllona, Ylonna.**

ILSA. *German variation of* **ELIZABETH.** Remembered as the radiant but tragic heroine of *Casablanca*. Spelled Ilse, it's having something of a European resurgence. **Ellsa, Elsa, Else, Illsa, Ilsae, Ilsaie, Ilse, Ilsey, Ilsie, Ilsy.**

ILUMINADA. *Spanish, 'illuminated'.* A distinctive, rhythmic and lovely Spanish name that suggests enlightenment. **Iluminada, Illuminata, Iluminata, Yluminata.**

IMA. *Japanese, 'present, now'; or variation of* **EMMA.** Frequently cited as an example of cruel baby naming, à la Ima Hogg.

♂ **IMAGINE.** *Word name.* If you like such uplifting New Age word names as Peace and Justice, the evocative and pretty Imagine should definitely be on your short list. **Imagination.**

IMALA. *Native American, 'strong-minded'.* Distinctive Native American choice with forceful meaning.

IMAN. *Arabic, 'faith'.* One of the best-known African names because of the Somali-born model and wife of David Bowie. **Aman, Eman, Imana, Imane, Imani.**

★**IMANI.** *Arabic, 'faith'.* Another strong Arabic name, this one is popular with parents throughout the Muslim world and would make a unique choice in other cultures.

IMARA. *Kiswahili, 'firm'.* Could make a hauntingly evocative name for an American child, striking the perfect

Names That Are Classic . . . but Not Boring

Beatrice

Celia

Cora

Cordelia

Delilah

Dorothea

Eliza

Flora

India

Julia

Juliet

Louisa

Nora

Patience

Serena

Sophia

Susannah

balance of the exotic and the familiar.

IMELDA. *Italian and Spanish from German, 'all-consuming fight'.* Saint's name made infamous by shoe-loving Philippine dictator's wife Imelda Marcos. **Amelda, Himaida, Imalda, Irmhilde, Melda, Ymelda.**

IMENA. *African, 'dream'.* Imani is a better choice in this vein. **Imee, Imene.**

IMMACULADA. *Spanish, 'immaculate'.* Even purer than Chastity . . . and as difficult, at least outside the Hispanic community. **Imacolata, Imaculada, Immaculata, Immacolata.**

★**IMOGEN.** *(IM-eh-jen) Celtic, 'maiden'.* Shakespearean name fashionable in England and strong in the Top 50; it lost its way in the US when spelled and pronounced *im-oh-GENE*. Said the British way, it's as pretty as it is distinctive. **Emogen, Emogene, Immy, Imogene, Imogenia, Imogine, Imojean, Imojeen, Innogen, Innogene.**

IMPERIA. *Latin 'imperial'.* Why not just name her Tyrannia? **Empress, Imperatrix.**

INA. *Latin, feminine suffix.* Used as an independent name, but doesn't your little girl deserve more? **Ena, Inanna, Inanne, Yna.**

INAYA. *Arabic, 'concerned'.* Unusual and exotic choice. **Anaya, Anayah, Enaya, Enayah, Inayah.**

INBAR. *(EEN-bar) Israeli, 'amber'.* Fashionable choice in Israel, also a place name there, not likely to succeed elsewhare.

★**INDIA.** *Place name.* One of the first and still one of the loveliest place names, exotic, euphonious and long stylish in England; it was used for a character in *Gone with the Wind,* and more recently it has been popular among trendy parents in urban areas. **Indea, Indeah, Indee, Indeia, Indeya, Indi, Indiah, Indian, Indiana, Indianna, Indie, Indieya, Indiya, Indio, Indy, Indya.**

♀ **INDIANA.** *Place name.* One of those American place names that sounds cooler than the place that inspired it. Instead consider India, which is at once simpler, more firmly rooted as a name, and more exotic.

★♂ INDIGO. *Colour name.* Colour names have joined flower and jewel names – in a big way – and this, a deep blue-purple dye from plants native to India, is particularly striking for both girls and boys.

INDIRA. *Sanskrit, 'beauty'.* Might have a more modern, exotic feel were it not for the somewhat middle-aged image of longtime Indian prime minister Indira Gandhi. **Indiara, Indeera, Indra, Indre, Indria.**

INDRE. *(IN-druh) Nature name.* The Indre is a river in France. Spelled Indra, it's the name of the supreme ruler (male, of course) of the Hindu gods. **Indra.**

INDU. *Hindi, 'moon'.* Truly unusual, though India or Indre might be easier-to-digest ways of getting a similar Eastern flavour.

INES, INEZ. *Spanish variation of* **AGNES.** This Spanish form of Agnes, the mother of Don Juan in the Byron poem, has a touch of mystery but has also been fully integrated into the British name pool. **International: Inesita, Inessa, Ynes, Ynesita, Ynez** *(Spanish),* **Inessa** *(Russsian),* **Annis, Annys** *(Greek).*

♂ INFINITY. *Word name.* A name that could have a long, bright future ahead of it. Spelled Infiniti, however, it's the name of a car.

INGA. *Norse, 'guarded by Ing'.* Ing was a powerful Norse god whose name inspired several modern variations – though this one has become a caricatured Scandinavian choice. **Ingaberg, Ingaborg, Inge, Ingeberg, Ingeborg, Ingela, Inngeborg. International: Inger** *(Slavic).*

★INGRID. *Norse, 'hero's daughter'.* The luminous Ingrid Bergman's appeal was strong enough to lend universal charisma to this classic Scandinavian name, which has been somewhat neglected elsewhere. **Inga, Ingaberg, Inge, Ingeborg, Inger.**

INOA. *Hawaiian, 'name chant'.* Evocative choice originating in the South Seas.

INOCENCIA. *Spanish, 'innocence'.* Few modern girls outside the Latino community would appreciate having to carry this name. **Innocencia, Innocenta, Inocenta, Inocentia, Ynocencia.**

INSPIRATION. *Word name.* Might inspire some as a middle name choice.

♂ INTEGRITY. *Word name.* Honor or True work better as names.

IO. *(ee-o or eye-o) Greek mythology name.* There aren't many two-letter names with as much substance as this Greek mythological example. **Eyo.**

IOANNA. *(yo-anna) Greek variation of* **JOANNA.** English-speaking tongues may have trouble wrapping themselves around three vowels. **Ioana, Ioanah, Ioani, Ioanna, Ioannah, Joanna, Yohanna.**

IOLA. *Greek variation of* **IOLE,** *'violet'.* Dated beyond redemption. **Iole, Iolee, Iolia.**

IOLANA. *Hawaiian, 'soaring like a hawk'.* Hip-swaying, melodic and unusual choice.

IOLANI. *Hawaiian, 'hawk of royalty'.* Feels quintessentially Hawaiian.

IOLANTHE. *(yo-lan-thuh) Greek, 'violet flower'.* Known through the Gilbert & Sullivan operetta of that name, could be a bit weighty; try Violet. **Iolanda, Iolande, Iolanta, Iolantha, Jolantha, Jolanthe, Yolanda, Yolantha, Yolanthe, Yolley, Yollie.**

IONA. *(eye-own-uh) Scottish place name.* This name of a small island off the coast of Scotland is trending upwards along with other *I* names.

IONE. *(eye-OWN) Greek, a violet-coloured stone.* This unusual Greek flower and colour name has gained attention via actress Ione Skye. **Ione, Ioney, Ioni, Ionia, Ionie, Iyona, Iyonna.**

IONIA. *(eye-own-ee-uh) Greek place name.* Also relating to the sea and the islands, this name is a bit more melodic than its cousins. **Eionia, Ionija, Ionya.**

IPHIGENIA. *(if-i-JEN-ee-uh) Greek, 'of royal birth'.* In mythology, Iphigenia was sacrificed by her father, Agamemnon – a difficult legacy to pass on to a daughter, and only one reason the name is hardly ever used. **Efigenia, Ephigenia, Ephigenie, Ifigenia, Iphigeneia, Iphigenie, Genia.**

♂ **IRA.** *Hebrew, 'watchful one'.* Ira for a girl? Yes, we consider it a good candidate for a gender switch, in light of tonal similarities with girl's names like Tyra and Keira. Annette Bening and Warren Beatty broke the ice by using this Old Testament male standard as the middle name of their daughter Isabel.

♂ **IRELAND.** *place name.* Kim Basinger and Alec Baldwin put this name on the map when they chose it for their daughter, saying that geographic names were a family tradition. Few have followed their lead.

IRENE. *Greek, 'peace'.* The name of the Greek goddess of peace was hugely popular in ancient Rome and again a hundred years ago, often pronounced then with three syllables. **Renie, Eirena, Eirene, Erena, Erene, Ireen, Iren, Irena, Irenee, Iriana, Iriena, Irin, Irine, Iryna, Reeni, Reeny, Rena, Rene, Reney, Reni, Renie.** International: **Eireen** *(Irish),* **Irenea** *(Spanish),* **Iren, Irenke** *(Hungarian),* **Irini** *(Romanian),* **Irenka, Irka** *(Czech),* **Arina, Arinka, Ira, Irena, Irina, Irini, Irisha, Iryna, Irya, Iryna, Jereni, Rina, Yarina, Yaryna** *(Russian),* **Eirene, Eirini, Ereni, Nitsa, Rena** *(Greek).*

IRIS. *Greek, 'rainbow'.* A faded flower name beginning to regain its appeal via celebrity power: Jude Law and Sadie Frost chose it for their daughter. **Irida, Iridianny, Irisha, Irissa, Irys, Iryssa.** International: **Irita** *(Spanish and Italian),* **Irisa** *(Russian).*

IRMA. *German, diminutive of several names, meaning 'universal, complete'.* Wears orthopedic shoes and support hose. **Erma, Ermengard, Irmgard, Irmgarde, Irmina, Irmine, Irminia.**

ISA. *German, 'strong-willed'; also diminutive of* **ISABEL.** With the new popularity of Isabel and Isabella, this form may become more familiar.

★**ISABEL, ISABELLE.** *Variations of* **ELIZABETH.** Both of these variations are staying firmly in the Top 50, a century after their first wave of success. Easy to see why: it's lady-like and melodic, traditional yet offbeat, and sounds smart as well as pretty. Only downside: so many other little Isabels, Isabelles, Isabellas, Belles and Bellas. **Bel, Belita, Bell, Bella, Belle, Ib, Ibbie, Ibby, Isa, Isabal, Isabele, Isabeli, Isabell, Issi, Issie, Issy, Izzie, Izzy, Sabella, Sabelle. International: Isibéal** *(Irish Gaelic),* **Iseabal, Iseabail, Ishbel, Isobel** *(Scottish),* **Isabeau, Isabelle** *(French),* **Isabella** *(Italian),* **Isabelita, Ysabel, Ysabella, Ysabelle** *(Spanish),* **Isa, Isobel, Isobella, Isobelle** *(German),* **Iza, Izabel** *(Polish),* **Bela, Bella, Izabela, Izabele, Izbel** *(Russian),* **Zobel** *(Armenian),* **Isibeal** *(Hebrew).*

ISABELLA. *Spanish and Italian variation of* **ELIZABETH.** Isabella is the real superstar

of the 'Isabel' group, and like Isabel and Isabelle, it has also made a strong appearance in the Top 50 in recent years. It's more feminine than Isabel, though some might find it too ornate.

★**ISADORA.** *Latin, 'gift of Isis'.* Why is Isabella megapopular while Isadora goes virtually ignored? Too close a tie with tragic modern dancer Isadora Duncan, perhaps, or with fusty male version Isidore. But we think it's worth reevaluating as an Isabella alternative. Quirky couple singer Björk and artist Matthew Barney did just that. **Isidora, Izadora, Ysadora.**

♂ **ISAK.** *(EE-sak) Scandinavian variation of* **ISAAC.** When the Danish author Karen Blixen chose Isak Dinesen as her male pseudonym, she set a precedent that could well be followed today.

ISAURA. *Greek place name.* This name of an ancient country may be too exotic. **Aura, Isa, Isaure.**

ISHA. *(eye-sha) Variation of* **AISHA.** One of the more

If You Like Isabella,
You Might Love . . .

Alessandra
Allegra
Anastasia
Angelica
Arabella
Christiana
Clementina
Cressida
Eliana
Engracia
Estella
Francesca
Gabriella
Julietta
Liliana
Mirabella
Raffaela
Tatiana

wishy-washy spellings. **Ishae, Ishana, Ishanaa, Ishanda, Ishanee, Ishaney, Ishani, Ishanna, Ishaun, Ishawna, Ishaya, Ishenda, Ishia, Iysha.**

Stellar Starbabies Beginning with *I*

Ida	Dolph Lundgren
Imogen	Julian Sands
India	Sarah McLachlan
Ireland	Kim Basinger & Alec Baldwin
Iris	Sadie Frost & Jude Law
Isa	Michael Bolton
Isabel	Annette Bening & Warren Beatty
Isabella	Nicole Kidman & Tom Cruise, Matt Damon, Lorenzo Lamas, Jane Leeves, Lou Diamond Phillips
Isadora	Björk & Matthew Barney
Iset	Wesley Snipes
Italia	LL Cool J

ISHANA. *Hindi, 'desire'.* Pretty Asian option. **Ishani.**

ISHI. *Japanese, 'stone'.* Connotes a strong, solid character. **Ishiko, Ishiyo, Shiko, Shiyo.**

ISIS. *Egyptian, 'supreme goddess'.* The name of the supreme Egyptian goddess of the moon and fertility is being revived by feminists and others willing to cross into arcane territory.

ISLA. *(eye-la) Scottish place name.* The name of a Scottish river, an island (spelled Islay), and hot actress Isla Fisher. It's now in the Top 100. **Isela, Islay.**

ISMAY. *Variation of* **ESMÉ.** The rise of the Isabel names may give a boost to this variation, which has a sunny, springtime feel.

ISOBEL. *Scottish variation of* **ISABEL.** Using this genuine old Scottish spelling might give this popular Top 100 name personal meaning.

ISOLDE. *Welsh, 'fair lady'.* Now that Tristan has been rediscovered, maybe it's time for his fabled lover in medieval legend and Wagnerian opera, a beautiful Irish princess, to be brought back into the light as well. **Iseult, Isold, Isolt, Isolte, Isottotte, Yseult, Yseuhe, Yseut, Ysolda, Ysolde, Ysotte.** **International: Esylit** *(Welsh),* **Isotta** *(Italian),* **Isolda** *(Spanish).*

ITA. *(ee-ta) Irish, 'thirst'.* Medieval saint's name used in Ireland but hardly worth importing.

★**ITALIA.** *Italian place name.* Authentic, exotic, melodic place name for the adventurous, chosen by rapper LL Cool J for his daughter. **Itali, Italie, Italina, Italy, Italya.**

ITHACA. *Place name.* The island home of Odysseus, and city site of Cornell University in the US, sounds soft and pleasant enough to make it a candidate for babynamehood.

ITZEL. *Spanish, 'protected'.* Surprisingly popular, primarily among Hispanic parents. **Itcel, Itchel, Itsesel, Itsel, Itssel, Itza, Itzallana, Itzayana, Itzell, Ixchel.**

IVANA. *Feminine variation of* **IVAN.** A rarely used Slavic name until the Czech-born ex–Mrs Trump took it over the top. Daughter's name Ivanka adds a dollop of charm. **Iva, Ivanah, Ivania, Ivanka, Ivanna, Ivannia, Ivany.**

IVARA. *German, 'yew tree, archer'.* Similar to Ivana but less personality-driven. **Ivernah.**

IVETTE. *French variation of* YVETTE. Feels more modern than the *Y* version but also less authentic. **Ivet, Ivete, Iveth, Ivetha, Ivett, Ivetta.**

IVONNE. *French variation of* YVONNE. The *I* freshens up this name. **Ivon, Ivona, Ivone, Ivonna, Iwona, Iwonka, Iwonna, Iwonne.**

IVORY. *Word name.* Ivory was last popular a hundred years ago – oddly, more for boys (à la Keenen Ivory Wayans) than girls. No serious comeback in sight for either sex. **Ivoory, Ivoreen, Ivori, Ivorie, Ivorine, Ivree.**

IVRIA. *Hebrew, 'from the land of Abraham'.* Perhaps to honour an ancestral Abraham, but presents a confusing image. **Ivriah, Ivrit.**

★**IVY.** *Nature name.* Quirky, offbeat, energetic century-old name enjoying the beginnings of a deserved revival. The clinging vine has an interesting history: ancient Greeks presented an ivy wreath to newly-weds as a symbol of fertility. And no, don't worry about 'poison ivy' teasing. **Ivee, Ivey, Ivi, Ivie, Ivye.**

IYABO. *African, Yoruba, 'mother has returned'.* Striking, but sounds a bit masculine.

IYANA. *Modern invented name.* A new name with an African accent and a New Age feel that's been on the popularity charts in the US, related to cousins Aiyana and Ayanna. **Aiyana, Aiyanna, Eiyana, Eiyanna, Iyania, Iyanla, Yanna.**

IZABELLA. *Variation of* **ISABELLA.** Parents seeking a way to differentiate their Isabella from all the others could consider this fresher spelling.

IZARA. *African, Hausa, 'section of tree'.* Attractive, rhythmic, exotic choice.

IZUSA. *Native American, 'white stone'.* Highly unusual; could be confused with the Isuzu automotive brand.

J *girls*

JACARANDA. *Spanish flower name.* Distinctive and charming nature name that blends elements of Jacqueline and Amanda. **Jacarannda, Jakaranda.**

JACELYN. *Modern invented name.* A possible, and not too successful, attempt to individualise Jocelyn or formalise Jacey.

JACEY. *Modern invented name.* Spelled-out combination of initials *J* and *C* doesn't make it much classier. **Jace, Jacee, Jaci,**

Jacie, Jacy, Jaice, Jaicee, Jaycee, Jayci, Jaycie.

★JACINTA. *(hah-SEEN-tah) Spanish for Greek flower name, 'hyacinth'.* This Spanish word for Hyacinth is a lot softer and sweeter than the English version. **Giacinda, Giacintha, Giacinthia, Hacinthia, Jacenda, Jacenta, Jacinda, Jacindia, Jacinna, Jacinta, Jacinth, Jacintha, Jacyntha, Jacynthe, Jacynthia, Jecinda. International: Hyacinthe, Jacinthe** *(French),* **Jacenty** *(Polish).*

JACOBA. *Hebrew, feminine variation of* JACOB. Now that Jacob has been the top boys' name for several years, this may come to the fore, the way Michaela did after Michael's long reign as a popular boy's name. **Jacobine, Jakoba, Jakobe. International: Jacobella** *(Italian),* **Diega** *(Spanish),* **Jakobe** *(Scandinavian),* **Jakobe, Jakube** *(Polish),* **Akiba, Akiva** *(Arabic).*

JACOBINA. *Hebrew, feminine variation of* JACOB. Another, more feminine, female form of Jacob sometimes heard in

Scotland. **Jacobetta, Jacobette, Jacobine, Jacobyna, Jakobina, Jakobine.**

JACQUELINE. *French, feminine diminutive of* JACQUES. To most people, this French name is reminiscent of the Kennedy era and its elegant First Lady, although it's lost much of its glamorous image and Gallic gloss. **Jacalin, Jacalyn, Jackaline, Jackalinne, Jackelyn, Jacketta, Jackette, Jacki, Jackie, Jacklin, Jacklyn, Jacklynn, Jacklynne, Jackqueline, Jacky, Jaclin, Jaclyn, Jacolyn, Jacqualine, Jacqualyn, Jacquel, Jacquelean, Jacquelin, Jacquella, Jacquelle, Jacquelyn, Jacquelynn, Jacquelynne, Jacquenette, Jacquette, Jacqui, Jacquine, Jaculine, Jakelyn, Jaquelin, Jaqueline, Jaquelyn, Jaquith, Zacqueline, Zakelina, Zhakelina, Zhaqueline. International: Jacquetta, Jacquie** *(French),* **Jaquetta** *(Italian),* **Jacquenetta** *(Swiss),* **Jakolina** *(East European).*

JADA. *(JADE-a) Spanish, 'jade'.* Long used in Spanish-speaking countries, it is a strong but feminine name. **Jadah,**

Jadeh, Jadia, Jaeda, Jaedah, Jaida, Jaidah, Jayda, Jaydah.

★JADE. *Jewel name.* As cool as the green stone said to transmit wisdom, clarity, justice, courage, and modesty, Jade rose in popularity when Mick and Bianca Jagger chose it for their daughter in 1971. Downside: the Big Brother celebrity. **Jada, Jadira, Jadra, Jaida, Jayda, Jayde, Jaydra, Zhade. International: Giada** *(Italian).*

♂ JADEN. *Spelling variation of* JADON. From obscure male biblical boy's name to unisex favourite, Jadon/Jaden, in all its variations, has had a meteoric rise in popularity, building on Jade and Jada, plus the trendy *en* ending. **Jadeen, Jadena, Jadene, Jadeyn, Jadin, Jadine, Jadyn, Jadynn, Jaeden, Jaiden, Jaidyn, Jaidynn, Jayden, Jaydyn, Jaydynn.**

JADINE. *Modern invented name.* Unusual and unfashionable name, found in Toni Morrison's novel *Tar Baby.* **Jadean, Jadeane, Jadeen, Jadeene, Jadyne.**

JADYN. *See* JADEN.

JAEDA. *Arabic, 'goodness' or 'long-necked beauty'.* Both an independent name and an alternate spelling of Jada. Jada, Jawda, Jaydra, Jayeda, Jaide.

♂ JAEL. *(yah-el) Hebrew, 'mountain goat'.* This attractive Old Testament option is the name of a place in northern Israel. Jaelle, Jayel, Jayil, Yael.

JAELYN. *Modern invented name.* An extremely feminised spelling of Jalen.

JAFFA. *(YA-fa) Hebrew place name, 'beautiful'.* A pleasant and adaptable place name for a part of Tel Aviv. Jafa, Jaffe, Jafit, Jafita, Joppa, Yafa, Yaffa, Yaffah, Yafit.

JAIDA. *See* JADA.

JAIDEN, JAIDYN. *See* JADEN.

JAILYN. *See* JALEN.

♂ JAIME. *Spanish variation of* JAMES. Though every Spanish student knows that the male classic is pronounced *HY-me,* for girls this is a straight homonym for Jamie, a favourite ambisexual

1970s nickname name. Another way to think of it is as a variation of the French 'J'aime' (I love). Jaimee, Jaimelynn, Jaimi, Jaimie, Jamee, James, Jamey, Jami, Jamia, Jamie, Jamilyn, Jayme, Jaymee, Jaymie.

JAKAYLA. *Modern invented name.* This name can be seen as either an elaboration of Kayla or a hybrid of Jacqueline and Makayla.

JALA. *Arabic, 'great, illustrious'.* Simple, pretty and delicate. Jalaa.

JALAJAA. *Hindi, 'a lotus'.* Intriguing, although vowel-intensive.

JALEESA. *Modern invented name.* Popular in the US since the 80s. Geleexa, Ja Leesa, Ja Lisa, Jaleisa, Jalisa, Jaliza, Jilleesa, Jilleisa, Joleesa, Joleisa.

♂ JALEN. *Modern invented name.* A current creation used far more for boys at this point. Jailen, Jalyn, Jalynn, Jaylen, Jaylin, Jaylinn, Jaylyn, Jaylynn.

JALILA. *Arabic, 'illustrious'.* The two *l*'s in this Arabic name give it a particularly rich

---

⊶━━◉

Truly Unisex Names

Alex

Brady

Casey

Devon

Dylan

Evan

Jaden

Jess

Jordan

Lane

Payton

Riley

Rory

Rowan

Sam

Taylor

---

rhythmic quality. Galīla, Galilah, Jalilah.

JALYN. *See* JALEN.

★JAMAICA. *Place name.* Among the least gimmicky, most appealing and colourful of all the names found in the atlas, Jamaica almost sings out the exotic rhythms of the West

Indies. Namesake: writer Jamaica (born Elaine) Kincaid. **Jamaeca, Jamaika, Jemaica, Jemayka.**

♂ **JAMES.** *Hebrew, 'supplanter'.* For a girl? Why not? This is one of the traditional male names most adoptable for girls – it's already been used as a pet name for some Jamies.

JAMESINA. *Feminine variation of* **JAMES.** Although it is more grown up than Jamie, it is still an awkward name to pronouce. If you don't like Jamie, try Jameson . . . or James. **Jamesetta, Jamesette.**

★**JAMESON.** *English, 'son of James'.* Stylish surname way to go if you want to name a girl after a James, and is more substantial than the passé Jamie; it was chosen for their daughter by Chynna Phillips and Billy Baldwin. **Jamison.**

♂ **JAMIE.** *Scottish, diminutive of* **JAMES.** Typical of the relaxed unisex names that seemed so cool in the 1960s after decades of Jeans and Joans, now pretty tepid. **Jaime, Jaimee, Jaimey, Jaimi, Jaimie, Jaimy,** Jama, Jamee, Jamei, Jamese, Jami, Jammie, Jayme, Jaymee, Jaymie.

JAMILA, JAMILLA. *Arabic, 'beautiful, graceful'.* Soft and appealing, with a whiff of vanilla. **Jameela, Jameelah, Jameila, Jamilah, Jamilla, Jamille, Jamillia, Jamillie.**

JAMISON. *See* **JAMESON.**

JAMYA. *Modern invented name.* A mysterious name found in fantasy fiction and climbing in popularity as a combination of Jamie and Tanya.

♂ **JAN.** *Feminine variation of* **JOHN.** Very *Brady Bunch*. **Jana, Janah, Janina, Janine, Jann, Janna, Jannah.**

JANA. *(YAH-nah or JAN-ah) Czech, feminine variation of* **JAN.** A sweet name with many cross-cultural ties, popular in the Slavic countries, Holland, Scandinavia and Ireland. **Iana, Janaya, Janayah, Janna, Jannah, Yana, Yanna.**

JANAE. *(Ja-NAY) American, modern elaboration of* **JANE** *or* **JAN.** Adds a soupçon of French flair to some old classics with the currently trendy *ae* ending. **Janay, Janea, Jenae, Jenay, Jenea, Jenee, Jennae, Jennay, Jinae, Jinnea.**

JANAN. *(jah-NAHN) Arabic, 'heart, soul'.* One of several similar unpretentious but undistinguished names. **Janaan, Jinan.**

★**JANE.** *English, 'God's gracious gift'.* Far from plain in this day of trendy Jadens and Jaylas, Jane has risen above its old generic status (Jane Doe, G.I. Jane) to become a standout. For a venerable and short one-syllable name, it still packs a surprising punch. **Jaine, Jainee, Jan, Jananelle, Janaya, Janaye, Janean, Janeane, Janee, Janeen, Janel, Janela, Janelba, Janella, Janessa, Janet, Janeta, Janeth, Janetta, Janette, Janey, Jani, Jania, Janice, Janicia, Janie, Janina, Janine, Janis, Janise, Jannette, Jayne, Jayni, Jaynie, Jennice, Joni, Jonni, Juanetta, Juanisha, Juanita.**

JANEANE. *Spelling variation of* **JANINE,** *a variation of* **JANE.** It could be pronounced *ja-NEEN*, which makes this one of the more confusing versions.

JANELLE. *American, modern elaboration of* **JANE.** Far cooler to drop the first syllable and go for Elle. **Janelba, Janell, Jannelle, Janely, Janiella, Janielle, Jenell, Jenelle, Jinella, Jinelle, Johnelle, Jonelle.**

JANET. *Diminutive of* **JANE.** Grandma Janet's knitting booties for baby Janae. **Janeta, Janetta, Janette, Jannet, Jannetta, Janit, Janot, Jenetta, Jenette, Jennet, Jennette, Jinnet, Jinnett.** International: **Janneth** *(Scottish),* **Sioned** *(Welsh),* **Gianetta** *(Italian),* **Zaneta** *(Russian).*

JANIAH. *See* **JANIYAH.**

JANICA. *Variation of Scandinavian* **JANNIK,** *'God is gracious'.* With its upbeat Slavic/Scandinavian air, it has the most potential of all the *Jan* names.

JANICE. *Variation of* **JANE.** For a minute or two this sounded more modern than Janet, now equally outmoded. **Janess, Janessa, Janiece, Janis,**

Jane's International Variations

Irish Gaelic	Sine, Siobhán, Sinéad
Irish	Shawn, Sheena, Shena, Shevaun
Scottish Gaelic	Sinéidin, Seónaid, Siubhan
Welsh	Siân
French	Jeanne, Jehanne
Italian	Gianna, Giannetta, Giannina, Giovanna
Spanish	Juana, Juanita, Nita
Basque	Jone, Yoana
Dutch	Johanna, Jonna
German	Hanne, Hansine, Johanna, Jutta
Danish, Norwegian	Jensine, Johanna
Finnish	Jaana, Janne
Polish	Jama, Janina, Jasia, Joanka, Joasta, Zannz
Hungarian	Janka, Zsanett
Romanian	Jenica
Czech	Hana, Ivana, Ivancka, Ivanka, Jana, Janica, Janka, Jenka, Johana, Johanka, Johanna
Russian	Ioanna, Ivanna, Zhanna
Slavic	Iva, Ivana, Ivanka
Latvian	Zanna
Greek	Ioanna
Armenian	Ohanna
Hebrew	Jans
Tongan	Seini

Janise, Jannice, Jannis, Janyce, Jenice, Jeniece, Jenise.

JANINE. *French variation of* **JANE.** Has lost all trace of its French accent.

JANIS. *Variation of* **JANE.** Its last moment of glory was in the Janis Joplin 1960s. **International: Janes** *(Dutch, Danish, Swedish, Norwegian and Finnish)*, **Januszy** *(Slavic)*.

JANIYA. *Modern invented name.* One of the newer names to appear on US African-American popularity lists. **Janiah.**

JANKA. *(YAHN-kah) Hungarian variation of* **JANE.** Not likely to succeed here because of the 'yanking' association. Ouch.

JANNA. *(YAH-neh) Dutch contraction of* **JOHANNA.** Could run into pronunciation confusion. **Jana. International: Jannat** *(Persian)*.

♂ **JANUARY.** *Word name.* If Afternoon, Early, Christmas and October are now seen as conceivable choices, why not January?

♂ **JANVIER.** *(zhan-vee-air) French word name, 'January'.* Used in France as a male name, this would make an appealing and unusual choice, as would two other Gallic month names, Avril and Mai. **Januaria, Janvière.**

JARAH. *Hebrew, 'honey'.* Possible alternative to Sarah, although the *jar* part might prove jarring.

JARITA. *Hindi-Sanskrit, 'mother' or 'legendary bird'.* Delicate and lacy, with less emphasis on the *jar* syllable.

JASMINE. *Persian flower name.* After the 1992 release of Disney's *Aladdin,* featuring Princess Jasmine, this delicate and aromatic flower name burst into popularity – highly unusual for an animated character. It's remained in the Top 50 in recent years, propagating a garden of spelling variations. **Jasmeen, Jasmina, Jasminda, Jasmyn, Jasmyne, Jassamayn, Jassi, Jazan, Jazmaine, Jazmin, Jazmina, Jazmine, Jazmon, Jazz, Jazzie, Jazzmin, Jazzmine, Jazzmon, Jazzmyn, Jazzmynn, Jessamina, Jessamine, Jessamyn,** Jessimine, Yashmine, Yasmeen, Yasmia, Yasminia, Yazmin, Yazz, Yazzi, Yazzie. **International: Jasmin** *(French)*, **Gelsomina** *(Italian)*, **Yasemin** *(Turkish)*, **Yasmin, Yasmina, Yasmine** *(Arabic)*, **Yasamin** *(Iranian)*, **Yasiman** *(Hindi)*.

♂ **JAY.** *Latin, 'jaybird'.* One of the boys' names newly appropriated for girls – either on its own, as a pet form of any *J* name or as a singular middle name. **Jae, Jai, Jaya, Jaycie, Jaye, Jey.**

JAYA. *Hindi-Sanskrit, 'victory'.* This exotic name of a Buddhist goddess, a possible alternative to the trendy Maya, was chosen for their daughter by Laura Dern and Ben Harper.

JAYCEE. *See* **JACEY.**

JAYDA. *See* **JADA.**

JAYDEN. *See* **JADEN.**

JAYLA. *Modern invented name.* Not quite as unusual as it might seem – there were a number of baby Jaylas born recently in the US.

JAYLEEN, JAYLENE. *Modern invented name.* The kind of countrified name that went out with ruffled gingham pinafores. **Jaleen, Jalene, Jaline, Jalynn, Jayelene, Jayleana, Jaylee, Jaylen, Jaylin, Jayline, Jaylyn, Jaylynn.**

JAYNE. *Variation of* **JANE.** Unplain (if dated) Jane.

JAZ. *Diminutive of* **JASMINE.** This abbreviated form chosen by tennis greats Steffi Graf and Andre Agassi couldn't be jazzier. **Jazz.**

JAZLYN. *Modern invented name.* One trendy syllable plus another trendy syllable does not usually, despite parents' best efforts, add up to a truly creative name.

JAZMIN, JAZMINE. *See* **JASMINE.**

JAZMYN, JAZMYNE. *See* **JASMINE.**

JEAN. *English and Scottish, from French variation of* **JOHANNA.** Jean was popular in Scotland long before it found favour elsewhere, and had its most shining moment elsewhere in the era of Jean Harlow, ultimate symbol of silver screen glamour, but now, though there are many grandmas and even mums with the name, it doesn't seem very baby-friendly. **Gene, Geni, Jeana, Jeane, Jeanee, Jeaneen, Jeanelle, Jeanene, Jeanetta, Jeanette, Jeanie, Jeanine, Jeannette, Jeannie, Jeanique, Jeanna, Jeanneen, Jeannine, Jeannique, Jenette, Jenica, Jennet, Jennetta, Jennine.** International: **Sina, Sine** *(Irish Gaelic),* **Jennice** *(Scottish Gaelic),* **Jeanne** *(French),* **Janne** *(Finnish),* **Jana, Janina, Janka, Janeska, Jasia, Jena, Jonna Nina** *(Polish),* **Ivana** *(Slavic),* **Jana** *(Latvian).*

JEANETTE. *French, diminutive of* **JEANNE.** Relic of a past period of French favourites, out to pasture with Claudette and Paulette. **Jeanett, Jeannette, Jennett, Jenette, Netti, Nettie.**

JEANNE. *French variation of* **JEAN.** *See* **JEAN.**

JEANNIE. *Diminutive of* **JEAN.** One-time girl next door – and dream girl – name has followed mama Jean down the ladder and out of the picture. **Jeanie.**

JEANNINE. *Variation of* **JEAN.** Passé. **Ganeen, Janene, Janine, Jannina, Jannine, Jeanine, Jeneen, Jenine, Jennine, Jineen.**

JELENA. *(yay-LAY-nuh) Russian variation of* **HELEN.** Pretty, but elsewhere it might simplify a child's life to use Helena or Elena. **Galina, Yelena.**

★**JEMIMA.** *Hebrew, 'dove'.* This name of a strong and beautiful Biblical daughter of Job has long been among the chicest choices of the aristocratic British – think Jemima Khan, rather than Jemima Puddle-duck. It is an excellent name, with its peaceful meaning. **Jamima, Jem, Jemi, Jemimah, Jemma, Jemmie, Jemmimah, Jemmy, Mima, Mimma.**

JEMINI. *Contemporary spelling of* **GEMINI.** *See* **GEMINI.**

JEMMA. *Spelling variation of* **GEMMA.** Jenna is overheated, but Jemma is still cool.

Russian Names

Alla	Mika
Amaliya	Mikhaila
Anastasia	Nadya
Dariya	Natalya
Dominika	Natasha
Duscha	Nelya
Fanya	Nika
Feodora	Olga
Galina	Roksana
Ivanna	Roza
Izabella	Sariya
Jelena	Stefanya
Jelina	Tatiana
Katarina	Valentina
Kira	Valya
Larisa	Varvara
Luiza	Viera
Marina	Viveka
Mariya	Yana
Marya	Zhanna
Masha	Zoya

JEMSA. *(HEM-sah) Spanish, 'gem, precious stone'.* One of the less euphonious of the international jewel cartel.

JENA. *(JAY-NAH) Sanskrit, 'patience'.* It can also be pronounced *jen-a;* either way it's a perfectly pleasant name. **Jenah, Jenai, Jenay, Jenea.**

JENELLE. *Variation of* **JEAN.** Combination of two long-popular syllables. **Janel, Janell, Jenella, Jennal.**

JENESSA. *Modern invented name.* This newer sounding coalition of Jennifer and Vanessa is gaining in popularity. **Gianessa, Janessa, Jenesa, Jenessia, Jennesa, Jennessa, Jinessa.**

JENICA. *Romanian variation of* **JANE.** If you can't decide between Jennifer and Jessica. **Jeneca, Jenika, Jenikka, Jennica, Jennika.**

JENIFRY. *Cornish variation of the Welsh name* **GWENFREWI,** *'white peace'.* This Celtic saint's name is the most offbeat *Jen* name of all.

JENNA. *English, diminutive of* **JENNIFER.** It was first noted on the 1980s TV series *Dallas,* and Jenna is still being used – however it no longer feels much fresher than Jennifer. **Jena, Jennah.**

JENNIE. *Diminutive of* **JANET, JANE, JEAN,** *and* **JENNIFER.** Long before the Jennifer Era, Jennie was a fashionable pet form of several names. It was replaced by the Jenny spelling in the 1960s, and the *ie* spelling is rarely seen today. **Jen, Jenee, Jeni, Jenne, Jennee, Jenney, Jenni, Jenny.**

JENNIFER. *Cornish variation of Welsh* **GUINEVERE.** There were thousands of baby Jennifers born in the 1970s, making it one of the top names of the decade – no wonder there are now online support groups for grown-up Jens who have suffered a lack of personal identity. These days it's no longer even in the Top 100. **Geniffer, Genn, Genna, Genni, Gennie, Gennifer, Genniver, Genny, Ginnifer, Jen, Jena, Jenae, Jenalee, Jenalyn, Jenefer, Jenessa, Jenetta, Jeni, Jenifer, Jeniffer, Jenita, Jenn, Jenna, Jennefer, Jenna, Jennee, Jennelle, Jenni, Jennica, Jennie, Jennika, Jennipher, Jennis, Jenniver, Jenny, Jinnifer. International: Genoveffa,**

Ginevra *(Italian)*, **Genoveva** *(Spanish)*, **Genowefa** *(Polish)*.

♂ **JENNISON.** *English surname.* Brings Jennifer into the twenty-first century.

JENNY. *Diminutive of* **JANET, JANE, JEAN** *and* **JENNIFER.** At the height of the Jennifer craze, many parents were cutting straight to the nickname and putting Jenny on the birth certificate, but now that Jennifer is the mum rather than the daughter, Jenny, which has been somewhat replaced by Jenna, has faded as well. **Jen, Jenee, Jennee, Jenney, Jenni, Jennie, Jeny.**

♂ **JENSEN.** *Scandinavian, 'son of Jens'.* The number one surname in Denmark could make a sophisticated and stylish girl's name.

JENSINE. *(YEN-seen) Danish, 'God is gracious'.* Sure to be mispronounced.

♂ **JERICHO.** *Biblical place name.* The scope of biblical names has expanded to include sacred place names, and this makes a plausible possibility,

although it does have a masculine feel.

♂ **JERSEY.** *Place name.* An established feminine place name that sounds more appealing when you attach it to the British Isles than to the American state.

JERUSHA. *(jeh-ROO-sha) Hebrew, 'the married one, a possession'.* Old Testament name with a Russian accent. **Jarusha, Jeruscha, Jerushah.**

JESS. *Short form of* **JESSICA.** Unlike Bess or Tess, rarely used on its own.

JESSA. *Short form of* **JESSICA.** Rare streamlined form of Jessica.

★**JESSAMINE.** *(JEH-sah-meen) French, 'jasmine flower'.* Charming name occasionally heard over here, that would really stand out elsewhere. **Jessamy, Jessamyn.**

JESSICA. *Hebrew, 'God sees,' 'wealthy'.* When Jennifer was ready to give up her throne, her crown was passed to Jessica, who reigned for not one but two decades – it was the top name

of both the 1980s and 90s, never sounding as trendy as its predecessor, maybe because of its classic Shakespearean pedigree. It is still a favourite, resting comfortably among the Top 5 in recent years. **Jennica, Jesica, Jesika, Jess, Jessa, Jessaca, Jessaka, Jessalin, Jessaline, Jessalyn, Jessca, Jesse, Jesseca, Jessey, Jessi, Jessicka, Jessie, Jessika, Jessiqua, Jesslyn, Jessy, Jessyca, Jessyka, Jezeka, Jezica, Jezika, Jezyca.** International: **Gessica** *(Italian)*, **Janka** *(Hungarian)*, **Iekika** *(Hawaiian)*.

JESSIE. *Diminutive of* **JESSICA.** Jessie has never been used as much as Jennie/Jenny, partly because it's a boys' name as well (spelled Jesse), but it does have a friendly and unpretentious, pioneer feel. **Jess, Jessa, Jesse, Jessee, Jessey, Jessi, Jessy, Jessye.**

JETHRA. *Hebrew, feminine variation of* **JETHRO.** Rare and ethereal.

JETTA. *English, 'jet'.* Although this is a legitimate name, most people would associate it with a line of Volkswagens – you'd be better off choosing a Mercedes. **Jet, Jeta, Jetia, Jette, Jettie.**

JETTE. *(YET-teh) German and Scandinavian, 'jet'.* If pronounced correctly, too similar to the unlovable Yetta.

JEUNE. *French word name, 'young'.* But what happens when Jeune grows *vieille?*

JEWEL. *Word name.* As Flora is for botanicals, Jewel is the generic gemstone name, not used much since the early twentieth century, when it was seen as a symbol of how precious a daughter could be. The French version, Bijou, feels more modern, as do Pearl and Ruby. **Jewell, Jewella, Jewelle, Juel, Jule.**

JEZEBEL. *Hebrew, 'impure, wicked'.* Biblical bad girl: not suitable for children. **Izavel, Jesibel, Jessabel, Jessabell, Jessebel, Jessebell, Jetzabel, Jez, Jezabel, Jezabella, Jezebela, Jezebell, Jezebelle, Jezibel, Jezibela, Jezibella, Jezibelle, Jezybell, Jezzybell.**

JILL. *Diminutive of GILLIAN or JULIANA.* Probably due to its nursery rhyme association, Jill has the perpetual air of a rosy-cheeked tot – even though its roots go back to the Middle Ages. Odds are against Jill making it back up the hill. **Jil, Jillane, Jillayne, Jilleen, Jillene, Jilli, Jillian, Jillianne, Jillie, Jilly, Jillyan, Jyl, Jyll.**

JILLIAN. *Phonetic spelling of GILLIAN.* This spelling is now four times more popular than the original. *See* **GILLIAN. Gillet, Gillette, Gilly, Jilan, Jilian, Jiliana, Jill, Jillana, Jillane, Jillet, Jillette, Jilliana, Jillianne, Jillie, Jilliyanne, Jilly, Jillyan, Jillyanna.**

JIMENA. *(hee-MAY-nah) Spanish variation of XIMENA, 'listener'.* Holds widespread popularity in the Latino community. **Ximena.**

JIN. *(JEEN) Japanese, 'tenderness, gentleness'.* Its similarity to the English name Jean could be a plus in a Japanese-British family.

♂ **JINĀN.** *(jih-NAHN) Arabic, 'garden, paradise'.* One of the most appealing Muslim names, both in sound and meaning.

JINJA. *African place name.* Gingery.

JINX. *Word name.* James Bond heroine name has ominous meaning but kinetic energy. **Jinxx, Jynx.**

JIVANTA. *Hindi, 'giver of life'.* A hauntingly lovely Indian name.

JO. *Diminutive of JOANNA, JOSEPHINE, etc.* Still evokes the spunky image of the character in Louisa May Alcott's *Little Women.*

JOAN. *English variation of JOHANNA.* Poor Joan. After being one of the most popular names throughout the 1930s, it has long lost its popularity and it would take a Joan of Arc to revive it today. **Joani, Joanie, Jone, Jonee, Jonette, Joni. International: Siobhán** *(Irish Gaelic),* **Seonag** *(Scottish Gaelic),* **Sion** *(Welsh),* **Jone** *(Basque).*

JOANNA. *Variation of JOHANNA.* The most usable name in her family, Joanna has been unobtrusively fashionable since the 1980s and continues to be appreciated for its New

Testament history and melodious three-syllable sound, though the simpler Anna ranks much higher. **Jana, Jo, JoAnn, Jo-Ann, JoAnne, Joan, Joanie, Joann, Joanna, Joanne, Joeann, Joeanna, Joeanne, Joni, Jonie, Ohanna.** International: **Siobhán** *(Irish)* **Shona** *(Scottish),* **Sion** *(Welsh)* **Hanne, Johannah** *(German),* **Jante, Johana** *(Dutch),* **Janne, Johanna** *(Scandinavian),* **Johanne, Joina, Jone, Jonella, Jonna** *(Danish),* **Joanka, Zana, Zanna** *(Polish),* **Hana, Johana** *(Czech),* **Ionna, Yannia** *(Greek),* **Johanna, Yochanna** *(Hebrew).*

JOANNE. *French variation of* **JOANNA.** Supplanted by Joanna.

JOAQUINA. *(wah-KEE-nah) Spanish, feminine variation of* **JOAQUIN.** As Joaquin enters the mainstream, his sister might just follow. **Joquina.**

JOBETH. *Combination of* **JO** *and* **BETH.** A *Jo*-plus name that sprang up in the 1940s.

JOBINA. *Hebrew, 'persecuted'.* Not many parents would inflict

the name Job on their baby, but the female version doesn't carry the same negative weight – in fact, few would get the connection. **Jobey, Jobi, Jobie, Jobina, Joby, Jobyna.**

JOBY. *Hebrew, 'persecuted'.* Reduces and lightens up the Job connection even further, sounding like a lively, Jody-like nickname name. **Jobey, Jobi, Jobie.**

★**JOCASTA.** *Greek mythology name.* Mythological name fashionably used over here, mostly ignored elsewhere. She was the mother of Oedipus, whom he (oops) married. If you can ignore that small error in judgment, you'll find an interesting and attractive *J* name that's neither overused nor terminally dated.

JOCELYN. *German, 'member of the Gauts tribe'.* The current passion for *lyn* endings has brought new life and popularity to what was – in medieval times – a male name. Now it couldn't sound more softly feminine. **Jocelin, Jocelinda, Joceline, Jocelyne, Joice, Joicelyn, Josalind, Josaline, Josalyn,**

Josalynn, Joscelyn, Joselina, Josiline, Josilyn, Joslin, Josline, Joslyn, Joss, Josselyn, Jossline, Josslyn, Joyce, Joycelin, Joycelyn, Josceline, Jozlyn.

JODIE. *See* **JODY.**

♂ **JODY.** *Diminutive of* **JOAN** *and* **JUDITH.** One of the cute and bouncy nicknames so popular in the 1960s and 70s, but that hasn't made a comeback in the way Eames chairs and bell-bottoms have. **Jodee, Jodey, Jodi, Jodie.**

JOELLA. *(yo-EHL-lah) Hebrew, 'the Lord is God'.* Most modern parents would drop the *Jo,* leaving the superpopular Ella. **Jola.**

JOËLLE. *Hebrew, 'the Lord is God'; French, feminine variation of* **JOEL.** A French name that's lost its chic. **Joela, Joelene, Joeliane, Joelin, Joeliyn, Joell, Joella, Joellen, Joellianna, Joelliane, Joellin, Joelly, Joely, Joelynn, Joetta, Jolene, Joline, Jowella, Jowelle.**

JOELY. *Feminine variation of* **JOEL,** *spelling variation of* **JOLIE.** Sounding both tomboyish and feminine at the same time, this name is mostly associated with actress Joely Richardson. **Jolie.**

♂ **JOEY.** *Diminutive of* **JOSEPH, JOANNA,** *or* **JOSEPHINE.** Tousle-haired and freckled, yet sexy in the way many boys' names are when used for girls.

JOHANNA. *Hebrew, 'God is gracious'.* Used in Holland, Germany and Scandinavia; the extra *h* makes this a slightly affected, more dignified version of Joanna. **Jo, Joanna, Johannah, Johnni, Jonni, Jonnie.**

JOIE. *French variation of* **JOY.** Pronounced as the English word *joy*, rather than as the French phrase *joie de vivre*, Joie might produce more complications than joy. **Joi.**

JOJO. *English, diminutive of* Jo-*beginning names*. Sprightly and engaging nickname for human, full name for pet.

JOLA. *Hebrew, 'God is willing'.* Could be used to honour a Joel.

JOLÁN. *(YO-lahn) Greek, 'violet'.* Various forms similar to this Hungarian one are used throughout Europe, so you might find one matching your own ethnicity. **International: Jolanda** *(Italian)*, **Jolanta, Jola** *(Polish)*, **Jolanka** *(Hungarian)*, **Jolana** *(Czech).*

JOLANDA. *Italian, 'violet'.* A sweet and feminine Italian name that is almost unheard of elswhere.

JOLANTA. *Polish, 'violet'.* A Slavic name that could easily blend in.

JOLENE. *Modern invented name.* Stuck in the image of the old Dolly Parton song. **Joeleen, Joeline, Jolean, Joleen, Jolena, Jolina, Joline.**

JOLIE. *French, 'pretty'.* As pretty as its literal meaning, nowadays also seen as a surname, via Angelina. **Jolee, Joleen, Joleigh, Jolena, Jolene, Joli, Jolien, Jolina, Joline, Jolleen, Jollene.**

JONET. *(zho-nay) Modern invented name.* A Frenchy name

that doesn't exist in France, probably inspired by Monet. **Jonette, Jonnette.**

JONI. *Spelling variation of* **JOANIE.** Only for hard-core fans of folksinger Mitchell. **Jonee, Jony.**

JONNA. *Feminine variation of* **JOHN.** Lacks personality or power.

JONQUIL. *Flower name.* Less outlandish than Daffodil and less common than Daisy, an unusual flower name that might appeal to parents seeking a singular botanical option. **International: Jonquille** *(French).*

JORA. *Hebrew, 'autumn rain'.* Unique possibility for a girl born between September and November.

♂ **JORDAN.** *Hebrew, 'flowing down'.* Originally used for children baptised in holy water from the river Jordan, it became one of the leading androgynous names of the 1990s. Not quite as sleek and shiny now, though it's still being used for both girls and boys. **Johrdan, Jordain, Jordanka, Jordann, Jordanna, Jordanne, Jordena, Jordenn, Jordie, Jordin, Jordyn, Jordynn, Jorey, Jori, Jorie, Jorrdan, Jorry, Jory, Jourdan, Yardena, Yordana.** International: **Jordane, Jourdaine** *(French),* **Giordana** *(Italian),* **Jordana** *(Spanish),* **Jordão** *(Portuguese),* **Jordaan** *(Dutch),* **Jardena** *(Hebrew).*

JORDANA. *Hebrew, 'flowing down'.* Used more before Jordan joined the girls' camp.

♂ JORIE. *Diminutive of* **MARJORIE** *or* **JORDAN.** Here is a fresh, spirited spin on the Cory-Tory-Rory group. The boys' Jory is a Cornish nickname for George. **Joree, Jorey, Jori, Jory.**

JORJA. *Modern American phonetic spelling of* **GEORGIA.** This simplified form of the lovely name Georgia has been used lately by some American celebrities to name their babies. Still, we'd opt for the traditional spelling.

JOSEFINA. *See* **JOSEPHA, JOSEPHINE.**

JOSELYN. *See* **JOCELYN.**

JOSEPHA. *Feminine variation of* **JOSEPH.** Less heard over here than in other parts of the world, seen as a slightly awkward feminisation à la Ricarda and Benjamina. **Hosefa, Josefa, Josepa, Josepha, Joseva, Josipha, Jozefa, Yosefa, Yosepha, Yosipha.** International: **Fifi, Josée, Josephe, Josette, Josiane** *(French),* **Chefa, Chepita, Josefa, Joseva, Peopa, Pepina, Pepita** *(Spanish),* **Pepita** *(Italian, Portuguese, Basque and Spanish),* **Joska** *(Basque),* **Josepha** *(German),* **Jozefa, Jozsa, Jozsefa, Jozsi, Jozska** *(Eastern European).*

★JOSEPHINE. *Feminine variation of* **JOSEPH.** Increasing numbers of parents think that, though not conventionally pretty, Josephine does have class and character and a gently offbeat quality – which adds up to style. Also boasts more than its share of lively nicknames, including Jo, Josie and Posey. **Feeney, Fifi, Fifine, Fina, Finetta, Finette, Jo, Joette, Joey, Jojo, Joline, Josana, Josanna, Josanne,**

If You Like Josephine,
You Might Love . . .

Alice

Amelia

Clara

Edith

Eugenia

Frances

Frederica

Helen

Imogen

Louise

Mae

Margaret

Pearl

Rosalind

Theodora

Josebe, Josee, Josefa, Josefena, Josefene, Josefine, Josepha, Josephe, Josephene, Josephina, Josephyna, Josephyne, Josetta, Josette, Josey, Josiane, Josianna, Josianne, Josie, Josy, Jozsa, Posey, Yosebe, Yosepha, Yosephina.

International: Seosaimhín (Irish Gaelic), Giuseppina (Italian), Hosefina, Josefana, Josefina (Spanish), Josefine (German), Józefina (Polish).

JOSETTE. French, diminutive of **JOSEPHINE.** One French form that is more down-market and froufrou than the original.

JOSIE. English, diminutive of **JOSEPHINE.** Jaunty and friendly; among the most winning of all nickname names. Josee, Josey, Josye, Josi, Josy.

JOSLYN. See **JOCELYN.**

♂ **JOSS.** English, diminutive of **JOCELYN.** A short form that could be used independently, à la singer Joss Stone.

JOURNEY. Word name. One of the new word names, appealing to parents attracted to the idea of a spiritual – or even an actual – voyage.

JOVITA. Spanish, feminine variation of **JOVE,** Roman king of the gods. Lively and joyful. Jovana, Jovena, Jovina.

JOY. Word name. From an older generation of word names, which also included Merry, Bliss and Glory – all of which exert personality pressure on a child. Gioia, Gioya, Jioia, Jioya, Joi, Joia, Joice, Joie, Joya, Joyann, Joye.

JOYCE. Latin, 'merry, joyous'. Once a boy-baby name, now a no-baby name. Joice, Joycie, Joyse. International: Joos, Joost (Dutch).

JUANA. (HWAHN-ah) Spanish, feminine variation of **JUAN.** Not nearly as popular as its male counterpart Juan outside Hispanic communities. Janina, Joanita, Juanita, Juanna, Juannia, Yuana.

JUANITA. Spanish, feminine variation of **JUAN.** Pervasive in all Spanish-speaking cultures, Juanita, like Juana, has not emigrated. Janita, Juanequa, Juanesha, Juanice, Juanicia, Juaniqua, Juanisha, Juanishia, Juanitia, Junita, Juwaneeta, Juwanita, Nita. International: Wahnita, Waneeta, Wanita, Wanna, Wenita, Wenitah (Native American, Cherokee and Sioux).

♂ **JUBA.** African, 'born on Monday'. This strong and resonant unisex name belonged to an ancient African king, is a city and river name, and is traditionally given to Ashanti (of Ghana) girls born on a Monday.

JUBILEE. Hebrew, 'ram's horn'. Joyous and jubilant aura, but not an easy name to carry. Jubalee.

♂ **JUDE.** Latin, diminutive of **JUDAH.** A rising boys' name that becomes a new version of Judith or Judy.

JUDITH. Hebrew, 'He will be praised', 'woman from Judea'. The biblical Judith, the fourth most popular name in 1940, may be getting ready for a comeback in its full, elegant, if somewhat solemn form. Joda, Jodee, Jodi, Jodie, Jody, Judah, Jude, Judee, Judey, Judi, Judie, Judite, Judy, Judye, Judyth, Judythe Jutta. International: Juditha, Judithe (French), Giuditta (Italian), Judeen, Judetta, Judina, Judit, Judita (Spanish), Jutka, Jutte, Juut (Dutch), Jutta, Jutte (German), Judit, Jytte (Scandinavian),

Judyta *(Polish)*, **Judit, Jutka**
(Hungarian), **Jitka, Judita**
(Czech), **Yudif, Yudita** *(Russian)*,
Hudes, Yehudah, Yehudit, Yidel,
Yudel, Yutke *(Yiddish)*.

JUDY. *Diminutive of* **JUDITH.**
Judy was the nickname of
choice for almost all the Judiths
born in the 1940s and 50s;
today's little Judiths are much
more likely to be called Judith –
or, possibly, Jude. **Judee, Judey,**
Judi, Judie, Judye.

♂ **JULES.** *Latin, 'youthful';*
Greek, 'soft, downy'. A middle-
aged male name that suddenly
seems young and fresh and
female, after having been an
off-the-radar-nickname for Julia
and Julie. Author and wife of
celebrity chef Jamie Oliver
spells her name Jools, and we've
also seen Joolz.

★ **JULIA.** *Latin, 'youthful'.*
An enduring classic, because
it has so much going for it:
ancient roots but a modern,
fashionable feel, simplicity and
sophistication, and connections
to both saints and celebs. One
of the least problematic choices
a parent could make. **Giulianna,**

Julia's International Variations

Irish	Iúile
Italian	Giulia, Giuliana
Spanish	Jovita, Julianita, Julienne, Julina, Julita
German	Juliana, Juliane, Juliann, Julianna
Polish	Jowita, Julita
Hungarian	Julea, Juli, Juliska
Romanian	Iulia, Iuliana
Czech	Julka
Lithuanian	Iulija
Bulgarian	Iulia
Russian	Iuliya, Julya, Ulana, Youlia, Yulia, Yuliya, Yulya
Ukrainian	Ulyana, Yulia
Latvian	Iuliya, Julija
Greek	Ioula, Ioulia
Armenian	Yulia
Hawaiian	Iulia

Guilie, Giulietta, Jiulia, Joleta,
Joletta, Jolette, Julee, Juleen,
Juley, Juliaeta, Juliaetta, Julianne,
Julie, Juliet, Julieta, Juliette,
Juline, Julinka, Julissa, Julitta,
Julyana, Julyanna, Julyet,
Julyetta, Julyette, Julyne, Ulya.

JULIANA. *Latin, 'youthful';*
feminine variation of **JULIAN.**
Long common in Europe, the
elegant and regal Juliana, also
spelled with two *n*'s, has become
popular, in tandem with
the more classic Julia. **Juliane,**
Juliann, Julianna, Julianne,

Stellar Starbabies Beginning with *J*

Jamison	James Belushi
Jasmine	Michael Jordan, Martin Lawrence
Jaya	Laura Dern & Ben Harper
Jaz	Steffi Graf & Andre Agassi
Jessie James	P Diddy & Kim Porter
Jolie	Keenen Ivory Wayans
Josephine	Linda Hamilton & James Cameron, Vera Wang
Judah	Ziggy Marley
Julianna	Emily *(Dixie Chicks)* Robison
Julie Rose	Eric Clapton
Juliet	Emily Watson

Julieana, Julieanna, Julliana, Julyana, Julyanna, Liana, Lianne, Lianna. International: Julienne *(French)*, Giuliana *(Italian)*, Juliane *(German)*, Julianja, Julesa, Julinka, Juliska *(Hungarian)*.

JULIANNE. *Latin, 'youthful'.* This variation on the Julia theme has spiked due to the popularity of Julianne Moore.

JULIE. *French variation of* JULIA. Wildly popular in the 1960s and 70s, Julie is no longer anywhere near as stylish

as the name's longer forms. Jule, Julea, Juleah, Julee, Juley, Juli, July.

JULIENNE. *French, feminine variation of* JULIEN. Pretty French name, although it does allude to vegetables sliced into thin strips.

★**JULIET.** *English from French, diminutive of* JULIA *or* JULIE. One of the most romantic names, the lovely and stylish Juliet seems finally to have shaken off her limiting link to

Romeo. In Shakespeare's play, it was Juliet who said 'What's in a name?' Julette, Juliett, Julietta, Juliette, Julyet. International: Juliette *(French)*, Giulietta *(Italian)*, Julieta, Julietta *(Spanish)*.

JULIETTA. *Spanish variation of* JULIET. Moves the name further from Romeo – which is a good thing.

JULIETTE *French variation of* JULIET. Same pronunciation, with a little something extra.

JULISSA. *Modern invented name.* This modern Julia-Alissa hybrid has been given to many American babies in recent years. Julis, Julisa, Julisha, Julyssa.

JULITTA. *Dutch variation of* JULIA. This fairly obscure saint's name was chosen by Oscar-winning actress Marcia Gay Harden for one of her twins.

JULITTE. *(ZHOO-LEET) Latin 'praised'.* Delicate and obscure version of this many-faceted name.

JULY. *Latin, month name.* Hotter than June. **International:**

Juillet *(French)*, Julia *(Spanish)*, Julha *(Portuguese)*, Yula *(Russian)*.

JUMANA. *Arabic, 'silver pearl'.* Rare and rhythmic. Jumanah, Jummanah.

JUNE. *Latin month name.* Locked in a time capsule with June Allyson. Junae, Junel, Junella, Junelle, Junette, Junia, Juniata, Junieta, Junina, Junine, Junya, Jyune. International: Juin *(French)*, Giugnia *(Italian)*, Junia *(Spanish)*, Junha *(Portuguese)*, Juni *(German and Scandinavian)*, Yuna *(Russian)*, Junia *(Greek)*, Yuni *(Hebrew and Arabic)*, Djuni *(Indonesian)*.

★♂ JUNIPER. *Latin plant name.* Fresh-feeling nature name – it's a small evergreen shrub whose berries make gin – with lots of energy.

★JUNO. *Latin, 'queen of the heavens'.* The name of the Roman mythological supreme female deity is a rare *o*-ending girl's name, which gives it an extra measure of strength. Juneau, Juneaux, Junot.

♂ JUSTICE. *Word name.* A fashionable word name, used almost equally for girls and boys, it has the distinction of being a virtue name without the religious implications of Faith or Grace. Justis, Justiss, Justisse, Justus, Justyce, Justys.

JUSTINA. *Latin, feminine variation of* JUSTIN. This was the pre-Justine feminisation of Justin, now a possible alternative to Christina. Justeena, Justine.

★JUSTINE. *Latin, feminine variation of* JUSTIN. A French name that's never reached the popularity we think it deserves. Like its far-more-fashionable brother Justin, it's sleek and sophisticated, but still user-friendly. Jestina, Jestine, Justa, Justeen, Justeene, Justene, Justicia, Justyn, Justyna, Justyne. International: Jestina *(Welsh)*, Giustina *(Italian)*, Justyna *(Polish)*, Justina *(Greek)*.

K *girls*

KACEY. *Variation of* CASEY *or combination of initials* K. *and* C. From the time when initial names seemed really cool. K.C., Kace, Kacee, Kaci, Kacie, Kacy, Kaicee, Kaicey, Kasey, Kasie, Kayce, Kaycee, Kayci, Kaycie, Kaysee, Kaysey, Kaysi, Kaysie, Kaysii.

KACIA. *Greek, diminutive of* ACACIA. Intriguing and unusual. Kaycia, Kaysia.

KADIDA. *Variation of* KHADIJAH. Anglicised Muslim or African name used by Quincy Jones and Peggy Lipton for their now-grown daughter.

KADY. *Irish, 'first'; variation of* KATY *or combination of initials* K. *and* D. Though it's more distinctive, everyone will just hear it as Katy. K.D., Kade, Kadee, Kadey, Kadie, Kadya, Kadyn, Kaidi, Kaidy, Kayda, Kayde, Kaydee, Kayden, Kaydey, Kaydi, Kaydie, Kaydy.

KAHLO. *Spanish artist name.* Cooler than Frida, though not everyone would get the artist connection.

KAIA. *Greek, 'earth'.* The new Maia, the next Kayla, Kaia has been becoming more popular in recent years. Kaiah, Kaija, Kaya, Kayah, Kya, Kyah.

KAITLYN. *Spelling variation of* **CAITLIN.** A huge name over the past few decades, this variation is still inching up the charts while others – the original Caitlin and Kaitlin, for instance – are moving down. No matter how you spell it, it's overused

and no longer even vaguely stylish. **Caitlin, Caitlyn, Kaetlyn, Kailyn, Kailynn, Kaitlan, Kaitland, Kaitleen, Kaitlen, Kaitlind, Kaitlinn, Kaitlinne, Kaitlon, Kaitlyn, Kaitlynn, Katelyn, Katelynn, Katelynne, Kathlin, Kathlinne, Kathlyn, Kaytlin.**

KALI. *Sanskrit, 'black one'; also nickname for several Greek names.* Cute name but be warned: Kali is the Hindu goddess of destruction, the fierce side of the goddess Devi. **Kala, Kalee, Kaleigh, Kaley, Kalie, Kallee, Kalley, Kalli, Kallie, Kally, Kallye, Kaly.**

★**KALILA.** *Arabic, 'beloved'.* Lilting name of a range of mythical mountains, with an extensive menu of spellings, and a more unusual way of fitting in with current favourites Lila and Lola. **Kahlila, Kailey, Kala, Kalah, Kaleela, Kalie, Kalilah, Kalilla, Kalla, Kallah, Kaylil, Kaylila, Kayllie, Kelila, Khalila, Khalilah, Khalillah, Kylila, Kylilah, Kylillah.**

KALINDA. *Hindi, 'sun'.* Exotic cousin of Belinda or Melinda.

Kaleenda, Kalindi, Kalynda, Kalyndi.

KALINDI. *Hindi, variation of* **KALINDA.** Lovely, rhythmic name that refers to one of the seven sacred rivers of India.

KALLAN. *Scandinavian, 'stream, river'.* Name with genuine roots that nevertheless feels synthetic. **Kalahn, Kalan, Kalen, Kallen, Kallon, Kalon.**

KALLIOPE. *Greek, 'beautiful voice'.* Original form of the more familiar Calliope, the muse of epic poetry. **Kalli, Kallie, Kallyope.**

KALLISTA. *Greek, 'most beautiful'.* Actress Flockhart popularised the *C* version, but this works, too. **Cala, Calesta, Cailie, Calia, Calista, Calli, Callia, Callista, Callisto, Cally, Kala, Kalesta, Kalista, Kallesta, Kalli, Kallia, Kallie, Kallisto, Kally, Kallysta, Kaysta.**

KAMA. *Hindi-Sanskrit, 'love, desire'; Hawaiian variation of* **THELMA.** This simple but exotic name – some might associate it with the Kama

Sutra – was chosen by heavy metal rocker Sammy Hagar for his daughter.

KAMALA. *Hindi, 'lotus'; Hawaiian, 'a garden'.* Soft and sinuous multicultural choice. **Kamalah, Kammala.**

KAMALI. *African, Mashona, 'spirit guide, protector'.* Spirit that protects babies from illness. **Kamali.**

KAMARIA. *Swahili, 'moonlight'.* Lush and unusual. **Kamar, Kamara, Kamarae, Kamaree, Kamari, Kamariah, Kamarie, Kamariya, Kamariya, Kamarya.**

★KAMILAH. *Arabic, 'perfect'.* One of the most adaptable of the Middle Eastern names, partly because of its similarity to the western Camilla. **Kameela, Kameelah, Kami, Kamila, Kamilla, Kamillah, Kammilah.**

KANIKA. *African, Mwera, 'black cloth'.* Energetic choice that bounces off the tongue. **Kaneeka, Kanica, Kanicka.**

KANYA. *Hindi, 'virgin'.*

Hindu goddess name used for children born under the sign of Virgo.

KARA. *Variation of* **CARA.** Once popular name now on the wane. **Cara, Carina, Carita, Kaira, Kairah, Karah, Karalea, Karalee, Karalie, Kari, Karina, Karine, Karita, Karra, Karrah, Karrie, Kera.**

KAREN. *Danish variation of* **KATHERINE.** This sweet good-girl Danish import was so popular during the baby boom in the 1960s that it's locked firmly into fashion limbo today. **Carina, Caron, Caronn, Carren, Carrin, Carryn, Carynn, Carynne, Kaaren, Kalina, Karaina, Karenna, Kari, Karna, Karon, Karra, Karren, Karron, Karryn, Karyn, Kerran, Kerrin, Kerron, Kerynne, Koren.** International: Ciarán *(Irish Gaelic),* Kieron, Kyran, Queron *(Scotch-Irish),* Caren, Carin, Caryn, Karan, Karena, Karin, Karine *(Scandinavian),* Kaarina *(Finnish),* Karina, Karine, Karyna *(Russian),* Keren, Keryn *(Hebrew),* Kalena, Kalina *(Hawaiian).*

KARENA, KARENNA. *Variation of* **KAREN.** Inspired by *Anna Karenina,* and modernises the middle-aged Karen that was overused in the 1960s.

KARINA. *Scandinavian variation of* **CARINA.** This sweet and loving name has been favoured in recent years by a mix of Hispanic-American parents and Bob Dylan fans.

KARLA. *German variation of* **CARLA.** Like many *K* versions, this one's rising while the original Carla-from-*Cheers* spelling is going down. **Karila, Karilla, Karlah, Karle, Karlene, Karlinka, Karlisha, Karlisia, Karlitha, Karlla, Karlon, Karlyn, Karrla.**

KARMA. *Hindi, 'destiny, spiritual force'.* Not even if you're planning on raising your baby in an ashram.

KASHMIR. *Sanskrit, Southwest Asian place name.* Soft and exotic, much like the similarly named cloth, but might have political implications. **Cashmere, Kashmear, Kashmere, Kashmia, Kashmira, Kasmir, Kasmira, Kazmir, Kazmira.**

Katherine's International Variations

Irish Gaelic	Caitlín, Caitrín, Caitríona, Catraoine
Irish	Kathleen
Scottish	Caitrona, Catriona, Catrona
Welsh	Catrin
French	Carine, Catant, Catherine, Trinette
Italian	Caterina, Cathe
Spanish	Catalina
Basque	Katarin
Portuguese	Catarina
Dutch	Kaatje, Katrien, Katrijn
German	Katarine, Katharina, Kathe, Katrina, Katrine, Katryn, Trina, Trinchen, Trine
Scandinavian	Karielle
Danish	Kari, Kasen
Swedish	Kolina
Finnish	Kaisa, Katja, Katri, Katrina
Polish	Kasia, Kasienka, Kasin, Kaska, Kassia, Katarzyna, Katine, Katrine, Katya
Hungarian	Kata, Katica, Katalin, Kati, Katica, Kato, Katoka, Koto
Czech	Kata, Katarina, Kateřina, Katica, Katka, Katuska

KATE. *English, diminutive of* **KATHERINE.** As pervasive as Kathy was in the 1950s and 1960s, Kate has been in more recent decades, both as a nickname for Katherine and Kaitlyn and as a strong, classic stand-alone name, with an image that's independent, smart, and energetic. However, it may have reached it's peak – it has recently slipped out of the Top 100. **Cait, Caitie, Cate, Catee, Catey, Catie, Kait, Kaite, Kaitlin, Kata, Katee, Katey, Kathe, Kati, Katica, Katie, Katka, Katy, Katya.** International: **Cáit** *(Irish Gaelic)*, **Ceit** *(Scottish Gaelic)*, **Käethe, Katja** *(German)*.

KATELL. *Breton variation of* **KATHERINE.** Original twist on this classic. **Caitlín, Caitriona.**

★**KATHERINE.** *Greek, 'pure'.* One of the oldest, most diverse, and all-round best names: it's powerful, feminine, royal, saintly, classic, popular, adaptable. Spellings, short forms and admirable namesakes abound. It's fallen out of the Top 100 only recently. **Cait, Caitie, Caity, Cass, Cassey, Cassi, Cassie, Casy, Cat,**

Cataleen, Cataleena, Catalin, Cataline, Catarine, Cate, Cateline, Cathaleen, Cathaline, Catharin, Catharina, Catharine, Catharyna, Catharyne, Cathee, Cathelina, Catherina, Catheryn, Cathie, Cathirin, Cathleen, Cathline, Cathlyne, Cathrine, Cathrinn, Kat, Kate, Katee, Kathann, Kathanne, Katharine, Kathereen, Katheren, Katherene, Katherenne, Katherin, Katherina, Katheryn, Katheryne, Kathi, Kathleen, Kathrine, Kathryn, Kathy, Kathyrine, Kay, Kitty.

Katherine's International Variations

Russian	Ekaterina, Katenka, Katerinka, Katia, Katinka, Katka, Katushka, Katya, Ketya, Kisa, Kiska, Kitti, Kotinka, Yekaterina
Estonian	Katharina, Kati, Rina
Greek	Kasienka, Kolena, Kolina
Yiddish	Reina
Hawaiian	Kakalina, Kalena

KATHLEEN. *Irish variation of* **KATHERINE.** The early Irish version that came between Katherine and Kaitlin, and which hasn't been used in so long it's almost beginning to sound fresh again. **Katheleen, Kathelene, Kathi, Kathileen, Kathlean, Kathleena, Kathleene, Kathlene, Kathlin, Kathlina, Kathlyn, Kathlyne, Kathlynn, Kathy, Katleen, Katline, Katlyn.**

KATHLYN. *Combination of* **KATHERINE** *and* **LYNN.** Annette Bening and Warren Beatty bestowed this name on their daughter in honour of his mother. **Kathlin, Kathlinn, Kathlinne, Kathlynn, Kathlynne.**

KATIA, KATYA. *Russian diminutive of* **EKATERINA.** One of the warm and earthy Russian nickname names now coming into style. Denzel Washington is the father of a Katia.

KATIE. *English diminutive of* **KATE.** This lively diminutive of Katherine is one of the top nicknames ranking at Number 13.

KATRINA. *German variation of* **KATHERINE.** The hurricane blew this one out of the realm of possibility. **Cat, Kat, Katreen, Katreena, Katrene, Katri, Katrice, Katricia, Katrien, Katrin, Katrine, Katrinia, Katriona, Katryn, Katryna, Kattrina, Kattryna, Katuska, Trina.**

KAY. *English diminutive of* **KATHERINE.** Cigarette-smoking, nightclubbing name of the 1930s that could be ready for a comeback along with cousins May/Mae and Ray/Rae. **Caye, Kae, Kai, Kaye, Kayla.**

KAYA. *Native American, Hopi, 'my elder sister'.* One of the currently trendy Kaia-Maya-Mia family, with a meaning that suggests wisdom.

KAYLA. *Arabic and Hebrew, 'laurel, crown'.* A name that appeared in the 1980s, giving birth to Mikayla. **Kaila, Kailah, Kailea, Kaileah, Kailee, Kailey, Kaylah, Kaylea, Kaylee, Kayleen, Kaylene, Kaylia, Keila, Keyla.**

KAYLEIGH. *English variation of* **KAYLA.** Was briefly a Top 100 name that pulls together something from Kayla and something from Hailey. **Kailee, Kalee, Kaleigh, Kaley, Kalie, Kayle, Kaylee, Kayley, Kayli, Kaylie.**

KAYLIN. *American variation of* **KAYLA.** Name on the rise in the wake of Kayla and Katelin, in several variations of nearly equal popularity. **Kaelan, Kaelen, Kaelin, Kaelyn, Kaelynn, Kaelynne, Kalyn, Kalynn, Kayleen, Kaylen, Kaylene, Kaylin, Kaylyna, Kaylyn, Kaylyne, Kaylynn, Kaylynne.**

KEARA. *Spelling variation of* **KEIRA.** One of many takes on the Keira/Kyra.

♂**KEEGAN.** *Irish 'son of Egan'.* One of several two-syllable surnames zooming up the ladder for boys, and poised to be grabbed by the girls.

KEELA. *Irish, 'so beautiful that only poets can describe her'.* Sounds more au courant than Keeley or Kelly . . . or even Kaylee. **Keeley, Keeli, Keely, Keila, Keyla, Kiela, Kyla.**

♂**KEELEY.** *Irish, 'slender'.* The one that's not Kelly or Kaylee. **Keeleigh, Keely, Keighley.**

KEELIN. *Irish, 'slender and fair'.* An obscure Irish choice poised for discovery. **Kealan, Kealen, Kealin, Kealyn, Kealynn, Keelan, Keelen, Keelyn, Keelynn, Keelynne, Keylyn.**

♂ **KEENAN.** *Irish, 'ancient'.* A lively boys' name that works well for girls.

KEIKO. *(keh-ee-ko) Japanese, 'happy child'.* Japanese classic with optimistic meaning. **Kei.**

♂ **KEIL.** *(keel) German, 'wedge'.* Simple, crisp name that works equally well for either gender.

KEIRA. *Irish, 'dark, black'.* Attractive name that has been given a huge boost from the meteoric rise of Keira Knightley. **Keaira, Keara, Kearah, Kearia, Kearra, Keera, Keerra, Keiara, Keiarah, Keiarra, Keira, Kera.**

KEISHA. *Spelling variation of* **KEZIAH.** African-American name first publicised by an American child actress a few decades ago, but it has faded in popularity in recent years.

KELDA. *Norse, 'spring, fountain'.* One of the few *K* names that sounds middle-aged. **Kellda.**

★**KELILA.** *Hebrew, 'laurel, crown'.* More distinctive and attractive Kayla relative. **Kayla, Kayle, Kaylee, Kelilah, Kelula, Kelulah, Kelulla, Kyla.**

KELIS. *(kul-EESE) Modern invented name.* Hot R & B singer Kelis Rogers's name is a combination of those of her parents' – Kenneth and Eveliss.

♂ **KELLY.** *Irish, 'war'.* Once the quintessential bouncy teenager name, Kelly helped launch the trend of unisex Irish names, but it now takes a backseat to more substantial surname names like Kennedy. **Keeley, Keely, Kellee, Kelley, Kelli, Kellie, Kellina, Kellye.**

♂ **KELSEY.** *English, 'island'.* Yesterday's favourite, now a teenager with best mate Chelsea. **Kelcey, Kelcie, Kelcy, Kelda, Kellsee, Kellsei, Kellsey, Kellsie,**

Kellsy, Kelsea, Kelsee, Kelsei, Kelseigh, Kelsi, Kelsie, Kelsy, Kelsye.

♀ **KENDALL.** *English, 'valley of the river Kent'.* This pleasantly boyish English surname has been rising in popularity for a number of years. **Kendal, Kendalla, Kendalle, Kendell, Kendelle, Kendera, Kendia, Kendyl, Kinda, Kindall, Kindi, Kindle, Kynda, Kyndal, Kyndall, Kyndel.**

KENDRA. *English, 'knowing'.* Kendra is sometimes seen as a feminisation of Kenneth. **Kandra, Keandra, Kenda, Kendrah, Kendre, Kendrea, Kendreah, Kendria, Kenna, Kenndra, Kentra, Kentrae, Kindra, Kinna, Kyndra.**

★♀ **KENNEDY.** *Irish, 'misshapen head'.* Attractive surname name still projects that Kennedy family charisma. **Kenedee, Kenedey, Kenedi, Kenedie, Kenedy, Kenidee, Kenidi, Kenidie, Kenidy, Kennadee, Kennadi, Kennadie, Kennady, Kennedee, Kennedey, Kennedi, Kennedie, Kennidee, Kennidi, Kennidy, Kynnedi.**

♀ **KENYA.** *African place name, Russian diminutive.* This name borrowed from the East African nation is now used exclusively for girls. **Keenya, Kenia, Kenja, Kenyah, Kenyana, Kenyatta, Kenyia, Kennya.**

KENZIE. *Scottish, 'light-skinned'; Irish, diminutive of* MACKENZIE. Freshens up Mackenzie. **Kenza, Kenzea, Kenzee, Kenzey, Kenzi, Kenzia, Kenzy, Kinzie.**

KERANI. *Hindi, 'sacred bells'.* A lovely Indo-Pakistani name that could be seen as the Karen of this multicultural century. **Kera, Kerah, Keran, Kerana.**

KEREN. *Hebrew, 'strength, power, ram's horn'.* Israeli-born singer Keren Ann introduced this traditional Hebrew name to other countries. It could well be mistaken for Karen. **Karin, Karnit, Kerena, Kerrin, Keryn, Koranit, Korenit, Korin.**

★ **KERENSA.** *Cornish, 'love'.* Forever exotic, a romantic Cornish name spelled with an *s* or *z*, the most modern of the Karen family. **Karensa, Karenza, Kerenza, Kerra.**

♀ **KERR.** *Scottish, 'living near wet ground'.* Simple, unusual unisex middle-name choice, can be pronounced either *car* or *kehr*.

KERRIS. *Welsh, 'love'.* Much easier phonetic spelling of popular and pretty Welsh name Carys or Cerys. **Karis, Karris, Karys, Keris, Kerys.**

♀ **KERRY.** *Irish, 'dark, dark-haired'.* The name of one of the most beautiful and lush counties of Ireland was a 1970s favourite. **Keary, Keiry, Kera, Keree, Kerey, Keri, Kerrey, Kerri, Kerria, Kerridana, Kerrie, Kerryann, Kerryanne, Kery, Kiera, Kierra.**

KESSIE. *African, Ashanti, 'chubby baby'.* Cute but slight. **Kess, Kessa, Kesse, Kessey, Kessi.**

★ **KETURAH.** *Hebrew, 'incense'.* The Old Testament name of Abraham's second wife is a possibility for anyone seeking a truly unusual and interesting biblical name; more distinctive than Abraham's first wife, Sarah. **Katura, Ketura.**

♂ **KEVYN.** *Irish, 'handsome'.* Using it for a girl breathes new life into this tired boys' name. **Keva, Kevan, Keven, Kevia, Keviana, Kevin, Kevina, Kevinna, Kevinne, Kevion, Kevionna, Kevon, Kevona, Kevone, Kevonia, Kevonna, Kevonne, Kevonya, Kevynn, Kevynne.**

♂ **KEW.** *Cornish, 'chick'.* Offbeat name of a saint from Cornwall with boyish appeal.

★**KEZIA, KEZIAH.** *Hebrew, 'cassia tree'.* Old Testament name – she was one of the three daughters of Job – widely used for slaves and still most common in the African-Caribbean community. This lovely, distinctive name – along with others like Jemima – deserves full emancipation. **Kazia, Kaziah, Kessie, Kessy, Ketzi, Ketzia, Ketziah, Kezi, Keziah, Kezzie, Kissie, Kizzie, Kizzy.**

KHADIJA. *Arabic, 'premature baby'.* The Prophet Muhammad's first wife and the first convert to Islam. **Kadaja, Kadeeja, Kadija, Kadiya, Khadaja, Khadajah, Khadeeja, Khadeejah, Khadeja, Khadejah, Khadejha, Khadijah,**

Khadije, Khadijia, Khadijiah, Khadiya, Khadyja.

KHALIDA. *Arabic, 'immortal, everlasting'.* Evocative Middle Eastern choice. **Kalida, Khali, Khalia, Khaliah, Khalidda, Khalita.**

KIA. *African, 'season's beginning'.* Sweet, simple name, now, unfortunately, associated with a Korean car label. **Kiah.**

KIANA. *Modern invented name.* The original polyester name. **Keanna, Keiana, Keyana, Keyona, Khiana, Khianah, Khianna, Ki, Kia, Kiah, Kiahna, Kiane, Kiani, Kiania, Kianna, Kiandra, Kiandria, Kiauna, Kiaundra, Kiyana, Kyana, Quiana, Quianna.**

KIARA. *(kee-AHR-a) Spelling variation of* **CHIARA.** Simba's daughter in *The Lion King*, Kiara fits in with stylish modern names like Keira and Kaia. **Keara, Keearra, Keyara, Kiarra, Kieara, Kiearah, Kiearra, Kiera, Kierra, Kyara.**

KIARIA. *Japanese, 'fortunate'.* Pretty but sure to prove confusing. **Kiarra, Kichi.**

KIERA. *See* **KEIRA.**

♂ **KIERAN.** *(keer-an) Irish, 'little dark one'.* Boys' name that could cross over, as an update of outmoded Karen. **Ciara, Ciarán, Kiaran.**

KIKI. *French and Spanish nickname.* One of the Coco-Gigi-Fifi-Lulu bohemian-type French names from the turn of the last century, which have endless energy and sparkle. Artist Kiki Smith is its most well-known contemporary representative.

KILEY. *See* **KYLIE.** **Kilea, Kilee, Kileigh, Kili, Kilie, Kylee, Kyley, Kyli, Kylie.**

♂ **KIM.** *English, diminutive of* **KIMBERLY.** The coolest name . . . of the 1960s. It was popularised by the sultry Kim Novak, and its energy is still maintained by rapper Lil' Kim, but it holds lil' or no appeal for new babies. **Kima, Kimana, Kimette, Kimm, Kym, Kymme.**

KIMANA. *Native American, Shoshone, 'butterfly'.* The name of a resort in the foothills of Mountain Kilimanjaro in Kenya would make an exotic path to the nickname Kim. **Kiman, Kimani.**

KIMBA. *Variation of* **KIMBERLY.** A name that is unlikely to take off – due to its simian feel. **Kimber.**

KIMBERLY. *English place name.* Though this South African diamond town name hasn't been stylish for decades there are still a number of parents that find it appealing today. **Cymberly, Cymbre, Kim, Kimba, Kimbely, Kimber, Kimbereley, Kimberely, Kimberlee, Kimberleigh, Kimberley, Kimberli, Kimberlie, Kimberlin, Kimberlyn, Kimbery, Kimblyn, Kimbria, Kimbrie, Kimbry, Kimmie, Kimmy, Kym, Kymberleigh, Kymberley, Kymberly, Kymbra, Kymbrely.**

KIMI. *Japanese, 'righteous'.* Barbie's Asian equivalent. **Kimia, Kimika, Kimiko, Kimiyo, Kimmi, Kimmie, Kimmy.**

KINSEY. *English, 'king's victory'.* Enjoyed popularity blip thanks to similarity to Lindsay, and because of Sue Grafton's

alphabet mysteries heroine, Kinsey Millhone. **Kinnsee, Kinnsey, Kinnsie, Kinsee, Kinsie, Kinsley, Kinza, Kinze, Kinzee, Kinzey, Kinzi, Kinzie, Kinzy.**

♀ **KINSLEY.** *English, 'king's meadow'.* Straddling the line between cute and classy. **Kingslea, Kingslee, Kingslie, Kinslea, Kinslee, Kinslie, Kinsly, Kinzlea, Kinzlee, Kinzley, Kinzly.**

KIONA. *Native American, 'brown hills'.* A New World alternative to Fiona. **Kionah, Kioni, Kionna.**

KIRA. *See* **KYRA.** **Keera, Kiera, Kierra, Kirah, Kiri, Kiria, Kiriah, Kiro, Kirra, Kirrah, Kirri, Kirya.**

♂ **KIRBY.** *English, 'church settlement'.* Unisex name around for several decades for boys and now ripe for girls. **Kirbee, Kirbey, Kirbi, Kirbie.**

KIRIAH. *(KIR-ee-ah) Hebrew, 'village'.* Unusual name that's close – possibly too close – to several more familiar choices. **Kiria, Kirya.**

KIRSI. *Hindi, 'amaranth blossoms'.* Most people will just hear Kirstie. **Kirsie.**

KIRSTEN. *Scandinavian variation of* **CHRISTINE.** Lovely, authentic name – but any Kirsten will be condemned to a lifetime of hearing 'Did you say Kristen?' **Karsten, Kearsten, Keerstin, Keirstan, Keirstin, Kersten, Kerstin, Kiersten, Kierstynn, Kirsteen, Kirsteni, Kirsta, Kirstan, Kirstene, Kirsti, Kirstie, Kirstin, Kirston, Kirsty, Kirstyn, Kirstynn, Kjerstin, Kristen, Kristin, Kristyn, Krystin, Kursten, Kyersten, Kyrsten, Kyrstin.**

KIRSTIE. *Anglicization of Ciorstag, the Gaelic nickname for* **CHRISTINE.** Actress Kirstie Alley popularised this short form that's been off the popularity register for a decade.

KISHA. *Spelling variation of* **KEZIAH.** Rather than simplifying matters, this spelling only complicates them.

KISMET. *Word name.* The next Destiny? Kismet seems fated for increased use.

K Versions of C Names

Kami	Klara
Kamilla	Klarissa
Kandace	Klaudia
Kari	Klementina
Karissa	Kloe
Karley	Klotild
Karlotta	Kody
Karmel	Kolby
Karmen	Konstance
Karol	Kora
Karolina	Koral
Karolyn	Korina
Karrie	Kornelia
Karsen	Kourtney
Kasey	Krystal
Kassandra	Kynthia
Kassidy	

KISSA. *African-Ugandan, 'born after twins'.* Affectionate sounding name that could have birth-order meaning.

♂ **KIT.** *English, diminutive of* **KATHERINE.** Crisp, old-time nickname that sounds fresh and modern today.

KITTY. *English, diminutive of* **KATHERINE.** Long out of fashion, we see this as a definite candidate for a comeback. **Ketter, Ketti, Ketty, Kit, Kittee, Kitteen, Kittey, Kitti, Kittie.**

KIZZY. *Variation of* **KEZIAH.** Keziah variations were widely used for slaves and this one starred in the American TV programme *Roots*. **Kizzey, Kissie, Kizzi, Kizzie.**

♂ **KOFFI.** *Swahili, 'born on Friday'.* Authentic African name with unfortunate coffee association, also too close to the male Kofi. **Kaffe, Kaffi, Koffe, Koffie.**

KOKO. *Japanese, 'stork'.* The Asian Coco.

KOSMA. *Greek, 'order, universe'.* Name from a 1950s science fiction movie. **Cosma.**

KRISTA. *Czech variation of* **CHRISTINA.** Long past its peak – along with all similar C-starting sisters. **Khrissa, Khrista, Khryssa, Khrysta, Krissa, Kryssa, Krysta.**

KRISTAL. *See* **CRYSTAL.**

KRISTEN, KRISTIN. *Danish variation of* **CHRISTIANA.** Two decades past its fashion moment, but forever crystalline clear. **Christen, Khristin, Krissie, Krissy, Krista, Kristan, Kristeen, Kristelle, Kristene, Kristiana, Kristien, Kristiin, Kristijna, Kristin, Kristina, Kristi Kristyn, Kristyna, Krysia, Krysta, Krysten. International: Karsten, Karste (Dutch), Kersten (Swedish), Kirsten, Kirsti, Kjersti (Norwegian), Kristi, Kristina, Krysta, Krystyn (Polish), Kriska, Kriszta, Krisztina (Hungarian), Krystin (Czech).**

KRISTIANA. *Greek, 'Christian, anointed'. See* **CRISTIANA.** **Khristian, Kristian, Kristiane, Kristiann, Kristi-Ann, Kristianna, Kristianne, Kristi-Anne, Kristienne, Kristyan, Kristyana, Kristy-Ann, Kristy-Anne.**

KRISTINA. *Scandinavian variation of* **CHRISTINA.** *See* **CHRISTINA.** **Khristina, Kristeena, Kristena, Kristina, Kristinka, Krystina.**

KRISTINE. *Scandinavian variation of* **CHRISTINE.** *See* **CHRISTINE.** **Kris, Kristeen,**

Kristene, Kristi, Kristie, Kristy, Krystine, Krystyne.

KYLA. *Feminine variation of* **KYLE;** *variation of* **KAYLA.** Kyle is stronger and sharper. **Khyla, Kylah, Kylea, Kyleah, Kylia.**

♂ **KYLE.** *Scottish, 'narrow spit of land'.* Not as popular for girls as Kylie or Kyla, but we prefer its simplicity. **Kial, Kiele, Kyall, Kyel, Kylee, Kyleigh, Kylene, Kylie.**

KYLIE. *Aboriginal, 'a boomerang'.* Popular name, inspired by the superstar Australian singer Kylie Minogue. **Keiley, Keilley, Keilly, Keily, Keyely, Kilea, Kiley, Kye, Kylee, Kyley, Kyli, Kyllie.**

KYOKO. *Japanese, 'mirror'.* One of the most familiar and attractive Japanese names, though rarely heard outside that culture.

KYRA. *Feminine variation of* **CYRUS.** Sounds like Keira/Kiera and just as popular, but has a different root. **Kaira, Keera, Keira, Kira, Kyrah, Kyreena, Kyrene, Kyrha,**

Kyria, Kyriah, Kyriann, Kyrie, Kyrina, Kyr.

L *girls*

LACEY. *English, 'from Lassy'.* A unique combination of a surname feeling and real femininity. The Lacey, Laci, Lacie, and Lacy spellings are all popular in the US. **Lace, Lacee, Laci, Lacie, Lacy, Laicee, Laicey, Laisey.**

LADONNA. *Modern elaboration of* **DONNA.** Typical of the practice of placing *La* in front of an

existing name, this one also relates to Madonna.

★**LAILA.** *Arabic, 'night, dark beauty'; spelling variation of* **LEILA.** Exotic and lovely, one of the lilting variations of Leila. **Laela, Lailah, Laily, Laleh, Lallie, Layla, Laylah, Leyla.**

LAINIE. *Diminutive of* **ELAINE.** Too flimsy for birth certificate name use. **Lainey, Laini, Lainy, Lanee, Laney, Lani, Lanie.**

♂ **LAKE.** *Nature name.* This body of water runs deep; the best of a group of new possibilities that includes Bay,

La Names

Ladasha

Ladawn

Lakaiya

Lakecia

Lakeisha

Lakendra

Lakenya

Laneisha

Lanita

Lashanda

Lashanna

Lashante

Lashauna

Lashonda

Latanya

Latara

Latasha

Latisha

Latoya

Lawanda

Ocean, River and the more established Brook. **Laiken, Laken.**

LAKEISHA. *Modern invented name.* Perhaps the best known of the *La* names that peaked in the 1980s, it stems from the biblical Keziah, plus the gallic *La* prefix that rose to prominence centuries ago among the Creole people and Free Blacks of New Orleans in the US. **Lakaysha, Lakecia, Lakeesha, Laketia, Lakeysha, Lakicia, Lakisha, Lakitia, Lekeesha, Lekeisha, Lekisha.**

♂ **LAKOTA, LAKOTAH.** *Native American, Sioux, 'friend to us'.* The name of one of the branches of the Great Sioux Nation has a strong, authentic feel, unlike many of the other *La* names.

LAKSHMI. *Sanskrit, 'a lucky omen'.* Often heard in India, this is the name of the Hindu goddess of abundance, beauty and prosperity, the embodiment of grace and charm – lucky omens indeed. **Laksmé, Laxmi.**

LALA. *Slavic, 'tulip'; Hawaiian, 'laurel'.* If it's possible for a name to be *too* musical, this one is. **Lalla, Lallah.**

LALAGE. *(la-LAH-yeh) Greek, 'to chatter'.* Interesting, but destined to be mispronounced. **Lala, Lalia.**

LALIA. *Latin, 'speaking well'.* Completely undiscovered name with an abundance of rhythmic charm. **Laelia, Lala, Lalah, Lali, Lallia, Lalya, Laylia, Lela, Lelea.**

LALITA. *Sanskrit, 'playful, charming'.* Lolita without the naughty implications.

LALLY. *Diminutive of any La-name.* Likable nickname name in the Callie, Hallie mode. **Lala, Lalla, Lallie.**

LANA. *Diminutive of* **ALANA.** Sexy sweater girl name of the 1940s that doesn't retain much power to attract today; Lane would be a stronger choice for a modern girl. **Lanae, Lanette, Lanna, Lannah, Lanny.**

♂ **LANE.** *English, 'from the narrow road'.* Though this is a rising name for boys, there's no reason why it can't be considered for a girl. **Laina, Laine, Lainey, Laney, Lanie, Layne.**

LANEY. *See* **LAINIE.**

♂ **LANGLEY.** *English, 'long meadow'.* This somewhat snobby-sounding surname popped onto the name map when Mariel Hemingway used it for one of her daughters. **Langlea, Langleah, Langly.**

LAPIS. *Persian, 'azure blue stone'.* Exotic gemstone name derived from lapis lazuli, which is said to enhance awareness and intellect, impart ancient wisdom and cure many ailments, making it an interesting possibility for a blue-eyed girl. Lazuli – or Azure or Blue – are other options.

LARA. *Russian, diminutive of* **LARISSA.** Laura or Lauren alternative made romantic by *Dr. Zhivago,* and sexy by video-game heroine Lara Croft. It's been a Top 100 name in recent years. **Larina, Larra.**

LARAINE. *Spelling variation of* **LORRAINE.** *See* **LORRAINE.** **Raina, Raine, Rayna, Reine, Reyna, Laraene, Larayne, Lareine, Larina, Larine.**

LARISSA. *Greek, 'cheerful, playful'.* Nymph name that's daintily pretty and a fresh alternative to Melissa or Alyssa. **Lara, Laressa, Larisa, Larissah, Larrissa, Larryssa, Laryssa, Laurissa, Laurissah, Lerissa, Lissa, Lorissa, Lyssa, Risa.**

LARK. *Nature name.* Lark is getting some new and well-deserved attention as a post-Robin bird name.

LATIFAH. *Arabic, 'kind and gentle'.* Singer-actress Queen Latifah – born Dana Owens – makes this North African Muslim name sing. **Lateefa, Lateefah, Lateifa, Lateiffa, Latifa, Latiffa.**

LATOYA. *Modern invented name.* Thanks to Ms Jackson, Latoya is one of the best-known *La* names, but names of this genre have been crowded out by newer favourites such as Destiny and Aaliyah. **Latoia, Latoyah, Latoyla, Letoya.**

★**LAURA.** *Latin, 'bay laurel'.* A hauntingly evocative perennial, never trendy, never dated, feminine without being fussy, with literary links stretching back to Dante, however it has been slipping its way down the Top 100 in recent years. **Laranca, Larea, Lari, Lauralee, Laurel, Lauren, Laureen, Laurella, Laurelle, Laurena, Laurence, Laurene, Laurentine, Laurestine, Lauretha, Lauretta, Lauri, Lauriane, Laurianne,** Lauricia, Laurie, Laurina, Lawra, Lollie, Lolly, Loree, Loreen, Lorelle, Loren, Lorena, Lorene, Loretta, Lorette, Lorey, Lori, Lorie, Lorinda, Lorine, Loris, Lorna, Lorretta, Lorette, Lorri, Lorrie, Lorry. International: **Laure, Laurette** (*French*), **Laurenza, Lorenza** (*Italian*), **Laureana, Laurensa, Laurentena, Laurentia, Laurinda, Laurita, Llora, Lorezza** (*Spanish*), **Laurice, Lauris, Lora, Lore, Lorita** (*German*), **Laurka** (*Polish*), **Lora** (*Bulgarian*), **Laurica, Laurissa, Lavra** (*Russian*).

LAUREEN. *Diminutive of* **LAURA.** Failed attempt to turn Laura into an Irish Colleen. **Laurene, Laurine, Lorene.**

★**LAUREL.** *Latin, 'laurel tree'.* Takes Laura back to its meaning in nature, resulting in a gentle, underused botanical option. **Laural, Lauralle, Laurell, Laurelle, Laurie, Lauryl, Laurylle, Loralle, Lorel, Lorelle.**

LAUREN. *English variation of* **LAURA.** More popular than Laura and also more trendy, Lauren – introduced by Lauren (born Betty) Bacall in 1944 – is still popular today and a member of the Top 50 list, chosen by parents seeking a gentle, not-too-extreme update of a Ralph Lauren–like classic. **Laren, Larentia, Larentina, Larenzina, Larren, Larryn, Larrynn, Larsina, Larsine, Laryn, Laureen, Laureena, Laurena, Laurence, Laurene, Laurentia, Laurentina, Lauri, Laurie, Laurin, Lauryn, Laurynn, Loreen, Loren, Lorena, Lorenn, Lorene, Lorenza, Lori, Lorin, Lorine, Lorne, Lorren, Lorrie, Lorrin, Lorrynn, Loryn, Lourenca, Lourence, Lowran, Lowrenn, Lowrynn.**

♂ **LAURENCE.** *Latin, 'from Laurentum'.* A feminine form in France, this boyish choice could make a fresh alternative to Lauren or Laura – or be an inventive way to honour Grandpa Larry.

LAURENZA. *Italian, feminine variation of* **LORENZO.** Unusual, exotic and appealing. **Laurenzia, Lorenza, Lorenzia.**

LAURETTA. *Diminutive of* **LAURA.** *See* **LORETTA.**

LAURIE. *English, originally a diminutive of* **LAURENCE.** Morphed into the more streamlined Lori in the 1960s, now uncool in either spelling.

LAURYN. *Spelling variation of* **LAUREN.** Given a new shot of style by singer Lauryn Hill, this spelling of the name is on the rise.

LAVANDA. *Italian, 'lavender'.* Cross between a colour name and a *La*-plus invention. **Lavenda.**

LAVENDER. *English herb and colour name.* Violet and Lilac are the up-and-coming purple shades – this might be a harder sell. **Lavendar.**

LAVERNE. *French, 'springlike'.* A name better left where is it, embroidered on a 1950s poodle skirt. **Laverine, Lavern, Laverna, LaVerne, Laverrne, Leverne, Loverna, Vern, Verna, Verne.**

LAVINIA. *Latin, 'woman of Rome'.* Prim and proper Lavinia dates back to Roman mythology, when it was the name of the mother of the Roman people. **Lavena, Lavenia,** Lavina, Lavinie, Levenia, Levener, Levinia, Lovina, Lovinia, Louvenia, Louvinia, Lovina, Lovinia, Vina, Vinia, Vinnie, Vinny. International: **Laia, Levina, Livinia, Luvena, Luvenia** *(Spanish).*

★**LAYLA.** *Arabic, 'dark beauty'; a variation of* **LEILA.** This lovely musical name (remember the old Eric Clapton song?) has seen a significant surge in popularity, no doubt through its kinship with hugely successful Kayla, recently entering the Top 100. **Laila.**

LEA. *Variation of* **LEAH** *or* **LEE.** More attractive than Lee, less meaningful than Leah.

♂ **LEAF.** *Nature name.* Hippy choice that, for girls, still retains an evergreen quality.

LEAH. *Hebrew, 'weary'.* For several years now, this serene biblical name – Leah was the sister of Rachel and first wife of Jacob – has been gaining a considerable following as a less common alternative to Sarah or Hannah, Rebecca or Rachel. It holds a firm spot in the Top 10. **Lea, Lee, Leigh, Lia, Liah.**

International: Leia, Léa *(French)*, Lia *(Italian)*, Leea, Leeah *(Finnish)*.

LEANDRA. *Latin, 'like a lioness'.* Two dated names – Leanne and Sandra – combine to make this far from a modern choice. **Leanda, Leanna, Leanne, Lelandra, Leyanne, Lianne.**

LEANNA. *Combination of* **LEE** *and* **ANNA.** A name that's gained some currency through its rhyming relationship to Breanna. **Leana, Leann, Leeann, Leyanna, Leyanne, Lianna, Lianne.**

LEATRICE. *Combination of* **LEE** *and* **BEATRICE.** Not quite Beatrice or Letitia, but still has a gently old-fashioned charm of its own.

LEDA. *Greek, 'happy'.* In classical Greek myth, Leda was a great beauty who mothered another great beauty, Helen of Troy. **Layda, Ledah, Leida, Leta, Leyda, Lyda. International: Lediana** *(Spanish),* **Lida, Lido, Lidochka** *(Russian).*

♂ **LEE.** *English, 'pasture, meadow'.* The original brief, breezy name, out of favour

now even as a middle name. **Lea, Leigh.**

LEELA. *Sanskrit, 'playful'.* See **LEILA.**

LEEZA. *Hebrew, diminutive of* **ALEEZA.** *See* **LISA. Leesa, Liza.**

LEIGH. *English variation of* **LEE.** This spelling adds a little more femininity to the neutral Lee.

LEILA. *Persian, 'dark beauty, night'.* The root name for a lush garden of similarly exotic examples, Leila was popularised by the poet Byron, who used it in a poem for a Muslim child. It's been chosen by such celebs as Greta Scacchi. **Laila, Layla, Leela, Leelah, Leilah, Leilia, Lela, Lelah, Leland, Lelia, Leyla, Lila, Lilah.**

LEILANI. *Hawaiian, 'a heavenly flower'.* A lovely Hawaiian name with a lovely meaning.

♂ **LEITH.** *Scottish, 'broad'.* Originally a male name, now a highly unusual, strong but soft, and intriguing girls' choice. **Leath, Leeth.**

LELIA. *(LEEL-ya) Contraction of* **EULALIA.** A rare and delicate choice. **Leelia, Leliah, Lellia.**

LENA. *English, Scottish, Dutch, German and Scandinavian, diminutive of various names ending in* lena. This pet form of Helena, long used as an independent name, is attracting notice again as an option both multicultural and simple. **Leena, Leina, Lina. International: Lene, Leni** *(German and Dutch).*

LENI. *German, diminutive of* **LENA;** *Spanish, diminutive of* **ELENA.** A foreign nickname name that has never been widely used here – possibly because of its similarity to the outdated male Lenny – it was chosen for her daughter by high-profile German supermodel Heidi Klum.

LENORA. *English, contracted form of* **LEONORA.** Used to be a modernised form of Leonora; now sounds more aged than the original. **Lennora, Lennorah, Lenorah.**

LENORE. *Greek, 'light';* *German variation of* **LEONORA.** A 'modernisation' of Leonora that no longer feels very modern. **Lenor, Lenora, Lenorah, Lenorr, Lenorra, Lenorre, Leonora, Leonore.**

LEOCADIA. *(lee-o-kay-dee-ah) Spanish, 'splendid brightness'.* A mix of sounds: the strength of a lion, with a rhythmic Latin ending. **International: Elocadia, Eleocaisa, Lacadia, Leokadia, Liocadia** *(Spanish),* **Llogaia** *(Catalan),* **Laocadia** *(Portuguese).*

LEONA. *Latin, 'a lioness'.* The most unfashionable of this pride of lion names. **Leeona, Leeowna, Leoine, Leola, Leonarda, Leone, Leonelle, Leonia, Leonice, Leontine, Leontyne, Leowna. International: Léonne, Léonie, Léonette** *(French),* **Leonida** *(Italian),* **Leonor, Leonita** *(Spanish),* **Lyonechika, Lyonya** *(Russian),* **Liona** *(Hawaiian).*

LÉONIE. *(LAY-o-nee) French, from the Latin, 'lion'.* Leona with a French accent that gives it a bit more flair. **Leoline, Leone, Leoni, Leonicia, Leonine, Leontine.**

LEONORA. *English, diminutive of ELEONORA or ELEANOR.* Its mellifluous sound makes this name, attached to the heroines of three major operas, a revival possibility. **Leanor, Leanora, Leanore, Lenora, Lenore, Leonore, Lionore, Nora, Norah, Ora. International: Leonara, Leonita, Lionora, Lioria, Nelida, Norita** *(Spanish).*

LEONTYNE. *English, 'lionlike'.* Almost exclusively associated with opera diva Leontyne Price. **Leontine.**

LEORA. *Hebrew and Greek, 'light'; diminutive of ELEANOR.* Somewhat dated Hebrew name that appears more modern when spelled Liora. **Leeora, Leorah, Leorit, Liora, Liorit.**

♂ **LESLIE.** *Scottish, 'garden by the pool'.* Leslie has a pleasant, heathery feel that keeps it consistently popular with parents; the Lesly and Lesley spellings are also frequently used. **Les, Leslea, Leslee, Leslei, Lesleigh, Lesley, Lesli, Lesly, Leslye, Lesslie, Lezlee, Lezley, Lezli, Lezlie.**

LETA. *Latin, 'glad, joyful'. See LITA.* **Leeta, Lelita, Lita.**

LETESHA. *Spelling variation of LETITIA.* Phonetic spelling of a Victorian-valentine name; it was chosen by rapper Ice-T. **Latesha, Lateesha, Leteesha.**

LETHA. *Greek, 'forgetfulness'.* Taken from Lethe, the mythological River of Oblivion, it now sounds as if it's missing a first syllable. **Leitha, Leithia, Lethe, Lethia.**

★**LETITIA.** *Latin, 'joy, gladness'.* Prim and proper sounding name whose staid image has been unbuttoned by numerous phonetic spellings. The original, often used in Spanish-speaking families, would still make an attractive, delicate choice. **Laetitia, Laetizia, Latia, Laticia, Latisha, Latticia, Leda, Leta, Letesha, Leteshia, Letha, Letice, Letichia, Leticja, Letisha, Letishia, Letisia, Letissa, Letiticia, Lettice, Lettie, Lettitia, Letty, Letycia, Letycja, Tish, Tisha. International: Letizia** *(Italian),* **Alaricia, Eleticia, Laiticia, Latisha, Leticia, Liticia, Ticha** *(Spanish),* **Letja** *(Dutch).*

LETIZIA. *(lat-TEET-zee-ah) Italian variation of LETITIA.* Pretty Latin variation of Letitia;

this was the first name of Napoleon's mother.

LETTICE. *English variation of* **LETITIA.** Although still occasionally heard in upper-class British families, we fear it could cause too much salad-lettuce teasing. **Lettie, Letty.**

LETTY. *English, diminutive of* **LETITIA.** Like Lottie, a nickname name not heard in over a century, giving it the patina of a treasured antique. **Letti, Lettie.**

LEXI. *Diminutive of* **ALEXANDRA.** Lexi and Lexie, pixieish offshoots of the prolific Alex family, have come into their own. **Lecksi, Leksi, Leksie, Lexey, Lexie, Lexy.**

LEXIA. *Greek, diminutive of* **ALEXIA.** *See* **ALEXIA.** **Lexa, Lexie, Lexina, Lexine, Lexya.**

LEXIS. *Greek, diminutive of* **ALEXIS.** A condensation of Alexis, or a wish to drive a Lexus? **Laexis, Lexuss, Lexius, Lexsis, Lexus, Lexuss, Lexxis, Lexxus.**

♂ **LEXUS.** *Greek variation of a diminutive of* **ALEXIS.** This automotive newcomer has recently taken off in the US – more because of its association, we fear, with the status symbol car than its relation to the name Alexis. **Lexuss, Lexxus, Lexyss.**

LEXY. *Diminutive of* **ALEXANDRA.** *See* **LEXI.**

LEYA. *(LAY-yeh) Spanish, 'the law'; Hindi, 'lion'.* A simple, attractive multicultural choice, but with some teasing peril. **Laia, Laya, Leia.**

LIA. *(LEE-uh) Italian variation of* **LEAH.** Used in Italy, Spain, Greece, Russia and Hawaii, Lia sounds just like Leah, but looks particularly pretty on paper. **Leeya. International: Liya (Russian).**

LIAN. *Chinese, 'graceful willow'.* Could be confused with the much less exotic Leanne.

LIANA. *French, 'to climb like a vine'.* Pretty and graceful name – it's a flowering tropical vine – that runs the risk of sounding as if its front end might have been cut off, as in Juliana or Eliana. **Leana, Leanna, Leiana, Liahna, Liane, Lianna, Lianne.**

Nouveau Names on the Rise

Ainsley
Aria
Ashton
Avery
Cadence
Cali
Campbell
Cheyenne
Elle
Essence
Genesis
Harley
Harmony
Haven
Heaven
Jaden
Kennedy
Lexi
Macy
Nevaeh
Presley
Skye
Skyla
Tayla
Trista

LIANNE. *Diminutive of* **JULIANNE.** Occasionally used independently, but fairly flimsy. **Leanne, LeeAnn, LeeAnne, LeighAnne, Liane.**

LIBBY. *English, diminutive of* **ELIZABETH.** Through all the years when Betty, Betsy, Beth, Liz and Lizzie were the Elizabethan nicknames of choice, Libby was set aside, but today it may be the most modern of all – it is firmly in the Top 100. **Lib, Libbey, Libbi, Libbie, Liby.**

LIBERTY. *Word name.* A 1970s hippy that is name now seeing something of a resurgence; chosen by sports superstar Ryan Giggs. **Lib, Libbey, Libbie, Liberti, Libertie.**

LIBRA. *Greek, 'scales, balance'.* Appropriate for a girl born between late September and late October, Libra suggests both balance and freedom.

LIDA. *Variation of* **LEDA.** *See* **LEDA.** (The similar but more mysterious **LIDDA** was the name of a character played by Kirsten Dunst.)

LIESL. *(LEEZ-el) German, diminutive of* **ELIZABETH.** Stuck in the Alps with Heidi. **Leesel, Leesl, Leezel, Leezl, Liesel, Liesl, Liezel, Liezl, Lisel.**

LIL. *Diminutive of* **LILLIAN** *and* **LILY.** Spunky old vaudeville era nickname name.

★**LILA.** *Arabic, 'night'; Hindi, 'the free, playful will of God'; Persian, 'lilac'; also diminutive of* **DELILAH.** Names with a double *l* sound – Lila, Lola and Lily – have recently caught on, particularly among the celebrity set (model Kate Moss and comedian Chris Rock both have little Lilas), and we must admit we recommend them all. Sultry and forceful, Lila has a slight Near Eastern tinge. **Layla, Leila, Lilah, Lyla, Lylah.**

LILAC. *English, from Persian, flower and colour name.* Bored by Lily and Rose? Consider this deeper hue as a cutting-edge but still sweet-smelling flower name. **International: Lilah, Lilas** *(French),* **Flieder** *(German and Yiddish),* **Suren, Syrin** *(Scandinavian),* **Siryen** *(Russian).*

LILEAS. *Scottish variation of* **LILY.** Adds some thorns to the smooth texture of Lily. **Lil, Lilas, Lilias, Lillas, Lilli, Lillias, Lillie, Lily.**

LILIA. *Latin, 'lilies'; Hawaiian, 'lily'.* Another pretty double *l* name, this one's more unusual and distinctive than some others. **International: Liliela, Liliosa** *(Spanish).*

LILIAN, LILLIAN. *English, from the Latin flower name, 'lily'.* Long dormant since its Lillian Russell–Floradora Girl heyday at the turn of the last century, Lillian is making a comeback, seen by parents as a more serious and subdued cousin of the megapopular Lily. **Lila, Liliann, Lilianne, Lilies, Lillia, Lillianne, Lillie, Lilly, Lillyan, Lillyanne, Lily, Lilyan, Lilyann, Lilyanne. International: Liliane** *(French),* **Liliana** *(Italian),* **Lilia, Liliana, Lilias, Liliosa** *(Spanish),* **Lili, Lilli** *(German),* **Lilja, Lilya** *(Finnish),* **Liljana** *(Polish),* **Lelya, Lilia, Liliya** *(Russian),* **Lilika, Lilis** *(Greek),* **Lilieana, Lilia** *(Hawaiian).*

LILIANA, LILLIANA. *Italian and Spanish variations of*

LILIAN. This melodious and feminine Latin variation of the Lily family is a favourite in the Hispanic community and would work beautifully with an Anglo surname as well. **Lillyana, Lilyana.**

LILIAS. *See* **LILEAS** *and* **LILLIAN.**

LILITH. *Assyrian, Sumerian, 'ghost, night monster'.* Lilith has been demonised since medieval times, with Jewish folklore portraying her as Adam's first wife, who was turned into a hideous bloodsucking night demon for refusing to obey him. So, in spite of its gently pleasant sound, Lilith is rarely heard. **Lillith.**

LILLA. *Italian, 'lilac'.* Three *l*'s may not be better than two. Consider Willa or Lila instead.

LILLY. *See* **LILY.**

LILO. *(LEE-lo) German, diminutive of* **LISELOTTE;** *Hawaiian, 'generous one'.* The little girl character in Disney's *Lilo & Stitch*.

★**LILY.** *English, from Latin, flower name.* One of the delicate century-old flower names making a return, Lily has many irresistible attributes: a cool elegance and a lovely sound, a symbol of purity and innocence, and a role in Christian imagery. It's a favourite of celebrity parents, including Kate Beckinsale and Johnny Depp. It has been zooming up the charts, recently entering the Top 10. **Leelee, Lil, Lila, Lilas, Lilian, Liliana, Lilias, Liliosa, Lilium, Lilla, Lilley, Lilli, Lillia, Lillianne, Lillika, Lillita, Lilly, Lilyan, Lilyanne.** International: **Lili, Liliane, Lys** *(French),* **Lili, Lilie** *(German),* **Lia, Lilia, Liliya, Liya** *(Russian),* **Lilike** *(Slavic),* **Liliah, Lilika** *(Greek).*

LINA. *Diminutive of* **ADELINA, EMELINA, CAROLINA, ANGELINA.** *See* **LENA. Leena, Leina.**

LINDA. *German, 'serpent'; Spanish, 'pretty'.* Linda will live forever in baby name history for toppling Mary from its reign as Queen of Names in the 1950s. Linda has fallen even further in favour than Mary today. **Lin,**

169
girls' names

> **If You Like Lily,**
> *You Might Love . . .*
>
> Camilla
> Delilah
> Ella
> Finlay
> Ivy
> Leila
> Libby
> Lila
> Lilac
> Liliana
> Millie
> Poppy
> Talullah
> Willa

Lindee, Lindi, Lindie, Lindey, Lindira, Lindka, Lindy, Linn, Linnie, Lyn, Lynda, Lynde, Lyndy, Lynn, Lynnda, Lynndie, Lynne.

♂ **LINDEN.** *Nature name.* The graceful, natural image of the verdant shade tree transcends any connection with Linda or

Lynn – though it could be an offbeat homage to someone with those names. **Lindenn, Lindon, Lynden.**

LINDSAY, LINDSEY. *English and Scottish, 'island of linden trees'.* In the early 1980s, Lindsay, riding in tandem with Courtney, were popular names, but while it deserves credit as a pioneering early unisex-last-name-first-name, its own currency has faded. **Lind, Lindsaye, Lindsea, Lindsee, Lindseigh, Lindsey, Lindsi, Lindsie, Lindsy, Lindzi, Lindzy, Linsay, Linsey, Linzee, Linzey, Linzi, Linzie, Linzy, Lyndsay, Lyndsey, Lyndsy, Lynsay, Lynsday, Lynsey, Lynsie, Lynzee, Lynzey, Lynzi, Lynzy.**

LINNÉA. *(lin-NAY-ah) Norse, 'lime tree, lime blossom'.* Popular Scandinavian name – first bestowed in honour of Swedish botanist Carl von Linné, a classifier of plants and animals – that could make an engaging choice. **Linea, Linnaea, Lynea, Lynnea, Nea.**

LINNET. *(LIN-et) French, 'flaxen haired'.* Although the accent is on the first syllable, it could be confused with the dated Lynette. **Lin, Linetta, Linette, Linnette, Linni, Linnie, Linny, Lynetta, Lynette, Lynnetta, Lynnette. International: Eluned** *(Welsh).*

♂ **LIONEL.** *French, 'young lion'.* Yet another traditional boy's name entering the girls' column, via prize-winning novelist Lionel (born Margaret Ann) Shriver, and gaining some new life from the move. **Lionell, Lionelle, Lyonel, Lyonell, Lyonelle.**

LISA. *English variation of LIZA, diminutive of ELIZABETH.* Elvis naming his daughter Lisa Marie and the hit song 'Mona Lisa' conspired to catapult this offshoot of Elizabeth towards the top in the 1970s. Its star barely twinkles now. **Leeza, Liesa, Liesebet, Liseta, Lisetta, Lisette. International: Elise, Lise, Lisette** *(French),* **Leesa, Liesja, Lissa** *(Dutch),* **Liese, Liesel** *(German),* **Lise** *(Danish),* **Lisza** *(Hungarian).*

LISBETH. *German, diminutive of ELIZABETH. See* **ELIZABETH. Lisbet, Lizbet, Lizbeth.**

LISETTE. *French, diminutive of LISE.* Although dated, it retains a certain dainty charm. **Lisette.**

LISSA. *African and Arabic mythology name; diminutive of* **MELISSA.** Might be an abbreviation of Melissa, but more substantial in its own right: it's the name of a supreme mother goddess in African mythology and an Arabic symbol of rebirth.

LITA. *Diminutive of* **ROSELITA, LOLITA, CARMELITA,** *etc.* Vivacious but lightweight.

LITZY. *Spanish nickname.* Inspired by the Mexican singer who uses it as her single name.

LIV. *Norse, 'life'.* The fame of actress and Aerosmith daughter Liv Tyler helped to infuse life into this short but solid Scandinavian name that was also chosen by Julianne Moore for her daughter.

LIVANA. *Hebrew, 'the moon, white'.* Pretty and unusual. **Leva, Levana, Liva, Livah, Livona.**

★**LIVIA.** *Latin, 'bluish'; Hebrew, 'crown'.* Though it sounds like a chopped-off variation of Olivia, the distinctively attractive Livia has been an independent name since ancient Rome, and is still commonly heard in modern Italy. Good Olivia alternative. **Levia, Liv, Livie, Livy, Livvy, Livya, Lyvia.**

LIZ. *Diminutive of* **ELIZABETH.** A girl given this name on her birth certificate could feel deprived of her full identity. **Lisette, Lizz, Lyz, Lyzz.**

LIZA. *Diminutive of* **ELIZA,** *diminutive of* **ELIZABETH.** Still tied to Ms Minnelli, who was named by her mother Judy Garland after a George Gershwin song. Step up to Eliza instead. **Lyza.**

LIZANNE. *Combination of* **LIZ** *and* **ANNE.** This does not sound as dated as other hybrids. **Lisann, Lisanne, Lizann.**

LIZBETH. *Short form of* **ELIZABETH.** For parents who are trying to cut down on their vowels and syllables. **Lisabet,** Lisabeth, Lisabette, Lisbet, Lizabeth, Lizabette, Lizbett, Lyzbeth.

LISETH. *Short form of* **ELIZABETH.** For parents who are trying to cut down on their vowels, consonants and syllables.

LISETTE. *See* **LISETTE.** Lisett.

LIZZIE. *Diminutive of* **ELIZABETH.** Commonly used as an independent name in the last half of the nineteenth century, today still one of the most stylish short forms of Elizabeth. **Lizzey, Lizzi, Lizzy, Lizy.**

LLIO. *(LEE-oh) Welsh, originally a diminutive of* **GWENLLIAN.** Looks unusual and almost on the brink of weird; sounds like a little lioness named Leo.

★♂ **LOGAN.** *Scottish surname, 'little hollow'.* With its appealing Scottish burr, this very hot boys' name would make a rich and resonant name for a girl.

LOIRE. *(Lo-AR) French river and region name.* The lovely sound and image of the French river and lush valley would make this a most distinctive and captivating choice. **Loir, Loirane.**

LOIS. *Greek, 'agreeable'.* The eternal fiancée of Superman turned sweet grey-haired lady who's always available to babysit her grandkids.

★**LOLA.** *Spanish, diminutive of* **DOLORES.** A hot starbaby name – chosen by Chris Rock, Charlie Sheen and Annie Lennox, and used as the nickname of Madonna's Lourdes – Lola manages to be sexy without going over the top, and has recently made it to the Top 100. Be warned, though: 'Whatever Lola wants, Lola gets'. **Loela, Lolita, Lolla.**

LOLITA. *Spanish, diminutive of* **LOLA** *and* **DOLORES.** Parents are beginning to ignore the adolescent sex kitten associations of the notorious Nabokov novel, seeing this as a charming, offbeat name with a good deal of style for those who defy convention.

LOLO. *Diminutive of* **CAROLINE.** One step up – or is it down? – from Lala.

LONA. *Diminutive of* **LEONA.** Unfashionable name, with the rather poignant *lone* sound. **Loni, Lonie, Lonna, Lonnee, Lonnie.**

★♂ **LONDON.** *English place name.* The capital makes a solid and attractive twenty-first-century choice, with a lot more substance than Paris. **Londen, Londin, Londun, Londyn, Londynn.**

LONI. *Variation of* **LEONA.** In baby name limbo along with Ronni, Connie, and Bonnie. **Lonni, Lonnie, Lonny.**

LORA. *German variation and spelling variation of* **LAURA.** Somewhat flat-footed form; go for the original. **Loree, Lorenna, Lorey, Lori, Loribelle, Lorra, Lorree, Lorrie, Lory.**

LOREEN. *English elaboration of* **LORA.** Superseded by Lauren. **Lorene.**

LORELEI. *German, 'alluring, temptress'.* A name that has been previously associated with the mythic seductive siren and the gold digger in *Gentlemen Prefer Blondes,* today it feels more modern and has recently been gaining in popularity. **Loralee, Loralei, Lorelai, Lorelie, Laurelei, Laurelie, Loralie, Loralyn, Lorilee, Lorilyn, Lura, Lurette, Lurleen, Lurlene, Lurline.**

LORELLE. *English elaboration of* **LORA.** Lorelei would make a cooler choice. **Lorella.**

♂ **LOREN.** *English spelling variation of* **LAUREN.** This version is more frequently used for boys.

LORENA. *(low-RAY-na) Spanish variation of* **LORRAINE.** A feminine name heard most often in the Hispanic community. **Laurena, Lorenita, Lorenna, Lorenza, Lorenya.**

LORENZA. *See* **LAURENZA.** **Laurencia, Laurenza, Lorencia.**

LORETTA. *English variation of Italian* **LAURETTA;** *diminutive of* **LAURA.** Long ago lost its Latin flair. **Laretta, Larette, Larretta, Lauret, Lauretta, Laurette, Leretta, Loret, Loreta, Lorette, Lorretta, Lowretta.**

LORI. *English spelling variation of* **LAURIE;** *diminutive of* **LAURA.** 1960s babysitter. **Lauri, Laurie, Loree, Lorri, Lorrie.**

LORINDA. *English elaboration of* **LORA.** Echoes of two dated names: Lori and Linda.

LORNA. *English literary name.* Invented for the 1869 novel *Lorna Doone,* and perpetuated as the name of a shortbread cookie, it doesn't make a very inspired choice. **Lorrna.**

LORRAINE. *French 'from the province of Lorraine'.* Sweet Lorraine is almost old enough to be ripe for reconsideration: aging hipster Jack Nicholson used it for his daughter. **Laraine, Larayne, Lareine, Lareyne, Larraine, Laurraine, Leraine, Lerayne, Lorain, Loraine, Lorane, Lori, Lorine, Lorrayne.**

LOTTIE. *English, diminutive of* **CHARLOTTE.** Nostalgic great-grandma name that conjures up lockets and lace, and – like Nellie, Josie, Tillie and Milly – has considerable vintage charm.

Lotie, Lotta, Lotte, Lottey, Lotti, Lotty.

LOTUS. *Greek, 'lotus flower'.* One of the most exotic and languorous of the flower names, with intriguing symbolic significance in several cultures.

LOUELLA. *English, combination of* **LOUISE** *and* **ELLA.** Combined names are rarely greater than the sum of their parts. **Luella.**

LOUISA. *Latinate feminine variation of* **LOUIS.** These days, old-style girls' names are more fashionable when they end with an *a* rather than with *e,* as in Julie/Julia, Diane/Diana – and this quaint eighteenth-century favourite is no exception. Another plus: the Louisa May Alcott reference. **Lou, Lu. International: Luisa** *(Italian and Polish),* **Aloisa, Aluisa, Loyisa, Luisetta, Luisianna, Luisina, Luiza, Lula, Lulita** *(Spanish),* **Aloisa** *(German),* **Lovisa** *(Swedish),* **Lovise** *(Danish, Norwegian),* **Lutza, Luyiza** *(Russian),* **Eloisia** *(Greek).*

LOUISIANA. *French place name.* A geographic spin on the

Louise theme; pretty, if a bit of a syllable overload.

LOUISE. *French and English, feminine variation of* **LOUIS.** This French form of Louisa is now seen as competent, studious and efficient – desirable if not dramatic qualities. **Loise, Lou, Louisetta, Louisette, Loulou, Lu, Lulie, Lulu. International: Aloyse, Eloise, Heloise, Louisiane** *(French),* **Eloisa** *(Italian and Spanish),* **Luise** *(German),* **Lovise** *(Danish and Norwegian).*

LOURDES. *(LURE-days) Basque, 'craggy slope'.* This name of the French town where a young peasant girl had a vision of the Virgin Mary in 1858 vaulted into the spotlight when Madonna chose it for her daughter, but few other families except for devout Roman Catholics have followed her lead (any more than they've used Rocco for their sons). **Lordes, Lourdette. International: Lourdecita, Lourdetta, Lurdes** *(Spanish).*

LOVE. *Word name.* Best left as a middle name, as in Jennifer

173
girls' names

Names Headed for Oxbridge

Anna
Beatrice
Caroline
Claire
Constance
Eleanor
Esther
Frances
Grace
Helen
Irene
Honor
Joanna
Louisa
Margaret
Martha
Portia
Rachel
Ruth

Love Hewitt. **Lovely, Lovey, Lovie, Lovy, Luv, Luvvy.**

LOWRI. *Welsh, from Latin, 'laurel'.* This unusual and appealing name is popular in

Anaelle
Armel
Axelle
Clea
Clemence
Elodie
Fabienne
Faustine
Flavie
Fleur
Ines
Isaline
Lea
Leonie
Lilou
Lou
Lucienne
Maelle
Maelys/Mailys
Maeva
Manon
Ophélie
Romane
Salome
Severine

sections of Wales. **Lowree, Lowrey, Lowrie, Lowry.**

LUANA. *Combination of* LOUISE *and* ANNA. The kind of vaguely exotic-sounding name used for Polynesian maidens in early movies. **Lewanna, Lou-Ann, Louanna, Louanne, Luane, Luann, Luanna, Luannah, Luanne, Luannie, Luwana, Luwanna.**

LUANDA. *African place name.* This name of Angola's capital city has occasionally been used for baby girls.

LUBA. *Russian, Slavic, 'love, lover'; Yiddish, 'dear'.* Its association with the word *liebe* gives this name an endearing, adored aura. **Liba, Lubah, Lyuba, Lyubah.**

♂ **LUCA.** *Italian variation of* LUKE. Very much a boy's name in Italy, it's beginning to be seen as a unisex possibility elsewhere.

LUCERNE. *Latin, 'lamp'; Swiss place name.* Projects the calm and pristine image of the picturesque Swiss lake and mountain town. **Lucerna, Luzerne.**

LUCETTA. *English elaboration of* LUCIA *or* LUCY. Lace-hankie name with Shakespearean pedigree.

★♂ **LUCIA.** *(loo-CHEE-a or LOO-sha) Italian, feminine variation of* LUCIUS. A lovely name with operatic connections that used to be given to babies born as daylight was breaking. **International: Lucinenne** *(French),* **Luciana, Luciella** *(Italian),* **Chia, Chila, Lusila** *(Spanish).*

LUCIE. *French spelling of* LUCY. *See* LUCY.

LUCIENNE. *(loo-see-EN) French, feminine variation of* LUCIAN. Soft and sophisticated French-accented option.

LUCILLA. *See* LUCILLE.

LUCILLE. *French variation of* LUCILLA *or* LUCY. A name overpowered by its long-lasting link to Lucille Ball, with an image of tangerine-coloured hair, big, round eyes and a tendency to stage daffy and desperate stunts. **Loucille, Lucila,**

Lucile, Lucilla, Lucyle, Luseele, Luselle, Lusile.

LUCINDA. *Variation of* **LUCIA** *or* **LUCY.** First found in *Don Quixote,* this is a pleasingly pretty embellishment of Lucy. **Cinda, Cindy, Loucinda, Lusinda, Sinda, Sindy. International:** Lucinde *(French).*

♂ **LUCKY.** *Word name.* Most parents would find it this name, though optimistic, not exactly substantial. **Lucki.**

LUCRETIA. *Roman family name.* Perfectly plausible Latin name that's gotten a raw deal through the years via a link to Lucretia Borgia, who, though mistakenly considered a demon poisoner, was actually a patron of learning and the arts. **Loucrecia, Loucresha, Loucrezia, Lucreecia, Lucreesha, Lucreisha, Lucresha, Lucrisha, Lucrishia. International:** Lucrèce *(French),* Lucrezia *(Italian),* Lucrecia *(Spanish).*

LUCY. *English, feminine variation of* **LUCIUS.** Consistently in the Top 10 in recent years, Lucy is slowly but surely gaining in popularity. It is an attractive name on so many levels: it's both saucy and solid, a saint's name and heroine of several great novels, and is associated with characters as diverse as the bossy little girl in *Peanuts* and the psychedelic 'Lucy in the Sky with Diamonds'. **Cindi, Cindie, Cindy, Lou, Loulou, Lu, Luce, Lucee, Lucetta, Lula, Lusita. International:** Luiseach *(Irish Gaelic),* Lleulu *(Welsh),* Lucida, Lucie, Lucienne, Lucette, Lucinde *(French),* Lucia, Luciana, Luciella, Luzia *(Italian),* Lucia, Luciana, Lucilla, Lucinda, Lucila, Luz *(Spanish),* Luzia *(Portuguese),* Luzi, Luzie *(German),* Lucya, Lucyna *(Polish),* Lizija *(Russian),* Luca, Luci, Lucika, Lucka *(Slavic).*

LUDMILA. *Slavic, 'beloved of the people'.* A Slavic name whose sound has never appealed to British parents. **Ludie. International:** Lidmila *(Czech),* Lyudmila, Lyuda, Lyuka, Myusya, Mika, Mila *(Russian).*

LUDOVICA. *Italian, feminine variation of* **LUDOVIC.** Old-fashioned name with a measure of continental style – an offbeat possibility for the bold baby namer.

LUELLA. *Spelling variation of* **LOUELLA.** *See* **LOUELLA.**

LUISE. *German variation of* **LOUISE.** *See* **LOUISE.**

LULU. *Arabic, 'pearl,' diminutive of* **LOUELLA** *and* **LOUISE.** A name with a firecracker personality, a singing and dancing extrovert. **Loulou, Lula, Lulie.**

LUMIÈRE. *French, 'light'.* Innovative French word name, suggesting illumination and clarity. **International:** Luminosa, Lumina *(Spanish).*

★**LUNA.** *Italian and Spanish, 'moon'.* This moonstruck name would make a daring, evocative choice. **Lune, Lunetta, Lunette, Lunneta, Lunnete, Luneth. International:** Lune, Lunette *(French).*

LUPE. *Latin, 'wolf'; Spanish, diminutive of* **GUADALUPE.** A nickname name heard in Spanish-speaking cultures, but be warned – it might lead to

Stellar Starbabies Beginning with *L*

Leila	Greta Scacchi
Leni	Heidi Klum
Liberty	Ryan Giggs
Lila	Kate Moss
Lily	Kate Beckinsale, Kathy Ireland, Greg Kinnear, Chris O'Donnell
Lillyella	Melanie (*All Saints*) Blatt & Stuart Zender
Liv	Julianne Moore
Lola	Denise Richards & Charlie Sheen, Chris Rock, Carnie Wilson, Lucy Pargeter, Sara Cox
Lorenza	Luciano Pavarotti
Lourdes	Madonna
Lydia	Bill Paxton

'loopy' jokes. **Lupelina, Lupi, Lupita, Pita.**

LURLEEN. *Modern variation of* **LORELEI.** Has a country and western twang. **Lura, Lurette, Lurline.**

LUX. *Latin, 'light'.* This name of a character played by Kirsten Dunst in the movie *Virgin Suicides* is more soapy than de luxe.

LUZ. *(LOOS) Spanish, 'light'.* This name that refers to the Virgin Mary – 'Our Lady of Light' – is well used in the Hispanic community. **Chitta, Lucecita, Lucelida, Lucelita, Lucha, Lucida, Lucila, Lusa, Luzana** *(Spanish).*

LYDIA. *Greek, 'woman from Lydia'.* An ancient place name, also seen in the New Testament and in Jane Austen, the once neglected Lydia is now beginning to be appreciated for its history and is now in the Top 100. **Liddie, Lidie, Lidya, Lyda.** International: **Lydie** *(French),* **Lidia** *(Spanish),* **Lida** *(Czech),* **Lida, Lidia, Lidija, Lidiya, Lydie** *(Russian).*

♂ **LYLE.** *French, 'from the island'.* Perfect example of a name that sounds old-fashioned for a boy, cool for a girl. **Lisle.**

LYNDA. *See* **LINDA.**

LYNDSEY. *See* **LINDSEY.**

LYNETTE. *Welsh, 'idol'; French elaboration of Lynn.* Dated name replaced by Lindsay. **Lanette, Linette, Lynett, Lynetta.**

LYNN. *Modern diminutive of* **LINDA.** Lynn arrived in the 1940s, spinning off from the wildly popular Linda, to become a top mid-century middle name. Now, Lynn's in limbo. **Lin, Linn, Linnell, Linnie, Lyn, Lynea, Lyndel, Lyndell, Lynell, Lynelle, Lynett, Lynette, Lynna, Lynne, Lynnelle.**

LYNWEN. *Welsh, 'fair image'.* A bit of a tongue-twister.

LYRIC. *Greek, 'lyre'.* A musical name with Greek roots that is given to several hundred babies a year in the US, appealing to parents who like such other names as Harmony, Melody and Cadence.

M *girls*

MAB. *Irish, 'joy, hilarity'; Welsh, 'baby'; Anglicisation of* **MAEVE.** Madcap Shakespearean name of queen of the fairies, if you want something both adventurous and simple. **Mabry, Mave, Mavis, Meave.**

MABEL. *Diminutive of* **AMABEL.** Victorian favourite still searching for its place in modern life. But if you love offbeat old-fashioned names like Violet or Josephine, only sassier, this is one for you to consider. **Amabel, Amable, Amaybel, Amaybelle, Amayble, Mab, Mabbs, Mabella, Mabelle, Mable, Mabyn, Maebell, Mabelle, Maible, Maybel, Maybeline, Maybelle, Mayble, Maybull. International: Máible** *(Irish Gaelic),* **Moibeal** *(Scottish),* **Mabilia** *(Italian).*

MABYN. *Cornish, from English, 'boy'.* This rare sixth-century saint's name has a modern, merry feel.

MACARIA. *Spanish from Greek, 'blessed'.* Unusual and rhythmic, but perhaps too reminiscent of the Macarena. **Macarisa, Macarria, Maccaria, Makaria, Makarria.**

MACHA. *(MOK-ha) Irish mythology name.* Irish goddess and saint name that's strong, to say the least.

MACHIKO. *Japanese, 'fortunate child'.* What parent wouldn't love this meaning? **Machi.**

♂ **MACKENZIE, McKENZIE.** *Scottish, 'son of the comely one'.* A number of today's parents, including *Harry Potter* creator J. K. Rowling, have flocked to this once male name, as well as other Mac choices. **Macenzie, Mackenna, Mackensi, Mackensie, Mackenze, Mackenzee, Mackenzey, Mackenzi, Mackenzia, Mackenzy, Mackenzye, Mackinsey, Mackynze, Makensie, Makenzie,** McKenzie, McKinzie, Mekenzie, M'Kenzie, Mykenzie.

♂ **MACON.** *Place name.* Fashionable-sounding name of cities in both France and Georgia, US, that seems distinctly boyish.

MACY. *English variation of* **MASSEY.** Singer Macy Gray has popularised this cute and upbeat choice, a modern replacement for Stacy and Tracy. **Macey, Macie, Maecy, Maicey, Maicy.**

MADEIRA. *Place name.* Madeira is an island off Morocco where the wine comes from. In general, we frown on alcoholic names, even one as theoretically attractive as this. **Madera, Madira.**

MADDISON. *Variation of Madison.* This double *dd* name is currently popular enough to be in the Top 100.

MADELINE, MADELEINE. *French variation of* **MAGDALEN.** The lovely, soft Madeline is an old-fashioned favourite that returned in the 1990s, combining a classic pedigree with a cute nickname option: Maddy. **Mada, Madalaina, Madaleine, Madaliene, Madalyn, Madalyne, Maddi, Maddie, Maddy, Madel, Madelayne, Madelena, Madelene, Madelina, Madelon, Madelyn, Madilyn, Madlen, Madline, Madlyn, Madoline, Madolyn, Mady, Magdalen, Magdalene, Magdaline, Magdalini, Maidel, Maighdlin, Malina, Marlean, Marlen, Marlyne.** International: **Madelaine, Madella, Madelle** (French), **Madalene, Maddalena** (Italian), **Madia, Madena, Madina** (Spanish), **Malena, Malin** (Dutch), **Madelina, Mahda** (Russian).

MADGE. Diminutive of **MARGERY** or **MARGARET.** Madonna's nickname. **Madgi, Madgie, Mady.**

♂ **MADIGAN.** Irish, 'little dog'. Unusual, energetic surname choice. Good Madison alternative.

♂ **MADISON.** English, 'son of the mighty warrior'. This is a trendy American import –

currently in the Top 40. It's inspired by the mermaid's name (she took it from a New York street sign) in the 1980s film Splash. **Maddison, Madisen, Madisson, Madisyn, Madsen, Madyson, Mattison.**

MADONNA. Latin, 'my lady'. There's only one. Okay, two. **Madona.**

MADRIGAL. Latin, 'song for unaccompanied voices'. Pretty choice for a child of a musical family.

MADRONA. Spanish, 'mother'. A bit grown-up for a tiny baby. **Madro, Madre, Madrena.**

★**MAEVE.** (MAYV) Irish, 'she who intoxicates'. Short but striking, this ancient Irish queen's name is now finding well-deserved favour. **Mab, Maevi, Maevy, Maive, Mave, Mayve, Meave.** International: **Madhbh, Maebh, Meadhbh, Medbh, Meibh** (Gaelic), **Maeva** (French).

MAGDA. German variation of **MAGDALEN.** On Sex and the City, she was the elderly nanny from the old country – which is

what this name sounds like. International: **Magdá** (Slavic).

MAGDALEN, MAGDALENE. Greek, 'high tower'. Biblical name forever associated with the fallen-yet-redeemed Mary Magdalen. **Mada, Magdaleen, Magdalene, Magdaline, Magdalyn, Magdalynn, Magdelane, Magdelene, Magdeline, Magdelyn, Magdlen, Magdolna, Maggie, Magola, Maighdlin, Mala, Malaine.** International: **Magdala, Magdalaine, Magdalen, Magdaleine** (French), **Maddalena** (Italian), **Magdalena** (Spanish, Portuguese, German, Dutch, Norwegian, Swedish, Polish, Czech), **Magda** (German and Czech), **Magdalone, Malene** (Danish), **Madzia** (Polish), **Magdolina** (Hungarian).

MAGENTA. Colour name. Vivid colour name, not for the reserved.

MAGGIE. Diminutive of **MARGARET.** Cute, earthy short form in style for a few decades now, sometimes used as an independent name. **Mag, Magali, Magge, Maggee, Maggey, Maggi, Maggia,**

Maggiemae, Maggy, Magi, Magie, Magli, Mags, Maguy, Meggy.

MAGNOLIA. *Latin, flower name.* Hothouse flower name. **Maggy, Nola.**

♂ **MAGRITTE.** *French surname.* Intriguing spin on Margaret or Maggie, for admirers of French surrealist René Magritte.

MAHALA. *(Ma-HAIL-ah) Hebrew, 'tender affection'.* Attractive Old Testament name best known in the form Mahalia, as in singer Jackson. **Mahalah, Mahalar, Mahalath, Mahaley, Mahalia, Mahaliah, Mahalie, Mahalla, Mahayla, Mahaylah, Mahaylia, Mahela, Mahelea, Maheleah, Mahelia, Mahila, Mahilia, Mahlah, Mahlaha, Mehala, Mehalah, Mehalia.**

MAHOGANY. *Spanish, 'rich, strong'.* Dark, woody name that's a bit heavy for a little girl. **Mahagony, Mahoganey, Mahogani, Mahoganie, Mahogney, Mahogny, Mohogany, Mohogony.**

MAI. *Japanese, 'dance'; French, 'the month of May'; Vietnamese, 'cherry blossom'; Navajo, 'coyote'.* Cross-cultural winner.

MAIA. *Greek, 'mother'.* Roman goddess of spring who gave her name to the month of May. Now more often spelled Maya. **International: Maiya** *(Russian).*

MAIDA. *English, 'maiden'.* Old English name as outmoded as the use of the word *maid* for a young girl. **Maddie, Maddy, Mady, Magda, Maidel, Maidie, Mayda, Maydena, Maydey.**

MAILE. *(my-lee) Hawaiian nature name.* Exotic and appealing name – a maile is a vine used to make leis – getting noticed via writer Maile Malloy.

♂ **MAINE.** *Place name.* Strong and spare American state name, maybe better in the middle – or for a boy.

MAIRE. *Irish variation of MARY.* Both Maire and Mare have begun making inroads with parents seeking novel yet authentic ways of honouring an ancestral Mary. **Mairi, Mare, Mayri. International: Mair** *(Welsh).*

MAIRÉAD. *(mawr-AID) Irish variation of MARGARET.* Common in its native habitat, and worth consideration by parents in search of an authentic Irish name, though a pronunciation challenge. **Maighread, Mairighead, Muiréad.**

★**MAISIE.** *Scottish diminutive of MARGARET.* A hundred-year-old favourite in perfect tune with today, currently in the Top 100. Spelled Maisy in a popular children's book series. **Maisey, Maisy, Maizie, Mazey, Mazie.**

MAIZE. *Colour name.* Would be more appealing if so many similar names – Maisie, Maeve, May – weren't even better.

MAJA. *Arabic, 'splendid'.* Whether you pronounce it *ma-zha* or *ma-ha*, it's an intriguing choice.

MAKALA. *Hawaiian, 'myrtle,' or variation of MICHAELA.* There are so many variations of this name in circulation, it makes it hard for any of them to feel as special as they might. **Makalae, Makalah, Makalai, Makalea, Makalee, Makaleh,**

Big in Britain

Alice

Amelia

Ava

Daisy

Ellie

Eve

Gracie

Keira

Libby

Lily

Lola

Maisie

Mia

Millie

Niamh

Phoebe

Poppy

Rosie

Scarlett

Sienna

Tilly

Makaleigh, Makaley, Makalia, Makalie, Makalya, Makela, Makelah, Makell, Makella.

MAKARA. *Hindi astrology name, 'Capricorn'.* Charismatic possibility for a January baby.

MAKAYLA. *Variation of* **MICHAELA.** This is now the best-selling version of this infinitely varied name, and it's still rising, leaving the original Michaela far behind.

MALAYA. *Filipino, 'free'.* Goes Maya one better. **Malayaa, Malayah, Malayna, Malea, Maleah.**

MALI. *Thai, 'jasmine flower'; Tongan, 'sweet'; Hungarian, diminutive of* **MALIKA.** Seems exotic, till you realise everyone will just hear it as Molly. **Malea, Malee, Maley.**

★**MALIA.** *Hawaiian variation of* **MARY.** Makes Grandma Mary or Maria's name fresh and modern.

MALINA. *Greek, 'from the high tower'; also Tabascan Mexican.* Feminissima name with a range of derivations. **Malin, Maline, Malinna, Mallana, Mallie.**

MALKA, MALKAH. *Hebrew, 'queen'.* Non-biblical Hebrew name used as an affectionate nickname since the Middle Ages. **Malcah, Malha, Maliah, Malke, Malkia, Malkiah, Malkie, Malkiya, Malkiyah, Milcah, Miliah, Milka, Milkie.**

MALLORCA. *(my-OR-ka) Spanish place name.* Trendy Spanish island makes for trendy girls' name. **Majorca.**

MALLORY. *French, 'unlucky'.* Early 1980s name that has been well used ever since, with an upbeat three-syllable sound and a slightly tomboyish edge. **Maliri, Mallary, Mallauri, Mallerey, Mallery, Malley, Malloree, Malloreigh, Mallorey, Mallorie, Malorey, Malorie, Malory, Malree, Malrie, Mellory.**

MALTA. *Place name.* One place name that sounds oddly stodgy.

MALU. *Hawaiian, 'peace'.* Charming Hawaiian name chosen by ex–Talking Head David Byrne for his daughter.

MALVA. *Greek, 'slender, delicate'.* Your zany neighbour, the one who's a potter and has five cats. **Melva, Melvina.**

MALVINA. *Scottish, 'smooth-browed one'.* An invention of an eighteenth-century romantic poet, sounds terminally dated today. **Mal, Malva, Malvie, Maveena, Mavina, Mel, Melva, Melvie, Melvina, Melvine.**

MAME. *Diminutive of* **MARY** *or* **MARGARET.** Has a dotty, antic feel via dotty, antic *Auntie Mame.*

★**MAMIE.** *Diminutive of* **MARY** *or* **MARGARET.** Now having lost its Mamie Eisenhower bangs, this insouciant and adorable nickname name is perfect if you want a zestier way to honour a beloved aunt Mary. **Maime, Mame, Mayme.**

MANDA. *Diminutive of* **AMANDA.** The full version is prettier. **Mandee, Mandie, Mandy.**

MANDARA. *Hindi, 'calm'.* Calm is certainly a quality worth courting in a child.

MANDOLINE. *Music name.* Better than Banjo. **Mandalin, Mandalyn, Mandalynn, Mandelin, Mandellin,** **Mandellyn, Mandolin, Mandolyn, Mandolynne.**

MANDY. *Diminutive of* **AMANDA.** Nickname left over from the last generation. **Mandee, Mandi, Mandie.**

♂ **MANET.** *(man-AY) French artist name.* Accessible, pretty name of Impressionist great; could be the next Monet.

MANETTE. *French, diminutive of* **MARIE.** Popular French Manon has more grace and heft.

★**MANON.** *French, diminutive of* **MARIE.** Well used in France; has the exotic yet straightforward feel that makes it a viable import. **Mannon.**

MANUELA. *(mahn-WEHL-lah) Spanish, feminine variation of* **EMMANUEL.** One feminine form that's more spirited than the male original. **Ammanuela, Chema, Emmanuela, Mannela, Manuala, Manuelita, Manuella, Manuelle, Manula, Melita, Nelia.**

♂ **MANZIE.** *Music name.* Woody Allen named his daughter after jazz drummer Manzie Johnson – a name not destined for widespread use. **Manzee, Manzey, Manzi, Manzy.**

MARA. *Hebrew, 'bitter'.* This evocative ancient root of Mary has a more modern appeal. **Mahra, Mar, Marae, Marah, Maralina, Maraline, Marra.**

MARCELLA. *Latin, 'warlike'.* Depicted as the world's most beautiful woman in *Don Quixote* (where it's spelled Marcela), this long neglected name seemed dated for decades but just might be ready for restoration. **Mairsil, Marca, Marce, Marceil, Marcele, Marcelen, Marcell, Marcellina, Marchella, Marchelle, Marci, Marcia, Marcie, Marciella, Marcile, Marcilee, Marcilla, Marcille, Marcy, Marella, Maricel, Marsalina, Marsella, Marselle, Marsellonia, Marshella, Marsiella. International: Marcelia, Marceline, Marcelle** *(French),* **Marcelina, Marcella** *(Italian),* **Marcela, Marcelina, Marquita** *(Spanish),* **Marzena** *(Polish),* **Marcela** *(Czech),* **Marcelina** *(Slavic).*

♂ **MARCH.** *Word name.* Never popular as a month name,

possibly because of its brisk, masculine beat.

MARCIA. *Latin, 'war-like'.* After a brief run of popularity in the mid-twentieth century, it was replaced by Marcy (now both are in limbo). **Mara, Marcelia, Marcena, Marcene, Marchia, Marchita, Marci, Marciale, Marciane, Marcie, Marcile, Marcille, Marcilyn, Marcilynn, Marcsa, Marcy, Marsha, Marseea, Marsia. International: Marzia** *(Italian),* **Marcina, Marcita, Marquita, Martia** *(Spanish).*

MARCIANA. *Latin, 'war-like'.* Cooler elaboration of Marcia.

MARCY. *Diminutive of* **MARCELLA** *or* **MARCIA.** As hip as bobby sox and saddle shoes. **Marcee, Marcey, Marci, Marcie, Marsee, Marsey, Marsy.**

MARDI. *French, 'Tuesday'.* Foreign word name that sounds like a home-grown nickname.

MARE. *Irish variation of* **MARY.** With this spelling, and one-syllable pronunciation, it sounds less like a whole

name than an equine animal. **Mair, Maire.**

MAREN. *Latin, 'sea'; Aramaic variation of* **MARY.** A twenty-first-century Mary; Marin spelling is preferable. **Marin, Marine, Marinn, Miren.**

MARGARET. *Greek, 'pearl'.* A rich, classic name used for queens and saints. It was replaced for decades by less starchy forms like Maggie and Molly, but some stylish parents are reviving it as an alternative to Elizabeth or Katherine. **Madge, Mag, Maggi, Maggie, Maggy, Mago, Maiga, Maisie, Maisy, Mamie, Marcheta, Marchieta, Maretha, Maretta, Margalo, Margaretha, Margarethe, Margarett, Margaretta, Margarette, Margarit, Margarite, Marge, Margeretta, Margerette, Margerie, Margery, Marget, Margetta, Margette, Margey, Marghanita, Margharita, Margherita, Marghretta, Margiad, Margies, Margise, Margred, Margreth, Margrett, Margrid, Marguita, Margy, Marjery, Marjey, Marji, Marjie, Marjorie, Markie, Markita,**

Meg, Meggi, Meggy, Metta, Meyta, Peg, Peggi, Peggie, Peggy.

MARGARITA. *Spanish variation of* **MARGARET.** Margaret, on tequila. **Margareta, Margaritis, Margaritta, Margharita, Margo, Marguarita, Marguita, Meta, Rita.**

MARGERY. *Medieval variation of* **MARGARET.** An old royal name in England and Scotland that's almost never used for babies today. **Marchery, Marge, Margeree, Margerey, Margerie, Margey, Margi, Margie, Margorie, Margy, Marje, Marjerie, Marjery, Marjie, Marjorey, Marjori, Marjorie, Marjory, Marjy.**

MARGIE. *Diminutive of* **MARGERY.** Prime pert-teenager name in the 1950s, now replaced by Maggie.

MARGO, MARGOT. *French, diminutive of* **MARGARET.** Adds a more dynamic *o* ending to Margaret, giving it a more streamlined, contemporary feel. Has creative ties to classic films and ballet. **Mago, Margaro, Margaux.**

MARGUERITE. *French variation of* **MARGARET**; *also a flower name.* Antiquated name with a remnant of old-fashioned Gallic charm; also a variety of daisy. **Margarete, Margaretha, Margarethe, Margarite, Margaruite, Margerite, Marghanita, Margherita, Marguaretta, Marguarette, Marguarite, Marguerette, Marguerite, Marguerita, Margurite.**

MARI. *Welsh and Spanish variation of* **MARY**. Turns a classic into a dated nickname name.

MARIA. *Latin variation of* **MARY**; *Aramaic variation of* **MIRIAM**. Imported from the Continent in the eighteenth century as a variation for the overused Mary. Today, as the most common name in all Spanish-speaking countries, it's more likely to be an ethnic name, retaining a timeless beauty. **Maie, Mara, Marea, Mareah, Mariabella, Mariae, Mariah, Marie, Mariesa, Mariessa, Mariha, Marija, Mariya, Mariyah, Marja, Marya, Mayra, Mayria, Moraiah, Moriah, Ria.** International: **Mali, Maritza** *(Spanish)*.

Margaret's International Variations

Irish	Mairead, Megan
Welsh	Marged, Meaghan, Megan, Meghan, Mared
French	Margaux, Margo, Margot, Marguerite
Italian	Margarita
Spanish	Marga, Margara, Margarita, Rita, Tita
Portuguese	Margarida
Dutch	Margarete, Margriet
German	Greta, Grete, Gretel, Gretchen, Margareta, Margarete, Margit, Margot, Margret, Margrete, Meta
Swedish	Margreta, Margrete
Finnish	Marjatta
Polish	Gita, Margisia, Margita, Rita
Hungarian	Gitta, Manci, Margit, Margita, Margo
Czech	Gita, Gitka, Gituska, Margareta, Margita, Marka, Marketa, Markit
Bulgarian	Marketa
Latvian	Grieta, Margrieta
Estonian	Marga, Margarete, Mari, Meeri, Reet
Greek	Margareta, Margaritis, Margaro
Armenian	Margarid
Hebrew	Penina
Yiddish	Gita
Tongan	Makelesi

MARIAH. *Latin variation of* **MARY;** *also related to the Hebrew* **MORIAH.** Thanks to Mariah Carey, everyone now knows this name – and is aware that it's pronounced with a long *i*. Reached a peak in the mid-1990s, but still a popular choice.

MARIAM. *Arabic variation of* **MARY.** Popular among parents with Arab roots. **Maryam.**

MARIAN, MARION. *French, medieval variation of* **MARIE.** If you can look past this name's middle-aged image to Robin Hood's romantic Maid Marian, you can see an attractive and now distinctive choice. **Mariam, Mariene, Marionne, Marrian, Marriann, Maryann, Maryanne, Maryon.** International: **Mariane, Mariann, Marianne** *(French),* **Mariana, Marianna** *(Spanish),* **Mariane** *(German),* **Marien** *(Dutch),* **Maryam** *(Greek).*

MARIANNA. *Spanish, combination of* **MARY** *and* **ANNA.** The more syllables you add, the better it gets. **Marianna, Marriana, Marrianna, Maryana.**

MARIANNE. *French, combination of* **MARY** *and*

ANNE. A mid-century Catholic classic that's not chosen by many stylish parents today. **Mariana, Mariane, Mariann, Maryann, Maryanna.**

MARIBEL. *French, combination of* **MARY** *and* **BELLE.** This modern name gathers some steam from the wildly popular Isabel. **Marabel, Marbelle, Mariabella, Maribella, Maribelle, Maridel, Marybel, Marybella, Marybelle, Meribel, Meribella, Meribelle.**

MARIE. *French variation of* **MARY.** Sounds more dated than either Mary or Maria at this point, though it once rivalled both. **Maree, Mariel, Marielle, Mariette, Marrie.**

MARIEL. *Dutch and French, diminutive of* **MARY.** Mariel Hemingway popularised this attractive and unusual variation. **Marelia, Marelle, Marial, Mariela, Mariele, Marietta, Marielle, Mariet.** International: **Marieke** *(Dutch).*

MARIELLA. *Italian, diminutive of* **MARIA.** Lilting and pretty, with the currently popular *ella*

ending, makes a good Marissa alternative. **International: Marielle** *(French).*

MARIETTA. *French, diminutive of* **MARIE.** Proper . . . and naughty. **Maretta, Maryetta.**

MARIGOLD. *Flower name.* Sometimes found in English novels; would be seen as wildly exotic here, though it does have a sunny, golden feel. **Maragold, Marrigold, Marygold.**

MARIKA. *Dutch variation of* **MARY.** Foreign variations of Mary are definitely the way to go; this one has a nice Dutch-girl feel. **Marica, Marieke, Marija, Marijke, Marikah, Marike, Marikia, Marikka, Mariska, Mariske, Marrika, Maryk, Maryka, Merica, Merika.**

MARILEE. *American, combination of* **MARY** *and* **LEE.** One of the cheeriest – if least substantial – combinations of Mary with another name. **Marili, Marilie, Marily, Marrilee, Marylea, Marylee, Merrilee, Merrili, Merrily.**

MARILYN. *English, combination of* **MARY** *and*

LYNN. When you realise that the iconic Marilyn would now be in her eighties, this name sounds anything but young and sexy. **Maralin, Maralyn, Maralyne, Maralynn, Maralynne, Marelyn, Marilee, Marilin, Marillyn, Marilyne, Marilynn, Marilynne, Marlyn, Marolyn, Marralynn, Marrilin, Marrilyn, Marrilynn, Marrilynne, Marylin, Marylinn, Marylyn, Marylyne, Marylynn, Marylynne.**

MARIMBA. *Music name.* Can you hear the beat?

★**MARIN.** *Place name.* It's a lovely county north of San Francisco in the US, and a lovely baby name on the rise. **Maren, Marena, Marinn, Marrin.**

MARINA. *Latin, 'from the sea'.* Pretty sea-born Shakespearean name, chosen for his daughter by Matt LeBlanc. **Mareena, Mareina, Marena, Marenka, Marinae, Marinah, Marinda, Marindi, Marine, Marinell, Marinka, Marinna, Marne, Marnetta, Marnette, Marni, Marnie, Marrina, Maryna, Merina, Mirena.** International: **Marine** *(French),* **Mareeba, Marna** *(Swedish),* **Marinochka** *(Russian)* **Mariná** *(Slavic).*

★**MARINE.** *Latin, 'from the sea'.* Extremely popular and fashionable name in France that's almost unknown elsewhere – and ripe for the plucking.

MARINI. *Swahili, 'healthy, pretty'.* It can be difficult to find African and Asian names that translate to the British culture – but this one manages it.

MARION. *See* **MARIAN.** **Marrian, Marrion, Maryon, Maryonn.**

MARIPOSA. *Spanish, 'butterfly'.* Rare, romantic choice. **Marriposa.**

★**MARIS.** *Latin, 'of the sea'.* Unusual and appealing, it comes from the phrase 'Stella Maris,' star of the sea, referring to the Virgin Mary, familiarised via the unseen character on *Frasier.* **Maries, Marisa, Marise, Marissa, Marisse, Marris, Marys, Maryse, Meris.**

MARISA. *Italian and Spanish variation of* **MARIS, MARISSA.**

A name that has been made famous by Marisa Tomei, never became as saturated as its cousin Melissa, so still a feasible choice. **Mareesa, Mareisa, Maresa, Mariesa, Mariessa, Marisela, Marissa, Mariza, Marrisa, Marrissa, Maryse, Marysia, Maryssa, Merisa, Moreisa, Morisa, Morysa.** International: **Marita** *(Spanish),* **Marijse, Marysa** *(Dutch),* **Maritza** *(German),* **Marisha** *(Russian).*

MARISKA. *Hungarian variation of* **MARIS, MARISSA.** This name makes a robust, energetic Slavic impression.

MARISOL. *Spanish, 'sea and sun'.* Puerto Rican favourite, and an excellent candidate for cross-culturisation. **Marise, Marizol, Marysol.**

MARISSA. *Variation of* **MARIS.** Recently popular name in the US, but it's not as fashionable here; Marisa spelling has more style. **Maressa, Marisa, Marisha, Marissah, Marisse, Marizza, Marrissa, Marrissia, Maryssa, Merissa, Meryssa, Morissa.**

MARIT. *Aramaic, 'lady';* *Norwegian and Swedish variation of* **MARGARET.** Unusual and straightforward: a winning combination. **Marita, Marite.**

MARJORIE. *Variation of* **MARGERY,** *diminutive of* **MARGARET.** Mid-century favourite that dates to medieval times – said to have faded with advent of the word 'margarine'. **Madge, Majorie, Marcharie, Marge, Margeree, Margerey, Margerie, Margery, Margey, Margi, Margie, Margorie, Margory, Margy, Marj, Marjarie, Marjary, Marje, Marjerie, Marjery, Marji, Marjorey, Marjori, Marjory, Marjy.** International: **Marjie** *(Scottish),* **Marjie, Marjo, Marjolaine, Marjolie** *(French).*

MARLA. *Variation of* **MARLENE.** A few semi-famous Marlas have kept this name alive. Barely. **Marlah, Marlea, Marleah, Marlla.**

MARLENE. *German variation of* **MADELINE;** *combination of* **MARY** *and* **MAGDALEN.** Marlene Dietrich made it famous when she condensed her first two names, Maria and Magdalena. Now more often pronounced with two syllables rather than three. **Layna, Lena, Marla, Marlaina, Marlaine, Marlane, Marlayne, Marlea, Marleah, Marlee, Marleen, Marleene, Marlen, Marlena, Marlenne, Marley, Marlie, Marlin, Marline, Marlyn, Marlyne, Marlynne.**

♂ **MARLEY.** *English,* *'pleasant seaside meadow'.* Reggae master Bob's surname is more popular for girls. **Marlea, Marlee, Marleigh, Marli, Marlie, Marly.**

MARLIN. *Combination of* **MARY** *and* **LYNN.** Sounds like Marlon (as in Brando) and looks like marlin (as in the fish). **Marlen, Marlenn, Marrlen, Marlinn, Marlyn, Marrlin.**

MARLO. *Modern invented name.* Perky nickname name that seems to have been invented by or for the American actress Marlo Thomas, who was born Margaret. **Marion, Marlon, Marlow, Marlowe.**

MARNIE. *Hebrew, diminutive of* **MARNINA,** *'causing joy'.* Short form that's much better known than the original, now dated to the era of the Hitchcock film that made it famous. **Marna, Marnay, Marne, Marnee, Marney, Marni, Marnina, Marnisha, Marnja, Marny, Marnya, Marnye.**

MARSHA. *Variation of* **MARCIA,** *diminutive of* **MARCELLA.** The most common version in the US, now found more often among mums and grandmas than babies. **Marcha, Marshae, Marshay, Marshel, Marshele, Marshell, Marshia, Marshiela, Marsia, Martia.**

MARTA. *Italian, Spanish, Scandinavian, and Eastern European variation of* **MARTHA.** Sounds perennially olde world. **Martica, Martina.**

MARTHA. *Aramaic, 'lady'.* Name with a prim, good girl aura – à la the New Testament Martha, patron saint of the helping professions – it has entered the Top 100 recently. **Maarya, Maret, Marit, Mart, Martaha, Martelle, Marth,**

Marthan, Marthena, Marthine, Marthini, Marthy, Marti, Martie, Martta, Marty, Martynne, Martyne, Marva, Mata, Matti, Mattie, Matty. International: Moireach *(Scottish)*, Martella, Marthe *(French)*, Marta *(Italian and Spanish)*, Maita, Martina, Martita *(Spanish)*, Martita, Marte *(Scandinavian)*, Marcia, Masia *(Polish)*, Marcsa, Martus, Martuska *(Hungarian)*, Martricka *(Czech)*, Martila, Martita *(Eastern European)*, Maata *(Maori)*.

MARTINA. *Latin, 'warlike'.* Tennis-related name popular throughout Europe that's never caught fire here. Marta, Marteena, Marteina, Martel, Martella, Martelle, Martene, Marthena, Marthina, Marthine, Marti, Martie, Martinia, Martisha, Martosia, Martoya, Martricia, Martrina, Marty, Martyne, Martunne, Tina, Tine. International: Martine *(French)*, Martimana *(Spanish)*, Martyna *(Polish)*, Martuska *(Hungarian)*, Martinka *(Czech)*.

MARTINE. *French, 'war-like'.* Sleek and sophisticated.

MARVEL. *English word name.* The miracle name of yesterday. Maravilla, Maraville, Marivel, Marivella, Marivelle, Marva, Marvela, Marvele, Marvella, Marvelle, Marvely, Marvetta, Marvette, Marvia, Marvina.

MARY. *Hebrew, 'bitter'.* The quintessential New Testament name was Number 1 for the last four hundred years. Today, it's used mostly for religious or family reasons. If it's style you're after, its diminutives and derivatives Maire, Mamie, May, Mitzi, Molly, Maura, Marietta and even Maria are all more fashionable. Mair, Mal, Malle, Mame, Mamie, Marabel, Marabelle, Maree, Marella, Marelle, Maren, Maretta, Marette, Mariam, Mariana, Mariann, Marianne, Maridel, Marietta, Marila, Marilee, Marilin, Marilla, Marilyn, Marin, Marla, Marlo, Marya, Maryann, Maryanna, Maryla, Marynia, Marysa, Marysia, Maurene, Maurine, May, Mayme, Maymie, Mayra, Mayria, Merrill, Millie, Milly, Mimi, Minette, Minnie, Minti,

Mirja, Moll, Molli, Mollie, Molly, Poll, Polli, Polly.

MARYA. *Arabic, 'purity, bright whiteness'.* The final *a* adds a lot of style. Maryah.

MARYANN. *English, combination of* **MARY** *and* **ANN.** *See* **MARIANNE.** Marian, Marryann, Maryan, Maryanne, Meryem.

♂ **MASON.** *English occupational name, 'stone-worker'.* Super-trendy name for boys that's just starting to cross over – Kelsey Grammer used it for his daughter. Creative speller's delight. Macen, Macin, Macyn, Maison, Maycen, Maycin, Maycyn, Maysen, Maysin, Mayson, Maysyn.

MASSIMA. *Italian, from Latin, 'greatest'.* Its meaning makes it a high-pressure boastful choice, even in Italian. Maxima.

MATALIN. *Surname name.* American politico Mary Matalin used her last name as her daughter's first, an idea any mum can adopt.

Mary's International Variations

Zuni	Malia
Irish	Maira, Maire, Mare, Moira, Maura, Maureen, Moira, Moire, Moya, Muire
Scottish	Mairi, Mhairie, Moira, Moire, Morag
French	Manette, Manon, Marie, Mariette, Marion, Maryse, Mérane
Italian	Maria, Marice
Spanish	Mari, Maria, Mariquita, Marita, Maruca, Maruja
Basque	Mendi, Molara
Dutch	Mariel, Mariela, Mariella, Marielle, Marika
German	Mitzi
Swedish	Mirjam
Finnish	Maija, Maijii, Maikki, Marja
Polish	Manka, Marjan
Hungarian	Mara, Marcsa, Mari, Maria, Marika
Czech	Marca, Marenka, Marienka, Mariska, Maruska
Lithuanian	Marija
Russian	Manka, Manya, Mara, Marika, Marinka, Marisha, Mariya, Masha, Mashenka, Mashka, Mura
Latvian	Mare
Estonian	Mayre

★MATILDA. *German, 'battle-mighty'.* Revived by Heath Ledger and Michelle Williams, Matilda's star is rising. It's the name of a charming Roald Dahl heroine and it has two great nicknames: Tillie for the bold, Mattie for the shy. **Mahilda, Makilde, Malkin, Mat, Matelda, Mathilda, Matti, Mattie, Matty, Maud, Maude, Maudie, Tilde, Tildie, Tildy, Tilli, Tillie, Tilly. International: Mathilde** *(French)*, **Mafalda, Matelda, Matilde** *(Italian)*, **Mati, Matilde, Matusha, Tilda** *(Spanish)*, **Mechtilde, Mette** *(German)*, **Macia, Mala, Matylda, Tila, Tylda** *(Polish, Czech)*.

MATTEA. *(ma-TAY-a) Italian, from Hebrew, 'gift of God'.* This pretty, exotic feminisation of Matthew would be a good choice to honour a Matthew in the family. **Matea, Mathea, Mathia, Matia, Matte, Matthea, Matthia, Mattia, Matya.**

★MAUD, MAUDE. *Variation of* MATILDA. This lacy, mauve-tinted name was wildly popular a hundred years ago, but has rarely been heard in the past fifty. Some stylish parents are starting to choose it again, especially as a middle. **Maudie, Maudine, Maudlin.**

MAURA. *Anglicised variation of* MAIRE. Somber, almost mournful name that still has a lovely sound. **Maurah, Maure, Maurette, Mauricette, Maurita, Mora.**

MAUREEN. *Irish variation of* MARY. Almost as popular in the 1950s among the Irish in Liverpool as it was with those back in Limerick; rarely used now. **Maura, Maurene, Maurine, Mo, Moreen, Morena, Morene, Morine, Morreen, Moureen.**

MAURELLE. *French, 'dark, elfin'.* New twist to the *Maur-* names, a bit cosmetic sounding. **Mauriel, Mauriell, Maurielle.**

♂ **MAURICE.** *French, 'dark-skinned'.* One of those old-mannish names that sounds a lot fresher for a girl. **Maurice, Maurisa, Maurissa, Maurita, Maurizia.**

MAUVE. *French, 'violet-coloured'.* Offbeat colour name whose spirit is conveyed by the name. **Maude.**

Mary's International Variations

Greek	Marika, Maroula, Roula
Hebrew	Miriam
Arabic	Maryam
Hawaiian	Malia
Tongan	Mele

MAVIS. *French, 'songbird'.* British World War II name, a friend of Beryl and Doris. **Mavies, Mavin, Mavine, Mavon, Mavra.**

MAXI. *German, feminine diminutive of* MAXIMILIAN. Better to go with Minnie. **Maxie, Maxy.**

MAXIMA. *French, feminine variation of* MAXIM. Just don't make her middle name Nissan.

MAXINE. *Latin, 'greatest'.* Playing mah-jongg down at the clubhouse with Bernice and Thelma. **Max, Maxa, Maxeen, Maxena, Maxene, Maxie, Maxima, Maxina, Maxna,** **Maxyne. International: Maxime** *(French).*

★**MAY.** *Diminutive of* MARGARET *and* MARY; *month name.* Sweet old-fashioned name that hasn't been used that much in the last fifty years, but is definitely sounding fresh and spring-like. One of the prettiest middle name options. **Mae, Maelea, Maeleah, Maelen, Maelle, Maeona, Maia, Maya, Mayberry, Maybeth, Mayday, Maydee, Maydena, Maye, Mayela, Mayella, Mayetta, Mayrene. International: Mai** *(French),* **Maggia** *(Italian),* **Maj** *(Scandinavian).*

MAYA. *Greek mythology name; Central American Indian empire* name; *Latinate variation of* **MAY**; *Spanish, diminutive of* **AMALIA**. A bourgeois-bohemian favourite, chosen by Uma Thurman and Ethan Hawke for their daughter, with an exotic, almost mystical image. It's made it into the Top 100 in recent years. **Maaja, Maia, Maiah, Maie, Maiya, May, Mayi, Mayja, Moia, Moja, Moya, Mya, Myah. International: Mayanita** *(Spanish),* **Maj, Maja** *(Scandinavian).*

McKAYLA. *Variation of* **MICHAELA.** Is this popular name really Michaela, or is it a combination of McKenna and Kayla? The real answer: it's a fusion of trends.

♂ **McKENNA.** *Irish, 'son of the handsome one'.* Mackenzie begat McKenna – a catchy but very trendy choice. **Mackena, Mackendra, Mackenna, Makena, Makenna.**

McKENZIE. *See* **MACKENZIE.**

♂ **MEAD.** *English, 'from the meadow'.* Sounds like an authentic upper-crust family

name – not necessarily a bad thing. **Meade, Meed.**

MEADOW. *Nature name.* How perfect is it that Tony Soprano's daughter's name is Meadow, suggesting the TV mobster was once a kinder, gentler young dad.

MEARA. *Irish, 'pool, lake'.* A name that has many close, more familiar relatives, like Mira and Myra.

MEDEA. *Greek, 'ruling'; Latin, 'middle'.* Mythological princess who killed her kids. Eternal no-no. **Medeia.**

MEDORA. *Greek, 'mother's gift'.* Sounds like the next weight-reduction tablet.

MEDRIE. *Meaning unknown.* We've only ever heard of one person with this name – painter Medrie McPhee – but it's a charming option.

MEENA. *Hindi, 'blue semi-precious stone, bird'; Greek, German, and Dutch variation of Mena. See* **MENA.**

MEG. *English, diminutive of* **MARGARET.** Still one of the *Little Women.*

MEGAN. *Diminutive of* **MARGED,** *Welsh variation of* **MARGARET.** One of the most popular of the Welsh names, it's long been in the British Top 20. **Maegan, Magan, Magen, Meagan, Meaghan, Maygan, Maygen, Meg, Megane, Megann, Megean, Megen, Meggan, Meggen, Meggie, Meghan, Megyn, Meygan.**

MEHIRA. *Hebrew, 'swift, energetic'.* An energetic ethnic choice. **Mahira.**

MEHITABEL. *Hebrew, 'God rejoices'.* Most famously, the name of a 1920s alley cat. **Hetty, Hitty, Mehetabel, Mehitabelle.**

MEHRI. *Persian, 'kind, lovable, sunny'.* Exotic, until you realise everyone will think it's Mary or Merry.

MEI. *(may) Chinese and Hawaiian, 'beautiful'.* Lovely name familiar in several Asian cultures.

♂ **MEL.** *Diminutive of* **MELANIE.** Balding-man name that's short and sweet for a girl.

MELA. *Hindi, 'religious service'; Polish variation of* **MELANIE.** Unlike Pamela and Melanie, Mela feels fresh and exotic.

MELANIA. *Spanish and Greek variation of* **MELANIE.** Saint Melania was an heiress who freed thousands of slaves, making this a name that is worthwhile of consideration – as well as pretty. **Mel, Melaina, Melainia.**

MELANIE. *Greek, 'black, dark'. Gone with the Wind* inspired a generation of Melanies, though it looks as though Scarlett will triumph in the end. **Malaney, Malania, Malanie, Meila, Meilani, Meilin, Mel, Melaina, Melaine, Melainie, Melane, Melanee, Melaney, Melanney, Melannie, Melany, Melayne, Melenia, Mella, Mellanie, Melli, Mellie, Melloney, Mellony, Melly, Meloni, Melonnie, Melony, Melya.** International: **Mélaine, Mélanie, Melani, Melaniu** *(French),* **Melania, Milena** *(Spanish),* **Melina** *(Italian and Spanish),*

Melain *(German),* **Ela, Mela, Melka** *(Polish),* **Melana, Melaniya, Melanka, Melanya, Melashka, Melasya, Milya** *(Russian),* **Melena** *(Slavic),* **Melania** *(Greek).*

MELANTHA. *Greek, 'dark flower'.* The *th* sound both softens and complicates this Melanie relative. **Mallantha.**

MELBA. *Modern invented name.* Australian opera singer Nellie Melba – self-named for her hometown of Melbourne – inspired this now-dated name more associated today with a peach dessert and dietetic toast. **Malva, Mellba, Melva.**

★**MELIA.** *Greek mythology nymph, also diminutive of* **AMELIA.** Rich, melodic shortening that can stand on its own. **Meelia, Melea, Meleah, Meleia, Meleisha, Meli, Meliah, Melya.**

MELINA. *Greek, 'quince yellow'.* This traditional Greek name feels somewhat more distinctive than Melissa. **Malina, Mallina, Melaina, Meleana, Meleena, Melena, Melibella, Melibelle,**

Meline, Melinia, Melinna, Mellina, Melynna.

MELINDA. *English combination name.* Once quasi-cool name that now feels mumish; most prominent modern bearer is philanthropist Melinda Gates, wife of Bill. **Linda, Lindy, Linnie, Lynda, Maillie, Malina, Malinda, Malinde, Mallie, Mally, Malynda, Mandy, Melina, Melinde, Melinder, Meline, Mellinda, Melynda, Melyne, Milinda, Milynda, Mylenda, Mylinda, Mylynda.**

MELIORA. *Latin, 'better'.* Unusual and lush Roman name adopted, improbably, by the Puritans. **Melior, Meliori, Mellear, Melyor, Melyora.**

MÉLISANDE. *French, from Greek, 'honeybee'.* Romantique French name invoking Debussy's haunting score for the opera *Pelléas and Mélisande.* **Lisandra, Malisande, Malissande, Malyssandre, Melesande, Melisandra, Melisandre, Melissande, Melissandre, Mellisande, Melysande, Melyssandre.**

MELISSA. *Greek, 'bee'.* Most parents today think of this as one of the fashionable names during *their* childhoods – it's recently slipped out of the Top 100. **Malissa, Mallissa, Mel, Melesa, Melessa, Meleta, Melicent, Melicia, Melisa, Melise, Melisenda, Melisent, Melisha, Mélissa, Melisse, Melissia, Melita, Melitta, Mellicent, Mellie, Mellisa, Mellissa, Melly, Melosa, Melyssa, Milissa, Milli, Millicent, Millie, Millisent, Millissent, Milly, Misha, Missie, Missy, Molissia, Mollissa, Mylissa, Mylissia. International: Mélisande, Melissande** *(French),* **Malisa, Melisa** *(Spanish).*

MELITA. *Greek, 'honey'.* Sounds like a brand name. **Malita, Malitta, Meleeta, Melida, Melitta, Melitza, Melletta, Melyta, Molita.**

MELODY. *Greek, 'song'.* Melodious choice big in the 1960s, now starting to pick up tempo again. **Meladia, Melodee, Melodey, Melodi, Melodia, Melodic, Melodie, Melodyann, Melodye.**

MELORA. *Greek, 'golden apple'.* Euphonic hybrid of the sounds of Melissa and Laura.

MELVINA. *Celtic, 'chieftain'.* Melvin doesn't deserve a feminine form. **Malvina, Melevine, Melva, Melveen, Melvena, Melvene, Melvonna.**

♂ **MEMPHIS.** *Place name.* Cool and bluesy American city name chosen by musician-activist Bono for his daughter.

MENA. *Spanish, diminutive of* **FILOMENA.** Actress Mena Suvari (named after an Egyptian hotel) made this name seem more appealing that it really is. **Meena, Menah.**

MERCEDES. *Spanish, 'gracious gifts, benefits'.* Although these days its first association is to the car, Mercedes is a legitimate Spanish appellation relating to the Virgin Mary – and an elegant choice. **Mercades, Mercadez, Mercadie, Merce, Merceades, Merced, Mercede, Mercedees, Mercedeez, Mercedez, Mercedies, Mercedis, Mercy, Mersade, Mersades.**

♂ **MERCURY.** *Roman, 'messenger of the gods, quicksilver'.* It's a car brand, a planet and the messenger of the gods – but we're not sure it's a usable name, especially for a girl.

★**MERCY.** *English, 'mercy'.* The quality of mercy makes this lovely Puritan virtue name undervalued today. **Mercey, Merci, Mercie, Mercille, Mersey.**

♂ **MEREDITH.** *Welsh, 'great ruler'.* Soft, gentle-sounding name that is used mainly for girls nowadays. **Meradith, Meredeth, Meredithe, Meredy, Meredyth, Meredythe, Meridath, Merideth, Meridie, Meridith, Merridie, Merridith, Merry.**

MERI. *Finnish, 'sea,' or diminutive of* Mer-*names.* Upbeat nickname name, somewhat flimsy.

MERIEL. *Irish variation of* **MURIEL.** Pleasant modernisation of dated original. **Meri, Merial, Merielle, Meriol, Merrill, Meryl.**

MERILEE. *English, combination of* **MERRY** *and* **LEE.** Merrily, we move on to more substantial names.

MERILYN. *English, combination of* **MERRY** *and* **LYNN.** All the names ending in-*lyn* seem sadly dated. **Merelyn, Merlyn, Merralyn, Merrelyn, Merrilyn.**

♂ **MERLE.** *French, 'blackbird'.* A sleek, smooth, understated name that last seemed creative a half century ago. **Merl, Merla, Merlina, Merline, Merola, Meryl, Murle, Myrle, Myrleen, Myrlene, Myrline.**

MERONA. *Aramaic, breed of sheep.* The name of a breed of Spanish sheep is hardly worthy as the name of a child. **Marona, Merrona.**

♂ **MERRILL.** *English, 'seabright'.* Once fairly common for males, it's rarely used for girls with this spelling. **Meril, Merill, Merrall, Merril, Meryl.**

MERRY. *English, 'light-hearted, happy'.* She'd better be. **Marrilee, Marylea, Marylee, Merie, Merree, Merrey, Merri, Merrie, Merrielle, Merrile, Merrilee, Merrili, Merrily, Merrilyn, Merris, Merrita.**

MERYL. *Variation of* **MURIEL** *via* **MERIEL.** Better known than it would otherwise be, thanks to Meryl (born Mary Louise) Streep. **Meral, Merel, Merrall, Merrell, Merril, Merrile, Merrill, Merryl, Meryle, Meryll.**

MESA. *(MAY-sa) Spanish, 'table'.* Mesa is the term for a flat-topped mountain. Better geologic choices: Sierra, Savannah, Lake, Ocean. **Maisa, Maysa.**

MESSIAH. *Aramaic, 'expected saviour or deliverer'.* Highly unusual – and audacious – choice. **Masai, Masaia, Masaiah, Massaia, Massaiah, Massia, Massiah, Massya, Massyah, Messaia, Messaiah, Messia.**

MIA. *Italian, 'mine,' shortening of* **MARIA.** Appealingly unfussy multicultural name that's enjoyed a meteoric rise up the charts, where it's firmly in the Top 25. Kate Winslet is the mother of Mia Honey. **Mea, Meah, Meea, Meeah, Meeya, Meya, Miah, Miya, Miyah.**

MIAMI. *Place name.* Miami – or Florida, for that matter –

Two-Syllable Standouts

Anna	Justine
Arden	Leah
Bridget	Lilac
Brontë	Lola
Chloe	Margot
Cora	Mercy
Dara	Milla
Delta	Nora
Flora	Patience
Gaenor	Poppy
Georgia	Ruby
Iris	Wylie
Jorie	Zoe

hasn't achieved the place name stardom of southern American sisters like Savannah and Georgia.

♂ **MIATA.** *(mee-AH-ta) Modern invented name.* Inspired by the Mazda sportscar. 'Nough said.

♂ **MICAH.** *(MY-ka) Hebrew, 'who is like the Lord?'* Long a traditional boys' name, now increasingly used for their sisters, as an alternative to the overused Michaela. Mecca, Meecah, Meica, Micha, Mika, Myca, Mycah, Myka, Mykah.

♂ **MICHAEL.** *Hebrew, 'who is like the Lord?'* An all-boy name that occasionally crosses over to the girls' side.

MICHAELA. *Feminine variation of* **MICHAEL.** This most proper form of the name shot up the charts in the 1990s, only to sink just as precipitously, supplanted by upstarts Makayla and McKayla ad infinitum. Macayla, Machaela, MacKayla, Maika, Makaela, Makaila, Makala, Makayla, Makyla, Mechaela, Meeskaela, Mekea, Mia, Michal, Michael, Michaelann, Michaelina, Michaeline, Michaila, Michalin, Michayla, Michaelia, Michaelina, Michaeline, Michaell, Michaella, Michaelyn, Michaila, Michal, Micheal, Micheala, Michelia, Michelina, Micheline, Michely, Michelyn, Micheyla, Mickee, Micki, Mickie, Mihaila, Mihalia, Mihaliya, Mikala, Mikhaila, Mikhayla, Mishaela, Mishaila, Miskaela, Mycala, Mychael, Mychal. International: Michèle, Micheline, Michelle *(French),*

Micaela *(Italian and Spanish),* Michele *(Italian),* Miguela, Miguelina, Miguelita *(Spanish),* Michielle *(Dutch),* Mikaela, Mikele *(Scandinavian),* Michala, Michalina *(Polish),* Mici, Mihálya, Mika *(Hungarian),* Michailya, Mikhailya, Misha, Mishenka *(Russian),* Mahail, Mahaila, Mahalia, Makis *(Greek),* Micaela, Micha, Michla *(Israeli).*

MICHAL. *(Mee-chahl) Hebrew, 'a brook'.* In the Bible, daughter of King Saul and wife of King David. Mica, Michala, Michalla, Michel, Mika, Miki.

MICHELINE. *French, feminine variation of* **MICHAEL.** One of those quintessentially French names still wearing a beret, also too tied to the image of tyres.

MICHELLE. *French variation of* **MICHAEL.** One-time superstar name that's now in steep decline. Chelle, Machealle, Machele, Machell, Machella, Machelle, Mashelle, M'chelle, Mechelle, Meechelle, Meichelle, Meschell, Meshell, Meshella, Meshelle, Mia, Micaela, Michaela, Michaelina, Michaeline, Michaella,

Michal, Michel, Michele, Michelina, Michell, Michella, Michellene, Michellyn, Micki, Mickie, Midge, Miguela, Mikaela, Miquela, Mischel, Mischelle, Misha, Mishael, Mishaela, Mishaelle, Mishayla, Mishell, Mishelle, Mitchele, Mitchelle, M'shell, Mychelle, Myshell, Myshella, Shelli, Shelly. International: Michéle, Micheline *(French).*

MICHIKO. *Japanese, 'the righteous way'.* One of the most familiar Japanese names thanks to the first commoner to become empress of Japan and to *New York Times* book empress Michiko Kakutani. Miche, Michee, Michi.

MICKI. *Diminutive of* **MICHELLE** *or* **MICHAELA.** Briefly cool in the 1950s, but now gone the way of Ricki and Nikki. Mickee, Mickey, Mickie, Micky, Mikki, Mikkie.

MIDORI. *Japanese, 'green'.* In Japan, colour names symbolise human qualities (in this case, fame); name of gifted violinist Midori, but also a Japanese melon liqueur.

MIEKO. *(Mee-eh-ko) Japanese, 'prosperous'.* Another of the better-known Japanese names. **Mieke.**

★**MIGNON.** *(meen-yawn) French, 'delicate, dainty'.* Charming French endearment, first used as a name by Goethe, that now makes an appealing choice. **Mignonette, Mignonne, Mingnon, Minnionette, Minnonette, Minyonne, Minyonell, Minyonette, Minyonne.**

MIGUELA. *Spanish, feminine variation of* **MIGUEL.** If you're looking for an unusual Michaela alternative, try this Spanish route. **Miguelina, Miguelita.**

MIKA. *(mee-ka or my-ka) Japanese, 'new moon'; Russian, 'God's child'; Hebrew variation of* **MICAH.** Multicultural name that has the shiny sparkle of the metallic mica. **Mikah, Mikka.**

MIKI. *(mee-kee) Japanese, 'flower stem'.* Attractive but slight Asian alternative, with a 1970s nickname feel. **Mikia, Mikiala, Mikie, Mikita, Mikiyo, Mikki, Mikkie, Mikkiya, Mikko, Miko.**

MIKKI. *See* **MICKI.** **Micki, Mickie, Mickey, Miki.**

MILA. *(mee-la) Diminutive of several European names.* Appealing continental short-form favourite. **Milah, Milla.**

MILADA. *Czech, 'my love'.* More unusual than attractive. **Mila, Miladi, Miladia, Milady.**

MILAGROS. *Spanish, 'miracles'.* Even in the Hispanic community, this name is very religious and very old-fashioned – this is definitely one that is best to avoid. **Mila, Milagritos, Milagro, Milagrosa, Miligrosa, Mirari.**

♂ **MILAN.** *Place name.* The sophisticated Italian city is not yet on the first name map, but certainly could be.

MILANA. *Italian, 'from Milan'; Russian variation of* **MELANA.** Makes Milan sound like less of a place, more of a name. **Milan, Milane, Milani, Milanka, Milanna, Milanne, Milano.**

MILDRED. *English, 'gentle strength'.* One grandma choice not slated for a comeback; in studies it's often picked as an example of an unappealing name. **Mil, Mila, Mildrene, Mildrid, Millie, Milly.**

MILENA. *Czech, 'love, warmth, grace'.* Popular name in the Czech Republic and in Italy that holds considerable continental appeal. **Mila, Milada, Miladena, Milana, Milanka, Milène, Milenia, Milenny, Milini, Milka, Millini, Mlada, Mladena.**

MILLAY. *English literary name.* Pretty and distinctive choice for poetry lovers.

★**MILLICENT.** *German, 'highborn power'.* Combining the mild and the innocent, this sweet and feminine name is worthy of a comeback, in the mode of Madeline and Cecilia. **Lissa, Mel, Melicent, Meliscent, Mellie, Mellisent, Melly, Milisent, Milissent, Millie, Millisent, Milliestone, Milly, Milzie, Missie, Missy. International: Mélisande, Mellicent, Melusine, Milicent** *(French),* **Melisenda** *(Spanish).*

MILLIE. *Diminutive of* **MILDRED** *or* **MILLICENT.** Fashionable again in London for

Cool Nickname Names

Bea	Libby
Billie	Lottie
Cleo	Lulu
Daisy	Maisie
Dixie	Mamie
Dottie	Millie
Dru	Minnie
Edie	Mitzi
Ellie	Nell
Emmy	Pippa
Evie	Rae
Fanny	Rosie
Gracie	Sadie
Izzy	Tally
Jorie	Tay
Josie	Tess
Kitty	Tillie

parents who like the offbeat, frilly, and old-fashioned – a regular in the Top 50. **Milly.**

MIM. *Diminutive of* **MIRIAM.** A hum of a name. Madame Mim was a villain in Disney's *The Sword in the Stone.*

MIMI. *Diminutive of* **MARY, MIRIAM,** *and others.* Flirty, flimsy name of the tragic heroine of *La Bohème* . . . and *Rent.* **Meemee, Mim.**

MIMOSA. *Latin plant name.* Adventurous parents are venturing deeper into the garden in search of fresh names, but this is also the American name for a Buck's Fizz.

MIN. *Chinese, 'sensitive' or 'quick'.* Puts the *-min* in diminutive.

MINA. *Scottish diminutive, also Hindu equivalent of Pisces.* Most famous as a Dracula victim, Mina is an all-purpose name lacking much character. **Meena, Mena, Min, Minna.**

MINDY. *Diminutive of* **MELINDA.** Time to go back to the original. **Mindee, Mindi, Mindie, Mindyanne, Mindylee, Myndy.**

MINERVA. *Latin, 'of the mind, intellect'.* The long-neglected name of the Roman goddess of wisdom and invention might appeal to adventurous feminist parents. **Merva, Min, Minivera, Minnie, Myna. International: Minerve, Minette** *(French),* **Minetta** *(Italian and Spanish).*

MINETTE. *French, 'faithful defender'.* Frenchified name rarely used in France. **Minnette, Minnita.**

MINNA. *German, diminutive of* **WILHELMINA.** One of those continental nickname names most popular these days in places like Finland. **Mina, Minetta, Minette, Minka, Minne, Minnie, Minny, Minta.**

MINNIE. *Diminutive of* **WILHELMINA.** Wildly popular in the early 1900s and completely obscure today. Blame Mickey's girlfriend. **Mini, Minie, Minne, Minni, Minny.**

MINTA. *English, diminutive of* **ARAMINTA.** An eighteenth century short form of a literary beauty that is still sometimes used here today. **Minty.**

MIRA. *(meer-a) Latin, 'admirable'; Hebrew, diminutive of* **MIRYAM.** Mira and Mirra have an arty aura. **Meara, Mirae, Mirah, Mirelle, Mireya, Mirieue, Miritta,**

Mirka, Mirra, Myra, Myrella, Myrene, Myritta.

★**MIRABEL.** *Latin, 'miraculous, beautiful one'.* Warning to modern mums: the author of *The Total Woman,* an antifeminist tract, was named Mirabel Morgan. Other than that, a wonderful name. **Meribel, Meribelle, Mira, Mirabell, Mirable. International: Mirabeau, Mirabelle, Mireille** *(French),* **Mirabella, Mirella** *(Italian and Spanish).*

MIRACLE. *Latin, 'wonder, marvel'.* A spiritual name that has recently become popular in the US.

★**MIRANDA.** *Latin, 'marvellous'.* Shimmeringly lovely Shakespearean name that's still a recommended choice even though its popularity peaked in the 1990s, perhaps as an antidote to Amanda. **Maranda, Marenda, Meranda, Mira, Miran, Miranada, Mirandah, Mirandia, Mirella, Mirinda, Mirindé, Mironda, Mirra, Mirranda, Muranda, Myra, Myranda, Myrella, Myrilla, Randa, Randi, Randie, Randy.**

MIREILLE. *(meer-AY) French, 'to admire'.* Pretty name that may pose pronunciation problems, but is well worth the effort. **Mircella, Mireil, Mirel, Mirella, Mirelle, Mirelys, Mireya, Mireyda, Mirielle, Mirilla, Myrella, Myrilla.**

MIRIAM. *Hebrew, 'bitter'; Aramaic, 'wished-for child'.* The oldest-known form of Mary, serious, solemn Miriam is most often used these days by observant Jewish parents. **Macia, Mairwen, Meriam, Meryam, Miram, Mirham, Miri, Miriain, Miriama, Miriame, Mirian, Mirjana, Mirriam, Mirrian, Miryam, Miryan, Mitzi, Mitzie, Miyana, Miyanna, Myriam. International: Mimi** *(French),* **Mirjam** *(Finnish),* **Mariam, Miri, Mirit** *(Hebrew/Israeli),* **Maryam** *(Arabic).*

♂ **MIRÓ.** *Spanish artist name.* If you love the colourful works of the Spanish abstractionist.

♂ **MISCHA, MISHA.** *Russian, diminutive of* **MIKHAIL.** This was a 100 per cent boys' name until recently, but is sometimes now being used for girls. **Meesha, Meescha, Mysha.**

MISSY. *English, diminutive of* **MELISSA.** A name that works until your daughter is, say, six. **Missi, Missie, Missy.**

MISTY. *English, 'mist'.* The *Play Misty for Me* jokes will get old really fast. **Missty, Mistee, Mistey, Misti, Mistie, Mistin, Mistina, Mistral, Mistylynn, Mystee, Mysti, Mystie.**

♂ **MITRA.** *Hindi, 'friend'; Persian, 'angel'.* This name of the Hindu god of the sun and of friendship sounds feminine enough to work for a girl. **Mita.**

MITZI. *German, diminutive of* **MARIA.** This spunky German nickname name might appeal to parents drawn to the genre of lively vintage chorus girl names. **Mitsi, Mitsie, Mitzee, Mitzey, Mitzy.**

MIUCCIA. *Italian, meaning unknown.* Influential designer Miuccia (nicknamed Miu Miu) Prada's surname is much better known than her first.

MOCHA. *Arabic, colour and coffee name.* Save this for your next run to Starbucks. **Moka.**

MODESTY. *Latin, 'modesty'.* Virtue name dating to Roman times, but never widely used, except for the 1960s film spoof heroine, Modesty Blaise. **Modesta, Modeste, Modestia, Modestie, Modestina, Modestine, Modestus.**

MOIRA. *(moy-rah) Irish, Anglicised variation of* **MAIRI.** Well-established name that is more popular in Ireland than elsewhere. **Moirae, Moirah, Moire, Moya, Moyra, Moyrah.**

MOLLY. *Diminutive of* **MARY.** Consistently popular as an independent name over the past few decades, although it's starting to slip down the Top 25. It is still an appealing option, with a spirited Irish feel. Mollie is also a Top 100 favourite. **Moli, Molie, Moll, Mollee, Molley, Molli, Mollie, Mollissa.**

MONA. *Irish, 'noble good'.* Moaner. **Moina, Monah, Mone, Monea, Monna, Moyna.**

MONDAY. *Word name.* Not most people's favourite day, but a pretty name.

MONET. *(mo-NAY) French artist name, from diminutive of* **SIMON.** A new favourite of the bohemian set, brought to light by actress Monet Mazur, daughter of the artist who designed the Rolling Stones' mouth logo. **Monae, Monay, Monee.**

MONICA. *Latin, 'advisor'.* Plummeted, especially after the demise of *Friends.* **Mona, Monee, Monia, Monic, Monice, Monicia, Monicka, Monise, Monn, Monnica, Monnie, Monya. International: Monca** *(Irish),* **Monike, Moniqua, Monique** *(French),* **Mónica** *(Spanish),* **Monika** *(German, Scandinavian).*

MONIQUE. *French variation of* **MONICA.** Passé.

MONSERRAT. *Catalan, place name.* This variation of Montserrat, the name of a mountain near Barcelona, is starting to be heard occasionally as a girl's name.

♂ **MONTANA.** *Spanish place name, 'mountainous'.* Overly trendy western place name in the US that is riding off into the sunset. **Montagne, Montaine, Montanna.**

MOON. *Word name.* The original oddball celebrity baby name, via Frank Zappa's daughter Moon Unit, who claims she's always liked it.

MÓR. *Scottish and Irish Gaelic, 'great one'.* Simple ancient name of a Celtic goddess, but her friends might sound like they were asking for more.

MORA. *Spanish, 'blueberry'.* Intriguing derivation, though people will assume it's a simplified form of Maura. **Morae, Morea, Moria, Morita.**

MÓRAG. *(MOHR-ahk) Scottish, 'the great one'.* A classic Gaelic name, but too hoary to be a hit elsewhere.

♂ **MORGAN.** *Welsh, 'circle' or 'sea'.* Early (i.e., 1970s) unisex name from Arthurian legend, now used more for girls than boys, and popular enough to make it into the Top 100 in recent years. We still find it a sophisticated choice. **Maughan, Morgain, Morgance,**

Morganetta, Morganette, Morganica, Morgann, Morganna, Morganne, Morgen, Morghan, Morgin, Morgyn, Morrigan. International: Morgaine, Morgana, Morgane, Muirgan *(French)*.

MORIAH. *Hebrew, 'the Lord is my teacher'.* Make life simpler and spell it Mariah. **Moraia, Moraiah, Moria, Moriel, Morit, Morria, Morriah.**

MORNA. *Irish and Scottish variation of* **MYRNA.** Poetic name that's terminally mournful.

♂ **MORNING.** *Word name.* There are many lovely day/month/seasonal names – and this is one of the best.

♂ **MOROCCO.** *Place name.* Rhythmic and exotic as the land itself, site of Casablanca and Marrakech.

♂ **MORVEN.** *English, poetic place name.* In the Ossianic poems, Morven is the hero's kingdom. Here, a harsher Morgan alternative. **Morvan, Morvin, Morvyn.**

MORWENNA. *Welsh, 'waves of the sea'.* Ancient Cornish name now being revived in Wales. **Medwenna, Morgan, Morwena, Morwina, Morwinna, Morwyn, Morwynna.**

MOSELLE. *Hebrew, 'drawn from the water'.* Feminine spin on Moses and European river name that's also the name of a wine. **Moiselle, Moisella, Mozelle.**

MOXIE. *English slang, 'aggressive energy, know-how'.* Give your daughter this name and you can have your own little brash babe.

MUGUET. *(moo-gay) French, 'lily'.* One of the few French words/names not attractive to the English-speaking person's ear. **Muguette.**

MURIEL. *Irish, 'of the bright sea'; Hebrew, 'bittersweet'.* A poetic Celtic name that now has a knitting-by-the-fire image. **Meriol, Merrial, Merriel, Merrill, Muire, Murial, Murielia, Muriell. International: Merial, Meriel, Muirgheal, Muiriol, Murielle** *(Irish),* **Muireall** *(Scottish).*

♂ **MURPHY.** *Irish, 'hound of the sea'.* Common Irish surname name once strictly male, now seen as a brisk and breezy possibility.

Art Names

Ansel

Calder

Christo

Georgia

Homer

Hopper

Jackson

Jasper

Kahlo

Klee

Leonardo

Magritte

Manet

Monet

O'Keeffe

Pablo

Picasso

Raphael

Sargent

Toulouse

Stellar Starbabies Beginning with *M*

Mabel	Neneh Cherry
Mackenzie	J. K. Rowling
Madelaine	Téa Leoni
Maggie	Jon Stewart
Makani	Woody Harrelson
Makena'lei	Helen Hunt
Malu	David Bryne
Manzie	Soon-Yi & Woody Allen
Manon	Helen McCrory & Damien Lewis
Marina	Matt LeBlanc
Martha	Ulrika Jonsson & Lance Gerrard-Wright
Mason	Kelsey Grammer
Mathilda	Molly Ringwald
Matilda	Elizabeth Perkins, Michelle Williams & Heath Ledger, Moon Unit Zappa
Mattea	Mira Sorvino
Maya	Uma Thurman & Ethan Hawke, Marlon Brando
Memphis	Bono
Mia	Kate Winslet
Molly	Marielle Frostrup
Moxie CrimeFighter	Penn Jillette

♂ **MURRAY.** *Scottish, 'from the land by the sea'.* An old-man name that sounds a lot cuter when used for a little girl. **Murry.**

MUSE. *Greek mythology name.* Remember, the Muse is passive: someone *else's* inspiration.

MUSETTA. *Latin, 'little muse'.* A musette is both a dance and an antique instrument, but the name is most associated with the classic opera *La Bohème.* **International: Musette** *(French).*

MUSIC. *Word name.* A musical name without much rhythm or harmony. **Musique.**

MYA. *Variation of* **MAYA.** This New Age spelling is catching up with the traditional one.

MYFANWY. *(muh-VAHN-wee) Welsh, 'my lovely little one'.* Intriguing Old Welsh name being revived, but would have major pronunciation problems elsewhere.

MYRA. *Greek, 'fragrant'; Latin, 'sweet-smelling oil'.* Most modern parents would probably prefer Mira or Mia. **Maira, Mayra, Mira, Myree, Myrena, Myria.**

MYRNA. *Irish, 'tender, beloved';*
Arabic, 'myrrh'. Myrna Loy,
Mrs *Thin Man,* was lovely –
but her name is not. **Meirna,**
Merna, Mirna, Moina, Morna,
Moyna, Muirna.

MYRTLE. *Greek botanical*
name. In Roman myth, a shrub
sacred to Venus; to us, an old-
fashioned 1940s name. **Mert,**
Mertice, Mertis, Mertie, Mertle,
Mirtle, Myrt, Myrta, Myrtia,
Myrtias, Myrtice, Myrtie,
Myrtilla, Myrtis.

MYSTERY. *Word name.* Pretty
sound, provocative meaning, but
a little over-the-top.

MYSTIQUE. *French word*
name. Better for a perfume.
Mistique.

N girls

NAAMAH. *(NAY-ah-mah)*
Hebrew, 'sweetness, grace, beauty'.
Interesting Old Testament name
that embraces many traditional
female attributes; also name of a
place in the Jordan Valley.
Naama, Naamana, Naami,
Naamia, Naamiah, Naamit,
Naamiya.

NAARAH. *(NAY-ah-rah).*
Hebrew, 'girl, maiden'. Another
rarely heard biblical name, with
some possible pronunciation
confusion. **Naara, Naarit.**

NABILA. *(nah-BEE-lah) Arabic,*
'honorable, noble'. Pretty and
feminine Muslim name popular
in Egypt. **Nabeela, Nabiha,**
Nabilah, Nabilia.

NADA. *Arabic, 'dew at sunrise'.*
Since it's also Spanish for
'nothing,' this name wouldn't be
great for a girl's self-esteem.
Nadda, Nadya.

NADIA. *Russian, Eastern*
European, 'hope'. Exotic but
accessible, this Slavic favourite,
which took on added energy and
charm when Romanian gymnast
Nadia Comaneci won the 1976
Olympics, is currently enjoying
a leap in popularity. **Nadea,**
Nadeen, Nadene, Nadiah, Nadie,
Nadija, Nadijah, Nadira, Nadja,
Nadjah, Nadya. International:
Nadége, Nadine *(French),*
Nadina, Nadine *(German and*
Italian), **Nadezhda, Nadzia, Nata**
(Polish), **Dusya, Nada, Nadenka,**
Nadina, Nadiya, Nadka, Nadya,
Nadyenka, Nadysha, Nadyuska
(Russian), **Nadina** *(Latvian).*

NADIDA. *Arabic, 'equal, a*
peer'. Light and rhythmic.
Nadeeda, Nadidah.

NADINE. *(nah-DEEN) French*
variation of **NADIA.** Part of the
vogue for French-sounding
names in the 1920s and 30s,
Nadine has been replaced by the
Russian sound of Nadia and
Natasha. **Nadean, Nadeen,**
Nadena, Nadene, Nadette,
Nadie, Nadien, Nadina, Nadyna,
Nadyne, Naideen, Naidene,
Naydeen.

NADIRA. *Arabic, 'precious,*
rare'. The *dir* syllable –
pronounced *deer* – is endearing,
but 'nadir' means the pits.
Naadira, Naarirah, Nadirah,
Nadra.

NAGIDA. *Hebrew, 'prosperous,*
successful'. Hebrew name with a
bountiful meaning but a less-
than-attractive sound. **Nagda,**
Nageeda, Nagia, Nagiah,
Nagidah, Nagiya, Najiah, Najiya,
Najiyan, Negida.

NAHARA. *Aramaic and Hebrew, 'light'.* Beguiling cousin of Sahara. **Nehara, Nehora.**

NAIA. *Hawaiian, 'dolphin'; Greek, 'to flow'.* Multicultural option, equally exotic as, but more unusual than, Maia. **Naiad, Naiah, Naiia, Naya, Nayah.**

NAIDA. *(NAY-dah), 'water nymph,' also diminutive of* ZENAIDA. Possibility for a girl born under one of the water signs – Cancer, Pisces or Scorpio. **Naiad, Nayad, Nyad.**

♂ **NAIRNE.** *Scottish, 'river with alder trees'.* Has a pleasant Scottish burr. **Naem, Naim.**

♂ **NAIROBI.** *African place name.* Kenya is fairly commonly heard as a girl's name, but its capital city makes a much more exceptional choice.

NAJA. *Arabic, 'success'; Navajo, 'silver hands'.* One of several similar feminine names often found in the Muslim world. **Najah.**

NAJIBA. *Arabic, 'wellborn'.* Rhythmic and exotic. **Nagiba, Nagibah, Najibah.**

NAJILA. *Arabic, 'bright eyes'.* Pretty and feminine Arabic name. **Naja, Najah, Najia, Najilah, Najja, Najla.**

♂ **NAKOTAH.** *Sioux, 'friend to all'.* This name of one of the three tribes in the Great Sioux Nation could provide an interesting alternative to Dakota. **Nakota.**

NALA. *African, meaning unknown.* A Disneyfied name – Nala was the friend who became the wife of Simba, hero of *The Lion King*. It was chosen for his daughter by Keenen Ivory Wayans.

NALANI. *Hawaiian, 'calm skies'.* Evocative of tranquil island escapes. **Nalanie, Nalany.**

NAN. *English, diminutive of* NANCY. *Bobbsey Twins*–era nickname name that could find new life via Nan, heroine of *The Nanny Diaries*.

NANA. *Diminutive of ANNA and* NANCY; *also Hawaiian, 'spring'.* The dog in *Peter Pan* and another name for Grandma.

NANCY. *Hebrew, 'grace'; diminutive of* ANN. Even if Nancy is now a middle-aged name, it still has a pleasantly light and airy feel. **Nan, Nana, Nance, Nancee, Nancey, Nanci, Nancie, Nanette, Nanita, Nann, Nanna, Nanncey, Nanncy, Nanni, Nannie, Nanny, Nanscey, Nansee, Nansey, Nusi, Nusa. International: Nainsí** *(Irish Gaelic),* **Nanine, Nannette, Nanou** *(French),* **Nanig** *(Breton),* **Nancsi, Nancsie** *(Hungarian),* **Nani** *(Greek),* **Nanée** *(Armenian).*

NANETTE. *Diminutive of ANN and* NANCY. There was a time when French names like Annette, Paulette – and Nanette – were chic, but now we'd have to say, 'No, no, Nanette'. **Nanelia, Nanelle, Nanetta, Nanon, Ninette. International: Nanée, Nanine, Nannette, Nynette** *(French).*

NANNA. *Scandinavian, 'daring'. See* NANA.

NANON. *French, diminutive of* ANN. Sweet and endearing, à la Mignon and Manon.

NAOMI. *Hebrew, 'my joy, my delight'.* This long-neglected Old Testament name seems to finally be finding favour with parents seeking a biblical name with a soft, melodic sound and a positive meaning, suddenly sounding fresher than the widely used Sarah, Rachel and Rebecca. Beautiful black model Naomi Campbell has helped the modernisation, and it's made an appearance in the Top 100 a few times recently. **Naoma, Naome, Naomee, Naomia, Naomie, Naomy, Neoma, Neomi, Nioma, Niomi, Noami, Nomi, Nyomi.** International: **Noémie** *(French),* **Noemi** *(Italian and Spanish).*

NARA. *Celtic, 'happy'; Japanese, 'thunderclap'.* Soft, simple and far more unusual than Tara or Farrah. **Narah, Narra.**

NARCISSA. *Greek, 'daffodil'.* This Greek flower and mythological choice doesn't make it into the pantheon of possibilities because of its association with narcissism. **Narcessa, Narcyssa, Narsissa.** International: **Narcisse, Narguise, Narqis** *(French),* **Narcisa** *(Spanish),* **Narkissa** *(Russian),* **Nergis** *(Turkish).*

NARDA. *Greek botanical name; Latin, 'fragrant'.* Too close to Nada.

NARETHA. *Aboriginal, 'a saltbush'.* As far-flung as the outback.

NARNIA. *Literary place name.* This Latin-sounding place name, created by C. S. Lewis for his *Chronicles,* will undoubtedly be adopted by a few admiring parents.

NARVA. *Modern invented name.* Though newly created, has a dated feel.

NASCHA. *Native American, Navajo, 'owl'.* Stick with Sascha.

NASHAWNA. *Contemporary blend of prefix na- with* SHAWNA. Variation on the more common Lashawna. **Nashana, Nashanda, Nashaun, Nashauna, Nashaunda, Nashawn, Nashuana.**

NASHOTA. *Native American, 'twin'.* Highly unusual possibility for a twin girl. **Nashoba.**

NASIA. *Hebrew, 'God's miracle'.* Too close to nausea. **Naseea, Naseeah, Nasiah, Nasiya, Nasya, Nsayah.**

NASIMA. *Arabic, 'breeze, fresh air'.* Associated with a spring festival, this exotic name is used by both Muslims and Christians. **Naseema, Naseemah, Nesima, Nesimah, Nessima, Nessimah, Nesimeh.**

NASTASSIA. *Variation of* ANASTASIA. A pleasing blend of Natasha and Anastasia, though there might be a Nasty nickname. **Nastasha, Nastashia, Nastasia, Nastasja, Nastassja, Nastassa, Nastassiya, Nastassya, Nastazia, Nastia, Nastiya, Nastya, Natasha.**

★**NATALIA.** *Russian, 'born on Christmas day'.* Heard frequently in Spain, Portugal and the Slavic countries, this is a distinctive, strong but feminine member of the Natalie/Natasha family, with the appealing short form Talia. **Nat, Nataleea, Natalie, Natalya, Natascha, Nataschenka, Natasha, Nattie, Talia, Tasha, Tasya, Tata, Tusya.** International: **Natalina, Nathalia,**

Supermodel Names

Alek	Karolina
Anouck	Laetitia
Coco	Liberty
Daria	Liya
Elle	Marija
Emina	Milla
Flavia	Natalia
Gisele	Snejana
Hana	Solange
Hannelore	Stam
Hye	Stella
Iselin	Tiuu
Jaunel	Tyra
Jelsa	Yasmin
Karmen	Yevgeniya

Natividad, Navidad *(Spanish)*, Nata, Nataliya, Nataly, Natella, Talya *(Russian)*.

NATALIE. *French variation of* **NATALIA.** This Franco-Russian name became Anglacised years ago; now a new generation is reviving it to join former canasta partners Sophie and Belle. Sometimes given to girls born on Christmas, Natalie was Cameron Diaz's character in *Charlie's Angels*. Newly popular spellings: Nataly, Nathalie, Natalee, and Nathaly. **Nat, Natalee, Natalene, Natalia, Natalina, Nataly, Nathalia, Nathaly, Natti, Nattie, Tallie, Tally, Tascha. International:** **Natalène, Nathalie, Tali, Talie** *(French),* **Natala, Natale** *(Italian),* **Natalia** *(Spanish),* **Natalya, Natascha, Natasha, Natashenka** *(Russian).*

NATANIA. *Hebrew, 'gift of God'.* This female form of Nathan can be pronounced with three syllables or four. **Nataniah, Nataniella, Natanielle, Natanya, Nathania, Nathaniella, Nathanielle, Natonya, Netaniella, Tania.**

NATASHA. *Diminutive of* **NATALIA.** The appealing, exotic Natasha is still in the Top 100, but it seems to have peaked in the 1990s. Singer Tori Amos came up with the unusual variation **NATASHYA** for her daughter. **Nastassya, Nastasya, Natasia, Natassia, Natascha, Nataschenka, Natashia, Natasya, Natosha, Tasha, Tasya, Tata, Tusya.**

NATIVIDAD. *Spanish from Latin, 'nativity'.* Traditionally given to girls born on the September birth date of the Virgin Mary. **Nati, Navidad.**

NAVA *(Nah-vah) Hebrew, 'pretty, pleasant, desirable'.* Hebrew name heard more frequently in Israel than elsewhere. **Navah, Naveh, Navice, Navit.**

NAVY. *Word name.* A highly original choice made by an American singer, who claimed to have thought of it in terms of the colour, not the seagoing armed service.

NAYANA. *Hindi, 'beautiful eyes'.* Hip-swayingly evocative.

NAYELI. *Zapotec, 'I love you'.* A name rarely heard outside the Latino community, which is strong enough in the US to propel it into their Top 400.

NAYO. *(NAH-yo) African Nigerian, 'she is our joy'.* A bit masculine in feel.

NAZARET. *Spanish, 'of Nazareth'.* Occasionally heard Spanish name referring to Christ's native village.

NAZIRA. *Arabic, 'equal'.* Striking, azure-tinted choice. **Nazirah.**

NAZY. *Persian, 'cute'.* Cute in Persian, verboten here. **Nazilla, Nazneen.**

♂ **NEAL.** *Irish, 'champion' or 'cloud'.* Instead of using an obscure feminisation like Neala, why not appropriate the boy's name itself? Like Sydney and Seth, Neal is more attractive after a gender switch. **Neel, Neil, Neill, Niall, Niallan, Niel.**

NEALA. Feminine variation of **NEAL.** *See* **NEAL. Neale, Neela, Neila, Neilla, Nelia. International: Neilina** *(Scottish).*

NEBULA. *Latin, 'misty'.* Too foggy.

NECHAMA. *(Neh-KAH-mah) Hebrew, 'comfort'.* Traditional Hebrew name that has never entered the mainstream elsewhere. **Nachman, Nachmanit, Nachmaniya, Nachmi, Nachum, Nachuma, Necha, Neche, Nechamit, Nehama.**

NEDDA. *Slavic, 'born on Sunday'.* Mid-century macramé-maker. **Nedra.**

NEEJA. *Hindi, 'lily'.* Sweet and feminine Eastern flower name.

NEEMA. *(neh-EH-mah or NEE-mah) Swahili, 'born during good times'.* Offbeat name sometimes heard in the African-Caribbean community.

NEESHA. *Modern invented name.* Has a truncated nickname feel. **Neisha, Niesha, Nisha, Nysha.**

NEFERTITI. *Egyptian, 'the beautiful one has arrived'.* This ancient Egyptian queen's name would be best saved for a cat.

NEHAMA. *Hebrew, 'comfort'. See* **NECHAMA.**

♂ **NEIL.** *Irish, 'champion' or 'cloud'. See* **NEAL. Neel, Neell, Neill.**

NEILA. *(Neh-ee-lah) Hebrew, 'locking, closing'.* This name of the final service on Yom Kippur, the Day of Atonement, is

sometimes given symbolically to girls born on that day. **Neala, Nealie, Neela, Neelie, Neely, Neilah, Neilia, Neilla, Neille, Nia, Nielsine.**

NEIMA. *(nee-mah) Hebrew, 'strong'.* One of the less attractive Hebrew choices. **Nima.**

NEITH. *Egyptian, 'divine mother'.* The name of the Egyptian goddess of home and femininity is beneath consideration.

NELDA. *English, 'one who lives by the alder tree'.* Occasionally heard in Ireland, small chance of success elsewhere.

NELIA. *Spanish, diminutive of* **MANUELA** *and* **CORNELIA.** Lively and appealing and able to stand on its own. **Neelia, Neelya, Nela, Nila.**

★**NELL.** *English, diminutive of* **HELEN, ELEANOR,** *et al.* Once a nickname for Helen, Ellen or Eleanor, Nell is a sweet old-fashioned charmer that is fashionably used today in its own right. **Nella, Nelley, Nelli,**

Nellie, Nelly, Neila, Nelma.
International: **Neila, Neile, Nela, Nialla** *(Irish)*, **Nelya** *(Russian)*.

NELLIE. *Diminutive, elongation of* **NELL**. This ready-for-revival name recalls the old Gay Nineties and bicycles-built-for-two era. **Neli, Nelley, Nelli, Nelly.**

NEMEA. *Greek place name.* The name of a famous valley in ancient Greece, with ties to the historic Nemean Games. **Nema.**

NEMY. *(NEE-mee) African, 'sweet'.* Friendly and energetic. **Neemy, Neemi, Neemie, Nemi.**

NEOLA. *Greek, 'the young one'.* Has an arty, creative image. **Neeola, Niola, Nyola.**

NEOMA. *Greek, 'new moon'.* Because of the many diseases that end in *oma,* this name has a vaguely medical feel. **Neomah, Neomea, Neomenia, Neomia.**

NEORAH. *Hebrew, 'enlightened'.* Soft and sensitive. **Neira, Nera.**

NERA. *(NEE-rah) Hebrew, 'candle, light'.* Because of its meaning, this is a symbolic name given to girls born on Hanukkah, the Festival of Lights. **Nerah, Neriah, Nerit, Neriya, Ner-Li.**

NERIAH. *Hebrew, 'light of Jehovah'. See* **NERA**. **Neria, Neriya.**

NERIDA. *Greek, 'sea nymph, mermaid'.* One of a group of Greek names connected to the sea. **Nereida, Nereyda, Neridah, Neried, Nerina, Nerine, Neris, Nerita.**

NERINE. *Greek mythology name.* A new brand of eye-drop? **Nereen, Nerice, Nerina, Nerita, Nissa.**

NERISSA. *Greek, 'from the sea'.* Offbeat possible replacement for the overused Melissa and Marisa, it was used by Shakespeare for Portia's witty confidante in *The Merchant of Venice.* **Narice, Narissa, Naryssa, Nerice, Nerisa, Nerise, Nerisse, Nerrisa, Nerrissa, Nerys, Neryssa, Nissa, Rissa.**

NERYS. *(NER-iss) Welsh, 'lady'.* Parents outside of Wales are just becoming aware of Welsh names like this one, similar to Carys, which was chosen by Welsh-born Catherine Zeta-Jones. **Neris, Neryss.**

NESSA. *Scandinavian, 'headlands, promontory'; also diminutive of* **VANESSA**; *Russian, diminutive of* **ANASTASIA**; *Scottish, diminutive of* **AGNES**. Like its cousin Tessa, Nessa – a shortening of Vanessa – is an attractive nickname that can stand on its own. **Nesa, Nesha, Neshia, Nesiah, Nessi, Nessia, Nessie, Netia, Neysa.**

NESTA. *Welsh variation of* **AGNES**. *See* **AGNES**.

NETTIE. *English, diminutive of names ending in* -ette *or* -etta. A knitting and crocheting great-grandma name that just might work as a relaxed choice for a contemporary little girl, perhaps to honour an ancestral Annette or Henrietta. **Neta, Netta, Netti, Nettia, Netty.**

NEVA. *Spanish, 'white snow'.* Has a pure, clean aura, but is also evocatively exotic. **Neeva, Neiva, Nevara, Nevia, Nieve, Niva, Nyva.**

♂ NEVADA. *Spanish place name, 'covered in snow'.* Named for its snowcapped mountains, Nevada is an American state name which, unlike Carolina, Montana and Dakota, has been relatively undiscovered. Warning: today's unvisited place name could become tomorrow's trampled tourist attraction.

NEVAEH. *Modern invented name.* One American singer had the idea of turning 'Heaven' around and using it as a baby name. Nevaeh has had phenomenal success in the US, where there are thousands of new little Nevaehs, and it was the top name for black baby girls born in Colorado.

NEVARA. *Spanish, 'to snow'.* Another snowy option, this one lacking a tie to a specific place: an asset.

★NEVE. *(nehv) Latin, 'snow'; Anglicised spelling of* **NIAMH.** Introduced by actress Neve Campbell — it was her Dutch-born mother's maiden name — Neve is an interesting and fresh new possibility worthy of consideration. **Nev.**

NEVES. *(NAY-vesh) Portuguese, 'snows'.* A name that refers to a title of the Virgin Mary – 'Maria des Neves', or Maria of Snows.

NEVIAH. *Hebrew, 'forecaster'.* All too likely to be confused with the ultratrendy Nevaeh. **Nevia.**

♂ NEVIS. *Place name.* Highly unusual name of a small, tranquil island in the Caribbean; chosen for her daughter by singer Nelly Furtado.

♂ NEWLYN. *Welsh, 'new pond'.* Male name that seems feminine enough to switch genders, if you're looking for a new *lyn* spin.

NGAIO. *(NYE-oh) Maori, 'reflections on the water'; also name of a New Zealand tree.* Anyone who has ever read the classic mysteries of New Zealand writer Ngaio (born Edith Ngaio) Marsh must have wondered about her name – and how to say it. It would certainly make an attention-grabbing if confusing choice.

NGOZI. *(n-GO-zee) African, Nigerian-Ibo, 'blessing'.* Dynamic and creative; common in Africa, challenging here.

NIA. *Swahili, 'resolve'; Welsh variation of* **NIAMH.** Short but energetic and substantial, Nia has special meaning and African roots, as it's one of the days of Kwanza. **Nea, Neya, Niah, Niya, Nya, Nyah.**

NIABI. *(nee-AH-bee) Native American, Osage, 'fawn'.* Strong and rhythmic American Indian name.

Spiritual Names

Amena

Angel

Destiny

Evangeline

Faith

Genesis

Heaven

Messiah

Miracle

Nevaeh

Praise

Trinity

207

girls' names

NIAMH. *(nee-av) Irish Gaelic, 'radiance, brilliance'.* An ancient Irish name that was originally a term for a goddess; rich in legendary associations, Niamh is in the Irish Top Ten. Here, where it is in the Top 100, the phonetic Neve would be simpler, if less intriguing. **Neve, Niam.**

NIANI. *Ancient capital of the kingdom of Mali.* Exotic place name that could find its place elsewhere.

NIARA. *Hindi, 'nebula, mist'.* More unusual alternative to Tiara.

NICHELLE. *American, contemporary variation of* **MICHELLE.** A modern twist on Michelle, spotlighted by *Star Trek* actress Nichelle Nichols. **Nachelle, Nichell, Nichella, Nischell, Nischelle, Nishell, Nishelle. International: Nichele** *(French).*

NICKI. *Diminutive of* **NICOLA, NICOLE, NICOLETTE.** Once the teenager, now more likely to be the mum who hires her. **Nickee, Nickie, Nickey Nicky, Niki, Nikkee, Nikkey, Nikki, Nikkie, Nikky, Niky.**

♂ **NICO.** *Italian, diminutive of* **NICOLA.** This is a much more dynamic nickname than Nicky for any of the *Nic*-names. **Neeco, Niko, Nyco.**

★**NICOLA.** *(NICK-oh-la) Greek; feminine variation of* **NICHOLAS.** Elegant Latinate feminisation of Nicholas, has long been standard issue for English girls but is currently out of favour, which we consider a pity, especially as Nicole's standing wanes. **Colletta, Collette. International: Colette, Nicholina** *(French),* **Niccola** *(Italian),* **Nicolina, Nicoline** *(Greek).*

NICOLE. *Greek, feminine variation of* **NICHOLAS.** One of the top girls' names of the 1980s and into the 90s, and it is still in the Top 100, although it has now lost most of its French flair. Substitutes to consider: Nico or Nicola. **Nicci, Niccole, Nichole, Nici, Nicki, Nickie, Nickole, Nicky, Nicol, Nik, Niki, Nikie, Nikki, Nikkie, Nikkole, Nikky, Nikole. International: Colette, Collette, Nichelle, Nicolette** *(French),*

Coletta, Niccola, Nicia, Nicola *(Italian),* **Coleta, Coletta, Nicanora, Nicolasa** *(Spanish),* **Kolenka, Kolya, Nikita** *(Russian),* **Nichola, Nichole, Nicholla, Nickoletta, Nicolla, Nikolla** *(Eastern European),* **Niki, Nikola, Nikoleta, Nikolia** *(Greek).*

NICOLETTE. *French, feminine variation of* **NICHOLAS.** Ultra-feminine name of an enchanting princess in a medieval French romance, has gotten stacks of publicity via *Desperate Housewives'* Nicollette Sheridan. **Nicholette, Nicki, Nicolett, Nicoletta, Nicollette, Nicki, Nikkolette, Nikolette.**

NICOLINA. *Diminutive of* **NICOLA.** Another light new twist in the Nicole family.

NIDIA. *Greek, 'she possesses sweetness and grace'.* Ear-catching alternative to Lydia. **Nidi, Nidya, Nydia.**

NIEVES. *(nee-A-bays) Spanish, 'snows'.* A name bestowed in honour of the Virgin Mary, *Nuestra Señora de la Nieves,* referring to a miracle she performed with unmelted snow in the August heat of Rome. **Neaves, Neives, Nieva, Nievas, Nievez, Nievis.**

NIGELLA. *Feminine variation of* **NIGEL,** *also flower name.* A name that sounded unthinkably priggish until it became attached to *Domestic Goddess* TV chef Nigella Lawson (named for her father), who gave it a big dollop of glamour.

♂ **NIK.** *Diminutive of* **NICOLE** *et al.* Modern, boyish, if self-consciously groovy nickname for Nicole or any of its variations. **Nic, Nick, Nikk.**

NIKA. *Russian, diminutive of* **VERONIKA.** Exotic modern nickname name possibility. **Nikka.**

♂ **NIKE.** *Greek, mythological goddess of victory.* Better than Adidas.

NIKEESHA. *Modern invented name.* A pretty but none-too-classy amalgamation of Nicole and Keesha. **Niceesha, Nici, Nickeesha, Nicki, Nickisha, Nickysha, Nicquisha, Niki, Nikisha, Nikki, Nikkisha, Nikysha, Niquisha.**

NIKI. *Greek, diminutive of* **NICOLE.** Streamlined version of outdated Nicki. **Nicki, Nicky, Nikki.**

♂ **NIKITA.** *Russian variation of* **NICOLE.** Nikita's image has come a long way from portly post-Stalin Soviet leader Khrushchev to the sexy spy/assassin in the movie and TV series *La Femme Nikita.* **Nakeeta, Nakeita, Nakita, Nickita, Nikeeta, Niki, Nikitah, Nikitia, Nikitta, Nikki, Nikkita, Nikyta, Niquita.**

NILEY. *Aboriginal, 'a shell'.* Could be seen as a stand-in for Riley, but not nearly as appealing.

NILLA. *African, 'glorious'.* Something slightly negative about that *Nil* beginning; more positive similar names would be Lilla or Willa, Lucilla or Priscilla. **Nila, Nile, Nilea, Nille.**

NIMA. *(Nee-mah) Hebrew, 'thread, hair'; Arabic, 'blessing'; Hindi, 'margosa tree'.* Multicultural name often heard in the Near East. **Neema, Neemah Nema, Niama, Nimah, Nimi.**

NINA. *Russian, diminutive of* **ANTONINA.** As multi-ethnic as you can get: Nina is a young girl in Spain, a common nickname name in Russia, a Babylonian goddess of the oceans and an Incan goddess of fire. At the moment, it's a stylish possibility that's been underused. 'Weird Al' Yankovic chose this decidedly nonweird name for his daughter. **Neena, Nena, Ninetta, Ninette, Ninna, Ninon, Nyna.** International: **Ninon** *(French),* **Neenah, Nenah, Neneh, Ninah, Niña, Ninita** *(Spanish),* **Niina** *(Finnish),* **Ninácska** *(Hungarian),* **Ninotchka, Ninacska** *(Eastern European).*

NINON. *French, diminutive of* **ANNE** *and* **NINA.** Sweet and charming à la Mignon.

NIOBE. *(NĪ-ah-BEE or nee-O-bee) Greek mythology name.* The mythological queen whose perpetual weeping for her slain children turned her into a stone has always cast a pall over this name.

NIRA. *(Nee-rah) Hebrew, 'light,' 'furrow, plowed field'.* Symbolic name given to girls born on

TuB'Shevat, the New Year of the Trees. **Neera, Nirela, Nirella, Niran, Nirel, Nirit, Nyra.**

NISHA. *Hindi, 'night'.* We don't see this translating too well. **Niasha, Nishay, Nishi.**

NISSA. *Hebrew, 'to test'.* Feels truncated, as though a first syllable was snapped off. **Nisse, Nissie, Nissy.**

NITA. *Hindi, 'friendly'; Hebrew, 'to plant'; Native American, Choctaw, 'bear'.* Although heard in several cultures, it still feels somewhat flimsy. **Neeta, Nitali.**

NIVA. *(Nee-vah) Hebrew, 'talk, expression'.* Also an Israeli place name, this is an unusual, feminine choice. **Neva, Nivi, Nivit.**

NIXI. *Latin, 'goddess of childbirth'.* Nix. **Nixie.**

NIXIE. *German, 'water nymph'; Latin, 'snowy'.* If you think Dixie, Trixie and Pixie are outlandish, this name of a mermaidlike sprite in German folklore is definitely not for you.

NIZANA. *Hebrew, 'a flower bud'.* Has a pleasantly fizzy, effervescent feeling. **Nitza, Nitzana, Zana.**

NOA. *Hebrew, 'movement, motion'.* This Old Testament female name, heard frequently in Israel, will be misunderstood elsewhere as an attempt to streamline and feminise the more familiar Noah.

♂ **NOAH.** *Hebrew, 'rest, comfort'.* The ark-builder's spelling of this name was brought into the realm of female possibility when country singer Billy Ray Cyrus gave it to his daughter.

♂ **NOEL.** *French, 'Christmas'.* The French word for Christmas has been given to both boys and girls born on that holiday since the Middle Ages. **Noela, Noelani, Noele, Noeleen, Noelene, Noeline, Noell, Noella, Noelle, Nowell.**

NOELIA. *Spanish, feminine variation of* **NOEL.** This Spanish variation of the holiday name has been picked up by hundreds of Hispanic parents.

NOELLE. *French, 'Christmas'.* Feminissima, with a French gloss. **Noël, Noele, Noell, Noella, Noellia, Novelia.**

NOEMÍ. *(no-ay-MEE) Spanish variation of* **NAOMI.** Right up there on the Hispanic popularity list. **Mimi, Naiomá, Naiomí, Neohmí, Neomi, Noemá, Noemé, Noemíe, Noemy, Nomi.**

NOÉMIE. *(no-AY-mee) French variation of* **NAOMI.** Particularly pretty ethnic version of the biblical standard.

NOLA. *Gaelic, 'white shoulder'; Latin, 'small bell'.* A name with a haunting, sensual quality, used for the much-pursued heroine of Spike Lee's breakout 1986 film, *She's Gotta Have It.* **Nolah, Nolana, Noli, Nolie.**

NOLITA. *Latin, 'unwilling'.* A saucy Latin name that could fit in with an Anglo surname. **Noleeta, Noleta.**

NOLWENN *(nohl-VEN) Welsh, 'shining, holy'.* Popular in Wales, not much chance elsewhere. **Nolwen, Nolwin, Nolwyn.**

NONA. *Latin, 'ninth'.* A name sometimes given to the ninth child – unlikely to serve that purpose today. **Non, Nonah, Nonia, Nonie, Nonita, Nonna, Nonnah, Nonya.**

NONN. *Welsh saint's name.* A non-name.

NOOR. *Hindi, 'light'.* Interesting name associated with the elegant American-born Queen Noor of Jordan. **Noora, Noura, Nur, Nura.**

★**NORA.** *Greek, 'light'; Irish, diminutive of* **HONORA.** This lovely, refined name conjures up images of Belle Epoch ladies in fur-trimmed coats skating in Central Park, the independent Ibsen heroine of *A Doll's House*, and the female half of the witty Nick and Nora Charles duo, adding up to a most desirable choice. **Norah, Norie, Norina, Norine, Norline, Norra. International: Noreen, Noreena** *(Irish),* **Norlene** *(Scottish),* **Norita** *(Spanish),* **Noora** *(Finnish),* **Neorah** *(Israeli).*

NORABEL. *English, 'beautiful light'; combination of* **NORA** *and* **BELLE.** Blended name sometimes heard in the early decades of the twentieth century.

NORAH. *Spelling variation of* **NORA.** The skyrocketing success of singer Norah Jones brought this spelling of the name onto the pop charts in 2003.

NORDICA. *Teutonic, 'from the north'.* Icy. **Nordika.**

NOREEN. *English, diminutive of* **NORA.** Noreen's in limbo, especially now that Nora has made a comeback. **Noreena, Noreene, Norena, Norene, Norina, Norine, Nureen, Nurine.**

♂ **NORI.** *Japanese, 'doctrine' or 'seaweed'.* Japanese name that would have no trouble assimilating. **Noriko.**

NORMA. *English, 'from the north'; Latin, 'the pattern'.* Invented for Bellini's opera, Norma had some star quality in the silent-screen and Marilyn Monroe days, but at this point it's a greying grandma in baby name limbo.

African Names

Abena
Afia
Amadi
Ebele
Eshe
Ife
Kamali
Kamaria
Kia
Marjani
Neela
Nemy
Nuru
Nyala
Panya
Salana
Subira
Taci
Taraja
Zuri

♂ **NORRIS.** *French, 'northerner'.* A British surname used only for males until Mrs Norman Mailer, Norris Church (born Barbara), came under the public eye.

Stellar Starbabies Beginning with N

Nala	Keenen Ivory Wayans
Natashya	Tori Amos
Nell	Vic Reeves & Nancy Sorrell
Nell Marmalade	Helen Baxendale
Neve	Conan O'Brien
Nevis	Nelly Furtado
Nico	Thandie Newton
Nina	'Weird Al' Yankovic
Ninna	Marlon Brando
Noah	Billy Ray Cyrus

NOVA. *Greek, 'new'; Native American Hopi, 'chasing butterflies'.* Astronomical term for a star that suddenly increases in brightness, then fades; probably works better for a TV science show than a child. **Nea, Novah, Novella, Novelle Novea, Novia.**

NUALA. *(NOO-la) Irish, 'white shoulders'.* Officially a shortening of the traditional and tricky Gaelic Fionnghuala/Fionnuala, Nuala makes a lovely choice all on its own. **Nula.**

NUNZIA. *Latin, 'messenger'.* A vivacious Italian name; also a diminutive of **Annunziata.** **Nunciata.**

NURIA. *Hebrew, 'fire of the Lord'.* Possible name . . . for a skin cream. **Nuri, Nuriel, Nurit, Nurita.**

NURU. *Swahili, 'light, born during the day'.* Related to the Muslim name Noor, which would be preferable. **Nor, Noor, Nur.**

NYA. *African, 'tenacity'.* A relatively new name on the scene. **Nia, Niah, Nyah, Nyia.**

NYALA. *(nee-YAH-lah) African, Ethiopian, 'mountain goat'.* The kind of name given to an exotic beauty in a 1940s movie.

NYASIA. *Meaning unknown.* Latina 'freestyle' singer Nyasia helped put this name on the popularity list in the US.

NYDIA. *Latin, 'nest' or 'home'.* Very rarely used, could provide a distinctive alternative to Lydia. **Needia, Nidia, Nidiah, Nyda, Nydiah.**

NYLA. *Arabic, 'winner'.* This name of an ancient Egyptian princess could make a fitting choice for a bicoastal child. **Nylah.**

NYOMI. *Hebrew spelling variation of* **NAOMI.** *See* **NAOMI. Nyome, Nyomee, Nyomie.**

NYREE. *New Zealand, Maori, 'flaxen'.* A variation on the unpronounceable Ngaire, this name is sometimes heard in New Zealand and very occasionally in England. **Niree.**

NYSSA. *(NYEH-sah) Greek, 'beginning'; Latin, 'goal'.* A fairly common Greek name that would fit in well elsewhere. **Nissa, Nisse, Nissie, Nisy, Nysa.**

NYX. *Greek mythology name.* In Greek mythology, Nyx was a powerful goddess and the embodiment of the night, but when spoken, its negative meaning can't be ignored.

O *girls*

♂ **OAK.** *Nature name.* Mighty, though mighty masculine.

♂ **OAKLEY.** *English, 'oak wood or clearing'.* Annie Oakley connection makes this a bit more girl-appropriate.

OBA. *Nigerian mythology name.* Intriguing name of the ancient goddess of rivers.

OBEDIENCE. *Virtue name.* It may have been used by the Puritans, but any modern child would chafe under this name.

OBELIA. *Greek, 'needle'.* Victorian feel.

♂ **OBERON.** *Literary name.* The name of the king of the fairies in Shakespeare's *A Midsummer Night's Dream;* could work just as well for your little sprite.

★♂ **O'BRIEN.** *Irish, 'child of the king'.* This kind of authentic Irish surname makes a memorable first name for either sex, following in the path of all the *Mac* and *Mc* names recently popular. See '*O*' Names' sidebar on page 496 for other possibilities.

OCEANA. *Greek, 'ocean'.* Great choice for the daughter of a beach lover. **Ocean, Oceananna, Oceania, Oceanna, Oceanne, Oceaonna, Oceon. International: Océane** *(French).*

OCÉANE. *(o-shay-ahn) French, 'ocean'.* Wildly popular name in France that could easily cross the Channel.

★**OCTAVIA.** *Latin, 'eighth'.* While there aren't many families large enough to have an eighth child anymore, this ancient Roman name has real possibilities as a substitute for the overused Olivia; recommended for its combination of classical and musical overtones. **Octabia, Octaviah, Octaviais, Octaviana, Octavianne, Octavice, Octavienne, Octavise, Octavya, Octiana, Octivia, Octoviana, Tavie, Tavy. International: Octava, Octavie** *(French),* **Ottavia** *(Italian),* **Otavia, Tavia** *(Spanish).*

♂ **OCTOBER.** *Word name.* So much more memorable and modern than April or May; chosen by innovative author/editor Dave Eggers.

ODEDA. *(oh-dehd-yah) Hebrew, 'to encourage'.* Virtually unknown in this country, the *dead* sound could be a problem.

ODELE. *English from Greek, 'song'.* Sounds a lot like the dated Adele. **Odela, Odelet, Odelette, Odelina, Odeline,**

Odell, Odella, Odelle, Odelyn, Udele, Udelia, Udilia.

ODELIA. *Hebrew, 'I will praise the Lord'.* Pretty Hebrew name that would create a strong but feminine impression. **Delia, Odeelia, Odele, Odeleya, Odelina, Odelinda, Odella, Odellia, Odelyn, Odila, Odilia, Udele, Udelia, Udilia. International: Odetta, Odette, Odile, Odilia** *(French),* **Oda, Odila, Odiel** *(German),* **Oda** *(Scandinavian).*

★**ODESSA.** *Russian place name.* This Ukrainian port city was given its name by Russia's Catherine the Great, who was inspired by Homer's *Odyssey,* and would make an original and intriguing choice. **Adesha, Adeshia, Adessa, Adessia, Odessia, Odissa, Odyssa, Odyssia.**

ODETTA. *German, 'wealthy'.* The memorable folk singer, an early single-name celeb, brought this into the spotlight.

ODETTE. *French, from German, 'wealthy'.* In the ballet

Swan Lake, she's the good swan; a sophisticated choice. **Oddetta, Odetta.**

ODILE. *French variation of German Otthild, 'prospers in battle'.* Odette's evil *Swan Lake* twin – gives the name a sinuous, sensuous appeal. **Odila, Odilia, Odolia, Udelia, Udile, Udilia.**

OFIRA. *Hebrew, 'gold'; also biblical place name.* Identified with a region famous for its gold, more attractive when spelled Ophira. **Ofarrah, Offir, Ophira.**

OFRA. *Hebrew, 'fawn'.* The name of a famous Israeli singer, Ofra Haza. **Ofrat, Ofrit, Ophra.**

♂ **OHARA.** *Japanese, 'small field'.* Could work for a blended Japanese-Irish family.

OKSANA. *Russian from Hebrew, 'praise to God'.* Ukrainian figure-skating champion Oksana Baiul made it known elsewhere. **Oksanna.**

OLA. *Scandinavian, feminine variation of* **OLAF.** Simple,

friendly, distinctive name heard in several cultures.

OLENA. *Russian variation of* **HELEN.** Alluring Eastern European name – though going straight to Lena might simplify things. **Alena, Elena, Lena, Lenya, Oleena, Olenka, Olenna, Olenya, Olinia, Olfauja, Olenya Olina, Olinia, Olinija, Olya.**

OLESIA. *Polish, diminutive of* **ALEKSANDRA.** Sounds a bit pharmaceutical. **Cesya, Ola, Olecia, Olessha, Oleishia, Olesha, Olesya, Olexa, Olice, Olicia, Olisha, Olishia, Olla, Ollicia.**

OLGA. *Russian, 'holy'.* Has lost whatever exotic oomph it once may have had. **Elga, Helga, Helsa, Olia, Olja, Ollya, Olva. International: Ola, Olenka** *(Polish),* **Olina, Olunka, Oluska** *(Czech),* **Olli, Olly** *(Estonian),* **Lelya, Lesya, Olenka, Olesya, Olka, Olya, Olyusha** *(Russian).*

OLIANA. *Polynesian, 'oleander'.* Lilting choice. *Oleanna* is the title of a David Mamet play. **Oleana, Oleanna, Olianna.**

OLIVE. *English, from Latin, nature name, 'olive tree'.* Though greatly overshadowed by the trendy Olivia, Olive has a quiet, subtle appeal of its own – if you just ignore the image of Olive Oyl, Popeye's steady. **Olie, Oliff, Oliffe, Olivet, Olivette, Ollie, Olly.**

OLIVIA. *Latin, 'olive tree'.* This lovely Shakespearean name, with its admirable balance of strength and femininity, is megapopular and hit the number one spot in 2006 – so don't say we didn't warn you. **Alivia, Alyvia, Liv, Liva, Livrie, Livvie, Livvy, Livy, Liwie, Liwy, Olevia, Olia, Oliff, Oliffe, Olive, Olivea, Oliveea, Oliveia, Olivet, Olivetta, Olivi, Olivianne, Olivija, Olivine, Olivya, Ollie, Olly, Oly, Olyvia. International: Olivette, Oliviane** *(French),* **Livia, Oliva, Olva** *(Spanish),* **Oliveria** *(Portuguese),* **Oliwa** *(Hawaiian).*

OLWEN. *Welsh, 'white footprint'.* Welsh favourite, the name of a legendary princess; a Bronwen alternative for those with a taste for the rare. **Olwenn, Olwin, Olwyn, Olwynne.**

★**OLYMPIA.** *Greek, 'from Mount Olympus'.* Beautiful name with an athletic, goddess-like aura: the perfect Olivia substitute. **Olimpe, Olimpiada, Olimpiana. International: Olympe, Olympiad, Olympienne** *(French),* **Olimpia** *(Spanish),* **Olympie** *(German).*

OMAIRA. *Arabic, 'red'.* Intriguing Middle Eastern possibility. **Omar, Omara, Omarah, Omari, Omaria, Omarra.**

♂ **OMEGA.** *Greek, 'last'.* Perfect choice for a youngest.

ONDINE. *Latin, 'little wave'.* Mythological spirit of the waters; spelled Undine, she was an Edith Wharton heroine. **Ondene, Ondyne, Undine. International: Ondina** *(Spanish).*

ONDREA. *Czech variation of* **ANDREA.** If you want people to pronounce Andrea with an *Ah* sound beginning, this spelling would guide the way. **Ohndrea, Ohndreea, Ohndreya, Ohndria, Ondraya, Ondreana, Ondreea, Ondreya, Ondria, Ondrianna, Ondriea.**

ONEIDA. *Native American, 'long awaited'; also a city and Shaker community.* One of the few familiar Native American choices, but now associated with several trade names in the US. **Onida, Onyda.**

ONEONTA. *Native American place name.* This town in central New York might make a rhythmic first name.

ONO. *Japanese surname.* Closely tied to the widow of John Lennon.

★ONÓRA. *Irish Gaelic variation of HONORIA.* Lovely variation of upstanding classic. **Onnora, Onoria, Onorine, Ornora.**

OONA. *Irish variation of UNA.* Name made famous by Eugene O'Neill's daughter, who became Charlie Chaplin's wife; the double-*o* beginning gives it a lot of oomph. **Ona, Onna, Onnie, Oonagh, Oonie, Una.**

OPAL. *Sanskrit, 'gem'.* Opal has lost its opalescence, but could return along with other vintage jewel names. **Opale, Opalina, Opaline, Opall.**

OPERA. *Word name.* Musical, yes, but be aware that everyone will think you've named your child Oprah.

OPHELIA. *Greek, 'help'.* This beautiful name has long been hampered by the stigma of *Hamlet*'s tragic heroine. **Availia, Ofilia, Ophelie, Ophelya, Ophilia, Ovalia, Ovelia, Phelia, Ubelia, Uvelia. International:**

Ofilia, Ophélie *(French)*, Filia, Ofelia *(Spanish)*.

OPHIRA. *Feminine variation of OPHIR, 'gold'; also biblical place name.* Ophir is an extraordinarily rich place, though the name doesn't rise to the same level. **Ofeera, Ofira.**

OPRAH. *Hebrew variation of ORPAH.* The misspelling that created an indelibly one-person name. **Ophra, Ophrah, Opra.**

ORA. *Latin, 'prayer'.* Short and slight. **Orabel, Orabelle, Orah, Orareeana, Orarariana, Orlice, Orra.**

ORABELLA. *Latin variation of ARABELLA.* Lacks the vintage charm of the original Arabella. **Orabel, Orabela, Orabelle.**

ORACIA. *Spanish, feminine variation of HORACE.* Rarely used aristocratic name with ancient roots and less than appealing sound. **Orasia, Oratia, Orazia.**

ORALIE. *French variation of AURELIA.* Better go to the original Aurelia or Aurelie. **Areli, Aurelie, Oralee, Orali, Oralia, Oralis, Oralit, Orelie, Oriel,**

Orielda, Orielle, Oriena, Orlee, Orlena, Orlene, Orli, Orly.

ORANE. *French, 'rising'.* Oriana's not-quite-as-pretty French cousin. **Orania, Oriane.**

ORANGE. *Fruit name.* Seems suddenly possible, in this era of Apple. But Clementine would be much better. **Orangetta, Orangia, Orangina.**

ORCHID. *Flower name.* Exotic hothouse bloom that has not been plucked by baby namers – yet. **International: Orquídea, Orquídia** *(Spanish)*.

ORELLA. *Latin, 'announcement from the gods, oracle'.* A pleasantly unfamiliar addition to the *ella* family of names. **Oreal, Orela, Orelle, Oriel, Orielle. International: Oreli** *(French)*.

★ORIANA. *Latin, 'dawn'.* Dashing medieval name with a meaning similar to Aurora. Strong and exotic. **Orane, Orania, Orelda, Orelle, Ori, Oria, Orian, Orianna, Orieana, Oryan. International: Oriane, Orianne** *(French)*.

ORIEL. *Latin, 'golden'.* Pretty Victorian-feeling cousin of Ariel; also, more prosaically, a kind of bay window. **Auriel, Auriella, Aurielle, Oriella, Orielle.**

ORINA. *Russian variation of* IRENE. Better: Irina. **Orya, Oryna.**

ORINDA. *place name.* Serene California town near San Francisco that could translate into a girl's name. **Orenda.**

♂ **ORINO.** *Japanese, 'worker's field'.* Not as familiar as some other Asian imports; has a strong unisex feel. **Ori.**

ORINTHIA. *Feminine variation of* ORIN. One of the frillier female forms of Oren. **Orenthia, Orna, Ornina, Orrinthia.**

ORIOLE. *Latin, 'golden'.* A not particularly graceful bird name. For a girl, better to consider feminized versions. **Auriel, Oreolle, Oriel, Oriell, Oriella, Oriola, Oriolle.**

♂ **ORION.** *Greek mythology name.* The Greek mythological hunter who was turned into a

constellation is much more often used for boys.

ORIT. *Hebrew, 'light'.* A bit blunt. **Ora, Orah, Orya.**

ORLA. *Irish, 'golden lady'.* Popular in Ireland and ripe for import. **Orlie, Orrla. International: Orfhlaith, Orflaith, Orlagh, Orlaith** *(Irish Gaelic),* **Aurla** *(Scottish),* **Orlee, Orly** *(French).*

ORLANDA. *Spanish and Italian, feminine variation of* ORLANDO. Orlanda is intriguing . . . but why not go all the way to Orlando? **Orlandia, Orlando, Orlantha, Orlenda, Orlinda.**

ORLEANNA. *Literary name.* Orleanna was the young heroine of Barbara Kingsolver's *The Poisonwood Bible.* **International: Orleane** *(French).*

ORLI. *Hebrew, 'light'.* Cute, nickname-y, and exotic, à la Romy or Demi. Spelling it Orly turns it into a busy French airport. **Orlice, Orlie, Orly.**

ORMANDA. *Latin, 'noble'; German, 'mariner'.* Has a

medieval, slightly fusty but romantic feel. **Orma.**

ORNA. *Irish, 'little pale green one'.* This Irish saint's name sounds like a lopped-off Lorna.

ORPAH. *Hebrew, 'a fawn'.* Old Testament name of the daughter-in-law of Naomi, now eclipsed by the originally misspelled Oprah. **Afra, Aphra, Ofrit, Ophrah, Oprah, Orpa, Orpha, Orphie.**

ORPHEA. *Greek mythology name.* The feminine form of Orpheus, the charming musician of Greek myth who descended to the underworld. **Orfeya, Orfia, Orphea, Orpheya, Orphia.**

ORSA. *Variation of* URSULA. Stick with Ursula. **Orsalina, Orsaline, Orse, Orsel, Orselina, Orseline, Orsola, Orssa, Ursa.**

ORTENSIA. *Latin variation of* HORTENSE. Slight improvement on Hortense. But then again, what isn't? **Ortensa, Ortensija, Ortensya.**

OSAKA. *place name.* With so many other places translating to

Stellar Starbabies Beginning with O

October	Dave Eggers
Olivia	Tim Henman, Beverly D'Angelo & Al Pacino, Julianne Moore, Eddie Vedder, Denzel Washington
Owen	Michelle Branch

first names, why not this major Japanese city – especially if it holds some personal significance.

OSANNA. *Latin, 'praise the Lord'.* May rise, along with other spiritually inclined names, but Westerners might find it too close to Osama. **Oksana, Osana.**

OTTHILD. *German, 'prospers in battle'.* Wears long blonde plaits, carries a spear and sings duets with Brunhilde. **Otthilda, Ottila, Ottilia, Ottille, Ottiline, Ottohne, Otyha.**

★**OTTILIE.** *French variation of* **OTTHILD.** How can we shun Otthild but love Ottilie? The *lie* ending makes it so much more feminine and friendly.

Odila, Otila, Otilia, Otka, Ottili, Ottalia, Ottalie Ottilla, Ottolie, Ottoline. International: **Ottorina** *(Spanish and Portuguese),* **Otylia** *(Polish),* **Otilie** *(Czech).*

OTTOLINE. *French and English, diminutive of* **OTTILIE.** Curiously appealing, in a hoop-skirted, wasp-waisted way.

OUIDA. *(WEE-da) English diminutive.* This Victorian pen name is the childish version of the novelist's real name, Louisa, but it has managed to gain a sophisticated image. Ouisa is a similar childhood nickname name.

♂ **OWEN.** *Welsh, 'wellborn'.* We hate to include this on the girls' list, since one of us has a son named Owen, however it's on crossover alert – along with other male hotties like Aidan and Jalen. **Owena.**

OZARA. *Hebrew, 'treasure, wealth'.* Striking and glamorous, though perhaps just plain Zara is exotic enough. **Ozari.**

P *girls*

♂ **PACE.** *Word name.* Unisex word and surname with an upbeat feel and a possible future as a more distinctive substitute for Grace or Page. **Pase.**

♂ **PACEY.** *English surname.* Although this is also a male name, it works much better for girls. **Pacee, Paci, Pacie, Pacy.**

PACIENCIA. *Spanish, 'patience'.* See **PATIENCE. Pacis, Pasencia.**

PACIFICA. *(pah-SEE-fee-cah) Spanish, 'tranquil'.* When properly pronounced, has an alluring sound and harmonious meaning. **Pacificia, Pasifica.**

★♂ PADGET. *English and French variation of* **PAGE.** This unusual offshoot of Page is an undiscovered gem, with lots of energy and charm. Equally effective spelled Paget. **Padgett, Padgit, Padgitt, Padgyt, Padgytt, Paget.**

PADMA. *Sanskrit, 'lotus'.* A name rich in Hindu tradition as the alternate name for the Goddess Lakshmi, the embodiment of beauty and charm.

PAGE. *French, 'page, attendant'.* Sleek and sophisticated single-syllable choice that's climbing the charts in the US. **Padget, Padgett, Paget, Pagett, Paige, Payge.**

PAIGE. *Spelling variation of* **PAGE.** More of a name, and more popular – in recent years it's made it into the Top 50.

PAILI. *(PAHL-ee) Irish variation of* **POLLY.** Authentic Irish choice, easy to spell, tricky to pronounce.

♂ PAISLEY. *Scottish, 'church, cemetery'.* Calls to mind the richly patterned fabric first made in Paisley, Scotland. **Paislee, Paisleigh, Paisli, Paislie, Paisly, Payslee, Paysley, Paysli, Payslie, Paysly.**

PAKUNA. *Native American, Miwok, 'deer jumping as she runs downhill'.* Unusual and lithe.

PALASHA. *Russian, diminutive of* **PELAGIA,** *'open sea'.* Friendly Slavic rarity.

PALILA. *(pah-LEE-lah) Hawaiian, 'a bird'.* Pacific island member of the currently-in-favour Lila/Leila family.

PALLAS. *Greek, 'wisdom'.* This rarified Greek name – in classical mythology Pallas Athena was the goddess of wisdom and the arts – might appeal to literary-minded parents.

PALMA. *Latin place name.* Appealing Latin name that's both geographical – it's the romantic city on the Spanish island of Majorca – and botanical, relating to the palm frond. Sometimes given to girls born on Palm Sunday. **Palmira, Palmyra.**

PALMIRA. *Latin, from Palmyra, ancient Syrian city.* Another place name relating to the tropical palm tree. **Palma, Palmer.**

★PALOMA. *Spanish, 'dove'.* Vibrant and ruby-lipped à la jewelry designer Paloma Picasso, but also suggesting peace, as symbolised by the dove, this is a highly recommended striking but soft name. **Aloma, Palometa, Palomita.**

PALOMINA. *Spanish, 'dove-coloured filly'.* Doubtful if a child would appreciate being given such a horsy name.

PAMELA. *English, invention of sixteenth-century poet Sir Philip Sidney.* A somewhat pampered beauty queen of the 1960s who was never called by her full name, which is a pity because Pamela is so mellifluous and rich in literary history. Rarely used now, Pamela might almost be ready for a revival. **Mela, Pam, Pama, Pamala, Pamalla, Pamelin, Pameline, Pamelita, Pamelja, Pamella, Pamelyn, Pamelynne, Pami, Pamila, Pamilla, Pamla, Pammeli, Pammi, Pammie,**

Moving Up Fast

Amelie

Daisy

Evie

Faith

Freya

Grace/Gracie

Isla

Keira

Lily

Lola

Poppy

Ruby

Scarlett

Sienna

Summer

Pammy, Permelia. International:
Paméla *(French),* **Pamelia,
Pamelina, Pamelita** *(Spanish).*

PAMINA. *Italian, meaning
unknown.* This operatic Italian
name – it appears in Mozart's
The Magic Flute – is a more
unusual route to the nickname
Pam. **Pam.**

♂ **PANAMA.** *place name.*
Sharing her name with a
country, a city, an isthmus, a
gulf, a canal and a hat might be
a bit much for a child to handle.

PANDARA. *Hindi, 'wife'.*
Pleasant-sounding exotic name.

PANDITA. *Hindi, 'learned,
scholarly'.* Might be a little too
close to *bandita.* **Dita.**

PANDORA. *Greek, 'all gifted'.*
Used by the horsy set but rarely
heard elsewhere, probably
because Pandora was the
mythological first woman
on earth whose curiosity
unleashed all the evils of the
world. **Dora, Doura, Pandorra,
Pandoura, Panndora.**

PANIA. *Maori, a mythological
sea maiden.* Possible alternative
to Tania, if you want to go the
Indonesian rather than Russian
route.

PANNA. *Hindi, 'emerald';
Hebrew, 'grace'.* A name with
many allusions – in addition to
those above, a serene and sacred
city in India and the Italian
word for cream. **Pana, Panah,
Pannah.**

PANSY. *English flower name
from French pensée, 'thought'.*
Early floral name that lost
credibility when it became a
derogatory slang term for
homosexuals. **Pansey, Pansie.**
International: Orvokki *(Finnish).*

PANTHEA. *Greek, 'all the gods'.*
Anthea is simpler and prettier.
Pantheia, Pantheya, Panthia.

PANYA. *African, Swahili, 'mouse,
tiny one'; Russian, diminutive of*
STEPHANIA, *'crowned one'.*
Multicultural possibility.

PAOLA. *(POW-lah) Italian and
Spanish variation of* **PAULA.**
Latinate version of Paula. Much
more appealing than the English
standard. **Pala, Paulana, Pauleta,
Paviana.**

PAQUITA. *Spanish, diminutive
of* **FRANCES.** Sassy but slight
nickname name.

PARADICE. *Modern invented
name.* Another side of Paradise.

PARASHA. *Russian, 'born on
Good Friday'.* Slavic possibility
for a girl born during the Easter
season. **Paraskeva, Pascha,
Praskovya.**

♂ PARIS. *French place name.* This one-time mythical and Shakespearean boys' name has been more acceptable as a girl's name, at least in part due to the highly publicised Paris Hilton. **Pariss, Parris, Parrish, Parriss, Parrys, Parryss, Parys, Paryss.**

♂ PARKER. *English occupational name, 'park keeper'.* Sophisticated surname that's still much more common for boys but rising for both sexes, unlike many of its other office mates.

PARMENIA. *Greek, 'studious'.* Very occasionally chosen by Latino parents.

PARTHENIA. *Greek, 'chaste maiden'.* A bit unwieldy, but does conjure up majestic images of the Parthenon. **Parthena, Parthenie, Parthenope.**

PARVATI. *Sanskrit, 'the daughter of the mountain'.* This Hindu goddess name is popular in India.

PASCALE. *French from Hebrew, 'Passover'.* Sophisticated, stylish feminine form of Pascal especially appropriate for girls born around Easter or Passover. **Pascala, Pascalette, Pascalle, Pascha, Paschale, Paschelle, Pasclina.** International: **Pascoe** *(Cornish),* **Pascalie, Pascaline, Pascasia, Pasquette** *(French),* **Pasquelina** *(Italian),* **Pascua, Pascuala** *(Spanish),* **Parasha, Pasha, Praskovia** *(Russian),* **Pesha** *(Greek).*

PASCUA. *Spanish from Hebrew, 'Easter'.* Occasionally used in the Latino community, another Easter-related name. **Pascuala, Pascualina, Pasqua.**

♂ PASHA. *Greek, 'of the ocean'; Russian, male diminutive of* **PAVEL.** Brings to mind a tubby Eastern potentate from an Arabian Nights movie. **Palasha, Pashka.**

♂ PAT. *Diminutive of* **PATRICIA.** An early and still quintessentially androgynous name, now supplanted by thousands of fresher options.

PATIA. *(pah-TEE-uh) Spanish Gypsy, 'leaf'; diminutive of* **PATRICIA.** An innovative way to honour Great-Aunt Patricia. **Pattia, Pattya, Patya.**

PATIENCE. *Latin virtue name.* A passive virtue turned engaging name, fresher than Hope, Faith or even Charity. **Patiencia, Patientia.** International: **Pazienza** *(Italian),* **Paciencia** *(Spanish).*

♂ PATRICE. *French variation of* **PATRICIA.** More modern-sounding and polished unisex alternative to Patricia. **Paddy, Pat, Patee, Patie, Patte, Patty, Patsie, Patsy, Trish, Trisha.**

PATRICIA. *Latin, 'noble, patrician'.* Patricia still sounds patrician, though its scores of nicknames definitely don't. Wildly popular from the 1940s through the 1960s, it has been fading ever since. **Paddy, Pat, Patee, Pati, Patie, Patrea, Patria, Patrisha, Patrisia, Patsy, Patti, Patty, Tricia, Trisa, Trish, Trisha, Trishia, Trisia.** International: **Pádraigín** *(Irish Gaelic),* **Patrice** *(French),* **Patrizia** *(Italian),* **Patrika** *(Scandinavian),* **Patryka** *(Polish),* **Padrika** *(Slavic).*

PATRIZIA. *(pah-TREET-zee-ah) Italian variation of* **PATRICIA.** Elegant Italian translation.

♀ **PATSY.** *English, diminutive of* **PATRICIA.** Sassy, spunky name used for the mostly Irish jump-roping pigtailed girls of the 1930s and 40s – and some Irish and Italian boys as well. **Patsey, Patsi, Patsie.**

PATTI, PATTY. *English diminutives of* **PATRICIA.** Replaced Patsy as the mid-century's popular, peppy teenager. **Pattee, Pattey, Pattie.**

PATZI. *Native American, Omaha, 'yellow bird'.* Would probably be taken as a fanciful spelling of Patsy.

PAULA. *Feminine variation of* **PAUL.** Seems stuck in the era of early rock and roll. International: **Paule, Paulette, Pauline** *(French)*, **Paola, Paolina** *(Italian)*, **Paoletta, Paolina** *(Portuguese)*, **Pola** *(Swedish)*, **Pauliina** *(Finnish)*, **Pawla, Pawlina, Pola** *(Polish)*, **Pasha, Pashenka, Pavlina, Polina** *(Russian)*.

PAULETTE. *French, feminine diminutive of* **PAUL.** Emigrated across the Channel in the 1930s; its passport is now long expired.

PAULE. *(POL-eh) French, feminine variation of* **PAUL.** This, the simplest French female version of Paul, was introduced internationally by novelist Paule Marshall, whose roots are in the West Indies.

PAULILLE. *French, feminine variation of* **PAUL.** Almost completely unknown outside France: an intriguing possibility if you want something a little different.

PAULINA. *Spanish, feminine variation of* **PAUL.** More stylish than either Paula or Pauline, it was given a glamour gloss by model Paulina Porizkova in the 1990s. **Pauleena, Paulena, Paulinia. International: Paolina** *(Italian)*.

PAULINE. *French, feminine variation of* **PAUL.** Pauline had its moment of glory almost a century ago, when film audiences were thrilling to

the silent serial *The Perils of Pauline;* a sweet and gentle name that just might be due for reconsideration. **Pauleen, Paulene, Paulyne, Polline.**

PAVANA. *Sanskrit, 'wind goddess'; Italian and Spanish, 'peacock'.* Too many Savannahs in your neighbourhood? Consider this.

PAVATI. *Native American, Hopi, 'clear water'.* Native American name with spiritual overtones.

PAVLA. *Czech, feminine variation of* **PAVEL.** Distinctive Slavic choice. **Pavliča, Pavlínka.**

♂ **PAX.** *Latin, 'peace'.* A cool unisex name, representing the Roman goddess of peace, recently given to their son by Angelina Jolie and Brad Pitt.

♂ **PAXTON.** *English, 'peace town'.* Set apart from other once-male-only surnames because of its peaceful element. **Paxten.**

PAYTON. *See* **PEYTON.**

★♂ PAZ. *(pahz) Hebrew, 'golden'; Spanish, 'peace'.* Would make a sparkling middle name choice. **Pax, Paza, Pazia, Pazit, Pazya.**

PAZIAH. *(pah-ZEE-ah) Hebrew, 'the gold of Jehovah'.* Often heard in Israel, spelled with or without the final *h*. **Paz, Paza, Pazia, Pazice, Pazit, Paziva, Paziya, Pazya.**

♂ PEACE. *Word name.* Spaniards use Pax and Paz, Hebrew speakers Shalom, for Greeks it's Irene, so why can't we make the English word a name?

PEACHES. *English fruit name.* Unlike the other fruit names coming onto the baby name menu, Peaches is an old-timey nickname previously reserved for showgirls, and now would be considered an outrageous – verging on hip – choice publicised by Peaches Geldof. Rose 2948 places in one year.

★PEARL. *Latin gem name.* Like Ruby, a gem name beginning to be polished up for a new generation of fashionable children after a century of jewellery box storage. The birthstone for the month of June would make it a cool name for a baby born in that month, or it could also make a fresher middle name alternative to the overused Rose. **Pearla, Pearle, Pearleen, Pearli, Pearlie, Pearlina, Pearline, Pearly, Perl, Perle, Perley, Perlie, Perlina, Perlline. International: Perle, Perlette, Perline** *(French),* **Perlezenn** *(Breton),* **Perla** *(Italian and Spanish),* **Perlita** *(Spanish).*

PEG. *English, from Greek, diminutive of* **MARGARET.** Nostalgic turn-of-the-last-century name, sociable but slight. **International: Peig** *(Irish).*

PEGEEN. *Irish, extended diminutive of* **PEG.** Infrequently used relic of the Maureen-Colleen-Kathleen era. **Peigin.**

PEGGY. *English, diminutive of* **MARGARET.** Still carries the perky, pug-nosed beauty-queen image it had from the 1920s into the 1950s; rarely used for babies today. **Peg, Pegeen, Pegg, Peggi, Peggie. International: Peigi** *(Scottish Gaelic).*

Names with Uplifting Meanings

Amity

Charity

Democracy

Free

Freedom

Honor

Integrity

Justice

Peace

Serenity

Sincerity

True

Verity

PELLA. *Hebrew, 'marvel of God'; Scandinavian, diminutive of* **PETRONELLA.** The power of the popular *ella* sound is sapped in this cross-cultural choice.

PENELOPE. *Greek, 'weaver' or 'duck'.* Image of elderly gardening lady in large-brimmed hat has of late been counterbalanced by the dramatic sensuality of Spanish actress Penélope Cruz. Chosen for his daughter by Taylor Hanson, of the group Hanson. **Pela, Pelcha, Pen, Peneli, Peni, Penina, Penna, Pennelope, Penney, Pennie, Penny. International: Pépélope, Pennelope** *(French),* **Penelopa, Peni** *(Spanish),* **Lopa, Pela, Pelcia** *(Polish),* **Pinelopi, Pipitsa, Popi** *(Greek),* **Peniel** *(Hebrew).*

PENINA. *(pay-NEE-nah) Hebrew, 'pearl, coral, ruby'.* Jewel-encrusted choice. **Peni, Penie, Peninah, Penine, Penini, Peninit, Peninna, Peninnah, Pnina, Pninit.**

PENNA. *Latin, 'feather'.* Occasionally heard in England, but rarely elsewhere.

PENNY. *English, diminutive of* **PENELOPE.** Like Peggy and Patsy, the kind of zesty moniker young Judy Garland would sport in her early let's-put-on-a-show flicks, rarely used today. **Penney, Penni, Pennie.**

PENSÉE. *French, 'thought'.* An interesting thought.

PENTHIA. *Greek, 'flower'.* Less than zero floral charm.

PEONY. *Latin, 'healing'; a flower name.* It may be the name of a beautiful flower, but it definitely could cause some teasing. **Peonie.**

PEPITA. *Spanish, diminutive feminine variation of* **JOSÉ.** Personification of pep. **Pepa, Peppie, Peppy, Peta.**

PEPPER. *English from Latin, 'the pepper plant' Sanskrit, 'berry'.* Parents are beginning to scan the whole spice shelf for inspiration, picking up on Saffron, Sage, and Cinnamon – and opening up a chance for this spiciest possibility of all. **International: Peppar** *(Swedish),* **Piper** *(Romanian),* **Biber** *(Turkish),* **Koshoo** *(Japanese),* **Pilipili** *(Swahili).*

PERDITA. *Latin, 'lost'.* Shakespearean invention for an abandoned baby in *The Winter's Tale,* its sense of loss has always been off-putting to parents. **Dita, Perdi, Perdie, Perdy.**

PERFECTA. *Spanish, 'flawless'.* Talk about pressure!

♂ **PERI.** *Greek, 'mountain dweller'; Hebrew, 'fruit'; Persian, 'fairy'.* Name used for both sexes in several cultures, quite popular in Israel.

PERIDOT. *(PEH-ree-doe) Arabic, 'a green gemstone'.* If you want a truly original gem name, consider this instead of Opal, Ruby or Diamond.

PERLA. *Spanish variation of* **PEARL.** Consistently popular Latina gem name.

PERNELLA. *French, from Greek, 'rock'.* One of the least appealing of the *ella*-ending names, especially if you check *pernicious* in the dictionary. **Parnella, Pernelle, Pernilla, Pernille.**

PEROUZE. *Armenian, 'turquoise'.* Interesting on paper, though most people would confuse it with the word *peruse.*

PERPETUA. *Latin, 'perpetual'.* Perpetually unwieldy. **International: Perpétue** *(French).*

PERRINE. *French, 'rock, stone'.* Sounds like either a feminisation of the dated Perry or a brand of eye-drops.

♂ **PERRY.** *English, 'pear tree'.* Relaxed male name occasionally used for girls; sounds novel compared to such shop-worn former favourites as Kerry and Sherry. **Perrey, Perri, Perrie, Perrin.**

PERSEPHONE. *(per-SEF-o-nee) Greek mythology name.* Name of the Greek goddess of spring, suited to a toga-wearing, lyre-playing ballerina. **Persephassa, Persephonia, Persephonie.**

PERSIA. *Place name, country now known as Iran.* Despite – or because of – the country's name change, still retains the brilliant colouration of an ancient Persian miniature. **Persis.**

PERSIS. *Greek, 'Persian woman'.* Parents seeking a distinctive New Testament name might consider this.

PESSA. *Yiddish, 'pearl'.* Old-fashioned and rife with teasing temptations. **Perril, Pesha, Peshe, Pessel, Pessye.**

PETA. *Native American, Blackfoot, 'golden eagle'; Greek, 'rock, stone'.* Too tightly tied to the acronym for the activist group People for the Ethical Treatment of Animals. **Petta, Peyta. International: Peita, Perette *(French)*, Petah, Petra, Petrea, Petrina, Petrine *(Danish)*.**

PETAL. *Greek word name.* Soft and sweet-smelling name of a character in the novel and film, *The Shipping News.*

♂ **PETER.** *Greek, 'rock'.* The current trend for appropriating male names rather than feminising them makes this a viable possibility.

PETRA. *Greek, feminine variation of* **PETER.** Soft sound, strong meaning. **Pedi, Pedie, Pella, Pernilla, Pernille, Perrine, Pet, Petee, Peterina, Peternella, Petria, Petronia, Petronilla, Petrova, Petrovna, Petta, Pieretta, Pierretta. International: Petrina *(Scottish)*, Pétronille, Pierra, Pierrette, Pierina *(French)*, Piera, Pietra *(Italian)*, Peitra, Peta, Petrona, Petronela, Petronila *(Spanish)*, Pedrine, Petrine *(Danish)*, Petronella**

(Swedish), **Petronela *(Polish)*, Petenka, Petya *(Russian)*, Peterke, Peti *(Slavic)*, Perrine, Petrina, Petrini, Petronella, Petronelle *(Greek)*.**

PETULA. *Modern invented name.* Swinging London songbird Petula Clark claims that this name was her father's invention; in any case it hasn't seen much copycat usage. **Bet, Betula, Pet.**

PETULIA. *Variation of* **PETULA.** Cross between Petula and Petunia that surfaced briefly as a 1960s British film title.

PETUNIA. *English, 'trumpet-shaped flower'.* **Pet, Pette, Petti, Pettie.**

♂ **PEYTON.** *English, 'fighting-man's estate'.* One unisex surname – now primarily female – that's not only survived but continues to grow in popularity because of its rich, Faulknerian softness. **Paiden, Paidyn, Payden, Paydon, Paydyn, Payten, Paytin, Payton.**

PHAEDRA. *(FAY-drah) Greek, 'bright'.* This name of a tragic figure in Greek mythology has a mysterious and intriguing appeal. **Faydra, Phaedre, Phaidra, Phedra, Phédre.**

PHEDORA. *Greek, 'supreme gift'.* A bit pharmaceutical, not to mention hat-like. **Fedora, Pheodora.**

PHILADELPHIA. *Greek place name, 'brotherly love'.* Place name mentioned in the New Testament and not yet on the name map. Philadelphia Thursday was the character played by Shirley Temple in John Ford's 1948 *Fort Apache*. **Delphia, Delphie, Phillie, Philly.**

PHILIPPA. *Greek, feminine variation of* **PHILIP.** Prime example of a boy's name adapted for girls that's as common as crumpets in England, but rarely used elsewhere. Its several lively nicknames add to its appeal. **Flip, Pelippa, Phil, Philippe, Phillie, Phillipa, Phillipina, Philly, Pippa, Pippi, Pippie, Pippy. International: Pelipa**

(Zuni), **Felipan, Filia, Filipa, Filippa, Philippine** *(French)*, **Fillippa, Filippina, Pippa** *(Italian)*, **Felepita, Felipa** *(Spanish)*, **Filipa, Filipina, Ina, Inka, Philipa, Philippine** *(Polish)*.

PHILIPPINE. *French, feminine variation of* **PHILIPPE.** In some countries this would be taken as an ethnic identification.

PHILLIDA. *Spelling variation of* **PHYLLIDA.** *See* **PHYLLIDA.**

PHILOMELA. *Greek, 'lover of songs'.* Name of a mythological Athenian princess who was transformed into a nightingale, rarely heard outside the Greek community. **Philomel, Philomella. International: Filomela** *(Spanish)*.

PHILOMENA. *Greek, 'lover of strength'.* Earthy Greek name now used in various Latin countries. **Filimena, Filomenia, Filomina, Filumena, Philomina. International: Philomène** *(French)*, **Filomena** *(Italian)*.

★**PHOEBE.** *Greek, 'radiant, shining one', goddess of the moon.* A mythological, biblical, Shakespearean and Salinger name, the warm and captivating Phoebe is a regular entrant in the Top 100. Bill and Melinda Gates used it for their daughter. **Febe, Pheabe, Pheby, Pheebe, Pheebee, Pheebey, Pheebi, Pheebie, Pheeby, Phoebee, Phoebey, Phoebi, Phoebie, Phoeboe, Phoeby. International: Phebe** *(Italian)*, **Pheobe** *(Greek)*.

♂ **PHOENIX.** *Greek, 'dark red' Arizona place name.* New Age name symbolising rebirth and immortality; Scary Spice chose it for her daughter. **Feenix, Fenix, Phenice.**

PHYLICIA. *Variation of* **FELICIA.** *See* **FELICIA.**

PHYLLIDA. *Greek variation of* **PHYLLIS.**

PHYLLIS. *Greek, 'green bough'.* Used by classical poets for the idealised pastoral maiden. **Fillis, Fillys, Fyllis, Philla, Philisse, Philys, Phylicia, Phylida, Phylie, Phylis, Phylla, Phyllicia, Phylliss, Phyllys.**

International: Filide, Philis, **Phillis** *(French)*, **Filide** *(Italian)*, **Filis** *(Spanish)*.

PIA. *Latin, 'pious'; diminutive of* **OLYMPIA.** Soft name in the Mia-Nia-Tia family, Pia is heard in both European and Hindi languages.

PIAF. *French surname, 'sparrow'.* Could be a possible musical tribute name to the waif-like, husky-voiced mid-century French singer who was given this last name because of her bird-like quality.

PIALA. *Celtic, meaning unknown.* This name of a saint martyred in Cornwall makes an unusual choice with traditional roots.

PICABIA. *Spanish artist name.* The name of the French surrealist, Francis Picabia, could make a lively, creative choice for the daughter of adventurous art-loving parents.

PICABO. *Native American, 'shining waters'; Idaho place name.* The name of Olympic skier Picabo Street is a one-of-a-

kind not recommended to others.

PIERETTE. *French, feminine diminutive of* **PETER.** Balletic, à la pirouette. **International: Péronelle, Perrette, Perrine, Pétronille** *(French)*, **Piera, Pierina, Pietra** *(Italian)*.

★**PILAR.** *Spanish, 'pillar'.* The nonvowel ending of this Spanish classic, which honours the Virgin Mary, gives it a special sense of strength, elegance and style, making it a worthy choice. Remembered as the valiant heroine of Hemingway's *For Whom the Bell Tolls.* **Pelar, Peleria, Pili, Piliar, Pillar, Piluca, Pilucha.**

PINK. *Colour name.* The singer known as Pink (born Alecia) brought this hue onto the name-possibility palette, especially as a middle choice. Could Pink be the next Blue?

PIPER. *English occupational name, 'pipe or flute player'.* A bright, musical name that's popular with American celebrities and cute for a child, but perhaps not viable as a future tax attorney. **Pyper.**

Bird Names

Alouette	Lark
Avis	Lonan
Aya	Manu
Bird/Byrd/Birdie	Merle
	Oriole
Deryn	Palila
Dove	Paloma
Eagle	Phoenix
Falcon	Raven
Finch	Robin
Gannet	Sparrow
Gull	Starling
Hawk	Talon
Heron	Teal
Jarita	Wren
Jay	

PIPPA. *English, diminutive of* **PHILIPPA.** Condensation of Philippa turns it from serious to sprightly.

PIPPI. *Norse variation of* **PHILIPPA.** Forever linked to the fictional childhood character of Pippi Longstocking.

Cool Middle Names

Bay

Belle

Dancer

Doe

George

Maeve

Max

Neve

Paz

Pearl

Plum

Poe

Rae

Snow

Teal

True

PLÁCIDA. *Spanish, 'tranquil, peaceful'; feminine variation of* **PLÁCIDO.** Familiar outside the Hispanic community through male opera singer Placido Domingo, this name has a calm, serene feeling. **Placi, Placide, Placidina, Placie.** International: **Placidie** *(French),* **Palacida, Placidia** *(Spanish).*

PLEASANT. *Word name.* An admirable quality to impart to your daughter; was used by Charles Dickens for a character in his novel *Our Mutual Friend*.

PLUM. *Fruit name.* British-born novelist Plum Sykes has taken this fruity name out of the produce section and put it into the baby name basket. More appealing than Apple, more presentable than Peaches.

♂ **PO.** *Italian river name.* The good news: the Po is Italy's longest river, flowing across the north. The bad news: Po is a manic, scooter-riding red Teletubby.

♂ **POE.** *English, 'peacock'.* Hip new middle-name choice, conjuring up the gothic tales of Edgar Allan.

POESY. *Word name, 'poetry'.* This old-fashioned word for poetry has some antiquated charm but doesn't exactly roll off the tongue.

♂ **POET.** *Word name.* A new name on the roster, used for

her daughter by the American celeb Soleil Moon Frye, who obviously appreciates the advantages of an unusual name.

♂ **POETRY.** *Word name.* A lyrical choice. **Poem.**

POLEXIA. *Meaning unknown.* Polexia Aphrodesia was the futuristic sounding name of the Anna Paquin character in the film *Almost Famous*.

POLINA. *Russian and Basque, feminine variation of* **PAUL.** *See* **PAULINA.**

★**POLLY.** *English variation of* **MOLLY.** An alternative to the no-longer-fresh Molly, the initial *P* gives it a peppier sound, combining the cozy virtues of an old-timey name with the bounce of a barmaid. **Poll, Pollee, Polley, Polli, Pollie, Pollyanna.**

POLLYANNA. *Combination of* **POLLY** *and* **ANNA.** Has become an adjective for being overly optimistic.

POMME. *French, 'apple'.* Une amie for Gwyneth Paltrow's little girl.

POMONA. *Latin, 'apple'; also California place name.* This name of the Roman goddess of fruit trees is also associated with a suburban town in Southern California.

★**POPPY.** *Latin flower name.* Most floral names are sweet and feminine, but this one packs a lot of punch; it's now reached Number 30. Jamie Oliver – the 'Naked Chef' – used it for his daughter. A good choice for a redhead. **Poppi, Poppie.**

PORSCHE. *Automotive name, also phonetic variation of* PORTIA. Chosen primarily by fans of sleek and spiffy German sports cars.

PORSHA. *Phonetic variation of* PORTIA. Chosen primarily by coveters of sleek and spiffy German sports cars. **Porcha, Porscha, Porsh.**

♂ **PORTER.** *French occupational name, 'doorkeeper' or 'carrier'.* One clubby surname that hasn't crossed to the girls' side – but could.

★**PORTIA.** *Latin, 'pig, hog' or 'doorway'.* A perfect role-model name, relating to Shakespeare's brilliant and spirited character in *The Merchant of Venice*. But some people will think you named your child for the car. **Porcha, Porchai, Porchea, Porscha, Porsche, Porschea, Porschia, Porsha. International: Porcie** *(French),* **Porcia** *(Spanish).*

POSY. *English, 'a bunch of flowers'; also diminutive for* JOSEPHINE. Fashionable in England, but this pretty bouquet-of-flowers name is rarely heard elsewhere. A possible alternative to Rosy? **Posey, Posie.**

★♂ **PRAIRIE.** *Nature name.* Unspecific place name with a wonderfully wide-open, spacious, western feel; used for a character in Thomas Pynchon's novel *Vineland*.

♂ **PRAISE.** *Word name.* Generally used in conjunction with another name to form a religious phrase – for instance, the daughter of rapper DMX is called Praise Mary Ella.

PRECIOSA. *Spanish, 'precious, valuable'. See* PRECIOUS.

PRECIOUS. *Latin word name, 'of great worth, expensive'.* Though many might find it too syrupy, hundreds of parents each year choose this name for their daughters to make them feel special. Precious Ramotswe is the engaging African sleuth in the popular *No. 1 Ladies' Detective Agency* series.

♂ **PRESLEY.** *English, 'priest's meadow'.* For those not ready to name their daughters Elvis. **Preslea, Preslee, Presleigh, Presli, Preslie.**

PRIMA. *Latin, 'first'.* Will assure your daughter she's *numero uno.* **Primalia, Primetta, Primina, Priminia.**

PRIMAVERA. *Italian, 'spring'.* A bit syllable-heavy, but a pretty name for a springtime baby. **Prima. International: Primevère** *(French).*

PRIMROSE. *English, 'first rose'; flower name.* Still found in British novels, such as *Watership Down,* but a bit too prim for today's babies. **International: Primarosa, Primorosa** *(Spanish).*

Stellar Starbabies Beginning with *P*

Paloma	Emilio Estevez
Paris	Michael Jackson
Pearl	Maya Rudolph & Paul Thomas Anderson
Penelope	Taylor Hanson
Pepper	Graham (Blue) Coxon
Petah	Ani DiFranco
Phoebe	Vernon Kay & Tess Daly
Phoenix	Melanie *(Scary Spice)* Brown
Piper	Gillian Anderson, Brian DePalma, Cuba Gooding Jr.
Poppy	Jamie *(The Naked Chef)* Oliver
Praise Mary Ella	DMX
Presley	Tanya Tucker

PRIMULA. *Flower name. See above.*

PRINCESS. *Word name.* Part of the trend for formerly canine royal names; this is one a little girl might love – up till the age of eight. **Princella, Princessa, Princesse, Principessa.**

PRISCILLA. *Latin, 'ancient'.* No way to get around the prissy part. **Cilla, Pris, Priscella, Prissie,** **Prissy, Prysilla. International: Prisca, Priscille** *(French),* **Priscila, Prisilla** *(Spanish),* **Piri, Piroska** *(Hungarian).*

PROMISE. *Word name.* Promising.

♂ **PROVENCE.** *(pro-VAHNCE) French place name.* One of the most picturesque and enchanting areas of France could become a distinctive baby name.

PRUDENCE. *Virtue name.* Like Hope and Faith, a Puritan virtue name with a quiet charm and sensitivity. Caveat: possible 'prude'-baiting during adolescence. **Pru, Prudentia, Prudi, Prudie, Prue, Pruie, Prudy. International: Prew, Prewdence, Prudencia, Prudentiane, Prudenzia, Prue** *(French),* **Prudencia** *(Spanish).*

PRUNELLA. *Latin, 'small plum'.* Most *ella* names are hot, but this is one that won't catch fire because of the disagreeable connotations of prunes. **International: Prune, Prunelle** *(French).*

PSYCHE. *Greek, 'breath'.* This name of the mortal girl loved by Cupid is too loaded with psyche/ psycho/psychic associations.

PUA. *(POO-ah) Hawaiian, 'flower'.* Overly teasable.

PUEBLA. *Spanish, 'the town'.* Sandy southwestern US feel.

♂ **PUMA.** *Animal name.* Lithe and leonine name chosen for her daughter by singer Erykah Badu, whose other child has the number name Seven.

PURITY. *Virtue name.* Only slightly less challenging than Chastity. **Pureza.**

Q *girls*

QADIRA. *Arabic, 'capable'.* This female form of Qadir represents one of the ninety-nine attributes of Allah. **Kadira.**

QITURAH. *Arabic, 'incense, scent'.* Exotic twist on the attractive and underused biblical name Keturah. **Qeturah, Quetura, Queturah, Quitara Quitarah.**

QUADEISHA. *American, a combination of* **QADIRA** *and* **AISHA.** Familiar-sounding hybrid name, made more unusual by virtue of the Q. **Quadaishia, Quadajah, Quadasha, Quadasia, Quadayshia, Quadaza, Quadejah, Quadesha, Quadeshia, Quadiasha, Quaesha, Qudaisha.**

QUANDA. *American, 'companion'.* A bit too close to 'quandary'. **Quandra.**

★ ♂ **QUARRY.** *Nature name.* Strong meaning, sweet but strong sound, fresh and earthy: a winner. **Quarree, Quarrey, Quarri, Quarrie.**

QUARTILLA. *Latin, 'fourth'.* Octavia has the same meaning and is much more user-friendly. **Quantilla, Quatilla.**

QUEEN. *Word name.* Not even when followed by Latifah. **Quanda, Queena, Queenette, Queenie, Quenna.**

QUEENIE. *English, 'queen'.* Name that is stuck in the 1950s. Started as nickname for girls named Regina – queen in Latin – now mostly a canine choice.

♂ **QUENBY.** *English, 'queen's settlement'.* Quirky and cute. **Quenbie, Quinbie, Quinby.**

QUERIDA. *(ker-ee-da) Spanish, 'dear, beloved'.* Loving choice.

QUESTA. *French, 'one who seeks'.* Sounds too much like the name of a minivan.

QUIANA. *(kee-AH-na) Modern invented name.* The first

synthetic name? Popular in the 1970s and 80s, along with the same-named form of polyester. **Qiana, Qianna, Quian, Quianah, Quiandah, Quiane, Quiani, Quianita, Quianna, Quianne, Quionna, Quiyanna.**

QUILLA. *English, 'quill, hollow stalk'.* A heroine in a Victorian novel written with a quill pen, has an unusual, offbeat charm. **Quylla.**

♂ **QUINCY.** *French, 'estate of the fifth son'.* Surname name that sounds both cute and strong when used for a girl. **Quincee, Quincey, Quinci, Quincia, Quincie, Quincy, Quinsy.**

★ ♂ **QUINN.** *Irish, 'descendent of Conn'.* One of the first Irish unisex surnames, a strong and attractive choice on the rise for both genders, though there are still more than three boy Quinns for every girl. **Quin, Quinna, Quinne, Quynn.**

QUINTANA. *Spanish, 'the fifth girl' Mexican place name.* Mexican place name famously

Boys' Names for Girls

Aidan
August
Austin
Barry
Claude
Curtis
Douglas
Eliot
Flynn
Gary
Harley
Ira
James
Jude
Keith
Lyle
Mason
Murray
Neil
Noah
Quincy
Raleigh
Roy
Sawyer
Spencer
Timothy
Wylie

used by Joan Didion for her daughter, Quintana Roo. **Quinntina, Quinta, Quintanna, Quintara, Quintarah, Quintia, Quintila, Quintilla, Quintina, Quintona, Quintonice.**

QUINTESSA. *Latin, 'essence'.* Sounds like a fictional rank of royalty. **Quintaysha, Quintesa, Quintesha, Quintessia, Quintice, Quinticia, Quintisha, Quintosha.**

QUINTESSENCE. *Word name.* Sounds pretty. But pretentious.

★QUINTINA. *Latin, 'fifth'.* The daintiest and most accessible of the many *Q* names for a fifth child, now used for girls situated anywhere in the birth order. **Quentina, Quintana, Quintessa, Quintona, Quintonett, Quintonice.**

QUIRINA. *Latin, 'warrior'.* Feminine form of the Roman god Quirinus; too close to the *queer* sound.

R *girls*

RAANANA. *(ray-ah-NA-na) Hebrew, 'beautiful, fresh'.* Lovely Hebrew name with distinctive double *a*'s, but beware of possible 'banana' teasing. **Raanan, Raananit, Ranana, Rananah.**

RABIAH. *Arabic, 'spring'.* Rhythmic name suitable for a girl born in a springtime month. **Rabi, Rabia.**

RACHEL. *Hebrew, 'ewe'.* Delicacy, softness and Old Testament importance made Rachel a top biblical choice from the 1970s on, after being a primarily Jewish name for centuries. **Rachael, Racheal, Rachelce, Racheli, Rachell, Rachella, Rachelle, Rae, Raquela, Raquella, Raquelle, Rashell, Rashelle, Ray, Raychel, Raychelle, Raschel, Shell, Shelley, Shellie, Shelly. International: Raghnailt, Ráichéal** *(Irish Gaelic),* **Raquel, Rachelle** *(French),* **Rachele** *(Italian),* **Raquel** *(Spanish),* **Rahel** *(German),* **Rakel** *(Swedish),* **Rachela, Rahel** *(Polish),* **Rahil, Rakhil, Rakhila, Rashel**

(Russian), **Rashka, Rashke, Rechell** (Israeli), **Rahel** (Hebrew), **Ruchel** (Yiddish), **Rahela** (Hawaiian).

RACHELLE. French variation of **RACHEL.** Elaboration of Rachel sometimes seen in France, but more rarely elsewhere.

RADA. Yiddish, 'rose'. Rose would be sweeter.

RADELLA. English, 'elfin advisor'. Extremely unusual ella-ending choice. **Radelle.**

RADEYAH. Arabic, 'contented'. One of several similar names with a pleasant, exotic sound. **Radeya.**

RADHIYA. (rahd-HEE-yah) Swahili, 'agreeable'. See **RADEYAH. Radhiyah, Radia, Radiah, Raziya, Raziyh.**

RADIAH. See **RADEYAH.**

RADINKA. (rah-DEEN-kah) Slavic, 'energetic, active'. Tinkly.

RADMILA. Slavic, 'industrious for the people'. Like cousin Ludmila, a Russian name rarely

heard in this country. **Radilla, Radinka, Radmilla, Redmilla.**

RAE. English, diminutive of **RACHEL.** One of today's coolest middle name choices. **Ray.**

RAEGAN. Spelling variation of **REAGAN.** An increasingly popular spelling as parents are responding more and more to the ae form of Braeden, Jaeden, Janae and Nevaeh.

RAFA. Arabic, 'happiness, prosperity'. Sounds a bit like a shortening of Rafael or a condensation of Rafaela. **Rafah.**

RAFAELA. Spanish, 'God has healed'. See **RAPHAELA. Raefaela, Rafaelia, Rafaelina, Rafaelita, Rafaila, Rafala, Rafalla, Rafeala, Rafela, Rafelia, Rafiela.**

RAI. Japanese, 'next child'. Distinctive and intriguingly exotic relative of Rae. **Raiko, Rayko, Reiko.**

RAIDAH. (rah-EE-dah) Arabic, 'leader'. Rhythmic choice sometimes heard in Muslim families. **Raaidah.**

RAIN. Word name. Among a small shower of rain-related names, this pure version can have, depending on how you look at it, a fresh or a gloomy image. **Raine, Rainnie, Reign. International: Chuva** (Portuguese), **Sade** (Finnish), **Yagmur** (Turkish), **Matar** (Arabic), **Ame** (Japanese).

RAINA. Slavic and German variation of **REGINA.** Strong and solid, with a touch of foreign intrigue, it's the most popular of the rain-related names, with a variety of pronunciations – ray-na, rah-ee-na, or ry-na. **Raenah, Raene, Rainah, Raine, Rainey, Raya, Rayna. International: Reina** (Spanish).

RAINBOW. Word name. Colourful, yes, but also the dippiest of hippy names. **Rainbeau, Rainbo, Rainboe, Reignbeau, Reignbo, Reignboe, Reignbow.**

RAINE. French, 'queen'. Attracted attention as the stepmother of Princess Diana. **Raina, Rana, Rane, Rayne, Reina, Reine, Reyna.**

RAINEY. *English, 'counsel power'; diminutive of* **REGINA.** Has an old-time country feeling, perhaps due to Ma Rainey, considered the 'Mother of the Blues'. **Rainee, Raini, Rainie, Rainy.**

RAINIE. *Spelling variation of* **RAINEY.** Singular spelling of Rainey used by Andie MacDowell for her daughter.

RAISA. *Russian, from Greek, 'easygoing'; Yiddish, 'rose'.* Known in Europe and the US via the wife of the former Soviet head Mikhail Gorbachev; a possibility for parents of Eastern European descent wanting to move beyond Natashia and Nadia. **Raissa, Raiza, Raisel, Raya, Rayzel, Rayzil, Razil.**

RAISEL. *Yiddish, 'rose'.* The most popular flower name in Israel, however it is a bit old-fashioned here. **Rayzil, Razil.**

RAJA. *Arabic, 'hope' or 'the anticipated one'.* Regal. **Rajaa, Ragaa, Rajya.**

RAJANI. *Sanskrit, 'dark, of the night'.* A name with lots of exotic charm.

RAKEL. *Scandinavian variation of* **RACHEL.** Apt to be confused with Raquel.

♂ **RALEIGH.** *English, 'meadow of deer'.* Attractive North Carolina unisex place name in the US, its soft sound is particularly appropriate for a girl. **Ralegh, Rawle, Rawleigh, Rawley, Rawling, Rawly, Rawlyn.**

RAMA. *Sanskrit, 'pleasing'; African, Hausa, 'restoration'; Hebrew, 'lofty'.* This name of a revered Hindu deity is heard in several cultures. **Ramah, Ramit, Romiya.**

RAMANA. *(rah-MAH-nah) Sanskrit, 'beautiful'.* Has a sound as lovely as its meaning.

RAMIRA. *Spanish, 'judicious'.* Pretty and unusual, worth consideration.

RAMONA. *Spanish, feminine variation of* **RAMÓN.** It is neither too trendy nor too eccentric, recently chosen by Maggie Gyllenhaal. **Raimonda, Ramonde, Raymonde, Raymondine** *(French)*, **Ramonda, Raymonda** *(German)*, **Romona** *(Slavic)*, **Rimona** *(Israeli).*

RANA. *Arabic, 'a beautiful object that catches the eye'; Hindi, 'queenly'.* A favourite in Near Eastern cultures with a charming meaning. **International: Ranee, Rania, Rani, Ranie** *(Sanskrit)*, **Raniyah, Ranya** *(Arabic).*

RANDA. *English, feminine variation of* **RANDALL;** *also Arabic, 'delicate desert tree'.* Sounds incomplete.

RANDI. *Feminine diminutive of* **RANDOLPH.** A relic of the mid-century Mandi-Sandi-Andi era. **Randa, Randie, Randy.**

RANI. *Hindi, 'queen'; Hebrew, 'she is singing'.* Cheerful. **Rana, Rancie, Ranee, Rania, Ranit, Ranica, Ranice, Ranita, Ranya.**

RANIELLE. *Modern invented name.* Ungainly hybrid of Randi and Danielle. **Rani, Raniel, Raniell, Ranyel, Ranyelle.**

RANITA. *Hebrew, 'song'.* Delicate embellishment of Rani. **Ranit.**

RANIYAH. *Arabic, 'gazing'.* Shy but sultry.

★**RAPHAELA.** *Hebrew, feminine variation of* **RAPHAEL.** Euphonious and exotic name with a dark-eyed, long-flowing-haired image, it might – like Gabriella and Isabella – be drawn into the mainstream. **Raefaela, Rafa, Rafaela, Rafaelia, Rafaelina, Rafaelita, Rafala, Rafella, Raffaela, Raffaele, Raphaëla, Raphaelia, Raphaelle, Raphayella, Raphella, Refaella, Refella, Rephaela, Rephayelle.** International: **Rafaella, Rafaila, Raffelle** *(French),* **Rafela, Rafelia, Rafiela** *(Spanish),* **Rafaly** *(Polish),* **Rafia, Raphia, Rafya** *(Hebrew).*

RAQUEL. *Spanish variation of* **RACHEL.** Attractive name popular in the Latino community, identified with half-Bolivian actress Raquel Welch.

RASHANDA. *Modern invented name.* One of several creations with the *anda* ending, this one drawing on the Muslim favourite Rashad. **Rashandah.**

RASHIDA. *Arabic, 'rightly advised'; Swahili, 'righteous'.* Evocative and alluring. **Raashida, Rasheda, Rasheeda, Rasheedah, Rasheida, Rashi, Rashidah, Rashyda.**

♀ **RAVEN.** *Word name.* Like Ebony, chosen by some parents in recent years to celebrate the beauty of blackness. **Raiven, Ravenne, Ravyn, Rayven, Rayvinn.**

★**RAVENNA.** *Italian place name.* An Italian city renowned for its Byzantine mosaics, and a name waiting to be discovered. **Ravena, Ravinia, Ravinna.**

RAY. *See* **RAE.**

RAYA. *Hebrew, 'friend'.* More unusual alternative to Maya. **Raea, Raia.**

RAYMONDA. *German, 'wise protector'.* More out of style than Raymond. **Rae, Raya, Raye.** International: **Réamonnie** *(Gaelic),* **Ramona** *(French, Italian, and Spanish),* **Raimona, Raimonda** *(Italian),* **Rajmundy** *(Danish and Eastern European),* **Raemonia** *(Greek).*

RAYNA. *Hebrew, 'song of the Lord'.* Also found in the Slavic and Scandinavian cultures. **Raina, Raine, Rana, Raynell, Raynette, Reyna, Reyne, Reyney.**

RAYSEL. *Yiddish, 'rose'. See* **RAISEL.**

♂ **RAZ.** *Aramaic, short for* **RAZIAH.** Could lead to razzing. **Razi, Razia, Raziah, Raziela, Razille, Razili, Razit, Raziye, Razzi, Razzy.**

RAZIAH. *Aramaic, 'the Lord's secret'.* More substantial form of this name. **Razel, Razi, Razia, Raziela, Raziella, Razilee, Razili, Razlee, Razli.**

RAZIELA. *Aramaic, 'the Lord's secret'.* Most graceful of the *Raz* names, relates to Graziella.

RAZILI. *Aramaic, 'the Lord's secret'.* Offbeat, exotic choice to honour a Grandma Rosalie.

RAZIYA. *Swahili, 'agreeable, pleasant'.* An appealing East African possibility. **Raziyah.**

REA. *Variation of* **RHEA.** Short but substantial. **Ria.**

Three-Syllable Standouts

Christina

Elena

Eliza

Flavia

Francesca

Gabrielle

India

Jacquetta

Juliet

Larissa

Lavender

Lilian

Livia

Louisa

Lucinda

Quintina

Sabina

Susannah

♂ **REAGAN.** *Irish, 'little king'.* A strong, straightforward Irish unisex surname, with a merry glint in its eye, Reagan has been leaping up the popularity lists in the US in recent years. **Reaghan, Regan, Raygen.**

REANNA. *Modern invented name.* Probably an offshoot of Deanna, lacking much identity of its own. **Reann, Reanne.**

REBA. *Hebrew, 'fourth born'; diminutive of* **REBECCA.** Tied to country singer/sitcom star Reba McEntire. **Rebah, Reyba, Rheba.**

REBECCA. *Hebrew, 'servant of God'.* A name representing beauty in the Bible, an Old Testament classic that reached the heights of revived popularity in the 1970s. However, it is still a pretty and prudent choice, and still popular – it is in the Top 50. **Becca, Beck, Becka, Beckee, Beckey, Becki, Beckie, Becky, Bekka, Bekki, Bekkie, Reba, Rebecka, Rebeckah, Rebekkah, Ree, Reeba, Riba, Ribecca, Riva, Rivah.** International: **Réba, Rébecca** *(French),* **Rebeca** *(Spanish),* **Rebeka, Rebekah, Rebekka** *(German),* **Rebecka, Rebeka** *(Nordic),* **Reveca** *(Romanian),* **Rebeka** *(Czech, Hungarian),* **Revekka** *(Russian),* **Reveka** *(Greek),* **Rive, Revka, Revkah** *(Israeli),* **Rifka** *(Yiddish).*

REBEKAH. *Spelling variation of* **REBECCA.** Many parents prefer this spelling used in the authorised version of the Bible.

REBEKKA. *Spelling variation of* **REBECCA.** A more creative spelling of the biblical favourite.

REECE. *See* **REESE.**

♂ **REED.** *English, 'red-haired'.* Sleek, unisex surname rarely heard for girls – which could be seen as an asset. **Read, Reade, Reid, Reida.**

♂ **REESE.** *Welsh, 'fiery, zealous'.* The sassy, steel magnolia appeal of Oscar-winning Reese (born Laura) Witherspoon has single-handedly propelled this formerly male name into unisex popularity over the past few years. **Reece, Rees, Rhys, Rice.**

♂ **REEVE.** *English occupational name, 'bailiff'.* Chosen by aviators Charles and Anne Lindbergh for their daughter, Reeve is another single-syllable surname waiting to be borrowed by the girls.

♂ **REGAN.** *Irish, 'little king'.* Like sister Reagan, a well-used Irish surname, despite negative Shakespearean and *Exorcist* connections. **Reagan, Reagann, Reagin, Reghan, Regin, Regyn.**

REGINA. *Latin, 'queen'.* A classic name with regal elegance. **Raina, Raine, Reggi, Reggie, Reggy. International: Regan, Regia, Régine, Reina, Reine, Reinette** *(French),* **Reina** *(Italian),* **Reina, Reyna** *(Spanish),* **Gina, Reinhilda, Reinhilde** *(German),* **Rane** *(Norwegian),* **Rana, Rania** *(Norse),* **Ina** *(Polish),* **Rani** *(Hindi).*

REGINY. *(reh-GEE-nee) Polish, from* **REGINA.** This sounds like a hillbilly take on Regina.

REIGN. *English word name.* Combines the look of royalty with the sound of nature.

REIKO. *(rah-ee-ko) Japanese, 'pretty child'.* Dainty and doll-like.

♂ **REILLY.** *Irish, 'courageous'.* Riley is the spelling of this lively Irish name most often picked for girls, but this version is occasionally used. **Riley, Rylee, Ryleigh, Rylie, Ryley.**

REINA. *Spanish, 'queen'.* An appellation for the Virgin Mary, 'Queen of the apostles'. **Reinella, Reinelle, Reinette, Reyna, Reynelle.**

♂ **REMEMBER.** *Word name.* No one will ever forget it.

♂ **REMINGTON.** *English, 'place on a river bank'.* Sharp, metallic image, thanks to Remington Steele and Remington razors.

REN. *Japanese, 'water lily, lotus'.* Though in Japan the lotus is the Buddhist symbol of purity and perfection, most Westerners would prefer Wren.

RENA. *Hebrew, 'song of joy'; African, Hausa, 'despised, disregarded, or refused'.* Conflicting meanings in two cultures; in Africa it's used to ward off evil spirits. **Reena, Rina, Rinah, Rinna, Rinnah.**

RENATA. *Latin, 'reborn'.* Widely used across Europe as a common baptismal name symbolising spiritual rebirth. **Renatia, Renatta, Renatya, Rennatta. International: Renate** *(French and German),* **Renátka, Renča** *(Czech),* **Rena, Nata** *(Russian).*

RENATE. *Latin, 'to be born again'.* Common French and German alternative to Renata. **Renata.**

RENÉE. *French from Latin, 'reborn'.* Chic in the 1950s, now kept in the public eye mainly by actress Zellweger; today's parents seek more moderne Gallic choices. **Ranae, Ranay, Ranée, Rena, Renae, Renai, René, Renell, Renella, Renelle, Renie, Rennay, Rennea, Rennie, Renny, Rhennae, Rhennay, Rinae, Rinee, Rinay. International: Renate** *(German).*

♂ **RENNY.** *Irish, 'little prosperous one'.* Offbeat Anglicised form of the intractable Gaelic Rathnait.

RESEDA. *Latin, 'the fragrant mignonette blossom'.* A town in the San Fernando Valley, California, slightly better than others like Encino or Tarzana.

RETA. *Greek, 'eloquent speaker';* *African, 'shaken'.* With a soft *e*, sounds like an affected pronunciation of Rita.

REUELLE. *(roo-EHL) Hebrew, 'friend of God'.* Spelling a bit elaborate and confusing. **Ruel, Ruelle.**

REVA. *(RAY-vah) Hindi river name; Hebrew, 'rain'.* Refers to one of the seven sacred rivers of India. **Revaya, Ravit.**

REXANNE. *Combination of* **REX** *and* **ANNE.** Stick to Roxanne. **Rexana, Rexanna.**

REYNA. *See* **REINA.**

♂ **REYNOLD.** *Scottish, 'powerful counsel'.* Used for girls in Scotland in the sixteenth century; this would make a bold but bonnie choice.

REZ. *(rehz) Hungarian, 'having copper-coloured hair'.* A beyond unusual choice for a little redhead.

RHEA. *Greek mythology name, 'a flowing stream'.* Old-style creative name of the Greek mythological earth mother of all

the gods. A lot better than the Roman equivalent: Ops. **Rea, Rhia, Ria.**

RHETA. *Greek, 'eloquent speaker'. See* **RETA.**

RHIAN. *(REE-an) Welsh, 'maiden'.* Popular in Wales, but likely to be mispronounced as Ryan elsewhere. **Rhiain.**

★**RHIANNON.** *(REE-an-on) Welsh, 'divine queen'.* A lovely Welsh name with links to the moon, associated with a 1970s Fleetwood Mac song; especially appropriate for a family with Welsh roots. **Reanna, Rheanna, Rhianna, Rhianon, Rianon, Rianna, Riannon.**

RHODA. *Greek, 'rose'.* A New Testament name now completely out of favour. **Rhodeia, Rhodia, Rhodie, Rhody, Roda, Rodi, Rodie, Rodina.**

RHONA. *Scottish, uncertain derivation.* Probably started life as a short form of Rhonwen, which we would definitely prefer. **Rona, Roana.**

RHONDA. *Welsh, 'noisy one'.* 'Help Me, Rhonda!' sang the

Beach Boys – help me convince my parents not to give me this 1960s name. **Rhondda, Rhondi, Rhondie, Rhondy, Rhonnda, Ronda, Ronna, Ronni, Ronnie.**

★**RHONWEN.** *Welsh, 'slender, fair'.* This delicate and haunting Welsh name is still a rarity. **Rhonwyn.**

RIA. *Spanish, 'small river'; diminutive of* **MARIA.** Rhythmic flow. **Rea.**

RIALTA. *Italian, 'deep brook'.* Unique choice, with a pleasant antique feel.

RIANA. *Contemporary American variation of* **RHIANNON.** In these days of ethnic authenticity, it's best to stick with the original. **Rhiana, Rhianna, Rhianne, Rian, Riane, Rianne.**

RIANE. *Feminine variation of* **RYAN.** Most modern parents would prefer the more straightforward Ryan. **Rhiane, Rhianna, Riana, Rianna, Rianne, Ryann, Ryanne.**

RICA. *Scandinavian, diminutive of* **FEDERICA** *or* **ERICA.** Pretty but slight. **Rhica, Ricca,**

Ricki, Rickie, Ricky, Rieca, Riecka, Rieka, Riki, Rikki, Riqua, Rycca.

RICHARDA. *(ree-SHAR-dah) Feminine variation of* **RICHARD.** Marginally better than Richardette or Richardina. **Rich, Richie, Richy, Ricki, Rickie, Ricky, Riki, Rikki, Rikkie, Rikky. International: Richarde, Richilde** *(French)*, **Ricciarda** *(Italian)*, **Ricarda** *(Spanish and Portuguese)*, **Rickarda** *(Scandinavian)*, **Ryszardy** *(Polish)*, **Rikárdy** *(Hungarian)*.

RICKI. *Diminutive of* **FREDERICA.** One of the earliest of the relaxed, unisex names, now relegated to oldies rock stations. **Ricki, Ricky, Ricquie, Rika, Riki, Rikki, Rikky, Ryckie.**

RIKKI. *See* **RICKI.**

♂ **RILEY.** *Irish, 'courageous'.* Red hot for girls (though still popular for boys), this upbeat, friendly Irish surname name is much more common in the US than here. **Reilley, Reilly, Rylea, Rylee, Ryleigh, Ryley, Rylie.**

♂ **RILIAN.** *German, 'small stream'.* A male character in *The Chronicles of Narnia*, but could conceivably be used for a girl. **Rilla, Rillie.**

RILLA. *German, 'small brook'.* Ripe for 'gorilla' teasing. **Rella, Rilletta, Rillette.**

RIMA. *Arabic, 'white antelope'.* Nature girl played by Audrey Hepburn in *Green Mansions*, it now has an old-style bohemian feel.

RIMONA. *Hebrew, 'pomegranate'.* Well used in Israel, likely to be confused with Ramona here.

♂ **RIO.** *Spanish, 'river'; Brazilian place name.* Sexy male name that might make an interesting middle name for a girl.

RIONA. *Irish, 'queenly'.* We'd opt for Fiona. **Rionach, Rionagh, Rionna, Rionnagh.**

♂ **RIPLEY.** *English, 'strip of clearing in the woods'.* Reflects powerful character played by Sigourney Weaver in the *Alien* films, chosen by actress Thandie Newton for her daughter.

RISA. *(REE-sah) Latin, 'laughing'.* Macramé-maker.

♂ **RISHI.** *(REE-shee) Sanskrit, 'sage'.* May be too exotic for a mainstream baby.

RISHONA. *Hebrew, 'first'.* A possible alternative to the better-known Shoshona.

RITA. *Diminutive of* **MARGARITA;** *Hindi, 'brave, strong'.* A hot name in the Rita Hayworth 1940s, rarely given to babies today. **Reeta, Reita, Rheeta, Riet, Rieta, Ritta. International: Reta, Rheta, Rhita** *(German)*, **Rida** *(Portuguese)*.

RIVA. *(REE-vah) Hebrew, 'maiden'.* A modernisation of the Hebrew Rivka, which doesn't sound so modern anymore. **Reba, Ree, Reeva, Revvabel, Reva, Rifka, Rivalee, Rive, Rivi, Rivka, Rivke, Rivkah, Rivy.**

RIVAGE. *French word name, 'shore'.* Unique, soft and flowing.

RIVKA. *Hebrew, 'young calf,' original form of* **REBEKAH.** Traditional name still used in Orthodox families. **Rifka,**

Rifke, Riki, Rivai, Rivca, Riveka, Rivi, Rivvy.

RIYA. *Indian, meaning unknown.* The growing popularity of this name among Indian parents may be due to the glamorous image of Bollywood star Riya Sen.

ROANNA. *Latin, 'sweet'; variation of* **ROSANNA.** Most modern parents would probably prefer the cooler Rowan. **Ranna, Roana, Roanne.**

ROBBIA. *Italian surname.* A creative alternative to the dated Robin, and also a reference to the famed Della Robbia family of Florentine Renaissance artists.

ROBERTA. *English, 'bright fame'; feminine variation of* **ROBERT.** Harks back to the day when Roberta sat around discussing the latest Sinclair Lewis novel with pals Lois and Lorraine. **Bertie, Berty, Bobbe, Bobbee, Bobbette, Bobbie, Bobbi, Bobby, Bobbye, Bobette, Bobi, Bobine, Bobinette, Reberta, Robbee, Robbey, Robbi, Robbie, Robbina, Robby, Robeena, Robella, Robelle,** Robena, Robenia, Robertena, Robertene, Robetta, Robette, Robettina, Robin, Robina, Robinett, Robinette, Robinia, Robyn, Robynn, Robynne, Robyna, Robynna, Rupetta. International: **Roba, Roberte, Robertina, Robine** *(French),* **Bertha, Bertunga, Ruperta** *(Spanish),* **Robertha, Ruperta** *(German),* **Erta** *(Polish),* **Berta, Bobina, Roba** *(Czech),* **Robia, Robi, Robie, Robya** *(Slavic).*

♂ **ROBIN.** *English, diminutive of* **ROBERT;** *also bird name.* Sounded bright and chirpy in the 1950s, but by now has lost much of its lilt. **Robee, Robbey, Robbi, Robbie, Robbin, Robby, Robbyn, Robene, Robenia, Robi, Robinet, Robinett, Robinette, Robinia, Robyn, Robyna.** International: **Robena, Robina, Robine** *(French).*

ROBINA. *Feminine variation of* **ROBIN.** Heard in Britain, but not elsewhere.

ROBYN. *See* **ROBIN.**

ROCHELLE. *French, 'little rock'.* Long-standing French name that retains a feminine, fragile and shell-like image.

Roch, Roche, Rochell, Rochella, Rochette, Roschella, Roschelle, Roshelle, Shell, Shelley, Shelly.

♂ **ROCIO.** *Spanish, 'dewdrops'.* This name, which refers to Mary as the Virgin of the Dew, is all but unknown in the Anglo community, but sometimes used in Hispanic families.

RODERICA. *German, 'renowned ruler'.* Unfashionably ornate female form of unfashionable Roderick. **Rica, Roddie, Roderiqua, Roderique, Rodriga.** International: **Roderiga** *(Spanish).*

ROHANA. *Sanskrit, 'sandalwood'.* Exotic alternative to Johanna? **Rohanna.**

RÓISÍN. *(roh-sheen) Irish Gaelic, diminutive of* **RÓIS,** *'rose'.* An authentic choice for your little Irish Rose, chosen by singer Sinead O'Connor for her daughter. **Rosaleen, Rosheen, Rois, Rosen.**

ROKSANA. *Polish and Russian variation of* **ROXANE.** This is a plausible name for parents with Slavic roots, known as the wife of Alexander the Great. **Ksana.**

ROLANDA. *German, 'famous in the land'.* Clunky. **Orlande, Rahlaunda, Ro Landa, Rolandah, Rollanda, Rollande, Rolline, Rollonda, Rolonda, Rolli, Rollie, Rolly.** International: **Roleen** *(Scottish),* **Rolande** *(French),* **Orlanda, Roldana** *(Spanish).*

ROMA. *Italian place name.* Never as popular as Florence; today's parents might prefer Venezia, Verona or Romy. **Romelle, Romilda, Romina, Romma.**

ROMAINE. *French, 'from Rome'.* Likely to conjure up visions of leafy lettuce. **Romane, Romayne, Romeine, Romene.**

ROMANA. *Latin, 'a roman'.* Romantic. **Roma, Romelle, Romia, Romola.** International: **Romaine, Romanade, Romance, Romanette, Romany, Romy** *(French),* **Romanadia, Romancia** *(Italian),* **Romantza, Romy** *(German),* **Romanka, Romi, Romka** *(Slavic),* **Romanadya, Romochka** *(Russian).*

ROMILLY. *English, 'spacious clearing'.* This English family name and French place name would make an interesting,

feminine choice; Emma Thompson used it as her daughter's middle name.

♂ **ROMNEY.** *Welsh, 'winding river'.* Brings to mind the romantic and elegant eighteenth century portraits of George Romney.

ROMOLA. *Latin, 'Roman woman'.* A literary name created by George Eliot, seems a bit ponderous. **Romala, Romella, Rommola, Romolla, Romula.**

♂ **ROMY.** *German, diminutive of* **ROSEMARY.** Exotic but friendly; like other *Ro*-names Roman, Rowan and Romeo, gaining favour with the celebrity set.

RONA. *Scottish spelling variation of* **RHONA;** *also Norwegian, 'might'.* Coined in Scotland in the late nineteenth century, has little appeal in the twenty-first. **Rhona, Ronella, Ronelle, Ronna.**

RONALDA. *Scottish, feminine variation of* **RONALD.** Not even if your husband is named Ron. **International: Ranalta, Ranalte** *(Irish Gaelic),*
Ronaldette, Ronaldine *(French),* Rinalda *(Italian and Spanish).*

Spanish Girls' Names Beyond Maria and Margarita

Aitana

Alba

Aniceta

Arcelia

Aroa

Blanca

Calida

Candela

Estela

Estrella

Jimena

Laia

Lorena

Marisol

Natalia

Nerea

Noa

Nuria

Pilar

Raquel

Soledad

RONJA. *Scandinavian, uncertain meaning.* This name of a character from an Astrid Lindgren children's book has a ninja feel.

RONNI. *English, diminutive of* **VERONICA.** Today's Veronicas would be called Veronica. **Ronee, Roni, Ronna, Ronnee, Ronney, Ronnie, Ronny.**

☿ **RORY.** *Scottish and Irish, 'red king'.* Buoyant, spirited name for a redhead with Celtic roots; still more often heard for boys, though for many modern parents that's a plus. **Roree, Rorey, Rori, Rorie.** International: **Ruaidri, Ruairí** *(Irish Gaelic),* **Ruaraidh** *(Scottish Gaelic).*

ROSA. *Latinate variation of* **ROSE.** One of the most classic Spanish and Italian names, also favoured by the upper-class here.

ROSAE. *Modern invented name.* Created by lovers of the *ae* vowel combo. **Rosai, Rosay, Rose, Rosee, Rosey.**

ROSALBA. *Latin, from the phrase rosa alba, 'white rose'.* One of many Spanish elaborations of Rosa.

ROSALEEN. *Irish, diminutive of* **ROSE.** The name of a sympathetic character in the best-selling novel *The Secret Life of Bees,* though as far out of style as Eileen or Colleen. **Rosheen, Rosealeen.**

ROSALIA. *Spanish, Latin ceremonial name.* A name commonly used in Spain and Italy, it refers back to the annual Roman ceremony of hanging garlands of roses on tombs. **Chala, Chalina, Lía, Rosaelia, Rosailia, Rosalá, Rosalya, Rosela.**

ROSALIE. *French variation of Latin* **ROSALIA.** Species of rose names popular from the 1920s to 40s, rarely used now. **Rosalea, Rosalee, Rosaleen, Rosaleigh, Rosaley, Rosalia, Rosalina, Rosaline, Rosalyne, Rozalie, Rozele, Rozelie, Rozella, Rozelle, Rozellia, Rozely.**

ROSALIND. *Spanish, 'pretty rose'; German, 'red dragon'.* With its distinguished literary history – as a lyrical name in early pastoral poetry, then as a charming heroine in Shakespeare's *As You Like It* – the long-dormant Rosalind might deserve a new look. **Ros,**
Rosalen, Rosaline, Rosalinn, Rosalyn, Rosalynd, Rosalynda, Roselin, Roselina, Roselind, Roselinda, Roselinn, Roselyn, Roslynn, Roslynne, Roz, Rozali, Rozalia, Rozalin, Rozlind, Rozalinda, Rozalynn, Rozalynne, Rozelin, Rozelind, Rozelinda, Rozelyn, Rozelynda, Rozlin, Rozlyn. International: **Rosaleen** *(Irish),* **Rosalin, Rosalina, Rosalinda** *(Spanish),* **Rosalinde** *(German).*

ROSALINDA. *Spanish, 'pretty rose'.* Rosalind feels fresher now. **Roslinda.**

ROSAMUND. *German, 'horse protection'.* Quintessentially British appellation, the name of a legendary twelfth-century beauty called 'Fair Rosamond'. **Ros, Rosamond, Rosamunde, Roz.** International: **Rosemonda, Rosemonde** *(French),* **Rosemund, Rosmunda** *(Italian),* **Rosemunda** *(Spanish).*

ROSANNA. *Combination of* **ROSE** *and* **ANNA.** One of the more mellifluous of the Rose-plus names. **Rosana, Rosanne.**

ROSARIO. *Spanish, 'rosary'.* Anglo parents are taking note of this Latina classic, thanks to Rosario Dawson. **Charo, Rosaria, Rosarita.**

ROSE. *Latin flower name.* This old-time sweet-smelling flower name has had a remarkable revival – as a middle name – with parents (including celeberity parents Teri Hatcher and Ewan McGregor) finding it the perfect connective, with more colour and charm than old standbys like Sue and Ann. **Rosie, Rosey, Rosy, Rozy. International: Roís, Roísín** *(Irish Gaelic),* **Roselle, Rosette, Rosine** *(French),* **Rosa, Rosana, Roseta, Rosetta, Rosina** *(Italian),* **Rosita** *(Spanish),* **Arrosa** *(Basque),* **Rasine, Roza, Rozalia, Rozycka** *(Polish),* **Ruza, Ruzena, Ruzenka** *(Czech),* **Ruza, Ruzha** *(Russian),* **Roza** *(Yiddish).*

ROSEANNE. *Combination of* **ROSE** *and* **ANNE.** Forever – or at least for a while – linked to the one-time 'Domestic Goddess' Roseanne Barr. **Roanna, Roanne, Rosana, Rosanna, Rosannah, Rosanne, Roseann, Roseanna, Rozan, Rozanna, Rozanne.**

ROSELLE. *Combination of* **ROSE** *and* **ELLE.** Most

contemporary parents would probably opt for the more streamlined Elle.

ROSELLEN. *Combination of* **ROSE** *and* **ELLEN.** Another of the *Rose*-plus names, now far out of fashion.

ROSELYN. *Combination name of* **ROSE** *and* **LYNN.** Takes Rosalind and makes it rosier.

ROSEMARIE *See* **ROSEMARY.**

ROSEMARY. *Latin, 'the rosemary plant'; combination of* **ROSE** *and* **MARY.** This amalgam of two classic names projects a sweet, somewhat old-fashioned sensibility; could come back as a herb name. **Rosemaree, Rosemarey, Rosemaria, Rose Marie, Rosmarie, Romy. International: Rosemarie** *(French).*

ROSEMOND. *Variation of* **ROSAMUND.** Elizabeth Taylor's middle name. **Rosemund.**

ROSETTA. *Persian, 'splendid'.* Associated with the ancient Rosetta stone, this is also the pretty Italian pet form of Rosa.

★**ROSIE.** *Diminutive of* **Rose.** Spunky, perky nickname name that is in the Top 100. **Rosey, Rosi, Rosy, Rozy.**

ROSITA. *Spanish, diminutive of* **ROSA.** Flamenco dancer.

ROSLYN. *Spelling variation of* **ROSALIND.** *See* **ROSALIND.** **Roslin, Roslinn, Roslynn, Roslynne, Rozlin, Rozlynn, Rozlynne.**

ROUX. *French, 'reddish brown'; also culinary term.* Possible middle name for your little auburn-haired babe.

★♂ **ROWAN.** *Irish, 'little red-haired one'.* Almost unheard of as a girl's name before Brooke Shields chose it for her daughter in 2003, now shows great promise as an appealing Celtic choice. **Roan, Roanna, Roanne, Rohan, Rowen.**

ROWENA. *Welsh, 'white spear' or 'famous friend'.* A fabled storybook name via the heroine of *Ivanhoe*, Rowena has some old-fashioned charm, though most modern parents seem to prefer Rowan. **Ro, Roe, Roweena, Roweina, Rowan,**

Precious Names

Amethyst

Beryl

Bijou

Copper

Coral

Crystal

Diamond

Emerald

Garnet

Gemma

Goldie

Ivory

Jade

Jet

Jewel

Mercury

Onyx

Opal

Pearl

Ruby

Sapphire

Silver

Steel

Topaz

Rowen, Rowina, Rowynna, Winnie.

ROXANA. *Persian, 'dawn' or 'little star'.* The name of the wife of Alexander the Great, more attractive than the better-known Roxanne.

ROXANNE. *Persian, 'dawn'.* Has a touch of the exotic from its Eastern origins, best known as the beautiful heroine to whom Cyrano de Bergerac says, 'Your name is like a golden bell'. **Roksanne, Roxan, Roxana, Roxann, Roxanna, Roxannia, Roxene, Roxey, Roxi, Roxiane, Roxianne, Roxine, Roxy, Roxyanna, Ruksana, Ruksane, Ruksanna.** International: **Roksana** *(Russian),* **Roxane** *(Greek).*

ROXIE, ROXY. *Diminutive of* **ROXANNE.** Audacious offshoot of Roxanne, the wayward heroine of the musical *Chicago.*

♂ **ROY.** *Scottish, 'red'.* If girls have adopted Ray, why not Roy?

♂ **ROYCE.** *English, 'son of the king'.* Upscale thanks to Rolls, and a contempo way to honour a grandparent Roy or Joyce.

ROZA. *Russian and Polish variation of* **ROSA.** Adds some zest to Rosa. **Rozi, Róży, Różyczka.**

RUBÌ. *Spanish, 'ruby'.* Perhaps worthy of considering if you're planning to move to Spain, otherwise the spelling would cause confusion.

★**RUBY.** *Latin, 'deep red, translucent precious stone'.* Unlike quiet gem names Pearl, Opal and Crystal, vibrant red Ruby is sassy and sultry and definitely on the rise, making it into the Top 5. An early rock classic – think 'Ruby Tuesday' – Ruby makes a cool yet warm choice. **Rubee, Rubetta, Rubette, Rubey, Rubi, Rubie, Rubina, Rubinia, Rubyna, Rubyr.**

RUE. *English, from Greek, 'aromatic medicinal plant'; also word name, 'regret'.* Unusual and mysterious choice you nevertheless may regret.

RUFINA. *Latin, 'red-haired'.* Might be too close to 'ruffian'. **Rufeena, Rufeine, Ruffina, Rufia, Ruphyna.** International: **Rufa** *(Spanish).*

RUMER. *English, 'a gypsy'.* Demi and Bruce made waves when they named their firstborn after novelist Rumer Godden; downside is its connection with the unpleasant word *rumour.* **Ruma.**

RURI. *(ROO-ree) Japanese, 'emerald'.* Naming babies after precious gems as a protection against evil spirits is an ancient Japanese tradition. **Ruriko.**

RUTH. *Hebrew, 'compassionate friend'.* With its air of calm and compassion, Ruth was the second most popular name in 1900, then faded away. Parents tiring of Rachel and Rebecca might want to give it a second thought. **Routh, Ruthanne, Ruthi, Ruthia, Ruthie, Ruthina, Ruthine. International: Rút** *(Gaelic),* **Ruthven** *(Scottish),* **Rut** *(Scandinavian).*

♂ **RYAN.** *Irish, 'little king'.* This ultrapopular boys' name is rapidly becoming a hot name for girls; admired for its buoyant Irish spirit. **Rian, Rianna, Rianne, Ryann, Ryen, Ryenne.**

RYANN. *Spelling variation of* **RYAN.** Increasingly used by

parents who want to make this name *really* unisex. **Riann, Rianne, Ryann, Ryanne.**

RYLEA. *Spelling variation of* **RILEY.** *See* **RILEY.**

RYLEE. *Spelling variation of* **RILEY.** This substitute spelling of Riley has been popular with parents for a decade: in the US, a few thousand little Rylees were born recently.

RYLEIGH. *Spelling variation of* **RILEY.** Another increasingly well-used form of Riley.

RYLIE. *Spelling variation of* **RILEY.** And another.

S *girls*

SABAH. *Arabic, 'morning'.* A popular Arabic name borne by a famed Lebanese actress and singer, could provide an exotic alternative to Sarah. **Saba, Sabaah, Sabba, Sabbah, Sheba, Shebah.**

SABINA. *(sa-BEE-na) Latin, 'Sabine'.* A sleek but neglected

Stellar Starbabies Beginning with R

Ramona	Maggie Gyllenhaal & Peter Sarsgaard
Renee	Rachel Hunter & Rod Stewart
Rhiannon	Robert Rodriguez
Ripley	Thandie Newton
Romy	Ellen Barkin & Gabriel Byrne, Sofia Coppola
Rowan	Brooke Shields
Ruby	Toby Maguire, Matthew Modine, Rod Stewart, Suzanne Vega
Rumer	Demi Moore & Bruce Willis

name (possibly due to *The Rape of the Sabine Women*) from an ancient Roman tribal name that's well worth consideration. The equally alluring Sabine is heard in France. **Byna, Sabeen, Sabena, Sabia, Sabin, Sabinna, Sabiny, Saby, Sabyna, Sahbina, Savine, Sebina, Sebinah.** International: **Sabienne, Sabine** *(French),* **Sabcia, Sabinka, Sabka** *(Polish),* **Bina** *(Czech),* **Sabinella, Sabyne, Savina, Savya** *(Russian).*

SABLE. *Animal name.* Soap opera name from the *Dynasty* days. **Sabel, Sabela, Sabella.**

SABRA. *Hebrew, 'prickly pear'.* Term for a native-born Israeli, first brought to notice in Edna Ferber's 1929 novel *Cimarron.* **Sabera, Sabira, Sabrah, Sabre, Sabrea, Sabreah, Sabree, Sabreea, Sabri, Sabria, Sabriah, Sabriya, Sebra, Sabrette, Sabrielle.**

★**SABRINA.** *Celtic mythology name.* The bewitchingly lovely Sabrina, the name of a legendary Celtic goddess, is best known as the heroine of the eponymous film, originally played by Audrey Hepburn, and later as a teenage TV witch; it would make a distinctive

alternative to the ultrapopular Samantha. **Brina, Sabre, Sabreena, Sabrinah, Sabrinas, Sabrine, Sabrinia, Sabrinna, Sabryn, Sabryna, Sebree, Sebreena, Sebrina, Subrina, Zabrina.**

SACHA. *See* **SASHA.**

SADA. *Hebrew variation of* **SARAH;** *also Japanese, 'chaste'.* An obscure but usable form of Sarah worthy as an alternative. **Saida, Saidah.**

SADE. *(shah-day) Nigerian, Yoruba, diminutive of* **FOLASHADE,** *'honour bestows a crown'.* The one-named singer clarified the confusing pronunciation on this one, but a number of parents have looked for more phonetic spellings. **Sáde, Sadé, Sadea, Sadee, Shaday, Sharday.**

SADIE. *Diminutive of* **SARAH.** Stylish along with its whole class of sweetly frumpy – or frumpily sweet – nickname names: think Josie, Milly, Tilly; this one has a lot more sass. Adam Sandler chose it for his daughter. **Sada, Sadah, Saddie, Sadee, Sadelle, Sadey, Sadi, Sadiey, Sady, Sadye, Saida, Saide,** **Saidee, Saidey, Saidi, Saidia, Saidie, Saidy, Sayde, Saydee, Saydie, Seidy, Syde, Sydella, Sydelle.**

SADIRA. *Persian, 'lotus tree'.* Intriguing name with great symbolic meaning in Eastern religions. **Sadra.**

SADIYA. *Arabic, 'lucky, fortunate'.* This female form of Sa'id is one of several eminently usable Arabic *S* names. **Sadi, Sadia, Sadiah, Sadiyah, Sadiyyah, Sadya.**

SAFFRON. *Flower and spice name.* Spice names are increasingly appealing to the senses of prospective parents, this one has a vaguely orange-scented-incense 1960s feel. **Saffran, Saffren, Saffronia, Safron, Saphron.**

SAFIYYA. *Arabic, 'confidante, best friend'.* The fact that this is pronounced *sah-FEE-yah* would cause Western ears to hear it as Sophia. **Safa, Safeya, Saffa, Safia, Safiyah.**

SAGA. *Word name.* Apt name for a little drama queen with a long future ahead of her.

♂ **SAGE.** *Latin, 'wise, healthy'; also herb name.* Simple, evocatively fragrant herbal name that also connotes wisdom, giving it a double advantage. **Sagia, Saige, Salvia, Sayge.**

SAHAR. *Arabic, 'dawn, morning, awakening'.* Muslim name commonly heard in the Middle East.

★**SAHARA.** *Arabic, 'desert'.* Beautiful and evocative place name that deserves wider use. **Sahar, Saharah, Sahari, Saharra, Saheer, Saher, Sahira, Sahra, Sahrah.**

♂ **SAILOR.** *Occupational name.* Supermodel Christie Brinkley launched an entire name genre when she picked this breezy occupational name for her daughter. **Sayler, Saylor.**

SALAMA. *African, Swahili, 'peace, safety, security'.* The three soft *a*'s make for a calm and rhythmic name, though some risk of salami jokes. **Sallama, Salma, Saloma, Soloma.**

♂ **SALEM.** *place name.* Would be more appealing if it weren't for the witch trials.

SALENA. *See* **SELENA.** Saleana, Saleen, Saleena, Salena, Salene, Salenna, Sallene, Salin, Salina, Salinah, Salinda, Saline.

SALIMA, SALIMAH. *(SAH-lee-mah) Arabic, 'healthy'.* Very popular throughout the Arab world. **Saleema, Salema, Salim, Salma, Selima.**

SALLY. *Diminutive of* **SARAH.** A cheerful, fresh-faced girl-next-door name long used independently but not heard as a baby name for years – though we can see Sally bouncing back. **Sal, Salaid, Salcia, Saletta, Sallee, Salletta, Sallette, Salley, Salli, Sallianne, Sallie, Sallyann.**

SALMA. *Arabic, 'safe'.* Mexican-born actress Salma Hayek lends a large dollop of glamour to this name that would otherwise resemble the middle-aged Selma.

♂ **SALMON.** *Word name.* Possibility for fish enthusiasts, but works better for a boy.

SALOME. *Hebrew, 'peace'.* Biblical dancer whose unseemly story has made parents shy away from her name, but the stigma seems to be fading. Ex-*ER* star

girls' names

Spice (& Other Food) Names

Amandine
Apple
Berry
Cayenne
Cherry
Cinnamon
Clove
Fennel
Honey
Olive
Pepper
Plum
Quince
Saffron
Sage
Yarrow

Alex Kingston named her daughter Salome Violetta. **Sahlma, Salima, Salma, Salmah, Salomey, Salomi, Selima, Selma, Selmah, Solome, Solomea. International: Salomé** *(French),* **Saloma, Salomea** *(Polish),* **Salama** *(Arabic).*

If You Like Samantha,

You Might Love . . .

Atlanta

Anastasia

Calista

Diantha

Georgiana

Marianna

Roxanna

Samara

Savannah

Selena

Susannah

Tabitha

Tamara

SALVADORA. *Spanish, feminine variation of* **SALVADOR.** Old-fashioned Latin.

SALVIA. *Latin, 'whole, healthy'.* Another name for the herb sage – which sounds younger and more modern than this version. **Sallvia, Salviana, Salviane, Salvina, Salvine.**

♂ **SAM.** *Diminutive of* **SAMUEL** *and* **SAMANTHA.** Yes, some parents – among them Denise Richards and Charlie Sheen – are cutting straight to the simple, unfussy unisex Sam, bypassing the trendy Samantha completely.

SAMALA. *Hebrew, 'requested of God'.* Sure to require lots of explanation. **Samale, Sammala.**

SAMANTHA. *Hebrew, 'told by God'.* Long-popular feminisation of Samuel, but finally fading along with other frilly girls' names. **Sam, Samana, Samanath, Samanatha, Samanitha, Samanithia, Samanta, Samanth, Samanthe, Samanthi, Samanthia, Samanthy, Samatha, Samentha, Samey, Sami, Sammanth, Sammantha, Sammee, Sammey, Sammi, Sammie, Sammy, Semantha, Semanntha, Simantha, Smantha, Symantha. International: Samanthée (French).**

★**SAMARA.** *Hebrew, 'under God's rule'; Latin fruit name; city in western Russia.* Exotic and lovely – and much more distinctive now than Samantha. **Saimara, Samaira, Samar, Samarah, Samari, Samaria, Samariah, Samarie, Samarra, Samarrea, Samary, Samera, Sameria, Samira, Sammar, Sammara, Samora, Semara.**

SAMARIA. *place name, ancient Palestinian city in present-day Jordan.* Similar to but distinct from Samara, this pretty name was chosen for his daughter by rapper LL Cool J.

SAMEH. *Hebrew, 'listener'; Arabic, 'forgiving'.* Unusual Samantha alternative with little aural appeal. **Samaiya, Samaya.**

SAMI. *Arabic, 'praised'; Hebrew, diminutive of* **SAMANTHA.** Cute, if overused in its more familiar Sammy form. **Samia, Samiah, Samiha, Samina, Sammey, Sammi, Sammie, Sammijo, Sammy, Sammyjo, Samya, Samye.**

SAMIRA. *Arabic, 'companion in evening conversation'.* Shiny cousin of Samara with an intriguing meaning. **Samirah, Samire, Samiria, Samirra, Samyra.**

SAMOA. *Place name.* Evocative of the beautiful South Pacific islands; we've also heard Samoan used as a name.

SAMUELA. *Feminine variation of* **SAMUEL.** Awkward, dated feminisation of Samuel we can't imagine anyone choosing over Samantha. **Samella, Samelle, Samuella, Samuelle.**

SANA. *Arabic, 'mountaintop, splendid, brilliant'.* One of the most easily imported Arabic names. **Sanaa, Sanáa, Sanaah, Sanah, Sane, Sanna.**

SANCIA. *(sahn-chee-ah) Italian, from Latin, 'sacred'.* Rarely heard outside Italy, could make an interesting import. **Sanceska, Sancharia, Sanchia, Sanchie, Sancie, Sancya, Santsia, Sanzia. International: Sancha, Santa, Santina** *(Spanish).*

SANDRA. *Diminutive of* **ALEXANDRA.** Mum name. **Sahndra, Sanda, Sandee, Sandi, Sandie, Sandira, Sandrea, Sandreea, Sandrella, Sandrelle, Sandretta, Sandrette, Sandria, Sandrica, Sandrina, Sandrine, Sandy, Sanndra, Sanndria, Sauhndra, Saundra, Sohndra,** Sondra, Sonndra, Wysandria, Zandr.

SANDRINE. *French variation of* **ALEXANDRA.** Sophisticated French choice? Or toxic petrochemical? **Sandreana, Sandrene, Sandrenna, Sandrianna, Sandrina.**

♂ **SANDY.** *Diminutive of* **SANDRA.** Nickname name hip in the era of *Grease.* **Sandee, Sandi, Sandie, Sandya, Sandye, Sanndi.**

SANIA. *(SAHN-ya) Hindi, 'pearl'.* Indian tennis sensation Sania Mirza is popularising this one. **Saneiya, Saniya, Sanya, Sanyia.**

SANNA. *Scandinavian, diminutive of* **SUSANNA.** If you're ready to move beyond Anna and Hannah, consider this, one of the most widely used names in Scandinavia. **Sana, Sanea, Saneh, Sanne, Sanneen, Zanna.**

SANNE. *(sah-na) Dutch, diminutive of* **SUSANNE.** Hugely popular in the Netherlands and almost unknown elsewhere – which makes it an interesting prospect for the parent in search of an unusual name.

SANTANA. *Spanish, condensed form of Santa Ana.* Saintly name . . . or Latin rock band. Santina might work better. **Santa, Santaniata, Santanna, Santanne, Santena, Santenna, Santina, Santinia, Shantana.**

SAOIRSE. *(sare-sha) Irish, 'liberty'.* Popular name in Ireland, used since the 1920s revolution as a statement of freedom, would have obvious pronunciation problems here.

SAPPHIRE. *Hebrew, jewel name.* Way beyond Ruby and Pearl, this September birthstone, occasionally used a century ago, might be worth a reappraisal. **Saffira, Saffire, Safira, Safire, Sapheria, Saphira, Saphire, Sapira, Saphyra, Saphyre, Sappha, Sephira. International: Sapphira** *(Greek).*

SARAH. *Hebrew, 'princess'.* Old Testament name – she was the wife of Abraham – that is truly a fashionable classic, as stylish as it is traditional and a regular in the Top 100. With such a range of images and variations any child can make it her own. Sadee, Sadeila, Sadelle, Sadellia, Sadie, Sadye, Sahra, Saidee, Sal, Sallee, Salley, Sallie, Sally, Sara, Saraha, Sarahann, Sarahi, Sarai, Saraia, Sarann, Saray, Sarely, Sarena, Sarette, Sarha, Sariah, Sarina, Sarine, Sayra, Sera, Serach, Serah, Serita, Shara, Zahra, Zara, Zarah, Zaria. International: Sarai, Saraid, Sorcha (Irish), Sarette, Sarotte, Zaidee (French), Saretta, Sarita, Zarita (Italian, Spanish), Chara, Charita (Spanish), Sarice (Swiss), Sassa (Swedish), Saara, Salli (Finnish), Salcia (Polish), Sari, Sarika, Sarolta (Hungarian), Sari, Sasa, Zsazsa (Eastern European), Sarka, Sarra (Russian), Saraqa (Persian), Sarit, Sarita (Israeli), Kala (Hawaiian).

SARAI. (sar-EYE) Hebrew, 'princess'. In the Old Testament, God changed Sarai's name to Sara, so this would make a very legitimate variation. **Sari, Sharai.**

SARDINIA. Italian place name. Beautiful Italian island, but as a baby name too redolent of sardines. **Sardegna.**

SARI. (SAH-ree) Arabic, 'noble'; also Finnish and Hungarian variation of **SARAH**. Cute spin on Sarah, though some may hear it as 'sorry,' and it is also an item of clothing worn in India. **Saree, Sareeka, Sareka, Sari, Sarika, Sarka, Sarri, Sarrie, Sary.**

SARIAH. Variation of **SARAH**. The perfect compromise name for when you say Sarah, and your spouse says Mariah.

SARITA. Italian and Spanish, diminutive of **SARA**. Delicately pretty name all but unknown elsewhere.

♂ **SASCHA, SASHA.** Russian, diminutive of **ALEXANDER**. Largely male in Russia, this name is really taking off for girls; it's been used for the daughters of Steven Spielberg, Jerry Seinfeld, and Vanessa Williams. **Sacha, Sahsha, Saschae, Saschenka, Sashae, Sashah, Sashai, Sashana, Sashay, Sashea, Sashel, Sashenka, Sashey, Sashi, Sashia, Sashira, Sashsha, Sashya, Sasjara, Sauscha, Sausha, Shasha, Shashi. International: Sasa, Zsazsa (Hungarian).**

★**SASKIA.** Dutch, uncertain derivation. One of those names that's been used in Europe (she was Rembrandt's wife) since the Middle Ages. Charming choice for the adventurous.

SASSANDRA. African place name. Sassy alternative to Cassandra – maybe too sassy.

♂ **SATCHEL.** English nickname, 'sack, bag'. Chosen by Woody Allen for his son with Mia Farrow (now renamed Seamus), honouring the great old-time baseball player Satchel Paige, and by Spike Lee for his daughter, but far too eccentric for ordinary use.

SATIN. French, 'smooth, shiny'. Sensuous to a fault. **Satinder, Satine.**

SAVANNAH. Spanish, 'flat tropical grassland'; place name. Once-obscure place name that shot to fame, with others of its genre, on the heels of the best seller *Midnight in the Garden of Good and Evil*, which was set in the Georgia city in the US. **Sahvannah, Savana, Savanah, Savanha, Savanna, Savannha, Savauna, Savonnah, Savonne,**

Sevan, Sevanah, Sevanh, Sevann, Sevanna, Sevannah.

SAVITA. *Hindi, 'sun'.* Popular Indian choice that could easily immigrate.

♂ **SAWYER.** *English occupational name, 'wood worker'.* Stylish, now unisex name used by the Steven Spielbergs for their daughter. **Sawyar, Sawyor.**

★**SCARLETT.** *English, 'scarlet'.* Scarlett Johansson is doing more for this seductively southern name than Scarlett O'Hara ever did. Sylvester Stallone's third *S* daughter is Scarlet, following Sophia and Sistine. A name that is rising quickly up the Top 50. **Scarlet, Scarletta, Scarlette, Scarlotte, Skarlette.**

♂ **SCHUYLER.** *(SKY-ler) Dutch, 'scholar, schoolteacher'.* This original spelling has been obscured by such phonetic upstarts as Skylar. **Schiler, Schuyla, Schuyler, Schuylia, Schylar, Schyler, Skila, Skilah, Skyela, Skyelar, Skyla, Skylar, Skyler, Skylia, Skylie, Skylin, Skyllar, Skylor, Skylyn, Skylyr, Skyylar.**

♂ **SCIROCCO.** *(shir-OK-ko) Italian, from Arabic, 'warm wind'.* Hot. **Cirocco, Sirocco.**

SCOTIA. *Latin term for Scotland.* Caledonia, Scotland's even earlier name, is better.

♂ **SCOTLAND.** *Place name.* Kim Basinger and Alec Baldwin's daughter Ireland opened up the map for names like this.

♂ **SCOTTY.** *Diminutive of SCOTT, or person from Scotland.* Cute but slight masculine nickname. **Scot, Scota, Scotia, Scott, Scottey, Scotti, Scottie.**

♂ **SCOUT.** *Word name.* This character nickname from *To Kill a Mockingbird* (her real name was Jean Louise) became a real-life possibility when Bruce Willis and Demi Moore used it for their middle daughter. **Scoutt.**

♂ **SEAN.** *Irish variation of JOHN.* Actress Sean Young brought this form into the girls' camp; much stronger than the feminised Shawn.

SEANA. *(SHAWN-a) Irish, feminine variation of SEAN.* One modern feminine spelling

with more credibility than the phonetic Shawna. **Seaana, Sean, Seane, Seann, Seanna, Seannae, Seannah, Seannalisa, Seanté, Sianna, Sina.**

SEASON. *Latin, 'time of sowing'.* A generic possibility if you don't want to specify Spring or Summer.

SEBASTIANE. *Latin, 'from Sebastia'.* Sebastian is a fine boy's name that doesn't really translate for girls. **Bastia, Sebastene, Sebastia, Sebastian, Sebastien. International: Bastienne, Bastina, Sébastienne, Seva, Sevastiane** *(French),* **Bastiana, Sebastiana** *(Italian and Spanish).*

SECRET. *Word name.* Mysterious.

SEDONA. *Place name.* Arizona city name renowned for its beauty and tranquility, could translate into an agreeable baby name. **Sadona, Sedonah, Sedonia.**

SEFARINA. *Spanish, from Greek, 'gentle wind'.* Exotic and feminine, but Serafina is far more commonly used. **Sefirina,**

Sepharina, Zefarina, Zepharina, Zephirina.

SELA. *(SEH-lah) Hebrew, 'rock';* *also Polynesian variation of* **SARAH.** Biblical place name – the original term for the city of Petra – finding new life through actress Sela Ward and also the young daughter of singer Lauryn Hill, who spells it Selah. **Saleet, Saleta, Selah.**

♂ **SELBY.** *English, 'manor village'.* This British surname has more substance than Shelby, which is now loosing ground. **Selbea, Selbee, Selbeigh, Selbey, Selbi, Selbie.**

SELENA, SELINA. *Latinised variation of Greek* **SELENE,** *'moon goddess'.* Smooth, shiny, and sensual, a nineteenth-century name that found new life in the Latino community. **Celene, Celie, Celinda, Cellina, Celyna, Saleena, Salena, Salina, Sela, Selana, Seleana, Seleena, Selen, Selenah, Selenia, Selenna, Selie, Selina, Selinda, Seline, Sena, Syleena, Sylena, Zelena.** International: **Célina, Céline** *(French),* **Celina, Celinka** *(Italian),*

Cela, Celek, Celina, Cesia *(Polish),* **Celena, Selene, Selia** *(Greek).*

SELIMA. *Hebrew, 'tranquil'.* Could be confused with Selina/Selena. **Saleema, Saleemah, Selema, Selemah, Selimah.**

SELMA. *German, 'godly helmet'.* Playing mah-jongg with her buddies Bernice and Myrna. **Anselma, Selima, Sellma, Sellmah, Selmah, Zelma.**

SEN. *Japanese mythology name.* Simple, Zen-like name of a mythological forest elf.

SENALDA. *Spanish, 'a sign'.* Nearly unknown elsewhere, with good reason. **Sena, Senda, Senna.**

♂ **SENECA.** *Latin surname and Native American, 'people of the standing rock'.* Both a Roman philosopher-statesman and a Native American Iroquois tribe; occasionally used for both girls and boys. **Senaka, Senecca, Seneka, Senequa, Senequae, Senequai, Seneque, Senneca.**

♂ **SENEGAL.** *African place name.* Unlikely to take over Kenya's spot as the dominant African place name.

SENGA. *Scottish variation of* **AGNES.** Spelling Agnes backwards is no great improvement.

SEPTEMBER. *Month name.* Parents are beginning to turn away from springtime months like April and June and are moving towards the cooler and crisper three-syllable September, October, November and December.

SEPTIMA. *Latin, 'seventh'.* Name for a seventh child, back when people had them.

♂ **SEQUOIA.** *Tree name.* This name of a giant tree, itself named for a nineteenth-century Cherokee who invented a way to write his tribe's language, makes a strong, stately statement. **Sacoya, Saquoia, Saquoya, Secoya, Seqoiyia, Sequouyia, Seqoya, Sequoi, Sequoiah, Sequora, Sequoya, Sequoyah, Sikoya.**

★SERAPHINA. *Hebrew, 'ardent'*. The highest-ranking angels, the six-winged seraphim, inspired this lovely name. **Fina, Sarafina, Serafine, Seraphe, Seraphin, Seraphita, Serapia, Serofina, Serophine. International: Séraphine** *(French),* **Serafina** *(Italian and Spanish),* **Fima, Fimochka, Seraphima, Sima** *(Russian).*

★SERENA. *Latin, 'tranquil, serene'.* Name used since Roman times, and given fresh life by tennis star Serena Williams, it's as calm and tranquil as its name implies. **Cerena, Reena, Sarina, Saryna, Seraina, Serana, Sereen, Sereina, Seren, Serenah, Serene, Serenea, Serenia, Serenna, Serina, Serenity, Serreana, Serrena, Serrenna, Seryna.**

♂ SERENADE. *Music name.* Peaceful and melodic, but a bit pretentious.

SERENDIPITY. *Word name, 'chance'.* It's doubtful that the child with this name will consider herself lucky to have it.

SERENITY. *Latin, 'peaceful'.* Pretty virtue choice, though the more conventional Serena works just as well. **Serenidy, Serenitee, Serenitey, Sereniti, Serenitiy, Serinity, Serrennity.**

♂ SESAME. *Word name.* If you're willing to name your daughter after a seed, Poppy would be preferable. Besides, in kids' minds, this would be overly associated with *Sesame Street.* **Sesamey, Sessame, Sessamee.**

♂ SETH. *Hebrew, 'placed, appointed'.* Although very rarely used for girls, its soft, gentle sound makes it a perfect candidate for crossing over to the female camp.

♂ SEVEN. *Numerical word name.* Seinfeld's George threatened to name his future child Seven – and then singer Erykah Badu actually did it.

★SEVERINE. *French, feminine variation of* SEVERUS; *Latin, 'stern'.* Long-popular name in France, sounds fresh and exotic here. **Séverine.**

SEVILLA. *(seh-VEE-yuh) Spanish place name.* This legendary Andalusian city, founded by Hercules, according to myth, is an undiscovered baby name destination. **Seville.**

SHADA. *Native American, 'pelican'.* Pretty and unusual bird-related name. **Shadae,**

Cool Saints' Names

Adela
Angelina
Antonia
Auria
Colette
Daria
Felicity
Flora
Gemma
Hyacinth
Joaquina
Lelia
Matilda
Maura
Natalia
Phoebe
Seraphina
Susanna
Tatiana
Verena

Shadea, Shadeana, Shadee, Shadi, Shadia, Shadiah, Shadie, Shadiya, Shaida.

♂ **SHADOW.** *English, 'shade'.* Better for a dog. **Shade, Shadoe.**

SHAFIRA. *Swahili, 'distinguished'.* Elegant African choice. **Shaffira.**

SHAINA. *Hebrew, 'beautiful'.* Despite its Irish sound, this commonly used word name has usually been confined to Jewish families. **Shaena, Shainah, Shaine, Shainna, Shajna, Shana, Shanee, Shani, Shanie, Shayna, Shayndel, Shayne, Sheina, Sheindel.**

SHAKILA. *Arabic, 'pretty'.* One of many similarly pretty names, this one identifiable as a female form of the familiar Shaquille. **Chakila, Shaka, Shakayla, Shakeela, Shakeena, Shakela, Shakelah, Shakilah, Shakyla, Shekila, Shekilla, Shikeela.**

SHAKIRA. *Arabic, 'woman of grace'.* The sexy Colombian-born singer inspired parents everywhere. **Shaakira, Shacora, Shaka, Shakeera, Shakeerah, Shakeeria, Shakera, Shakiera, Shakierra, Shakir, Shakirah, Shakirat,** Shakirea, Shakirra, Shakora, Shakuria, Shakyra, Shaquira, Shekiera, Sheira, Shikira.

SHALOM. *Hebrew, 'peace'.* Supermodel Shalom Harlow glamorised this name, which is heard as a greeting every day in Israel. **Shalome, Shalva, Shalvah, Shelom, Shilom, Sholome.**

SHALONA. *Modern invented name.* One of the sha-la-la sisters. **Shalon, Shalone, Shálonna, Shalonne.**

SHALONDA. *Modern invented name.* Sha-la-la-la-la-la-la . . . **Shalonde, Shalondie, Shalondra, Shalondria.**

SHALYN. *Modern invented name.* . . . sha-la. **Shalin, Shalina, Shalinda, Shaline, Shalyna, Shalynda, Shalyne, Shalynn, Shalynne.**

SHAMARA. *Arabic, 'ready for battle'.* The *M* and the *R* add welcome strength. **Shamar, Shamarah, Shamare, Shamarea, Shamree, Shamari, Shamaria, Shamariah, Shamarra, Shamarri, Shammara, Shamora, Shamori, Shamorra, Shamorria, Shamorriah.**

SHAMIRA. *Hebrew, 'he who defends'.* Hebrew name with a bright sheen. **Mira, Shameera, Shamir, Shamirah, Shamiran, Shamiria, Shamyra, Shemira.**

SHANA. *Diminutive of* **SHOSHANA** *or* **SHANNON,** *variation of* **SHAINA.** Part of a group of similar mid-century names rarely given to babies today. **Shaana, Shaina, Shan, Shanae, Shanah, Shanda, Shandi, Shane, Shania, Shanna, Shannah, Shauna, Shawna, Shayna.**

SHANELLE. *Spelling variation of Chanel.* French design meets Asda. **Schanel, Schanell, Shanel, Shanell, Shanella, Shanelly, Shannel, Shaney, Shannell, Shanilly, Shanisse, Shanita, Shenel, Shenela, Shenell, Shenelle, Shenelly, Shinella, Shinelle, Shonelle, Shynelle.**

SHANI. *Hebrew, 'scarlet'.* It would be easy to dismiss this girlish name, if you didn't know it refers to the 'scarlet thread' or theme of a story.

SHANIA. *(shan-EYE-a) Ojibway, 'I'm on my way'.* This obscure Native American name owes its very life to country singer Shania Twain, who dropped her original name, Eileen, for it. **Shaniya.**

SHANICE. *(sha-NEES) Modern invented name. Sha* name, by way of Janice. **Chenise, Shanece, Shaneese, Shaneice, Shanese, Shanicea, Shaniece, Shanise, Shanneice, Shannice, Shanyce, Sheneice.**

SHANIQUA. *Modern invented name.* Unfortunate name that's become a caricature, like Muffy, say, or Bruce.

SHANNON. *Irish, 'old, ancient river'.* Irish place name – it's a river, a county and an airport – once popular but now slipping towards the bottom of the Top 100 and being supplanted by Aidan and Maeve. **Channa, Shana, Shanan, Shanandoah, Shandy, Shane, Shani, Shann, Shanna, Shannae, Shannan, Shanneen, Shannen, Shannie, Shannin, Shannyn, Shanon.**

SHANTAL, SHANTEL. *American variation of* **CHANTAL.** Yet another phrase of the *sha* chorus. **Seantelle, Shanntell, Shanta, Shantal,** Shantae, Shantahl, Shantale, Shantalle, Shantay, Shante, Shanteal, Shanteil, Shantele, Shantell, Shantella, Shantelle, Shantrell, Shantyl, Shantyle, Shauntel, Shauntell, Shauntelle, Shauntrel, Shauntrell, Shauntrella, Shentel, Shentelle, Shontal, Shontaile, Shontalla, Shontalle, Shontel, Shontelle.

SHANY. *Swahili, 'marvelous, wonderful'.* Peppy teenager with African roots. **Shaney, Shannai, Shannea, Shanni, Shannia, Shannie, Shanny, Shanya.**

SHAQUILLA. *Feminine variation of* **SHAQUILLE.** For die-hard Shaq fans. **Shaqeela, Shaquila, Shaquilia.**

SHARAI. *Hebrew, 'princess'. See* **SARAI.**

SHARDAE. *Punjabi, 'charity'; Yoruba, 'honored by royalty'; Arabic, 'runaway'.* Whatever its derivation, best known now in the version used by the jazz singer, Sade. **Sade, Shadae, Sharda, Shar-Dae, Shardai, Shar-Day, Sharde, Shardea, Shardee, Shardée, Shardei, Shardeia, Shardey.**

SHARI. *Anglicised variation of Hungarian Sári, variation of* **SARAH.** This once-cool nickname name now belongs to the grandma generation. **Shara, Share, Sharee, Sharia, Shariah, Sharian, Shariann, Sharianne, Sharie, Sharra, Sharree, Sharri, Sharrie, Sharry, Shary.**

SHARLENE. *Variation of* **CHARLENE.** Dates from when Charlene was hot enough to have spelling variations. **Scharlane, Scharlene, Shar, Sharla, Sharlaina, Sharlaine, Sharlane, Sharlanna, Sharlee, Sharleen, Sharleine, Sharlena, Sharleyne, Sharlina, Sharline, Sharlyn, Sharlyne, Sharlynn, Sharlynne, Sherlean, Sherleen, Sherlene, Sherline.**

SHARON. *Hebrew, 'a plain'.* This Old Testament place name was popular fifty years ago; now Sharon's off on a cruise with cousin Karen. **Charin, Cheron, Shaaron, Shara, Sharai, Sharan, Shareen, Sharen, Sharene, Shari, Sharie, Sharin, Sharla, Sharna, Sharolyn, Sharona, Sharonda, Sharone, Sharran, Sharren, Sharreni, Sharrin, Sharron, Sharrona, Sharronne, Sharyn,**

Sharyon, Sheran, Sheren, Sheron, Sherri, Sherry, Sherryn, Sheryn, Sherynn.

SHARONA. *Elaborated form of* **SHARON.** Limited appearances inspired by hit 1979 song *My Sharona* by The Knack. Sharonah, Sharone, Sharonia, Sharonna, Sharrona, Shirona.

SHAUNA. *Hebrew, 'God is gracious'; or feminine variation of* **SEAN.** More modern options: Shaw, Shay or even Sean. Shaun, Shaunah, Shaunda, Shaune, Shaunee, Shauneen, Shaunelle, Shaunette, Shauni, Shaunice, Shanicy, Shaunie, Shaunika, Shaunisha, Shaunna, Shaunnea, Shaunta, Shaunua, Shaunya.

SHAVONNE. *Phonetic variation of* **SIOBHAN.** Many of the parents who choose this name may not even be aware of the lovely Irish Gaelic name that spawned it. Shavanna, Shavon, Shavondra, Shavon, Shavonn, Shavonna, Shavonni, Shavonnia, Shavonnie, Shavontae, Shavonte, Shavonté, Shavoun, Shevon, Shevonne, Shivaun, Shivawn, Shivonne, Shyvon, Shyvonne.

♂ **SHAW.** *English, 'lives by the thicket'.* Streamlined Shawn.

♂ **SHAWN.** *Hebrew, 'the Lord is gracious'.* Feminisation of Sean; it was cool thirty years ago but now rarely heard – but Sean still has some unisex punch. Sawna, Sean, Seana, Seanna, Shana, Shanna, Shaun, Shauna, Shaunee, Shaunie, Shaw, Shawna, Shawnae, Shawnai, Shawnea, Shawnee, Shawneen, Shawneena, Shawnell, Shawnette, Shawnna, Shawnra, Shawnta, Sheona, Siân, Siana, Sianna.

SHAWNEE. *Native American tribe name.* Eastern tribe that migrated westwards; makes an unusual name, if a little dated à la Tawnee. Shawney, Shawni, Shawnie, Shawny.

★♂ **SHAY, SHEA.** *Irish, 'fine, stately'.* Ditch all the girly forms – Shayla, Shayna and so on – and go for this stronger, more straightforward name. Schae, Shae, Shaelee, Shaelyn, Shay, Shaye, Shayla, Shaylee, Shaylyn, Shealy, Shealyn, Sheann, Sheannon, Sheanta, Sheaon, Shearra, Sheatara, Sheaunna, Sheavon.

SHAYLA. *Variation of* **SHEILA.** Stick to Shay. Shaela, Shae-Lynn, Shaila, Shailagh, Shaylah.

SHAYNA. *Variation of* **SHAINA.** American name losing ground, now that country music's Shania is the hot variety. Shaina, Shaynae, Shaynah, Shayne, Shaynee, Shayney, Shayni, Shaynie, Shaynna, Shaynne, Shayny, Sheana, Sheanna, Sheina.

SHAYNE. *Femininised variation of* **SHANE.** This distinctive variation was chosen for their third daughter by the Eddie Murphys.

SHEBA. *Hebrew, short variation of* **BATHSHEBA.** Exotic biblical place name for the region now known as Yemen is given to puppies and kittens more often than babies. Saba, Sabah, Scheba, Shebah, Sheeba, Shieba.

SHEENA. *Anglicization of* **SINE;** *Irish variation of* **JANE.** Animated Irish-American name popularised by singer Sheena Easton. Sheenagh, Sheenah, Sheenan, Sheeneal, Sheenika, Sheenna, Sheina, Shena, Shiona, Shionagh, Sina, Sine.

SHEHERAZADE. *Arabic, 'dweller in cities'.* The tale-spinning heroine of *The Thousand and One Nights* has too extravagantly elaborate a name for a little girl. **Sharazad, Sharizad, Sheherazade.**

SHEILA. *Irish variation of* CECILIA. Peaked in popularity in the 1930s, along with Maureen and Colleen; parents today would probably go back to the original Cecilia. **Seelia, Seila, Selia, Shaila, Shayla, Shaylah, Sheela, Sheelagh, Sheelah, Sheilagh, Sheilah, Sheileen, Sheiletta, Sheilia, Sheillynn, Sheilya, Shela, Shelagh, Shelah, Shelia, Shiela, Shila, Shilah, Shilea, Shyla.** International: **Sile** *(Irish Gaelic).*

♂ **SHELBY.** *English, 'estate on the ledge'.* Trendy, ten years ago. **Chelby, Schelby, Shel, Shelbe, Shelbee, Shelbey, Shelbea, Shelbee, Shelbeigh, Shelbey, Shelbi, Shelbie, Shelbye, Shellby.**

SHELL. *Word name.* Might be cool, were it not for the outdated Shelley. **Chelle, Sheila, Shelle.**

SHELLEY. *English, 'clearing on a bank'.* The Shirley of the 1950s. Shelley Winters was born a Shirley. **Schelley, Shelee, Shell, Shella, Shellaine, Shellana, Shellany, Shellee, Shellene, Shelli, Shellian, Shelliann, Shellie, Shellina, Shelly.**

♂ **SHERIDAN.** *Irish, 'searcher'.* Upper crust surname gains some energy when used for a girl. **Sheredon, Sherida, Sheridane, Sheridawn, Sherideen, Sheriden, Sheridian, Sheridon, Sherridan, Sherriden, Sherridon, Sherrydan.**

SHERRY. *Phonetic variation of French* CHERI; *also a Spanish fortified wine.* Peppy teenager name of the 1960s and 70s that's sure to evoke the Four Seasons song of that name. **Cheray, Shame, Sharee, Shari, Sharie, Sherae, Sherale, Sheray, Sheree, Sherey, Sheri, Sherice, Shericia, Sherie, Sherina, Sherissa, Sherita, Sherree, Sherrey, Sherri, Sherria, Sherriah, Sherrie, Sherryn, Sherye, Sheryy, Sh'rae.**

SHERYL. *Variation of* CHERYL. Somehow, the *S* versions are even more passé than the *C*'s. **Cheralin, Cheralyn, Cheralynne, Cherilynn, Sharel, Sharil, Sharilyn, Sharyl, Sharyll, Sheral, Sheralyn, Sheralin,** Sherell, Sheriel, Sheril, Sherileen, Sherill, Sherily, Sherilyn, Sherilynne, Sherissa, Sherita, Sherleen, Sherral, Sherrell, Sherrelle, Sherril, Sherrill, Sherryl, Sheryll, Sherylly.

SHEVONNE. *American, phonetic spelling of* SIOBHAN. Proof that a name can be pretty and tacky at the same time. **Shevaun, Shevon, Shevonda, Shevone.**

SHILOH. *Hebrew, 'he who is to be sent'; biblical place name.* Cool meets Born Again meets Brad and Angelina, who made this name an instant star when they chose it for their daughter. **Shilo, Shylo.**

SHIRA, SHIRI. *Hebrew, 'my song'.* Popular Israeli choice, ripe for adoption here. **Shirah, Shiray, Shire, Shiree, Shirit, Shirk, Shyra.**

SHIRLEY. *English, 'bright meadow'.* All Shirleys were born in 1937, when Shirley Temple was America's princess – or at least sound as if they were. **Sherlee, Sherleen, Sherley, Sherli, Sherlie, Sherrlie, Sheryl, Shir, Shirely, Shirl, Shirlea, Shirlee, Shirleen, Shirleigh, Shirlene,**

Armenian Girls' Names

Anoush

Arda

Arpina

Azni

Caroun

Garin

Lucine

Nadalia

Nairi

Nazelli

Ohanna

Sera

Shirin

Shoushan

Siran

Taline

Yulia

Zarouhi

Shirlie, Shirlinda, Shirline, Shirlley, Shirly, Shirlly, Shirlyn, Shurlee, Shurley.

SHIVANI. *Hindi, 'life and death'.* Fresh and powerful. **Shiva, Shivana, Shivanie, Shivanna.**

SHONA. *Anglicised variation of* **SINE.** Unusual and appealing Irish name, but it may be too close to the ubiquitous *Sha* names. **Shiona, Shonagh, Shonah, Shonalee, Shonda, Shone, Shonee, Shonette, Shoni, Shonie, Shonna, Shonnah, Shonta, Shuna, Shunagh.**

SHOSHANA. *Hebrew, 'lily'.* Exotic and lovely form of Susannah. **Shoshan, Shoshanah, Shoshane, Shoshanha, Shoshann, Shosanna, Shoshannah, Shoshauna, Shoshaunah, Shoshawna, Shoshona, Shoshone, Shoshonee, Shoshoney, Shoshoni, Shoushan, Shushana, Sosanna, Sosannah, Sosha, Soshana. International: Xuxa** *(Basque),* **Shosha** *(Yiddish).*

SHULA. *Hebrew, diminutive of* **SHULAMIT.** A short form often used on its own in Israel. **Shuala, Shulah, Shuli.**

SHULAMIT, SHULAMITH. *Hebrew, 'peace'.* Serious-sounding Old Testament name that appears in the *Song of Songs.* **Shula, Shulamil, Sula, Sulamith, Sulamuth.**

SIAN. *(shahn) Welsh variation of* **JANE.** Simple and pretty and user-friendly, this Welsh choice was used by U2's Dave 'the Edge' Evans for his daughter.

♂ **SIBLEY.** *Variation of* **SYBIL.** Meet my sibling, Sibley. **Sybley.**

SIBYL. *Greek, 'seer, oracle'.* The original but less common spelling of the ancient mythological name, now used mostly for fictional witches. **Cybil, Cybill, Cybilla, Libby, Sabilla, Sabylla, Sib, Sibbell, Sibel, Sibell, Sibella, Sibelle, Sibilla, Sibyll, Sybel, Sybella, Sybelle, Sybill. International: Sibéal** *(Irish Gaelic),* **Cybele, Sibylle, Sybilla, Sybille** *(French),* **Sibylla** *(Dutch and Swedish),* **Sybilla** *(Swedish),* **Sibilia** *(Slavic).*

SICILY. *Place name.* Lilting Italian place name that sounds like the elegant Cicely – which you might consider a plus or a minus. **Sicilia, Sicillia, Sicilly.**

SIDDA. *Literary name.* Name made famous by the heroine of *The Ya-Ya Sisterhood,* it probably started life as a nickname. **Siddalee.**

SIDNEY. *See* **SYDNEY.**

SIDONIA. *Dutch variation of* **SYDNEY**; *variation of* **SIDONIE**. Exotic spin on the now-trendy Sydney. **Sydania, Syndonia.**

SIDONIE. *Latin, 'from Sidon (in modern Lebanon)'.* Appealing and chic French favourite – its problem is likely confusion with Sydney. **Sedona, Sidaine, Sidanni, Sidelle, Sidoine, Sidona, Sidonae, Sidonia, Sidony, Sydona, Sydonah, Sydonia, Syndonia.**

SIDRA. *Latin, 'like a star'.* Uncommon name shared by a gulf off the coast of Libya. **Sidrah, Sidras.**

★**SIENA, SIENNA.** *Italian place name.* Soft and delicate Tuscan town name given a big fashion boost by lovely young actress/gossip column staple Sienna Miller. A real up-and-comer and in the Top 100.

♂ **SIERRA.** *Spanish place name, 'saw'.* Name borrowed from the western mountain range in the US, with Latin rhythm and cowboy charm, that has led to many offshoots, it's now probably past its peak. **Ciera, Cierra, Seara, Searria, Seera, Seirra, Siara, Siearra, Siera, Sierrah, Sierre, Sierrea, Sierriah, Syerra.**

SIGNE, SIGNY. *Scandinavian, 'new victory'.* Offbeat alternative to Sydney, with Norse roots.

SIGOURNEY. *French, 'daring king'.* Actress Sigourney – born Susan – Weaver made this unusual name (which she found in *The Great Gatsby*) famous, if not popular. **Signe, Sigornee, Sigournee, Sigournie, Sigourny.**

SIGRID. *Norse, 'fair victory'.* Forever Scandinavian. **Siegrid, Siegrida, Sigred, Sigritt.**

SÍLE. *(SHEE-la) Irish Gaelic variation of* **SHEILA**. Simple spelling complicates pronunciation.

SILENCE. *Word name.* The Puritans used it as a virtue name, but today it would just be considered weird: silence is no longer golden.

SILKEN. *Word name.* Smooth and evocative, but not very name-like. **Silk, Silke, Silki, Silkie, Silky, Silkya.**

♂ **SILVER.** *Word name.* Among the first wave of word names used in the hippie era, it actually

Celebrity-Inspired Names

Aaliyah	Kyra
Angelina	Liv
Ashanti	Macy
Audrey	Mariah
Beyoncé	Mariska
Bryce	Milla
Calista	Mischa
Cameron	Natalie
Charlise	Neve
Edie	Paris
Eva	Parker
Evangeline	Reese
Gwyneth	Scarlett
Halle	Shakira
Isla	Sienna
Jada	Téa
Jolie	Tyra
Keira	Venus

is a legitimate girl's name with a lot of lustre. **Silverey, Silverie, Sylver.**

SILVIA. *Latin, 'from the woods'.* This original form of the name – the more familiar Sylvia spelling came later – seems more modern now. **Silvanna, Silvija, Silvy, Silvya, Sylvana, Sylvia, Zilvia, Zylvia. International: Silvie, Sylvette, Sylvianne** *(French),* **Silva, Silvana, Silvia** *(Italian),* **Silvana, Silveria, Silvina** *(Spanish),* **Silwia** *(Polish).*

★**SIMONE.** *French, feminine variation of* **SIMON.** This classy French feminisation of Simon strikes that all-important balance between unusual and familiar, and it's oozing with Gallic sophistication. **Samone, Shimona, Shimonah, Simeona, Simina, Siminie, Simmi, Simmie, Simmona, Simmone, Simoane, Simon, Simonia, Simonina, Simonna, Simonne, Somone, Symona, Symone. International: Simonette** *(French),* **Simona, Simonetta** *(Italian),* **Cimona, Jimena** *(Spanish),* **Ximene, Ximenia** *(Basque).*

SIMPLICITY. *Word name.* Sound contradicts its meaning.

♂ **SINCERE.** *Word name.* Does it really work as a name? Apparently a number of iconaclastic American parents have thought so.

SINCERITY. *Word name.* Strikes more of a name-like rhythm than its sister Sincere.

♂ **SINCLAIR.** *English, 'from the town of St. Clair'.* The most famous Sinclair was the (male) writer Lewis, but these days the name works at least as well for a girl. **Sinclaire, Sinclare.**

SÍNE. *(SHE-neh) Irish Gaelic variation of* **JEAN.** Another case where the more authentic spelling complicates matters; most parents outside Ireland would opt for Sheena.

SINÉAD. *(shih-NADE) Irish Gaelic variation of* **JANE** *or* **JANET.** Popular Irish name brought here by singer Sinead O'Connor, could make a striking choice for a child with deep Irish roots. **Shinead, Seonaid, Sina, Síne.**

SIOBHÁN. *(zhuh-VAHN) Irish Gaelic variation of* **JOAN.** Lovely Irish name whose perplexing spelling has inspired many phonetic variations, but using the original form preserves the integrity of one of the most beautiful Gaelic girls' names. **Chavonne, Chevonne, Chivon, Chyvonne, Shavaun, Shavon, Shervan, Shevon, Shevonne, Shibahn, Shibani, Shibhan, Shioban, Shirvaun, Shivahn, Shivaun, Shobana, Shobha, Shobhana, Shovonne, Shyvonne, Sh'vonne, Siobahn, Sioban, Siobhana, Siobhann, Siobhian, Siobhon, Siovaun, Siovhan, Syvonne.**

SIRENA. *Greek, 'entangler'.* Sounds like Serena, but refers to the mythological sirens – half woman, half bird – who virtually sang men to death. Not a great role model for your little girl. **Sireena, Sirene, Sirine, Syrena, Syrenia, Syrenna, Syrina.**

SIRI. *Norse, diminutive of* **SIGRID.** Charming and lively Scandinavian name that strikes a positive chord for a modern girl.

SIRIA. *Spanish from Persian, 'sun-bright, glowing'.* Would undoubtedly be confused with the geographical Syria. **Seeria, Sirius, Syria.**

SISSY. *Diminutive of* **CECILIA;** *pet name for 'sister'.* Old-fashioned nickname for a sister, almost never heard today. **Cissey, Cissi, Cissie, Cissy, Sisi, Sisie, Sissee, Sissey, Sissie.**

SISTINE. *place name.* Sylvester Stallone used the name of the Vatican chapel, the site of Michelangelo's magnificent frescoed ceiling, for one of his daughters – an imaginative choice.

♂ **SKY.** *Nature name.* Hippyish, but bright and sunny nonetheless, and popular in the US.

SKYE. *Scottish place name.* The *e*-ending version deserves its own listing as the name of the picturesque island off the coast of Scotland, and it's by far the more popular spelling in the Top 100. **Ski, Skie, Skii, Skky, Sky, Skya, Skyy.**

SKYLA. *Variation of* **SKYLER.** Skyler meets Kayla

meets Kylee, making Skyla one supertrendy name.

♂ **SKYLAR, SKYLER.** *Spelling variations of* **SCHUYLER.** Newer, simpler forms of the Dutch surname Schuyler, stylish for both genders, and used by several celebs, including Sheena Easton. **Schuyler, Schyler, Skila, Skilah, Skye, Skyeler, Skeylur, Skyla, Skylar, Skylee, Skylena, Skyli, Skylia, Skylie, Skylin, Skyllar, Skylor, Skylyn, Skylynn, Skylyr, Skyra.**

♂ **SLATE.** *Word name.* Sleek colour name, though a bit flinty for a little girl.

♂ **SLOANE.** *Irish, 'raider'.* Upscale surname that would make a Ralph Laurenish choice. **Sloan, Sloanne.**

★**SNOW.** *Word name.* Brisk, fresh, evocative, strange – and magical. Haunting middle name choice. **Snowdrop.**

SOCORRA. *Spanish, 'one who helps'.* Popular Spanish choice that refers to the Virgin Mary, Our Lady of Perpetual Help – or *Perpetuo Socorro*. **Secora, Secorra, Socaria, Soccora, Sucorra.**

SOFIA. *Greek, 'the one who possesses wisdom'.* This name of a Greek saint and queens of Russia and Spain made a brief appearance in the Top 100. It's the choice of several celebs, including Felicity Huffman and William H. Macy. **Sophia.**

SOLANA. *Spanish, 'sunshine'.* Bright and warm. **Solande, Solanna, Solatia, Solenne, Soleil, Solena, Soley, Solina, Solinda, Soline, Souline, Soulle.**

SOLANGE. *(so-LAHNZH) French, 'with solemnity'.* Soignée French name that has never made it elsewhere, but would make a striking, sophisticated choice. **Souline, Zeline.**

SOLEDAD. *Spanish, 'solitude'.* Strong Spanish name that refers to the Virgin Mary (Our Lady of Solitude), it can combine well with the right Anglo surname. **Saledá Saledad, Soladá, Sole, Soleda, Soletá, Solitá.**

SOLEIL. *(so-LAY) French, 'sun'.* An attractive French word name that could be a sophisticated choice.

Names for Winter Babies

Christmas

December

Frost

January

March

Neva

Nevada

Neve

Neves

Nixie

Noel/Noelle

North

Snow

Valentine

Winter

Yule

SOLITA. *Variation of* **SOLEDAD.** A lace-hankie version that's not as fresh sounding as the original.

SOLVEIG. *Scandinavian, 'woman of the house'.* Terminally Nordic. **Sotvag, Solve.**

SONATA. *Music name.* Undiscovered musical form melodious enough to be a hit on the name charts.

SONDRA. *Variation of* **SANDRA.** Considered distinctive back when Sandra was stylish. **Saundra, Sohndra, Sondre, Sonndra, Sonndre, Zohndra, Zondra.**

SONIA, SONJA. *Russian and Scandinavian variation of* **SOPHIA.** Early continental import, well known in the 1940s via Norwegian skating movie star Sonja Henie, that has sailed back across the Channel, despite the rising popularity of other Russian names. **Sohnia, Sohnnja, Sondja, Sondya, Sonica, Sonida, Sonita, Sonna, Sonni, Sonnia, Sonnie, Sonnja, Sonny, Sonnya, Sonya, Sonyae, Sunya.** **International: Sonje** *(German).*

SONNET. *Word name.* Could there be a more poetic name? Actor Forest Whitaker chose it for his daughter.

SONOMA. *Place name.* This beautiful northern California wine-growing region in the US might inspire some parents. **Senoma, Sonohma.**

SONORA. *Place name.* More unusual and melodic choice than Sierra, but this Mexican state name may sound too much like Senora to work as a name.

SONYA. *See* SONIA.

★**SOPHIA.** *Greek, 'wisdom'.* Ancient name with a sensuous sound and high-minded meaning, chosen by several celeb parents, and heading up the Top 100 without losing any – okay, much – of its sophisticated beauty. A real winner. **Saffi, Soph, Sophee, Sophey. International: Sophie** *(French),* **Sofía** *(Italian and Spanish),* **Chofa, Chofi, Fifi, Sofi, Soficita** *(Spanish),* **Sofi** *(Swedish),* **Sonja** *(Norwegian),* **Sohvi** *(Finnish),* **Zocha, Zofia, Zosha, Zosia** *(Polish),* **Zsófia, Zsófika** *(Hungarian),* **Zofia, Zofie, Zofka** *(Czech),* **Sofija** *(Serbian, Croatian),* **Sofiya, Sofka, Sofya, Sonia, Sonya, Sonyuru, Sonyusha** *(Russian,*

Ukrainian), **Sofi, Sophoon, Sophronia** (*Greek*), **Safa, Safiyah** (*Arabic*), **Sofya** (*Turkish*), **Tzophiah** (*Hebrew*), **Sofie, Sophi, Sophy** (*Persian*).

★**SOPHIE.** *French variation of* **SOPHIA.** Sophie's the choice of many parents today (including Eric Clapton and Luke Perry), as Sophia's cuter, more irreverent near-identical twin – it's in the Top 10.

SOPHRONIA. *Greek, 'sensible, prudent'.* Way too weighty spin on Sophia. **Soffrona, Sofronia.**

SORAYA. *Persian, 'princess'.* The last empress of Iran made her exotic name famous in the Western world. **Suraya.**

SORCHA. (*SOR-ra*) *Irish, 'bright, shining'.* Popular Irish name unknown elsewhere – with a pronunciation that's far from obvious.

♂ **SORREL.** *Botanical name.* Fragrant herbal name that could make a sensitive, distinctive choice. **Sorel, Sorelle, Sorrell, Sorrelle.**

SOSIE. *Diminutive of* **SUSAN.** Kyra Sedgwick and Kevin Bacon chose this unusual diminutive for their daughter.

♂ **SPENCER.** *French, 'keeper of provisions'.* Yes, Spencer makes a plausible and powerful female choice these days, though still thought of as primarily for boys. **Spence, Spenser.**

SPIRIT. *Word name.* Spiritual names – Peace, Destiny – are becoming more popular, but this may be taking it too far.

SPRING. *Word name.* Doesn't sound half as contemporary as Summer. **Spryng.**

♂ **SPRUCE.** *Nature name.* Call us traditional, but for girls we still prefer flower names to trees.

♂ **STACY, STACEY.** *Diminutive of* **ANASTASIA.** A key peppy teenager in the 1970s, Stacy is now the mum. Consider Stacia, or the original Anastasia. **Stace, Stacee, Stacey, Staceyan, Staceyann, Staci, Stacia, Stacie, Staicy, Stasa, Stasee, Stasey, Stasia, Stasie, Stasey, Stasha, Staska, Stasy, Stayce, Staycee, Staycey, Staysie, Staysy, Steacy,**

Tacy, Taisie. International: **Stasya** (*Russian*).

STAR. *Word name.* Most parents today would prefer the softer Stella. **Staria, Starisha, Starla, Starleen, Starlene, Starlet, Starletta, Starlette, Starley, Starlight, Starly, Starr, Starre, Starri, Starria, Starrika, Starrsha, Starry, Starsha, Starshanna, Shatrish.**

STARLING. *Bird name.* Odd choice that was the original name of children's illustrator Tasha Tudor.

♂ **STEEL.** *Word name.* Strong, but cold and soap opera-ish. **Steele.**

★**STELLA.** *Latin, 'star'.* Following on the heels of Ella, Gabriella, Isabella et al., Stella manages to be both celestial and earthy at the same time. It's a popular choice among US celebs, and its star may rise higher here. **Estelle, Estella, Estretla, Steile, Stela, Stelle, Stellina.**

STEPHANIE. *Greek, feminine variation of* **STEPHEN.** Had more staying power than most female forms of a boy's name, managing to be feminine without being frilly, but is now fading fast from the Top 100. **Fania, Fanya, Phanie, Phanya, Stef, Stefany, Stefenney, Stefeia, Steffa, Steffaney, Steffanie, Steffenie, Steffi, Steffie, Stefinney, Stepahnie, Stepfanie, Steph, Stephana, Stephane, Stephanee, Stephani, Stephania, Stephanida, Stephanina, Stephanine, Stephann, Stephannie, Stephany, Stephene, Stepheney, Stephenie, Stephianie, Stephine, Stephney, Stephoney, Stevana, Stevena, Stevanee, Stevie, Stevey, Stevonna, Stevonne.** International: **Etienette, Stéfhanie** (French), **Stefania** (Italian, Greek, Polish, Russian), **Estafania** (Spanish), **Stefani, Stefanie, Stephanine** (German), **Stefa, Stefcia, Szczepanike** (Polish), **Stefka** (Czech), **Panya, Stepa, Stepania, Steanyda, Stesha, Steshka** (Russian), **Stefaniá** (Slavic), **Stefania, Stavra, Stamatios** (Greek).

♂ **STERLING.** English, 'of the highest quality'. One of those names, like Tiffany or Cash,

that's infused with money, but doesn't necessarily convey class.

STINA. Diminutive of **CHRISTINA.** Not-so-attractive short form of a lovely name. **Steena, Stena, Stine, Stinna.**

STOCKARD. English, 'tree stump'. Stockard Channing picked this strong, first name over her original, Susan.

♂ **STORM.** Word name. Asking for trouble. **Storme, Stormee, Stormey, Stormie, Stormm, Stormy.**

★ ♂ **STORY.** Word name. Imaginative choice with an uptempo Cory/Rory/Tori sound, perfect for the child of a writer – or anyone with a good story to tell.

SUE. Diminutive of **SUSAN.** Much-used mid-century diminutive, now fallen far from favour even as a middle name. **Sioux, Su.**

SUKEY. Diminutive of **SUSAN.** Eighteenth-century nickname that still appears occasionally as an alternative to

Suzy. **Soki, Sokie, Sukee, Suki, Sukie, Suky.**

SUKI. Japanese, 'loved one'. One of the most familiar and usable Asian names. **Sukie.**

♂ **SULLIVAN.** Irish, 'dark eyes'. Stylish and boyish but could work for a girl – especially one with brown eyes – though Sully is not the most appealing of nicknames. **Sully.**

SUMI. Japanese, 'elegant, refined'. Simple and, yes, elegant – until you think of the wrestlers. **Sumiko.**

SUMMER. Word name. First-wave word name, temperature (and rating) rising. **Somer, Sommers, Sumer, Summar, Summerbreeze, Summerann, Summerhaze, Summerine, Summerlee, Summerlin, Summerlyn, Summerlynn, Summers, Sumrah, Summyr, Sumyr.**

SUN. Korean, 'obedient'. But to Westerners, it just means that huge glowing orb in the sky. **Sundance, Sundee, Sundeep, Sundi, Sundip, Sundrenea, Sunta, Sunya.**

SUNDAY. *Word name.* Among the best of the day names, with its sunny opening syllable.

SUNNY. *English nickname.* Short form too reductive for a fully dimensional human. **Sonny, Sunnee, Sunni, Sunnie, Sunshine.**

SUNSHINE. *Word name.* A teenager would make you pay for this one. **Sunshyn, Sunshyne.**

SURI. *Persian, 'rose'; Hebrew, 'talk to the hand'; and a Nubian tribe name.* This once obscure exotic name hit the big time when chosen by Katie Holmes and Tom Cruise for their daughter. It also means 'the sun' in Sanskrit, and is the name of the Andean Alpaca's wool.

SURYA. *Hindi, 'sun god'.* Graceful Indian choice. **Suria, Suriya, Surra.**

SUSAN. *Hebrew, 'lily'.* Hugely popular mid-century name, common among mums and new grandmas now but rare for babies and way too early for a revival. Think Susannah instead. **Sawsan, Shu Shu, Sioux, Siouxsie, Siusan, Soosan,** Soosanna, Sosan, Sosana, Sosanna, Suanny, Sue, Suesan, Suesann, Suesonne, Sueva, Suezanne, Suisan, Suke, Sukee, Sukey, Sukie, Sonel, Sunel, Susanetta, Susanka, Susanna, Susannagh, Susannah, Susee, Susen, Susette, Susi, Susie, Suson, Susy, Suzan, Suzane, Suzanna, Suzannah, Suze, Suzee, Suzetta, Suzie, Suzon, Suzy, Suzzanne, Zanna, Zanne, Zannie. International: Suzanne, Suzette *(French)*, Susana *(Italian, Spanish, Portuguese)*, Susanita *(Spanish)*, Susanne, Suse *(German)*, Susann *(German, Swedish)*, Zuzanna *(Polish, Latvian)*, Zsazsa, Zsuzsa, Zsuzsanna, Zsuzsi *(Hungarian)*, Zuzana *(Czech)*, Syuzanna *(Russian)*, Suzana *(Slavic)*.

★**SUSANNAH, SUSANNA.** *Hebrew, 'lily'.* By far the most stylish form of the classic name now that Susan has retired. Susannah has New Testament and musical pedigrees, is impervious to trends, and has an irresistible, flowing rhythm. Can be spelled with or without the final *h*. **Sanna, Sannah, Shanna, Shoshanna, Shu Shu, Sonel, Sosana, Sue, Suesanna, Susana,** Susanah, Susanka, Susannagh, Susette, Susie, Suzanna, Zanna, Zannie.

SUSIE. *Diminutive of* **SUSAN.** In the 1950s and 60s, the name every little girl wanted for her very own. **Siouxsie, Susey, Susi, Susy, Suzee, Suzey, Suzi, Suzie, Suzy, Zuzey, Zuzi, Zuzie, Zuzu, Zuzy.**

SUZANNE. *French variation of* **SUSAN.** Became popular along with Susan, but has faded and almost disappeared. Wait a generation (or two). **Suesana, Susanna, Susanne, Suzane, Suzannah, Suzette, Suzzanne, Zanne, Zannie.**

SUZETTE. *French diminutive variation of* **SUSANNAH.** The name of the sexy French maid in a 1950s film – so kitsch it's almost cool again. **Susette.**

SVETLANA. *Russian, 'star'.* Popular Russian name, familiar elsewhere via author Svetlana Stalin, the dictator's daughter. **Lana, Sveta, Svetlanna, Svetochka, Svjetlana, Swetlana.**

SWANHILD. *Saxon, 'battle swan'.* This one will cause

Stellar Starbabies Beginning with *S*

Sadie	Joan Allen, Adam Sandler
Saffron	Simon Le Bon
Sage	Lars *(Metallica)* Hendrikson
Sailor	Christie Brinkley
Salome	Alex Kingston
Sam	Denise Richards & Charlie Sheen
Sameria	LL Cool J
Sascha	Jerry Seinfeld
Savannah	Marcia Cross
Scarlet	Jennifer Flavin & Sylvester Stallone
Scarlett	Jack White & Karen Elson
Scout	Tom Berenger, Demi Moore & Bruce Willis
Selah	Lauryn Hill & Rohan Marley
Shayne	Eddie Murphy
Shiloh	Angelina Jolie & Brad Pitt
Sistine	Jennifer Flavin & Sylvester Stallone
Skyler	Montell Jordan
Sofia	Felicity Huffman & William H. Macy
Solita	Geraldo Rivera
Sophie	Eric Clapton, Luke Perry, Gary Sinise
Spencer	Kelsey Grammer

trouble in secondary school. **Swanild, Swanilda, Swanilde, Swanhilda, Swanhilde, Swannie, Swanny.**

SWEDEN. *Place name.* Unlikely to make it on to the name map.

SYBIL. *Variation of Sibyl.* The most common spelling of a now-dowdy name, which the ancient Greeks used as the generic word for a prophetess. **Cybill, Sib, Sibbel, Sibbie, Sibbill, Sibby, Sibel, Sibell, Sibilla, Sibyl, Sibylline, Sybel, Sybella, Sybelle, Sybill, Syble. International: Sibéal** *(Irish Gaelic),* **Cybele, Sibylle, Sybilla, Sybille** *(French),* **Sibylla** *(Dutch and Swedish),* **Sybilla** *(German),* **Sybilla** *(Swedish),* **Sibilia** *(Slavic).*

♂ **SYDNEY.** *French, 'St. Denis'.* Anorak boy Sidney has become polished, poised, creative, elegant girl Sydney. On the rise since the 1990s and still popular. **Cidney, Cydney, Cydnie, Siddeny, Sideny, Sidneigh, Sidnee, Sidney, Sidni, Sidnie, Sy, Syd, Sydel, Sydelle, Sydna, Sydnee, Sydni, Sydnie, Sydny, Sydnye, Syndona, Syndonah. International:**

Sidaine, Sidonie *(French)*, Sidonia *(Dutch)*, Tzidoni *(Israeli)*.

SYLVANA. *Latin, 'from the forest'.* Sleek, woodsy European choice. Silvaine, Silvana, Silvanna, Silviane, Sylva, Sylvaine, Sylvanah, Sylvania, Sylvanna, Sylvie, Sylvina, Sylvinnia, Sylvonah, Sylvonia, Sylvonna.

SYLVIA. *Latin, 'from the forest'.* The musical, sylvan qualities of Sylvia have faded over the years, and the name is seen as middle-aged or older. The French Sylvie is a more attractive option. Silvaine, Silvania, Silvanna, Silvianne, Silvie, Sylva, Sylvana, Sylvee, Sylvian, Sylviana, Sylvine, Zilvia. International: Sylvette, Sylvianne, Sylvie *(French)*, Silva, Silvana *(Italian)*, Silvana, Silveria, Silvia, Silvina *(Spanish)*, Silwia *(Polish)*, Silivia *(Hawaiian)*.

SYMPHONY. *Word name.* Name that makes an overblown musical statement. Symfoni, Symphanie, Symphany, Symphanée, Symphoni.

SY'RAI. *Variation of SARAH.* This unusual name, created by the singer Brandy for her daughter, uses punctuation in an inventive way – a trend that takes creative spelling to a new but sometimes confusing level.

T *girls*

TABIA. *East African, Swahili, 'talents, gifts'.* Has a feminine feline feel.

TABITHA. *Aramaic, 'gazelle'.* Though never a popular choice, Tabitha has its own quirky charm – but be warned, it's also a common feline name. Tab, Tabatha, Tabbee, Tabbey, Tabbi, Tabbie, Tabbitha, Tabby, Tabetha, Tabi, Tabita, Tabotha, Tabytha. International: Tabea *(German)*.

TACI. *(TAH-shee) African, Zuni, 'washtub'.* One African choice that might be easier to understand if spelled phonetically. Tacee, Tacey, Tacie, Tacy, Tahcee, Tahcey, Tahci, Tahcie, Tahcy, Tahsee, Tahsi, Tahsy.

TACITA. *Latin, feminine variation of TACITUS, 'silence'.* This Roman mythology name for the goddess of silence has the ancient Roman feel now coming into fashion, as boys begin to have names like Atticus and Aurelius. Tace, Tacey, Tacia, Tacie, Tacy, Tacye.

TADITA. *Native American, Omaha, 'to the wind'.* Feminissima. Tadeeta, Tadeta.

Invented T Names

Tabora

Taisha

Taleesa

Talisha

Talitha

Taliyah

Tamia

Tamika

Tamiqua

Tamisha

Tamya

Tamyra

Tanesha

Tanika

Taquanna

Tashawna

Tawanna

Teesha

Terranda

Tianna

Tonika

Tonique

Tonisha

Tyana

Tyeesha

TAFFETA. *English, from Persian, word name.* A few boys have adopted fabrics like Denim and Suede; here's a singular one for the girls, with a distinctively silky sheen.

TAFFY. *Welsh, diminutive of* **DAVID.** This name has a hard time projecting anything but sweetness, sexiness and empty calories. **Taafe, Taffi, Taffie, Tavi, Tavita, Tevita.**

TAHIRA. *Arabic, 'pure and chaste'.* A pretty Arabic virtue name.

TAHITI. *Polynesian place name.* One of the most evocative geographical possibilities, conjuring up swaying palms and the brilliant palette of Gauguin.

TAHNEE. *Spelling variation of* **TAWNY.** Sounds Native American, but probably just an imaginative spelling of Tawny; used by Raquel Welch for her daughter. **Tahni, Tahnie, Tahny.**

TAIMA. *(tah-EE-mah) Native American 'crash of thunder'.* Traditionally given to children born during a thunderstorm.

♂ **TAJ.** *(tahzh) Sanskrit, 'crown'.* Cool new name with ancient Eastern roots.

TAJA. *(TAHZH-ah) Arabic, 'crown'; also Kiswahili, 'to mention, to name'.* Soft, sultry resonance. **Tajah, Talajara, Tejah, Tejal.**

TAKALA. *(TAH-ka-la) Native American, 'corn tassel'.* A name found among the Hopi people that could appeal to a wider audience. **Takalah.**

TAKARA. *Japanese, 'treasure, jewel'.* A lovely Asian relative of Tamara.

TALA. *Native American, 'wolf'.* Name with a creative, dark-haired image. **Talah, Talla.**

TALI. *Hebrew, 'dew'.* Friendly and relaxed choice used by singer Annie Lennox for her daughter; **Tal** is a unisex Hebrew version. **Tal, Talee, Talei, Taleigh, Taley, Talia, Talie, Talle, Tallee, Tallei, Talleigh, Talley, Talli, Tallie, Tally, Taly, Talya, Talye, Tylea, Tylee, Tyleigh, Tyli.**

★**TALIA.** *Hebrew, 'gentle dew from heaven'.* In tandem with its longer-form Natalia, this pretty Russian-flavoured name has been bounding up the popularity charts. **Tal, Tahlia, Taliah, Talila, Talja, Talya.**

♂ **TALIESIN.** *(tahl-YES-in) Welsh, 'shining brow'.* A name only an architecture-minded parent could love, because of its close association with Frank Lloyd Wright.

TALISA. *Modern invented name.* A new addition to the Tali family, associated with actress Talisa Soto. **Talicia, Talise, Talisha, Telisa.**

★**TALLULAH.** *Native American, 'leaping waters'.* With memories of the outrageous actress Tallulah Bankhead fading, this hauntingly euphonious Choctaw name has re-entered the public domain; used by Demi and Bruce and by rocker Simon (Duran Duran) Le Bon, plus other celebs. **Lula, Lulu, Tali, Talley, Talli, Tallie, Tallula, Tally, Talula, Talulla.**

TALLY. *Diminutive of* **TALIA.** Nickname sometimes heard on its own, sort of an updated Sally and playmate of Hallie. **Tali, Tallee, Talley, Talli, Tallie.**

TALMA. *Hebrew, 'hill, mound'.* A not particularly happy marriage of Thelma and Alma. **Talmah, Talmit.**

TALULA. *Native American, Choctaw, 'leaping water'.* See **TALLULAH.**

TALULLAH. *Irish, Anglicised variation of* **TUILELAITH,** *'lady of abundance'.* This old Irish name of two early saints is almost identical to the Native American Talula or Tallulah. **Tallula.**

TALYA. *Russian, diminutive of* **NATALYA;** *also spelling variation of* **TALIA.** *See* **TALIA.**

TAMAH. *Hebrew, 'innocent, honest'.* Gentler and much less frequently heard than Tamar. **Tama, Tamara, Tamora.**

TAMAKO. *Japanese, 'jewel child'.* Two similarly delicate names, Tamako and Tamaki, can be found in the Japanese community. **Tamaki.**

TAMALA. *African, 'dark tree'.* Would you really want to name your child after a Japanese anime film called *Tamala 2010: A Punk Cat in Space?*

TAMAR. *Hebrew, 'date palm tree'.* A rich, strong Old Testament name sometimes given to girls born on the holiday of Sukkoth, as palm branches were used to make the roof of the sukkah. **Tama, Tamah, Tamara, Tamarah, Tamer, Tammi, Tammie, Tammy, Tamor, Tamour, Tayma, Temira, Thama, Thamar, Thamer, Timi, Timora, Tmarah.**

TAMARA. *Hebrew, 'date palm tree'.* Adding a final *a* to Tamar lends it a more sensual Slavic tone, making it a more popular choice than the original. **Tamar, Tamarah, Tamarra, Tamary, Tamera, Tami, Tamma, Tammara, Tammi, Tammie, Tammy, Tamora, Tamra, Tamrah, Tamryn, Tamyra, Thamar, Thamara, Thamarra, Toma, Tomka. International: Mara** *(Czech),* **Tama, Tamarka, Tomochka** *(Russian).*

TAMARIND. *Arabic, 'date from India'.* Though spice names are in – Cinnamon, Saffron, etc. – this Indian spice from the pods of the tamarind tree would prove too cumbersome for a daily diet. **Tamarinda.**

♂ **TAMAYO.** *Japanese, 'generation jewel'.* Japanese name with a special crossover/creative touch via its association with the colourful paintings of acclaimed Mexican artist Rufino Tamayo.

TAMMY. *English, diminutive of* **TAMARA.** Made famous in 1950s movies as a wholesome backwoods gal, Tammy has now retired back to the woods. **Tami, Tamie, Tammee, Tammey, Tammie.**

TAMORA. *Meaning unknown.* Exotic name associated both with a queenly character in Shakespeare's *Titus Andronicus*.

TAMRA. *Indian mythology name.* Sounds as if you might have swallowed the middle *a* in Tamara.

★**TAMSIN.** *English, contracted form of* **THOMASINA.** Offbeat name formerly confined to Cornwall, now being revived, though beware that dated Tammy nickname. **Tamasin, Tamasine, Tammy, Tamsine, Tamsinne, Tamsyn, Tamzen, Tamzin.**

TANA. *Greek, 'fire or star goddess'; Ethiopian place name; Slavic diminutive.* Lots of multicultural meanings but little substance.

★**TANAQUIL.** *(tan-a-KEEL) Latin, meaning unknown.* This intriguing name of an ancient Etruscan queen is also associated with the prima ballerina Tanaquil LeClerq.

TANDY. *Native American, 'flower'.* Fresher sounding than Mandy or Brandy, but Thandie might be a more original way to go. **Tandee, Tandie, Thandee, Thandey, Thandie, Thandy.**

TANGERINE. *Word name.* We've had Apples, Plums, Peaches, Cherries and Berries added to the fruit basket: you could be the first to pick a Tangerine. **Tangerina.**

TANGIER. *place name.* Evocative of exotic Moroccan bazaars. **Tangiers.**

TANIA. *Spelling variation of* **TANYA,** *diminutive of* **TATIANA.** *See* **TANYA.**

TANIS. *Spanish, 'camp of glory'.* Obscure name found in Sinclair Lewis's *Babbitt,* a bit hipper than most other *is*-ending names like Janis and Doris. **Tanisha, Tannis.**

TANITH. *Irish, 'estate'.* Lispy. **Tanita, Tanitha.**

TANIYAH. *Modern invented name.* Synthetic name that's popular in the US.

TANSY. *Greek, 'immortal'; English flower name; diminutive of* **ANASTASIA.** A flower name rarer than Rose, livelier than Lily and less teasable than Pansy. **Tansi, Tansie, Tanzey, Tanzi, Tanzie, Tanzy.**

TANWEN. *Welsh, 'holy fire'.* A far more singular and colourful alternative to Bronwen. **Tanwyn.**

TANYA. *Russian, 'praiseworthy'; diminutive of* **TATIANA.**

Long integrated into the British name pool but still retaining some Slavic flavour, Tanya feels a bit tired; it's ready for replacement by cooler Russian choices like Sasha, Mischa or parent name Tatiana. **Tana, Tanazia, Tahnee, Tahnya, Taneea, Tania, Tanita, Tannia, Tarnia, Tarnya, Tawnya, Tonnya, Tonya, Tonyah.** International: **Tahnia, Tanja** (German).

TARA. *Irish, 'rocky hill'.* Despite a rich history in Irish myth preceding its plantation appearance in *Gone with the Wind,* widespread use in the 1970s caused Tara to lose its Irish accent. **Tarah, Tarra, Tarrah.** International: **Teamhair** (Gaelic).

TARAJA. *African, Kiswahili, 'hope'.* The *raja* sequence of sounds gives it a regal feel.

TARANA. *Hindi, 'one who uplifts'; Nigerian, 'born during the day'.* Both graceful and melodious.

★♂ **TARIAN.** *Modern invented name.* A distinctive name that could be an updated tribute to Grandma Marian.

♂ **TAROT.** *French, fortune-telling cards.* A unique New Age possibility with a pleasing sound.

TARRAGON. *Latin herb name.* Aromatic but also problematic.

TARYN. *Modern invented name.* An offshoot of Tara created in the Karen-Sharon Era that still appeals to some parents. **Taran, Taren, Tarin, Tarina, Tarnia, Taron, Tarren, Tarryn, Taryna, Tarynn, Tarynne, Teryn.**

TASHA. *Diminutive of* NATASHA. *See* NATASHA. **Tahsha, Tashey, Tashina, Tasia, Tasenka, Taska, Tasya.**

TASMINE. *Possible variation of* JASMINE. Probably better to stick with Jasmine – this one's a little too Tasmanian devil. **Tasmeen, Tasmeena, Tasmin, Tasmina, Tasmyne.**

♂ **TATE.** *Norse, 'cheerful'.* Though almost exclusively used for boys, we can see it as a stronger surname alternative to Kate. **Tait, Taite, Tayte.**

★**TATIANA.** *Russian from Latin family name.* A longtime popular name in Russia and starting to catch on elsewhere, this delicate and feminine name has a pleasing touch of the exotic about it. **Tania, Tanya, Tasha, Tata, Tati, Tatianna, Tatie, Tatijana, Tatiyana, Tatiyanna, Tatjana, Tatyana, Tiahna, Tiane, Tianna, Tiauna, Tionna, Tonya, Tusya.** International: **Tanja** (German), **Taina** (Scandinavian).

TATUM. *English, 'Tate's homestead'.* Strong, distinctive, energetic, and recommended, especially if your last name is as congenial as O'Neal.

TATYANA. *Spelling variation of* **TATIANA.** This alternate spelling definitely has its followers.

TAURA. *Latin, 'like a bull'.* A possibility for a girl born between mid-April and mid-May, but, if a name is destiny, its meaning does suggest stubbornness. Consider Laura, Flora or Honora instead.

Colour Names

Amber	Moss
Aqua	Navy
Ash	Raven
Auburn	Red
Azure	Roan
Blue	Rose
Burgundy	Russet
Cerulean	Sage
Citron	Silver
Green	Slate
Grey	Sterling
Indigo	Teal
Magenta	Umber
Mahogany	Violet
Maise	

TAVORA. *Hebrew, feminine variation of* **TAVOR**, *'break, fracture'.* An attractive option, based on the name of a mountain in northern Israel.

TAWNY. *English word name, 'golden brown'.* Y-ending colour adjectives like Tawny and Rusty are nowhere near as stylish as the more sophisticated Lilacs

and Violets. **Tawnee, Tawney, Tawni, Tawnia, Tawnie.**

TAYA. *Japanese, 'young'.* Has recently jumped into the mainstream name pool, perhaps because of kinship with Maya and Kaya.

TAYLA. *Spelling variation of* **TAYLOR.** Recipe for sudden – if brief – new name success: take two of the trendiest choices, Taylor and Kayla, stir, and voilà . . . Tayla, which started to become popular in the mid-1990s.

♂ **TAYLOR.** *English occupational name, 'tailor'.* One of the prime unisex surnames used for girls at the end of the twentieth century, Taylor is now oh so 1990s. **Tae, Taelor, Tahlor, Tai, Tailor, Tay, Taye, Taylar, Tayler.**

TAZU. *Japanese, 'rice-field stork'.* Has a certain snazzy appeal.

TÉA. *(TAY-a) Greek variation of* **THEA.** Brought into the mix by actress Téa (born Elizabeth Téa) Leoni, an attractive feminine option in the Mia/Lea mode.

♂ **TEAGAN, TEGAN.** *(TAY-gun or TEG-han) Irish, 'little poet'.* As Meghan/Megan and Reagan/Regan show signs of wilting, along comes Teagan to take up the slack: this is definitely one to consider. **Taegen, Taygan, Teegan, Tegin, Tiegan, Tigan.**

★ ♂ **TEAL.** *Bird and colour name.* One of the prettiest and most straightforward of the new colour names – an ideal middle name choice. **Teale.**

TEGAU. *(TEG-ay) Welsh, 'fair, pretty'.* This name of one of the most virtuous women in King Arthur's court is overpowered by pronunciation problems.

TEGWEN. *Welsh, 'fair, lovely, shining'.* Nowhere near as pretty as its meaning.

TEHILA. *Hebrew, 'praise song'.* Danger: might tend to sound like a mispronunciation of tequila. **Tehilla.**

TEMPERANCE. *Virtue name.* Unlike Hope, Faith, Amity and even Prudence, this is one early-American virtue name we don't ever expect to see again.

TEMPEST. *Word name, 'turbulent, stormy'.* Storm warning. **Tempeste, Tempestt.**

♂ **TEMPLE.** *English, 'dweller near the temple'.* Has gained some recent notice as a girls' name via autistic writer Dr Temple Grandin.

♂ **TENZIN.** *Tibetan, 'protector of Dharma'.* A name with special significance for Buddhists, being the first name of the Dalai Lama; it was chosen for his daughter by Beastie Boy Adam Yauch.

TEODORA. *(tay-o-dor-ah) Italian, Spanish, Swedish and Polish variation of* **THEODORA.** An extremely attractive and exotic choice, with several equally attractive, user-friendly nicknames. **Dora, Teda, Téo, Tey. International: Teodara, Tiodora, Tiodoria** *(Spanish),* **Teda, Teodory, Theadora** *(Polish).*

TERENCIA. *Roman clan name, feminine variation of* **TERENCE.** Let's leave this one packed away in the attic. **Tareena, Tarena, Tarina, Terancia, Terantia, Tereena,** Terenia, Terenne, Terentia, Terentila, Terentina, Terentine, Terenzia, Terocencia, Terrancia, Terrantia, Terrena, Terrentia, Terriell, Terriella, Terina, Terrena, Terrene, Terrentia, Terrin, Terrina, Terry, Teryl, Teryll, Teryna, Therena.

TERESA. *Italian and Spanish variation of* **THERESA.** *See* **THERESA.**

TEREZA. *Portuguese, Czech, and Romanian variation of* **THERESA.** A favourite in Brazil, with the *z* adding extra zest.

TERI. *See* **TERRY.**

TERRA. *Latin, 'earth'.* A video game *(Final Fantasy IV)* character with green hair, and a name that brings the outmoded Terry and Tara into the postmodern age. **Tera, Terah, Teralyn, Terrah, Tiera, Tierra.**

TERRI. *English, diminutive of* **THERESA.** *See* **TERRY.**

♂ **TERRY.** *English, diminutive of* **THERESA.** Terry was popular in the 1950s; it was seen then as a cool, sleek gender-neutral name, but it's long since lost that edge. **Terall, Terea, Teree, Tereigh, Terell, Terella, Terelynn, Teri, Terie, Terree, Terreigh, Terrey, Terri, Terrye.**

TERRYL. *Modern invented name.* Made-up name that tried to feminise Terry and copycat Sheryl. **Terelle, Teril, Terril, Terrill, Terryll, Teryl.**

TERTIA. *(TER-sha) Latin, 'third'.* An unconventional possibility for the third child in a family. **Tercia, Tersia, Tersha. International: Terza** *(Italian).*

★**TESS.** *English, diminutive of* **THERESA.** With its solid Thomas Hardy background, Tess has a lot more substance, strength and style than most single-syllable names, with an efficient yet relaxed image. **Tessa, Tessie, Tesza.**

TESSA. *Diminutive of* **THERESA.** Appreciated for its touch of the bohemian, Tessa is given to many babies each year. **Tess, Tessie, Tessy, Teza.**

TESSIE. *English, diminutive of* **THERESA.** With Tillie a new favourite of avant-garde parents, Tessie might conceivably follow. **Tessee, Tessi, Tessy.**

TETTY. *English, diminutive of* **ELIZABETH.** Commonly heard in the eighteenth century, but could cause secondary-school titters today. Consider Letty or Tessie instead. **Tetti, Tettie.**

TEVY. *Cambodian, 'an angel'.* A unique choice for your little angel. **Texanna.**

THADDEA. *Feminine variation of* **THADDEUS.** Although Thaddeus has long been used in this country, Thaddea is almost unknown and, with its air of mystery, could make a distinctive choice. **Tada, Tadda, Taddie, Thada, Thadda, Thadee, Thaddie, Thadine.**

THAÏS. *(THA-ees) Greek, 'beloved'.* A paramour of Alexander the Great and the heroine of a Massenet opera, this name is nothing if not dramatic. **Tais, Taisa, Taisse, Thaisia, Thaisis. International: Taisiya** *(Russian).*

THALASSA. *Greek, 'the sea'.* Another rarely used Greek name, this one with mythological roots. **Talassa.**

THALIA. *Greek, 'to flourish'.* One of the Three Graces in Greek mythology, and also the Muse of Comedy, this is a Hellenic choice well worthy of consideration. **Talia, Talie, Talley, Tally, Thaleia, Thalie, Thalya.**

THANA. *Arabic, 'praise'; Greek, 'death'.* Though the Greek meaning sounds ominous, the mythological god Thanatos was actually a jolly winged creature living in the underworld, so it shouldn't deter you.

THANDIE. *South African, Xhosa, diminutive of* **THANDIWE, *'loving one'.*** A captivating and sprightly name that makes a fresher alternative to the old-fashioned Mandy.

★**THEA.** *Greek, 'goddess, godly'; diminutive of* **ALTHEA** *and* **DOROTHEA.** Whether pronounced *THEE-a* or *THAY-a* or *TAY-a,* this name of the Greek goddess of light and the mother of the sun, moon and dawn presents an appealing artistic image, sensitive and serene. **Tea, Teah, Theia, Theolan, Thia, Tia, Tiah.**

THEDA. *German, 'people'.* The quintessential silent-film vamp name, rarely heard today. **Theida, Thida, Theta.**

THEKLA. *Greek, 'fame of God'.* New Testament name – Thekla was the first virgin martyr – with an unappealing sound. **Tecla, Tekla, Tekli, Telca, Telka, Thecla.**

THELMA. *Literary invention for a Norwegian character.* If you're desperate to honour an ancestor named Thelma, think Thea instead. **Telma, Thellma.**

★**THEODORA.** *Feminine variation of* **THEODORE.** One of the most revival-worthy of the charmingly old-fashioned Victorian valentine names, softly evocative but still substantial. **Dora, Ted, Tedda, Teddi, Teddy, Tedra, Tedre, Thaddea, Thadine, Thea, Theodora, Thekla, Theo. International: Feodora, Teodora** *(Italian and Spanish),* **Teodory, Teodozji** *(Polish),* **Fedora, Fedosia, Feodora, Theda, Theodosia** *(Russian).*

THEODOSIA. *Feminine variation of* **THEODORE.** Dig deeper in the attic and you'll find this even more antiquated name of several early saints, which has its own distinctive charm. **Docia, Dosia, Feodosia, Teodi, Theda, Tossi, Tossia.**

THEONE. *Greek, 'godly'.* A solid, somewhat serious Greek name. **Teofanie, Teofila, Teophania, Teophanie, Teophila, Theofania, Theofila, Theona, Theoni, Theonie, Theophanie, Theofila, Theophila, Theophile.**

THEORA. *Greek, 'a thinker or watcher'.* Soft and gentle, but feels like a less meaningful contraction of Theodora.

THERESA. *Greek, 'to reap, to gather'.* The popular appeal of the strong, intelligent Saint Teresa, combined with the selfless compassion of the more recent Mother Teresa, have fused to give this name a somewhat noble, religious image. It reached its peak in the 1950s and 60s. **Tassos, Tera, Terasa, Terecena, Teresse, Terezita, Teri, Terosina, Terri, Terrie, Terrill, Terry, Tersia,** Teskia, Tess, Tessa, Tessia, Tessie, Tessy, Thera, Tosia, Tracee, Tracey, Traci, Tracy, Treska, Tressa, Tressella, Zita, Zyta. International: **Treasa** *(Irish Gaelic)*, **Toireasa** *(Irish)*, **Tereson, Terez, Terezie, Thérèse** *(French)*, **Tereza** *(Breton)*, **Teresa, Terina, Tersa** *(Italian)*, **Techa, Tere, Teresita, Tete** *(Spanish)*, **Teressa, Tereza** *(Portuguese, Brazilian)*, **Resel, Resi, Therese, Theresia, Tresa, Trescha** *(German)*, **Terese** *(Scandinavian)*, **Teresia** *(Swedish)*, **Terese** *(Norwegian)*, **Renia, Terenia, Tereska, Tesa, Tesia** *(Polish)*, **Rezi, Riza, Rizus, Teca, Tercsa, Terez, Tereza, Terezia, Terike, Teruska, Treszka** *(Hungarian)*, **Tereza, Zizi** *(Romanian)*, **Reza, Rezka, Terezia, Terezie, Terezka, Terinka, Terka** *(Czech)*, **Terezilya, Zilya** *(Russian)*.

THÉRÈSE. *(tay-REHZ) French variation of* **THERESA.** Last popular outside of France from the 1920s to the 1950s, it now seems more modern than Theresa.

THIRZA. *Hebrew, 'delightful'.* This rarely used Old Testament name will inevitably set off a connection to thirst. **Terza,** Thersea, Therza, Thirsa, Thursa, Thurza, Thyrza, Tirtza, Tirza, Tirzah.

THISBE. *Greek mythology name.* This name of a beautiful but tragic lover in Greek mythology is thistly and prickly.

THETIS. *Greek, 'dogmatic'.* This name of the mythological mother of Achilles might suffer from its rhyming association to the word foetus.

THOMASA. *English, feminine variation of* **THOMAS.** One of those feminisations used in the seventeenth century but that has been lost ever since.

THOMASIN. *English, feminine variation of* **THOMAS.** Pre-Thomasina female form of Thomas, now seen as more literary and upscale.

THOMASINA. *English, feminine variation of* **THOMAS.** Rarely used now that many parents would rather appropriate men's names than sweeten them with feminine endings, but Thomasina does have some vintage appeal. **Tamanique, Tamasin, Tamasine,**

Names That Sound
Creative

Abra

Allegra

Anaïs

Brontë

Calliope

Dharma

Djuna

Electra

Gaia

Ianthe

Isadora

Magritte

Musetta

Story

Tessa

Thea

Thisbe

Zandra

Tami, Tammie, Tamsin, Tamzin, Tamzine, Tamzon, Thoma, Thomasa, Thomasin, Thomasine, Thomassine, Thomson, Tommi, Tommianne, Tommy, Tomsina. International:

Tamerlaine, Tamlane, Tammy *(Scottish)*, Thomasette, Thomasine, Thomassia, Tomasa, Tomasina, Tumajina *(French)*, Toma, Tomassa *(Italian)*, Tomasine, Tomasina *(Spanish)*, Tomsia *(Polish)*, Tamasa *(Eastern European)*.

THORA. *Norse, 'thunder goddess'.* Much softer and gentler than its meaning suggests. **Thodia, Thordis, Thyra, Tora, Tyra.**

♂ **THYME.** *(time) English herb name.* Not yet time for Thyme.

TIA. *Spanish, 'aunt'; diminutive of* **TIANA** *and* **TIARA.** A popular short and pretty name that has been in the Top 100 in recent years. **Thia, Tiana, Tiara.**

TIANA. *Slavic, 'fairy queen'; contemporary American variation of* **TATIANA.** Feminine name favoured by some parents over the past few decades. **Tia, Tiane, Tianie, Tianna, Tianne.**

TIARA. *Latin, 'crown, jewelled headdress'.* The perfect name-accessory for a little princess,

though its popularity is waning. **Teara, Tiarra.**

TIBBY. *Diminutive of* **ELIZABETH.** Cute and unusual as a nickname, but lacking the legs to stand on its own. **Tibbee, Tibbey, Tibbi, Tibbie.**

★♂ **TIERNEY.** *Irish, 'descendent of a lord'.* An uncommon Irish-accented surname that seems particularly well suited to a girl, as is the related Tiernan. **Tiernan, Tierneigh, Tiernie.**

TIERRA. *Spanish, 'earth'.* Earthy but ethereal Spanish word name that sounds a lot fresher than its sister Sierra.

TIFFANY. *Greek, 'God's appearance'.* One of the first luxury brand names, and the quintessential Booming Eighties status-conscious moniker; used by Donald Trump for his daughter, Tiffany has plummeted from its high since. **Teffan, Teffany, Thefania, Theophaneia, Theophania, Theophanie, Tifara, Tifaine, Tifany, Tiff, Tiffan, Tiffaney, Tiffani, Tiffanie, Tiffeny, Tiffney, Tiffy,**

Tiphanie, Tiphara, Tiphenie, Tipheny, Tyffany, Tyffenie.

TIJUANA. *(TEE-wan-a) Mexican place name.* There are more charming places – and place names – for your child.

TIKVAH. *Hebrew, 'hope'.* Appreciated by religious Jews for its connection to 'Hatikva,' the Jewish national anthem. **Tiki, Tikva.**

TILDA. *Estonian, diminutive of* **MATILDA.** Actress Tilda Swinton injected this dated nickname name with some modern charm. **Thilda, Thilde, Thildie, Tilde, Tildy, Tillie, Tilly.**

★**TILLIE, TILLY.** *English, diminutive of* **MATILDA.** A surprise recent hit revival and just nudging into the Top 100; Tillie is cute, frilly and sassy all at once.

TIMOTHEA. *Greek, feminine variation of* **TIMOTHY.** A tarnished relic not worth bothering to polish up. **Thea, Timaula, Timmey, Timmi, Timmie, Timotheya, Timothia.**

TINA. *Persian, 'clay'; diminutive of* **CHRISTINA** *and* **MARTINA.** Despite its petite and tinkly image, these days Tina is apt to be replaced by the more elegant originals. **Teena, Teenie, Teina, Tena, Tine, Tiny.**

TIPPER. *Irish, diminutive and variation of Irish surname* **TABAR.** The nickname of Mrs Al Gore (born Mary Elizabeth), bestowed because her favourite childhood lullaby was 'Tippy Tippy Tin', should remain her exclusive property.

TIRA. *Hebrew, 'small village'.* Tyra would be a more modern pick.

TIRZAH. *(teer-zah) Hebrew, 'cypress tree,' 'delight'.* A fairly common Hebrew name without much crossover potential. **Thersa, Thirsa, Thirza, Thirzah, Thursa, Thurza, Thyrza, Tierza, Tierzah, Tirza, Tyrzah. International: Tirsa** *(Spanish).*

TISA. *African, Swahili, 'ninth born'.* Tisa's too teasable.

TISH. *Diminutive of* **PATRICIA** *or* **LETITIA.** Tissue-thin. **Tisha, Tysh, Tysha.**

TITA. *English, diminutive of* **MARTITA** *et al.* A diminutive diminutive, too tease-worthy. **Teeta, Tyta.**

TITANIA. *(tit-TAHN-ya) Greek, 'giant, great one'.* This name of the queen of the fairies in *A Midsummer Night's Dream* has a delicate, lacy charm similar to Tatiana's. **Tania, Tita, Titaniya, Tiziana.**

♂ **TITIAN.** *(TISH-un) Italian artist name, also colour.* A creative choice, suggesting the Venetian Renaissance painter (born Tiziano), and the brownish orange red hue that was featured on his palette. It's a possible choice for a ginger baby.

TIVONA. *Hebrew, 'lover of nature'.* Hebrew name not often heard in other communities, but would have no trouble fitting in. **Tibona, Tiboni, Tivoni, Tivonit.**

♂ **TOBY.** *Diminutive of* **TOBIAS.** Early unisex name with a Shakespearean pedigree; when used for a girl it retains its tomboyish quality. **Taube, Taubey, Taubie, Thobey, Thobie, Thoby, Toba, Tobe, Tobee, Tobey, Tobi, Tobiah, Tobie, Tova, Tovah, Tove.**

TOINETTE. *(twon-et) French, diminutive of* **ANTOINETTE.** Tongue-twister.

TONI. *Diminutive of* **ANTONIA.** In the 1940s, Toni began to surpass its progenitor, Antonia, but today's parents would be better advised to reconsider the pioneer strength of the original. **Toinette, Toinon, Tola, Tona, Tonee, Toney, Tonia, Tonie, Tonina, Tony, Tonya, Twanette.**

TONIA. *(TOE-nee-ah) Diminutive of* **ANTONIA.** A more interesting and unusual shortening of Antonia than Toni. **Toni, Tonie, Tonisha.**

TONYA. *(TOHN-yah) Variation of* **TANYA.** This common variation of Tanya makes it less exotic and more ordinary. **Tonea, Tonia, Toniah, Tonisha, Tonja, Tonnia, Tonnya, Tonyia.**

TOPANGA. *Native American, 'where the mountain meets the sea'.* This name of a beautiful Southern California canyon in the US does have an unconventional aura.

TOPAZ. *Latin gem name.* As a name, it's sophisticated and sultry; as a golden gem, it's said to have soothing properties; and being the birthstone for November could make it perfect for a baby born in that month. **Topaza.**

TORA. *Japanese, 'a tiger'; Norse, 'thunder'.* Stands apart from other *ora* names like Nora and Flora via its aural association with the Jewish Torah. **Toril, Torill, Torille, Torez.**

TORDIS. *Norse, 'thunder'.* One of the less-likable feminisations of Thor, the Norse god of thunder, and perhaps a little to close to *Dr Who*'s Tardis.

TORI. *Japanese, 'bird'; English, diminutive of* **VICTORIA.** A more modern nickname for Victoria than Vicky, Tori is used fairly frequently on its own, kept in the public eye by singer Tori Amos. **Torey, Torie, Torree, Torrey, Torri, Tory.**

TORIL. *Norse, 'thunder'.* An unknown, strong Scandinavian name that would fit in perfectly elsewhere. **Torril, Torrill, Torryl, Torryll, Toryl.**

TORY. *English, diminutive of* **VICTORIA.** *See* **TORI.**

TOSCA. *Italian, 'from Tuscany'.* Tosca is one operatic heroine that has never taken off as a baby name.

TOTTY. *Diminutive of* **CHARLOTTE.** Too close to Potty. **Tottie.**

TOVA. *Hebrew, 'good, pleasing'.* Lively modern Hebrew name with a positive meaning. **Toba, Tobit, Tovah, Tovat, Tove, Tovit, Tuvit. International: Gittel** *(Yiddish).*

♂ **TRACY.** *French, 'of Thracia'; or diminutive of* **THERESA.** A popular choice in the unisex

1970s, these days Tracy would more likely be Gracie. **Trace, Tracee, Tracey, Traci, Tracie, Trasey, Treacy, Treasa, Treasey.**

♂ **TRAVELLER.** *Occupational name.* The kind of occupational name with an inspirational feel that's new now. **Traveler.**

TREASURE. *Latin, 'highly valued possession'.* Doting parents have begun to use names like Precious and Treasure, which are sweet for a baby, but might not hold up over the years. **Tesora, Tresor.**

TREENA. *English, modern spelling variation of* **TRINA.** *See* **TRINA.**

TRESSA. *Cornish, 'third'.* More unusual than Tessa, would make an interesting, meaningful choice for a third child. **Treasa, Tesa.**

TREVA. *Welsh, 'large homestead'; feminine variation of* **TREVOR.** Trevor with a New York accent. **Trevia, Trevina.**

TRICIA, TRISHA. *Diminutives of* **PATRICIA.** Back in Patricia's

mid-century heyday, Patty/Patti was the plebeian nickname while Tricia/Trisha and Tish/Trish carried a snobby-yet-insubstantial image. **Treasha, Trichia, Tris, Trisa, Trish, Trisha, Trisia, Trissina, Trysh, Trysha.**

TRILBY. *Coined by writer George du Maurier, 1894.* Literary character that fell under the hypnotic power of Svengali: not the best choice for an independent and self-determining daughter. **Trilbea, Trilbee, Trilbeigh, Trilbey, Trilbie, Trillby.**

TRINA. *Scandinavian, diminutive of* **KATRINA.** Nickname name that retains an Old Country feel. **Treena, Treina, Trena, Trine, Trinette, Trinita, Trinnette. International: Tríona** *(Irish and Scottish Gaelic).*

♂ **TRINIDAD.** *Spanish, 'holy trinity'; also place name of Caribbean island.* Rhythmic name with both religious and geographical ties, commonly heard in Latin countries. **International: Trini** *(Spanish),* **Trindade** *(Portuguese).*

TRINITY. *Latin, 'triad'.* It has gained in popularity after the release of *The Matrix,* whose heroine was called Trinity. Despite its spiritual meaning and euphonic sound, it's far from unique. **Trini, Trinidad, Trinidade, Trinita, Trinitee, Trinitey, Triniti, Trinitie.**

TRISHA. *English, phonetic respelling of* **TRICIA,** *diminutive of* **PATRICIA.** *See* **TRICIA.** **Tish, Tisha, Trish, Trycia, Trysh, Trysha, Tysh, Tysha.**

TRISTA. *Celtic mythology name, 'riot, tumult'.* This female form of Tristan has been a popular choice in the US as a new millennium Trisha. **Triste, Trysta.**

♂ **TRISTAN.** *Celtic mythology name, 'riot, tumult'.* Though Tristan was the male figure in the romantic legend and his name has become trendy for boys, it's used now for girls, too, much more often than the harder-sounding Isolde. **Tris, Tristain, Tristen, Tristin, Tristyn, Tristynne, Trystan, Trysten, Trystin, Trystyn, Trystynne.**

Names from Films

Amelie

Bonanza

Cadence

Chase

Clover

Domino

Elle

Ines

Jinx

Jude

Nola

Petal

Samara

Satine

Storm

Toula

Trinity

Zee

TRISTANA. *Celtic mythology name, 'sorrowful'.* A more substantial but less-popular feminisation of Tristan. **Tristanah, Tristanna, Tristannah, Tristen, Tristina, Tristine, Tristyn, Tristyna, Tristyne, Trystana, Trystanna.**

TRIXIE. *Latin, diminutive of* **BEATRIX.** Sassy, spunky name for the bold parent. **Trixee, Trixey, Trixi, Trixy.**

TRUDY. *German, 'spear of strength'.* Innocent, sincere, and bright-eyed, and as outdated as its mother name, Gertrude. **Trudi, Trudie.**

♂ **TRUE.** *Word name.* Inspirational, aspirational word name that would work especially well as a middle name; it was used by Forest Whitaker for his daughter. **Truely, Truly, Truth.**

TULIA. *Latin, 'destined for glory'.* Evokes colourful springtime tulips.

TUESDAY. *English, 'Tiu's Day,' for ancient Indo-European sky god.* When actress Susan Ker Weld changed her name to Tuesday, she opened up a whole calendar of possibilities. **Tuesdee, Tuesdy. International: Mardi** *(French),* **Martedi** *(Italian),* **Martes** *(Spanish),* **Kwayubi** *(Japanese).*

TULA. *Choctaw, 'mountain peak'; Hindi, 'a Libra'; Kiswahili,* *'to be tranquil'.* Polyethnic name which, spelled Toula, was used for the heroine of the hit film *My Big Fat Greek Wedding.* **Toola, Toolia, Toolya, Toula, Toulya, Tuliana, Tulya. International: Tulla, Tullia** *(Irish).*

TULIP. *Turkish flower name.* One of the most unusual flower names, cute but tough to pull off.

♂ **TULSA.** *American place name.* Unlike many other western city names in the US, Tulsa has not proved attractive to parents.

♂ **TUNDRA.** *Geographical name.* Icy. **Tunndra.**

TURQUOISE. *French, 'Turkish stone'; also a colour name.* Similar in hue to Aqua, which is one of the cool new colour names on the palette. **Turquois.**

TWILA, TWYLA. *English, 'woven with a double thread'.* Creative name largely associated with choreographer Twyla Tharp, it also has a pleasant tie to the word twilight. **Tuwyla, Twilla.**

♂ **TYLER.** *Occupational name, 'maker of tiles'.* Once-trendy name starting to fade for girls as well as boys. **Tyla, Tylah, Tyller.**

TYNE. *English river name.* Compact and creative. **Tyna.**

TYRA. *Scandinavian, feminine variation of* **TYR,** *an ancient Indo-European god.* High profile supermodel/entrepreneur Tyra Banks has put this name in the spotlight, endowing it with her confident, super-attractive image. **Thyra, Tyria.**

♂ **TYSON.** *English, 'firebrand'.* Appealingly boyish a decade ago, less so now.

TZOFIA. *(zo-FEE-ya) Hebrew, 'a scout of Jehovah'.* There are any number of Hebrew *Z* names beginning with a silent *T,* but, in this case, as with most others, it's an unnecessary complication. **Tzadika, Tzafra, Tzahala, Tzefira, Tzeira, Tzeviyam Tzila, Tzili, Tzina, Tzioira, Tzippora, Tzipporah, Tzofi, Tzofiya, Tzuria, Tzuriya, Zofia, Zuria.**

U girls

UDA. *Teutonic, 'wealthy'.* One of several three-letter *U-a* names – Uda, Ula, Uma, Una – take your pick. **Udele, Udella, Udelle, Yewdelle, Yudella, Yudelle.**

ULA. *Celtic, 'gem of the sea'.* See **UDA. Eula, Uli, Ulla, Ulli, Yula, Yulla.**

ULIMA. *(oo-LEE-mah) Arabic,* *'astute, wise'.* Unusual, exotic and just a little bit diagnostic. **Uleema, Ulema, Ullima.**

ULLA. *(OO-lah) Norse, 'will, determination'.* Ulla, the beautiful, tall, sexy, blond Swedish secretary in *The Producers* (played by Uma Thurman in the film) who purrs, 'Ven you got it, flaunt it,' has changed the image of this name forever. **Oula, Ula, Ulli.**

ULRICA. *Scandinavian, feminine variation of* **ULRIC.**

Doesn't exactly roll off the tongue. **Rieka, Rica, Ricka, Uhlrike, Ulka, Ullrica, Ullricka, Ulrika, Ulrike, Uulrica.**

ULTIMA. *Latin, 'end, farthest point'.* Name of a cosmetics brand, and sounds it. **Ulltima, Ultimata.**

UMA. *Sanskrit, 'light, peace, flax, turmeric'; also Hebrew, 'nation'.* A throaty, exotic name for a Hindu goddess . . . and a Hollywood one, whose father is a professor of Eastern religion. But as popular as Uma Thurman is, other parents have not picked up on her name. **Ooma.**

♂ **UMBER.** *Colour name.* A rich brown hue, but can be misheard as Amber, said with a pretentious accent.

UMBRIELLE. *Latin, 'one in the shadow'.* Pretty French sound, but there might be a lot of 'umbrella' cracks.

UMEKO. *Japanese, 'plum-blossom child, patient'.* Unfamiliar Asian choice. **Ume, Umeyo.**

UNA. *Latin, 'one'; also 'lamb'.* In an epic poem, the personification of truth, beauty, and unity; this ancient name is popular in Ireland but rarely heard elsewhere. The Oona spelling has more oomph. **Euna, Oona, Oonagh, Unah, Unna, Uny.**

UNDINE. *Latin, 'little wave'.* Mythological water spirit with the more common spelling of Ondine, heroine of an Edith Wharton novel. **Ondina, Ondine, Undeen, Undene, Undina.**

UNICE. *Variation of* **EUNICE.** Eunice is problematic enough. **Uniss.**

♂ **UNIQUE.** *Word name.* Finding a really distinctive name is a better way to stamp your daughter as a true individual. **Uinita, Unika, Uniqia, Uniqua, Uniquia, Unita, Unite, Unitee, Unitey.**

★**UNITY.** *English, 'oneness'.* Like Verity and Amity, this virtue name used by the British Mitford literary family is ready to join its more popular peers Hope, Faith and Grace.

URANIA. *Greek, 'heavenly'.* The name of one of the Greek Muses would be really difficult to bear here on earth. **Ourania, Ouranie, Urainia, Uranie, Uraniya, Uranya.**

♂ **URBAN.** *Latin, 'of the city'.* This name of eight popes might appeal to confirmed city-dwellers, but Urbana would be more feminine. **Urbana, Urbanah, Urbanna.**

URIELA. *Hebrew, 'God's light'.* That difficult *Ur-* sound cancels out the feminine appeal of the rest of the name. **Uriella, Uriyella.**

URSA. *Greek, diminutive of* **URSULA.** Better to stick with the name in full, as this sounds a bit too much like a crossword puzzle clue for a body part. **Ursey, Ursi, Ursie, Ursy.**

URSULA. *Latin, 'little female bear'.* Today's kids will probably associate this with the campy, corpulent octopus in Disney's *The Little Mermaid*, while their parents might consider it too Germanic, though it has a noteworthy literary background. It was recently chosen by novelist Plum (born Victoria) Sykes for her daughter. **Irsala, Irsaline, Orsa, Orsala, Orsel, Orsola, Ursa, Ursala, Urse, Ursela, Ursella, Ursely, Ursie, Ursilla, Ursillane, Ursley, Ursola, Ursulette, Ursuline, Ursy.** International: **Ursule** *(French)*, **Ursulina** *(Spanish)*, **Ulla, Urse** *(German)*, **Ursule** *(Romanian)*, **Vorsila** *(Czech)*, **Sula, Ulli, Urmi** *(Estonian)*, **Urzula** *(Latvian)*.

UTA. *(OO-ta) German, 'prosperity, riches'.* Medieval name that still hasn't crossed over elsewhere, perhaps because it's a bit harsh sounding. **Ode, Ude, Utako, Ute, Utte, Yuta.**

V girls

♀ **VAL.** *Diminutive of* **VALENTINA, VALERIE,** *etc.* Occasionally used as an independent name, but why?

VALA. *German, 'singled out'.* Mystical overtones. **Valla.**

VALDA. *German, 'battle heroine'.* Seventies comic-book-heroine-style name. **Val, Valdis,** **Vallda, Valma, Velda.**

★**VALENCIA.** *Spanish, 'brave, strong'.* Lovely orange-scented Spanish place name.

VALENE. *Modern invented name.* Downscale name with no history or character.

★**VALENTINA.** *Feminine variation of* **VALENTINE.** More exotic and artistic ballerina-type successor to Valerie; a pretty, recommended choice. **Teena, Teina, Tena, Tina, Val, Vale, Valeda, Valen, Valena, Valencia, Valene, Valensia, Valenteen, Valentia, Valenzia, Valera, Valida, Valina, Valja, Vallatina, Valli, Vallie, Vally, Velora, Valyn.** International: **Valentine** *(French)*, **Valentijne** *(Dutch)*, **Walentyna** *(Polish)*, **Bálintka** *(Hungarian)*, **Valya** *(Russian)* **Valeska** *(Slavic)*.

VALERIA. *Latin, 'strong, vigorous'.* This original form of the name, used by early Christians, more distinctive than the Franco-American Valerie. **Valeriana, Valerya.**

VALERIE. *French variation of* **VALERIA.** Valerie peaked in the 1960s, but still doesn't sound terminally dated; association with the word *valour* gives it a sense of boldness. **Val, Valaree, Valarey, Valari, Valaria, Valarie, Vale, Valeraine, Valere, Valeree, Valeri, Valerye, Vallarie, Valleree, Vallerie, Vallery, Vallorey, Vallorie, Vallory, Vallrie, Valora, Valorie, Valri, Valry.** International: **Valérie** *(French)*, **Valeria** *(Italian)*, **Valeriana** *(Spanish)*, **Valery, Valeska, Wala, Waleria** *(Polish)*, **Lera, Lerka, Valka, Valya** *(Russian)*.

VALESKA. *Slavic variation of* **VALERIE.** Strong, Slavic and spirited. **Valesca.**

VALETTA. *Latin place and surname.* This name of the major Maltese city has an air of attractiveness via model Amber Valletta, making it an appealing alternative to the overexposed Valerie and Vanessa. **Valeda, Valeta, Valletta.**

♀ **VALI.** *Norse mythology name.* Although a bold male figure in Scandinavian legend, this is

Names That Mean Brave or Powerful

Althea

Audrey

Baldwin

Bernadette

Briana

Bridget

Drusilla

Imara

Isa

Keren

Matilda

Maude

Neima

Rainey

Rita

Valencia

Valeria

more appropriate for a girl. **Valli, Vallie.**

♂ **VALLEY.** *Word name.* A natural phenomenon that makes a plausible baby name. **Vali, Vallee, Valli, Vallia, Vallie, Valonia, Vallonia, Valonya.**

VALORA. *Latin, 'courageous'.* Amazonian. **Vallora, Valoria, Valorie, Valory, Valorya, Valoura, Valouria.**

VANDA. *German variation of* **WANDA.** Brings to mind phrases like 'I vanda new bike' or 'I vanda go home'. **Vahnda, Vannda, Vanora, Vohnda, Vonda.**

VANESSA. *Literary invention; also a species of butterfly.* One of the ultrafeminine three-syllable hits of the 1980s, originally invented by writer Jonathan Swift, Vanessa has had more staying power than others like Tiffany, Kimberly and Melissa, due to its classic beauty. **Nessa, Nessie, Nessy, Van, Vana, Vanesha, Vanessah, Vanesse, Vanetta, Vania, Vanija, Vanna, Vannessa, Vannetta, Vanni, Vannie, Vanny, Vanya, Venesa, Venetta, Vinessa, Vonessa, Vonesse, Vonnessa.** International: **Vanesa, Venessa** *(Spanish).*

VANILLE. *(van-EEL) French, 'vanilla'.* While Vanilla might be too bland, the French version is more flavourful.

VANITA. *Modern invented name.* You're so vain, I bet you think this name is about you.

VANJA. *(VAHN-yah) Scandinavian, feminine variation of* **VANYA.** Russian Uncle Vanya becomes niece Vanja in Sweden: an intriguing switch. **Vania, Vanya.**

VANNA. *Diminutive of* **VANESSA** *or* **IVANNA.** Flimsier than either of the originals. **Vana.**

VARANA. *Hindi, 'a river'.* Soft and rhythmic.

VARDA. *Hebrew, 'rose, pink'.* Commonly heard in Israel, but elsewhere it could be an unusual way to honour Grandma Rose. **Vardia, Vardice, Vardiel, Vardiell, Vardina, Vardis, Vardit, Vardith, Vardiya.** International: **Vardar** *(French).*

VARSHA. *Hindi, 'rain'.* This Indian name with a Slavic sound definitely has potential.

VARVARA. *Russian, Greek, and Czech variation of* **BARBARA.** An interesting and appealingly exotic spin on Barbara, with a lot of charm and energy. **Vara, Varenka, Varina, Varinka, Varka, Varya, Vava, Vavka, Vavra. International: Várvara, Várvera** *(Spanish)*.

VASHTI. *Persian, 'lovely'.* This Persian name with an Old Testament pedigree has a warm Sasha-like feel. **Vashtee.**

VASILIA. *Greek, 'royal, kingly'.* Sweet, dainty name that's the feminine of Basil. **Vaseelia, Vasilija, Vasiliya, Vasillia, Vasilliya, Vasya, Vazeelia, Vazeeliya. International: Vasilisa** *(Russian)*.

VEDA. *Sanskrit, 'knowledge'.* A name with religious resonance, as the Vedas are the most sacred texts of Hinduism. **Vedis, Veeda, Veida, Veta, Vida.**

VEDETTE. *French, 'star, leading actor'.* In France, this would be like naming your child Star. **Vedetta.**

♂ **VEGA.** *Arabic, 'swooping eagle'.* Another astral name, this one relating to one of the largest and brightest stars in the heavens, is popular in Scandinavia. **Vaga, Vaiga, Vayga.**

VELDA. *Variation of* **VALDA.** *See* **VALDA. Vellda.**

VELMA. *Origin disputed, possibly diminutive of* **WILHELMINA.** Out playing bridge with Thelma and Selma. **Vehlma, Vellma, Vilma.**

VELOUTÉ. *French word name, 'velvety'.* An affected way of saying 'velvet' *en français.*

VELVET. *English word name.* Could a name possibly be softer or more luxuriant? But it does sound a bit like a favourite pony – or a high-class hooker. **Vellva, Velva, Velveina, Velvetta, Velvette, Velvina.**

VENDELA. *Scandinavian, meaning unknown.* Unusual name associated with gorgeous Swedish-Norwegian single-named model.

★ ♂ **VENETIA.** *Italian place name.* The name of the region encompassing Venice has a radiant, picturesque authenticity. **Vanecia, Vanetia, Venecia, Veneta, Venetta, Venezia, Venice, Venitia, Venise, Venita, Venise, Vennice, Vinetia, Vonitia, Vonizia.**

VENICE. *Italian place name.* The name of one of the most romantic cities in the world could easily find its way onto a British baby girl's birth certificate, one of the more enticing place names. **International: Venise** *(French)*, **Venezia** *(Italian)*.

♂ **VENTURA.** *Spanish 'good fortune'.* A California place name that could travel.

VENUS. *Latin, Roman mythology name.* The name of a heavenly planet and the Roman goddess of beauty and love was an intimidating no-no until tennis champ Venus Williams put an athletic, modern spin on it. **Venisa, Venita, Venusa, Venusette, Venusina, Venusita, Vinita. International: Venera** *(Russian)*.

VERA. *Russian, 'faith'; Latin, 'truth'.* The height of exotic fashion in 1910, but now almost impossible to picture embroidered on a baby blanket. Verity would be a better expression of truth today. **Veera, Verene, Verina, Verine. International: Varena, Veira, Ver, Véra, Verana, Vérane, Verania,**

Vériane, Veranina, Vere, Verena, Vreni *(French)*, Veradis, Veradisia *(Latin)*, Verana, Verbena, Verena *(Spanish)*, **Wera** *(Swedish)*, **Veera** *(Finnish)*, **Wiera, Wiercia, Wierka** *(Polish)*, **Verka, Verunka, Verushka, Viera** *(Czech)*, Verasha, Verinka, Verka, Verochka, Verusya, Vjera *(Russian)*. Vere, Verla, Verra *(Slavic)*.

VERBENA. *Latin, 'sacred foliage'.* This name of a showy, lemony plant makes an unusual entry into the name garden. **Verbeena, Verbeina, Verbina, Verbyna.**

♂ **VERDAD.** *Spanish, 'truth'.* A modern virtue name possibility.

♂ **VERDE.** *Spanish, 'green'.* Would it be easy being Verde? Easier than being Green. **Verda.**

♂ **VERDI.** *Latin, 'green'.* Embodies both colour and operatic style. **Verda, Veridian, Verne, Vernee, Vernie, Vernique, Vernita, Vernona, Virida, Viridis. International: Viridienne** *(French)*, **Viridiana** *(Spanish)*.

VERENA. *Latin, 'integrity'.* Pleasant but outdated. **Varena, Varina, Vereena, Verene,** Veruchka, Veruschka, Veryna, Vrini. International: **Verandia** *(Dutch)*, **Verina, Verine, Verinka, Verochka** *(Russian)*.

★**VERITY.** *Latin, 'truth'; virtue name.* If you love Puritan virtue names and want to move beyond Hope and Faith and even Charity, this three-syllable option is an interesting alternative to the New Age-y True and has great potential. **Veretie, Verety, Verita, Veritie.**

♂ **VERMILION.** *Colour name.* This vivid reddish-orange colour name is an undiscovered possibility – kind of a female equivalent of Cerulean for boys. **Vermillion.**

VERNA. *Latin, 'springtime'.* Verna may mean 'springtime,' but May or Spring is fresher. **Verda, Verne, Verneta, Vernetta, Vernette, Vernice, Vernie, Vernis, Vernise, Vernisse, Vernita, Virna.**

VERONA. *Italian place name.* Scenic place name with the added attraction of a Shakespearean connection. **Varona, Veron, Verone, Verowna.**

VERONICA. *Latin, 'true image'.* Veronica is both saintly (patron of photographers) and sensuous (Veronica Lake, *Archie* comics), and has been out of style so long it's beginning to sound new and novel. **Rana, Ranna, Roni, Ronica, Ronika, Ronna, Ronnee, Ronni, Ronnica, Ronnie, Ronny, Veera, Veira, Vera, Veranica, Veranique, Verinique, Vernice, Vernicka, Vernika, Verohnica, Verohnicca, Veronice, Veronicka, Veroniqua, Veronqua, Vonnie. International: Verenice, Verone, Véronique** *(French)*, **Veronika, Veronike** *(German)*, **Weronikia** *(Polish)*, **Verona, Veronika** *(Hungarian)*, **Verona, Veronika, Veronka** *(Czech)*, **Berenike, Veronike** *(Greek)*.

VÉRONIQUE. *French variation of* **VERONICA.** The seductive French version of Veronica has considerable class and chic. **Véro, Véron, Verona, Verone, Veronik, Veronika.**

VERVE. *English from French word name.* Vibrant and vital noun name recently chosen by one actress for her daughter.

VESPERA. *Latin, 'evening star'.* Said to refer to either Jupiter or

Venus, either of which would be preferable as a name. **Vespa, Vesperia, Vespira.**

VESTA. *Latin, 'pure'.* The name of the Roman goddess of the household is not recommended for your little goddess.

VEVINA. *Scottish, 'sweet lady'.* This unusual name found in Scottish poetry would make a distinctive Gaelic pick.

VIANNE. *French, blend of* **VIVIAN** *and* **ANNE.** A smooth and velvety Gallic choice first heard here as the heroine of the movie *Chocolat.* **Viane, Vianna.**

VICA. *(VEE-kah) Hungarian variation of* **VITA.** A particularly distinctive and dainty example of the life-affirming family of names. **Vicuka, Vicus, Vicuska.**

VICENZA. *(vee-CHEN-za) Italian place name.* This name of an architecturally glorious Italian city makes a romantic and evocative possibility. **Vicensa, Vicenzia, Vichensa, Vichensia, Vichenza.**

VICKY. *Diminutive of* **VICTORIA.** This once vivacious mid-century nickname is rarely used for modern babies. **Vicci, Vickee, Vickey, Vicki, Vickie, Vicqui, Vikkey, Vikki, Vikky, Viqui.**

VICTOIRE. *(vic-TWA) French, 'victory'.* Adds French flair to the somewhat tired Victoria.

VICTORIA. *Latin, 'victory'.* The epitome of gentility and refinement, reflecting the image of the long-reigning British queen, Victoria is a steadily used regal classic. **Tori, Toria, Torie, Tory, Toya, Vic, Vicci, Vickee, Vickey, Vicki, Vickie, Vicky, Victorie, Victory, Vikkey, Vikky. International: Bhictoria** *(Scottish Gaelic),* **Victoire, Victoriana, Victorin, Victorine, Victrice** *(French),* **Vittoria** *(Italian),* **Victoriana, Victorina, Vitoria** *(Spanish, Portuguese),* **Viktoria** *(German, Norwegian, Swedish, Bulgarian),* **Viktorie, Viktorka** *(Czech),* **Tora, Vika, Viktoria** *(Russian),* **Nike** *(Greek),* **Vika, Viki** *(Serbian).*

♀ **VIDA.** *Spanish, 'life'; diminutive of* **DAVIDA.** One of several life-affirming names, this one has been tied to several health products. **Veda, Veeda,** Videtta, Vidette, Vieda, Vita, Vitia.

VIEIRA. *Spanish, 'scallop'.* A vivacious Latin alternative to the super-popular Sierra.

★**VIENNA.** *Place name: the capital of Austria.* One of the most promising of the newly discovered European place names, with a particularly pleasant sound. Possible substitute for the rapidly climbing Siena/Sienna.

VIGDIS. *Norwegian, 'war goddess'.* Charmless. **Vigdess.**

VILLETTE. *French, 'small town'.* Charming Gallic name uncommon in France, and unknown here, with literary credibility as the title of a Charlotte Brontë novel.

VILMA. *Russian, diminutive of* **VILHELMINA;** *a Polish place name.* Not much to recommend this relative of Wilma; consider Willa or Willow instead. **Wilma.**

VINA. *Spanish, 'vineyard'; diminutive of* **DAVINA, LAVINIA,** *etc.* Occasionally

Cool Flower Names

Azalea

Bryony

Daisy

Delphine

Fleur

Flora

Iris

Ivy

Jacinta

Jasmine

Leilani

Lilac

Lily

Poppy

Primrose

Violet

Zahara

Zinnia

heard in the 1920s and 30s, along with siblings Bina and Mina; Vienna would be a more modern choice. **Veena, Veina, Vena, Vinetta, Vinette, Vinia, Vinica, Vinita, Vinya, Vyna, Vynetta, Vynette.**

VINCENTIA. *Feminine variation of* **VINCENT.** Vincenza would be a more user-friendly form in this country. **International: Vincence, Vincentine, Vinciane** *(French),* **Vincenza, Vinceta** *(Italian).*

♂ **VINNIE.** *English, diminutive of* **LAVINIA.** A winning, gold locket nickname name of the turn of the last century, though also a common nickname for Vincent.

VIOLA. *Latin, 'violet'.* Has several positive elements going for it: the rhythm of the musical instrument, the association with the flower, and its leading role in Shakespeare's *Twelfth Night.* **Vi. International: Viole, Yolande** *(French),* **Jolanta** *(Polish),* **Violka** *(Czech).*

VIOLANTE. *Greek and Latin, 'purple flower'.* Too close to violent. **Violanthe.**

★**VIOLET.** *Latin, 'purple'.* Soft and sweet but not shrinking, the Victorian Violet, one of the prettiest of the colour and flower names, was chosen by high-profile parents Jennifer Garner and Ben Affleck; has

begun a sure-to-be rapid climb to popularity. **Eolande, Iolande, Iolanthe, Jolanda, Jolande, Jolanta, Jolantha, Jolanthe, Vi, Violaine, Violanta, Violanthe, Viole, Violeine, Viollet, Violletta, Viollette, Vyolet, Vyoletta, Yolande, Yolane, Yolantha. International: Violette, Vyolette, Yolanthe** *(French),* **Viola, Violetta** *(Italian),* **Violante, Yolanda** *(Spanish),* **Orvokki** *(Finnish).*

VIOLETTA. *Latin variation of* **VIOLET.** A more vibrantly coloured, operatic form of Violet.

VIONNET. *(vee-oh-nay) French designer name.* This name of a famous Parisian fashion designer known for her sophisticated 1920s and 30s style could translate into a pretty British baby name.

VIRGILIA. *Feminine variation of* **VIRGIL.** This Shakespearean name is even more out of step than its male counterpart, but it may possibly be so far out it could make its way back in.

VIRGINIA. *Latin, 'virginal'; American place name.* The American state was named in honour of Elizabeth I, the 'Virgin Queen'. Literary influences include Virginia Woolf. **Geena, Geenia, Geenya, Genia, Genya, Ginella, Ginelle, Ginger, Gingia, Ginnee, Ginni, Ginnie, Ginny, Ginya, Jenell, Jenella, Jenelle, Jinia, Jinjer, Jinnie, Jinny, Vergie, Verginia, Verginya, Virge, Virgenya, Virgie, Virgine, Virginnia, Virgy.** International: *Gigi, Virginie (French),* **Gina, Ginata, Ginia** *(Spanish),* **Vegenia, Wilikinia** *(Hawaiian).*

VIRTUE. *Latin, 'moral excellence'.* The mother of all virtue names.

VITA. *Latin, 'life'.* Vital and vivacious, but not very much alive at this time. **Veeta, Vitel, Vitella, Vitia, Vitka.** International: **Vicuska** *(Hungarian).*

VITTORIA. *Italian variation of* **VICTORIA.** An appealing Italian alternative.

VIVA. *Latin, 'alive, living'.* Viva la bébé with this life-affirming name! **Veeva, Viveca, Vivva.**

★**VIVECA.** *Scandinavian, 'alive'; Teutonic, 'place of refuge'.* This is the most exotic and feminine of the *v* names meaning life. **Vivecka, Viveka, Vivica, Vivika.** International: **Vibeke** *(Danish).*

VIVI. *English, diminutive of* VIVIAN. This nickname name has more sass than substance. The Italian form Vivia has a bit more heft. **International: Vivia** *(Italian).*

VIVIAN. *Latin, 'alive'.* From the enchantress of Merlin in Arthurian legend to Julia Roberts's hooker in *Pretty Woman*, Vivian has a long and varied history; always strong, never overused. **Bibi, Bibiane, Bibyana, Vevay, Vi, Vibiana, Viv, Vivean, Vivee, Vivi, Vivianna, Vivianne, Vivie, Vivien, Vivyan, Vivyana, Vivyanne, Vyvyan, Vyvyana, Vyvanne.** International: **Bibianne, Viviane, Vivienne** *(French),* **Vivia, Viviana** *(Italian),* **Bibiana, Bibianna** *(Spanish),* **Viivi** *(Finnish).*

★**VIVIANA.** *Latin, 'alive'.* Lively and rhythmic version of Vivian heard in Italy and Spain. A vivid choice. **Bibiana, Bibiane, Viv, Vivianna.**

VIVICA. *Spelling variation of* **VIVECA.** Brought into the mix by American actress Vivica A. Fox.

VIVIEN. *Latin, feminine variation of once-male* **VIVIAN.** Vivien (Scarlett O'Hara) Leigh was born Vivian. *See* **VIVIAN.**

VIVIENNE. *French variation of* **VIVIAN.** An elaborated Gallic version of the name, chosen by Rosie O'Donnell for her daughter.

VIVIETTE. *French variation of* **VIVIAN.** Embroidered lace hankie of a name, used in a Thomas Hardy novel.

★ ♂ **VRAI.** *French word name, 'true'.* A happy combination of several desirable genres: it's a word name, it has a foreign accent and it has a highly virtuous meaning. And few other parents will be bold enough to choose it.

W *girls*

WALBURGA. *German, 'strong protection'.* Not even if you were certain your daughter would be gorgeous, popular and very, very self-confident. **Walberga, Wallburga, Walpurgis.**

WALDA. *German, 'ruler'.* Where's Walda? Out of the running. **Waldena, Waldette, Waldina, Waldine, Walida, Wallda, Welda, Wellda.**

♂ **WALKER.** *English occupational name, 'cloth walker'.* A name on the rise for boys, but it hasn't hit yet for girls. **Wallker.**

WALLIS. *Variation of* **WALLACE.** Famously borne by the woman for whom an English king sacrificed his throne, it has the force of a masculine name with a distinctive spelling to set it apart from the boys. Anthony Edwards revived it for his daughter. **Walless, Wallie, Walliss, Wally, Wallys.**

WANDA. *Slavic, 'shepherdess'; German, 'wanderer'.* Rarely heard, and when it is, usually attached to a witch. **Vanda, Wahnda, Wandah, Wandely, Wandie, Wandis, Wandy, Wandzia, Wannda, Wenda, Wendaline, Wendall, Wendeline, Wendy, Wohnda, Wonda, Wonnda.**

WANETA. *Native American, 'charger'.* Try Juanita. **Waneeta,** Wanita, Wanite, Wanneta, Waunita, Wonita, Wonnita, Wynita.

♂ **WAVERLY.** *English, 'meadow of quivering aspens'.* With literary resonance and a lilting three-syllable sound, this could ride the next wave of unisex names. **Waverley, Waverli, Wavierlee.**

♂ **WELCOME.** *Word name.* Warm and open, but way too much teasing potential. **Wellcome.**

WENDY. *Literary name.* Famously coined for the heroine of *Peter Pan,* Wendy's heyday was once upon a time; it's now seen as bouncy and peppy – the perfect name for a babysitter. **Wenda, Wendaline, Wende, Wendee, Wendeline, Wendey, Wendi, Wendie, Wendye, Windy, Wuendy.**

★ ♂ **WEST.** *Word name.* Straightforward yet romantic, this is one newly minted name with long-term appeal, especially as a middle name. It was used as such for Téa Leoni and David Duchovny's Madelaine, whom they call West. **Wester, Westerlee, Westerleigh, Westerly.**

♂ **WHARTON.** *English, 'farm near the river'.* Stuffy banker name that becomes creative as a middle name choice for lovers of the novels of writer Edith.

WHITLEY. *English, 'white meadow'.* Eighties spin on megapopular Whitney. **Whit, Whitelea, Whitely, Whitlea, Whitlee, Whitleigh, Whitlie, Whittley.**

♂ **WHITNEY.** *English, 'white island'.* Yesterday's sensation that rose with the popularity of Whitney Houston. **Whiteney, Whitne, Whitné, Whitnea, Whitnee, Whitneigh, Whitni, Whitnie, Whitny, Whitnye, Whittaney, Whittany, Whittney, Whittnie, Whytne, Whytney, Witney.**

WHIZDOM. *Spelling variation of* **WISDOM.** Outlandish configuration used by one American celeb.

WILFREDA. *English, 'purposeful peace'.* A hopeless anorak. **Wilfridda, Wilfrieda.**

WILHELMIINA. *German, feminine variation of* **WILHELM.** Burdened with the Old Dutch opera-singer image of thick blond plaits and clunky wooden clogs. **Billa, Billee, Billey, Billi, Billie, Billy, Min, Minnie, Minny, Welma, Wilhelma, Willa, Willabella, Willabelle, Willamine, Willeen, Willene, Willemina, Willetta, Willette, Williamina, Willie, Williebelle, Willmina, Willmine, Willy, Willybella, Wilmette, Wilmina, Wilna, Wimina, Wylma.** *International:* **Willamina, Wilma** *(Scottish),* **Guillaumette, Guillaumine, Guilette, Mimi, Minette, Wilhelmine** *(French),* **Guillerma, Guillermina, Guilla, Ilma, Mini, Vilma** *(Spanish),* **Helma, Helmine, Mina, Minchen, Minna, Wilhelmine** *(German),* **Vilhelmina** *(Swedish),* **Mini, Valma** *(Finnish),* **Mina, Minka** *(Polish),* **Vilma** *(Czech, Hungarian, Russian, Swedish).*

★**WILLA.** *Feminine variation of* **WILLIAM.** Increasingly fashionable, with its combination of Willa Cather-like pioneer strength and the graceful beauty of the willow tree.

WILLOW. *Nature name.*

Names Sure to Shock Grandma

Ace	Lucida
Adecyn	Macen
Annistyn	Merrigan
Brycin	Raiden
Brylie	Ramses
Capri	Ryo
Clor	Snow
Colt	Tequila
Cyder	Tycen
Explorer	Vegas
Golden	Wellesley
Grande	West
Jantzen	Whizdom
Kodiak	Xen
Legend	Zeus

Elegant and charming nature name chosen for their daughter by Will Smith and Jada Pinkett Smith. **Willo, Willough, Willoughby.**

WILMA. *Diminutive of* **WILHELMINA.** Eternally fossilised in Bedrock as Fred Flintstone's wife. **Valma, Vilma, Williemae, Wilmanie, Wilmayra,**

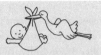
Wilmetta, Wilmette, Wilmina, Wilmyne, Wylma.

WINDY. _English, 'windy'._ And her sisters, Stormy and Sunny. **Windee, Windey, Windi, Windie, Wyndee, Wyndy.**

WINIFRED. _Welsh, 'holy peacemaking, gentle friend'._ One of those once prissy-sounding names that's just far out enough to be in, with the sassy nickname Winnie to further enliven it. **Fred, Freda, Freddie, Freddy, Fredi, Fredy, Wenfreda, Wennafred, Win, Wina, Winafred, Winefred, Winefride, Winefried, Winfred, Winfreda, Winfrieda, Winiefrida, Winifreda, Winifrid, Winifrida, Winifryd, Winnafred, Winne, Winnefred, Winnie, Winniefred, Winnifred, Winnifrid, Wynafred, Wynette,** Wynifred, Wynn, Wynne, Wynnifred.

WINNIE. _English diminutive of_ **WINIFRED.** This pet form of such names as Winifred and Edwina has a lot of vintage charm, à la Milly and Maisie; but also has the Winnie the Pooh association. **Wina, Winne, Winney, Winni, Winny, Wynnie.**

WINOLA. _German, 'charming friend'._ Native American feel via similarity to Winona. **Wynola.**

WINONA. _Sioux Indian, 'firstborn daughter'; Minnesota place name._ Rode two rockets to fame, with actress Winona Ryder. **Wanano, Wenona, Wenonah, Winnie, Winnona, Winoena, Winonah, Wynnona, Wynona.**

WINSOME. _English, 'agreeable, lighthearted'._ Sweet, modern descriptive name, but perhaps a little too cute for its own good. **Wynsome.**

♂ **WINTER.** _Word name._ Fresher than Summer or Autumn. But we like Snow even more. **Wintar, Wintr, Wynter.**

♂ **WISDOM.** _Virtue name._ Better than Whizdom _(see above),_ but still a bit too self-congratulatory. Exceedingly rare.

WISTERIA. _Flower name._ Frilly flower name with less potential than many other floral choices. **Wistaria.**

♂ **WREN.** _Bird name._ This lilting songbird name could be the next Robin, and for architects there's the link to the great Sir Christopher Wren. **Wrenn.**

★ ♂ **WYLIE.** _Scottish, diminutive of_ **WILLIAM.** One Celtic surname with as much appeal for girls as for boys.

★ ♂ **WYNN.** _Welsh, 'fair, pure'._ Attractive unisex Welsh name, especially worth considering as a winning middle name. **Win,**

Winn, Winne, Winnie, Winny, Wyn, Wynette, Wynne.

♂ **WYOMING.** *Place name.* A possibility for your li'l cowgirl.

X *girls*

Note: as a general rule, most names starting with *X* are pronounced with a *Z* sound.

XABRINA. *Spelling variation of* **SABRINA.** *See* **SABRINA.**

XANDRA. *(ZAN-dra) Spanish, diminutive of* **ALEXANDRA.** Like most *X* names, pronunciation would surely be a problem for other kids – at least until they're able to say and spell *xylophone.* **Zandra.**

XANTHE. *(ex-AHN-theh or ZAN-theh) Greek, 'golden, yellow'.* This Cynthia-equivalent conjures up an image of an exotic, otherworldly being. **Xantha, Xanthia, Xanthipe, Zanthe.**

XANTHO. *(ZAN-tho) Greek, 'golden-haired one'.* The ethereal name of a Greek mythology sea nymph.

XAVIERA. *(zah-vee-AIR-ah) Feminine variation of* **XAVIER.** Will have spicy associations for the older generation via author of the 1972 bestseller, *The Happy Hooker.* **Exaviera, Exavyera, Xavienna, Xavierre, Xavyera, Xevera, Xeveria, Zaveeyera, Zaviera.** International: **Xaverie, Xavière** *(French),* **Javiera** *(Spanish),* **Xabiera** *(Basque).*

XENA. *(ZEE-na) Greek, 'guest'.* Still projects the potent allure of television's warrior princess.

XENIA. *(ZEEN-ee-ah) Greek, 'hospitable, welcoming'.* The name of a Christian saint and a city in Ohio in the US, one of the more accessible *x* names. **Xeenia, Xene, Xia, Xiomara, Zeena, Zenam, Zina, Zyna.** International: **Chimene** *(French),* **Aksiniya, Ksenia, Oksanochka** *(Russian),* **Oksana, Xena, Zena, Zenda, Zene, Zenia, Zenina, Zenna** *(Ukranian).*

XENOBIA. *Greek, 'of Zeus'.* As long as nobody connects it with xenophobia – the fear of strangers and the unknown.

Unusual International Choices

Antonella
Apollonia
Aziza
Cai
Chiara
Cylia
Daru
Eliana
Eluned
Faizah
Federica
Fiorella
Graziella
Iman
Inaya
Izara
Kalila
Kalindi
Ottoline
Romane
Saskia
Savita
Siri
Xanthe
Xia

XIA. *(ZEE-uh) Chinese dynastic name.* This name of the first recorded dynasty of ancient China is short and simple enough to make a possible Asian-British alternative to Mia and Tia.

XIAMARA. *(zee-ah-MAH-ra) Aramaic, 'joyful deer'.* The longer form of Xia is more rhythmic but also more problematic. **Tzia, Xia. International: Tziamara** *(Eastern European),* **Tziamarnit** *(Hebrew).*

XIMENIA. *Spanish nature name.* For any parents out there searching for a nature name starting with *x* – and we doubt there are many – this one, named for a Spanish monk called Ximenes, is a small tropical plant bearing wild limes. **Chimene, Ximena.**

XIN. *(Shing) Chinese, 'beautiful, elegant'.* A lovely name, but unfathomable outside the Chinese community.

XUXU. *(SHOO-sha). Portuguese diminutive of* **SUSAN.** Made known in South America by a popular children's TV show presenter; cute but prohibitive here.

XOIS. *(zoh-us) African place name.* This name of the capital of an ancient Egyptian dynasty makes Lois X-rated.

Y *girls*

YADIRA. *Hebrew, 'friend'.* Feminine name consistently popular in the Latino community. **Yadirah, Yadirha, Yadyra.**

YAEL. *(yah-ehl) Hebrew, 'mountain goat'.* Old Testament name often heard in Israel that could work well elsewhere: just remember that it's pronounced with two syllables . . . and ignore the goat connection. **Jael, Yaala, Yaalat, Yaalit, Yaeli, Yaella, Yale, Yeala, Yeela.**

YAFFA. *Hebrew, 'beautiful'.* A modern Hebrew translation of Shayna, the Yiddish word for 'beautiful,' and commonly heard in Israel. **Yafa, Yafeal, Yaffit, Yafit.**

YALENA. *Greek and Russian variation of* **HELEN.** Exotic Slavic twist on a classic.

YAMINA. *Arabic, 'right, proper'.* Attractive Middle Eastern choice used in a variety of spellings. **Yaminah, Yamini, Yemina, Yeminah, Yemini.**

YANA. *Slavic variation of* **JANA.** A Slavic classic, as common as Jane or Joan here. **Yanae, Yanah, Yanay, Yanaye, Yanesi, Yanet, Yaneth, Yaney, Yani, Yanik, Yanina, Yanis, Yanisha, Yanitza, Yanixia, Yanna, Yannah, Yanni, Yannica, Yannick, Yannina.**

YASMEEN. *Persian, 'jasmine flower'.* One of the less frequently seen spellings of this popular name. **Jasmeen, Jasmin, Jasmine, Yasiman, Yasmine.**

YASMIN. *Persian, 'jasmine flower'.* This name, whose sweet and fragrant floral essence has always been widespread across the Near Eastern world has been in the Top 100 in the UK in recent years. **Yashmine, Yasiman, Yasimine, Yasma, Yasmain, Yasmaine, Yasmeen, Yasmina, Yasminda, Yasmine, Yasmon, Yasmyn, Yazmin, Yesmean, Yesmeen, Yesmin, Yesmina, Yesmine, Yesmyn.**

♂ **YEARDLEY.** *English, 'fenced meadow'.* Yeardley (born Martha) Smith is the unusual name of the voice of Lisa Simpson; not advised unless your surname is Smith or Jones. **Yardley.**

YEHUDIT. *Hebrew variation of* **JUDITH.** Stuck in the Old Country. **Yudit, Yudita, Yuta.**

YEKATERINA. *Russian variation of* **KATHERINE.** An overly elaborate version for use in this country. **Katya, Katinka, Katusha.**

YELENA. *Russian variation of* **HELEN.** One of many exotic versions of this classic. **Nelya, Yeleana, Yelen, Yelenna, Yelenne, Yelina, Ylena, Ylenia, Ylenna.**

YESENIA. *Arabic, 'flower'.* Hispanic favourite popularised by a character on a Spanish-language soap opera. **Yasenya, Yecenia, Yesinia, Yesnia, Yessenia.**

YETTA. *Yiddish, 'light'.* Too close to *yenta.* **Yette, Yitta, Yitty.**

YNEZ. *(ee-nez) Spanish variation of* **AGNES.** *See* **INEZ. Ynes, Ynesita.**

YOKO. *Japanese, 'good girl'.* There are many in Japan, but for most British people there's only one Yoko. **Yo.**

YOLANDA. *Greek, 'violet flower'.* Conjures up visions of mid-century films like *Yolanda and the Thief,* complete with gauzy veils, harem pants and invisible navels. **Yalanda, Yolaine, Yolana, Yoland, Yolane, Yolanna, Yolantha, Yolanthe, Yolette, Yolie, Yolonda, Yorlanda, Youlanda, Yulanda, Yulonda.** International: Iolanthe, Yolande *(French),* **Jolanda** *(Italian and Danish),* **Iola, Iolanda, Jolan, Jolana, Jolanta, Yola, Yoli** *(Spanish),* **Jolande, Yolande** *(Swedish),* **Jolante** *(Norwegian),* **Jolanta, Jola** *(Polish),* **Jolana, Jolanta** *(Czech),* **Jolán** *(Hungarian),* **Jólan, Jolanka, Joli** *(Eastern European),* **Iolanda, Iolande** *(Greek).*

YORI. *Japanese, 'reliable'.* An appealing, usable Japanese choice, since there are so many familiar *ori/ory*-ending Western names. **Yoriko, Yoriyo.**

YOSHI. *Japanese, 'good, respectful'.* Popular name in Japan, wouldn't work too well outside that culture. **Yoshie, Yoshiko, Yoshiyo.**

YSABEL. *Spanish variation of* **ISABEL.** Original spelling of this ever-more-popular name. **Ysabell, Ysabella, Ysabelle, Ysbel, Ysbella, Ysobel.**

YSEULT. *(ee-solt) Irish, 'fair, light-skinned'.* Variation of Isolde, the name of a great Celtic heroine. **Isolde, Isolt, Iseult, Yseulte, Ysolt.**

YUDITA. *Russian variation of* **JUDITH.** The original is so out of style that this old-fashioned version sounds almost cool. **Yudit, Yudith, Yuditt.**

YUKI. *Japanese, 'snow'.* An appealing Asian name with a nickname feel. **Yukie, Yukiko, Yukiyo.**

YVETTE. *French variation of Yvonne.* Sixties sexpot name not ready for a comeback. **Yavette, Yevett, Yevetta, Yevette, Yvet, Yveta, Yvett, Yvetta.**

YVONNE. *French, 'yew wood'.* Conjures up visions of green eye shadow and leopard-printed polyester. **Evon, Evonne, Vonni,**

Vonnie, Vonny, Yavanda, Yavanna, Yavanne, Yavonda, Yavonna, Yavonne, Yveline, Yvon, Yvone, Yvonna, Yvonnah, Yvonnia, Yvonnie, Yvonny. International: Ibane, Ibona (*Basque*), Ivone (*Portuguese*), Iwona, Iwonka (*Polish*), Ivona (*Russian*).

Z girls

ZABANA. *Native American, 'meadow'*. Has a nice exotic but outdoorsy, beachy cabana feel.

ZADA. *(ZAH-dah) Arabic, 'fortunate, prosperous'*. An exotic choice, popular in Syria. In Yiddish, pronounced *ZAE-dah*, this is a term for grandfather. Zadah, Zadie, Zaida, Zayda, Zayeeda.

ZADIE. *Variation of* SADIE. When aspiring writer Sadie Smith decided to change her name to Zadie at the age of fourteen, this attention-magnet name was born.

ZAFIRA. *Arabic, 'to succeed'*. Has a gem-like glow, as in Sapphire. Zafira.

ZAGORA. *North African place name; also Swahili*. If you're looking for an African place name, this one belongs to the main town in eastern Morocco.

★ZAHARA. *Hebrew, 'to shine'; Swahili, 'flower'*. This delicate but strong multicultural name came into the spotlight when Angelina Jolie bestowed it on her Ethiopian-born daughter, and we predict many other parents will adopt it as well. Zaha, Zahar, Zahari, Zaharit, Zaher, Zahir, Zahira, Zahra, Zakit.

ZAHAVA. *Modern Hebrew name*. This is a Hebrew word name, created from the word *zahav*, meaning gold. Zachava, Zachavah, Zahavah, Zechava, Zehavah, Zehavit.

ZAHIRA. *Arabic, 'shining' or 'flower'*. A pretty choice, sometimes heard in Latin countries, related to Zahara. Zaheera, Zahirah, Zahirita.

ZAHRA. *Arabic, 'flower'*. Abbreviated form of Zahara that was used by Chris Rock for his daughter and as a middle name by both Eddie Murphy and

David Bowie. Zahara, Zaharah, Zahirah, Zahrah, Zara, Zuhra.

ZAIDA. *(zah-EE-dah) Arabic, 'properous'*. Could be some disconnection between spelling and pronunciation. Zahida, Zayda, Ziada, Ziyada.

ZAINA. *(zay-nah) Swahili, 'beautiful'*. Simplified form of Zainabu, the name of the eldest daughter of Muhammad. Zainabu, Zayna, Zaynabu.

ZAIRA. *(ZARE-ah) Irish literary creation*. Would make a truly original alternative to the overused Sarah.

ZAKIA. *(za-KEE-a) Arabic and Hebrew, 'pure'*. Strong cross-cultural name that could be a feminine spin on the Zachary family. Zachya, Zachyah, Zaki, Zakiah, Zakiyya, Zakiyyah.

ZALA. *African, Ethiopian, 'a people from southwest Ethiopia'; also Hungarian place name*. Simple but sultry.

ZALIKA. *Arabic, Swahili, 'wellborn'. See* ZULEIKA. Zaliki, Zuleika.

ZALTANA. *Native American, 'high mountain'.* Has an evocative gypsy feel. **Zaltana.**

ZAMORA. *Spanish place- and surname.* Heard in Spain more as a last name, but would work here as an exotic Latin first.

ZÀN. *(TSAN)* or *(CHAN) Chinese, 'support, favour, praise'.* Confusion with English male name Zan could cause pronunciation problems.

ZANA. *Polish variation of JANE; Hebrew, diminutive of SUSANNA.* An international possibility, heard from England and Israel to Poland, Latvia and Albania. **Zaina, Zanna.**

ZANDRA. *Variation of SANDRA and ALEXANDRA.* When unconventional British fashion designer Zandra Rhodes changed her first initial from *S* to *Z*, she transformed a diminutive of Alexandra into a legitimate name – one that is still rarely heard and might be worth considering. **Xandi, Xandie, Xandra, Xandrah, Zahndra, Zandi, Zandie, Zandrah, Zandy, Zanndra, Zohndra, Zondra.**

ŻANETA. *Russian variation of JANET.* See **JANET.**

ZANIAH. *Astronomical name.* This name of a triple star system in Virgo has a New Agey astral feel.

ZANNA. *Diminutive of SUSANNA; Polish variation of JANE.* A feminine multicultural nickname name perfectly able to stand on its own. **Zana, Zanne, Zannie.**

ZARA. *Hebrew and Arabic, 'eastern brightness, dawn'.* This evocative name, often used in early films and novels for a sultry character from the East, was chosen by Princess Anne for her daughter in the 1980s and is now rising in the Top 100. **Zahara, Zahra, Zaira, Zarah, Zareena, Zaria, Zarina, Zarinda, Zayeera.**

ZARELA. *Spanish variation of SARAH.* Rhythmic, tangoish name quite popular in Spanish-speaking cultures. **Zarita.**

ZARIA. *Arabic, 'rose'; also African place name.* Nigerian capital city inspires an exotic spin on Daria. **Zariah.**

Short & Strong Names

Alex

Asa

Bree

Bryn

Chan

Claire

Dane

Eve

Greer

Jade

Kate

Maeve

Petra

Quinn

Tamar

Tess

Zea

ZARINA. *Persian, 'golden one' or 'a golden vessel'.* Indian name fit for your own little *tsarina.*

ZARIZA. *Hebrew, 'gold, brilliantly bright'.* Glitzy gold-bangle name. **Zehara, Zehari,**

Zehavi, Zehavit, Zehuva, Zohar, Zohere.

ZARYA. *Slavic mythology name.* In Slavic myth, this exotic name belonged to the water priestess and protector of warriors. **Zaria, Zariah.**

ZATHURA. *Derivation and meaning unknown.* Exotic name kids will relate to the space adventure book and family film of that name.

ZAYNA. *Arabic, 'beauty, ornament'.* Name for a future fortune-teller.

ZAZA. *Hebrew, 'movement'.* Zaza-zoom. **Zazu.**

ZEA. *(ZAY-uh) Latin, 'grain'.* An unusual possibility; Zea would fit right in with schoolmates named Téa and Leya.

ZEBORAH. *(ZEB-ah-rah) Modern invented name.* Zippier Deborah.

ZEHAVA. *Hebrew, 'gold, golden'.* The more dignified and attractive Hebrew equivalent of

Golda or Goldie. **Zahava, Zahavah, Zehave, Zehavi, Zehavit, Zehovit, Zehuvit.**

ZEILA. *African place name.* This name of a port town in Somalia has cultural resonance and an appealing sound. **Saylah, Zeilah.**

ZELA. *African variation of* ZOE. *See* **ZELLA.**

ZELDA. *German, diminutive of* **GRISELDA**; *also Yiddish, 'luck'.* Since 1986, Zelda has been a prime Nintendo name, as in the *Legend of Zelda: Twilight Princess.* May be wise to wait until this fever cools down. Or longer. **Selda, Zelde, Zellda.**

ZELENA. *Greek variation of* **SELENA.** *See* **SELENA.**

ZELENIA. *Greek variation of* **SELENA.** *See* **SELENA.** **Zelaina, Zelenya.**

ZELENKA. *(zeh-LAIN-ka) Czech, 'green, new, fresh, innocent'.* Has a certain twinkle.

ZELIA. *Hebrew, 'zealous, ardent'.* An appealing name almost unknown in our culture

but with roots in several others; worldlier than cousins Celia and Delia. **Solina, Soline, Souline, Soulle, Zalia, Zailie, Zaylia, Zelene, Zelina, Zeline. International: Zele, Zélie** *(French).*

ZELLA. *African, Bobangi, 'lacking nothing, one who knows the way'; also Libyan place name.* This is an African name that would fit into any culture. **Zela, Zellah.**

ZELMA. *German, diminutive of* **ANSELMA,** *'God helmet'.* The Selma-Thelma-Velma connection dates it. **Zellma.**

ZEMORA. *Hebrew, 'branch, extension'.* Rarely, if ever, heard in this country, and unlikely to appeal to many British people; sounds slightly like a product you might put in your coffee. **Zemorah, Zmora.**

ZENA. *Greek variation of* **XENA.** Familiar through the similarly pronounced TV Warrior Princess, but the original Xena spelling is cooler. **Zeena, Zeenia, Zeenya, Zenia, Zenya, Zina.**

ZENAIDA. *(zay-NAY-dah) Greek, 'the life of Zeus'.* This name of a daughter of Zeus has an intriguing air of antiquity. **Cenaida, Cenaide, Cenanida, Naida, Sanaida, Seneida, Seniada, Sinayda, Xenaida, Zenaide, Zeneida, Zina. International: Zénaïde** *(French),* **Zinaida** *(Russian).*

ZENDA. *Persian, 'sacred'.* Anyone who remembers the classic novel or film *The Prisoner of Zenda* would find this an odd choice.

ZENOBIA. *Greek, 'power of Zeus'.* With historical roots as a beautiful and intelligent ancient queen and literary ties to Hawthorne and Edith Wharton novels, this rarity could appeal to adventurous parents seeking the exotically unusual. **Cenobie, Zeba, Zeena, Zenaide, Zenayda, Zenda, Zenina. International: Zenaida, Zenia, Zenna, Zenobie** *(French),* **Cenobia, Senobia** *(Spanish),* **Zenovia, Zinovia** *(Russian).*

♂ **ZEPHYR.** *Greek, 'west wind'.* Zephyrus was the Greek god of the west wind, and all names associated with him have a pleasantly gentle, breezy feel. **Zefir, Zephira, Zephirem, Zephirine, Zephrine, Zephyra, Zephyrine, Zyphire. International: Zéphyrine** *(French),* **Cefariana, Cefernia, Sefarina, Seferina, Zaferina, Zefarabam Zeferuba** *(Spanish),* **Zefiryn** *(Polish),* **Zephyra** *(Greek).*

ZERA. *(ZAY-rah) Hebrew, 'seeds, beginnings'.* More than zero, but too close to the unfashionable Vera. **Zerah.**

ZETA. *Greek, 'born last'.* A final letter of the Greek alphabet, popularised by Welsh actress Catherine Zeta-Jones – Zeta was her grandmother's first name.

ZETTA. *Hebrew, 'olive'; diminutive of* **ROSETTA.** Too reminiscent of the universally disliked Yetta. **Zeta, Zetana.**

ZHANE. *Modern invented name.* Mix a bit of old-fashioned Jane with the male-inflected Zane, et voila! Zhane. **Zhana, Zhané.**

ZHEN. *Chinese, 'a treasure'.* A striking choice, but might possibly be taken for Jen. **Zhin.**

ZIA. *Latin, 'grain'; Arabic, 'light, splendor'; Italian, 'aunt'.* Nontraditional name that has a certain minimalist appeal, though in an Italian-British family it would be strange to have a baby named Aunt. **Zea.**

ZILLA. *Hebrew, 'shadow'.* Although this Old Testament name is soft and delicate, it runs the risk of conjuring up the monstrous Godzilla. **Zila, Zilah, Zillah, Zylla.**

ZINA. *African, Nsenga, refers to a child's secret spirit name; Russian, related to Zeus.* Old-style arty. **Zinah.**

ZINAIDA. *(zee-nah-ee-dah) Russian, from Greek, related to Zeus.* This unusual name belonged to a character played by Kirsten Dunst in an early film. **Ida, Zina.**

★**ZINNIA.** *Latin flower name.* A floral choice with a bit more edge and energy than most. **Zinia, Zinnya, Zinya.**

ZIPPORA. *Hebrew, 'bird, a sparrow'.* This upstanding Old Testament name of the wife of Moses would almost inevitably provoke some tricky *zipper* teasing. **Tzippa, Tzzipporah, Zipora, Ziporah, Zipporah.**

ZITA. *Greek, 'seeker'; Arabic, 'mistress'.* A thirteenth-century Tuscan saint, patron of homemakers, Zita is the kind of name that sounded really creative in an earlier era. **Zeeta, Zyta.**

ZIVA. *(ZEEV-uh) Hebrew, 'brilliance, brightness'.* Relates to the month of Israeli independence. **Zeeva, Zivanit, Zivi, Zivit.**

ZIVANKA. *Slavic, 'full of life'.* Life-affirming name with a Russian accent. **Zivka.**

♂ **ZIZA.** *Hebrew, 'splendor, abundance'.* This was the name of two men mentioned in the Bible; Aziza might be a better choice.

ZIZI. *African, Kiswahili, 'animal shelter'; Hungarian, diminutive of* **ELIZABETH**; *Romanian, diminutive of* **TEREZA**; *Hebrew, 'pledged to God'.* Despite its varied cultural ties, Zizi still sounds like a cancan dancer or a fluffy lapdog. **ZsiZsi.**

★**ZOE.** *Greek, 'life'.* Zoe (or Zoë) has been zooming up the popularity lists and is in the Top 100. It was chosen by celebs from Rosanna Arquette to Woody Harrelson; it makes a perfect fitting in/standing out choice. **Zoee, Zoelie, Zoeline, Zoie, Zooey, Zoya.** **International: Zoa, Zoelle, Zoey, Zoia, Zoyechka, Zoyenka** *(Russian).*

ZOEY. *Spelling variation of* **ZOE.** Lea Thompson chose this phonetic spelling for her daughter. Its kinship with Joey gives it a tomboyish feel. Zoie is rising in popularity, too. **Zoie.**

ŽOFIA. *Czech, Polish, and Ukrainian variation of* **SOPHIA,** *'wisdom'.* See **SOPHIA.** **Žofie, Žofinka, Žofka.**

ZOHARA. *Hebrew, 'light, splendor'.* See **ZAHARA.** **Zahara, Zaharira.**

ZOIA. *Slavic variation of* **ZOE.** See **ZOE.**

ZOILA. *Greek, feminine variation of* **ZOILO.** One of the less enchanting Zoe-related names. **Chola, Soilla, Zaila, Zalia, Ziola, Zolla. Zoyla.**

♂ **ZOLA.** *African, Congolese, 'productive'; Italian, 'lump of earth'; also literary name.* When the Eddie Murphys named their fourth daughter Zola, it affirmed the up-and-coming status of the name. **Zoela, Zoila, Zolah.**

ZONA. *Latin, 'belt, girdle'.* This name of a constellation in Orion's belt has an astral feel; it also belonged to the first woman to win a Pulitzer prize in drama, Zona Gale. **Zonia.**

♂ **ZOOEY.** *Literary name.* Readers who remember J. D. Salinger's *Franny and Zooey* have probably forgotten that the character was male (nee Zachary). Nowadays the somewhat loopy spin on Zoe is associated with actress Zooey Deschanel.

ZORA. *Slavic, 'dawn's light'.*
Meaningful literary heroine
name honouring Zora Neale
Hurston, an important
American black writer. **Zorah,
Zorana, Zorina, Zorine, Zorra,
Zorrah, Zorya.**

ZORAH. *Biblical place name.*
Zorah, the Old Testament home
of Samson, is both soft and
substantial.

ZORAIDA. *(zo-RYE-duh)
Arabic, 'captivating woman'.* This
name of a beautiful Moorish
woman character in *Don
Quixote* is rarely heard. **Saraida,
Soraida, Soraita, Zaraida,
Zarida, Zeraida, Zorida.**

ZORINA. *Slavic, 'golden dawn'.*
Both a first and last name,
Zorina has a pretty, ballerina-
like quality. **Sorina, Zora,
Zorah, Zorana, Zori, Zorie,
Zory.**

ZOYA. *Russian and Greek
variation of* **ZOE.** *See* **ZOE.**
Zoia, Zoyenka, Zoyya.

ZSA ZSA. *Hungarian,
diminutive of* **SUSAN.** Though
she's left the large and small

Stellar Starbabies Beginning with Z

Zahara	Angelina Jolie
Zahra	Chris Rock
Zara	Princess Anne & Mark Phillips
Zelda	Robin Williams
Zoe	Rosanna Arquette, Woody Harrelson, Darcey Bussell
Zola	Eddie Murphy

screens, Zsa Zsa (born Sári)
Gabor is not forgotten, and this
name will forever be associated
with her. **Zsuzsa, Zsuzsanna.**

ZUELIA. *Arabic, 'peace'.* An
occasionally heard African name,
hobbled by a zoolike sound.

ZULA. *English, derived from
Zulu, South African tribal name.*
Related to the powerful South
African warrior people,
sometimes chosen by those with
African roots to celebrate their
heritage.

ZULEIKA. *Arabic, 'brilliant and
lovely'.* A high wire act of a
name: only for the intrepid. Has
a striking literary association

to Max Beerbohm's *Zuleika
Dobson,* a heroine so gorgeous
that the entire student body of
Oxford University killed
themselves for love of her.
Zulaica, Zuleica, Zulekha.

ZULMA. *Arabic, 'healthy and
vigorous'.* Unappealing. **Sulema,
Zulema, Zulima.**

ZUWENA. *African, 'good'.* More
original than any made-up name.

ZUZANNA. *Slavic variation of*
SUSANNAH. A nice, energetic
twist on Susannah.

ZUZELA. *Native American,
meaning unknown.* This exotic

Sioux name belonged to one of Sitting Bull's many wives.

ZUZI. *Swiss variation of* **SUSAN.** Effort to make Susan or Susie more exotic.

ZUZU. *Czech, diminutive of* **SUSAN.** Heard every Christmas as the name of Jimmy Stewart's little girl in *It's a Wonderful Life*.

A boys

AAKIL. *Hindi, 'intelligent, smart'.* If meaning were destiny, this would start a boy off on the right foot.

♂ AALTO. *Scandinavian surname.* The last name of Finnish moderne designer/ architect makes an original, creative choice.

AARON. *Hebrew, 'exalted, enlightened'.* This name of Moses' brother has been in the last two decades and it still has an attractive, timeless quality. Variant Arran, as in the Scottish Isle, is popular in Scotland. **Aahron, Aaran, Aaren, Aarron, Aeron, Ahron, Aran, Aren, Arin, Aron, Arron, Arun. International: Aronne** *(Italian, German),* **Aarão** *(Portuguese),* **Arek** *(Polish),* **Aronoa** *(Russian),* **Aharon** *(Hebrew),* **Haroun** *(Arabic).*

AART. *Dutch, 'eagle-like'.* That double *a* invests the old Arthur nickname with fresh life.

AARU. *Egyptian, 'peaceful'.* Egyptian mythology place name with an intriguing sound.

♂ ABACUS. *Greek word name.* A mathematical possibility. **Abacas, Abakus.**

ABÁN. *Persian, 'clearer'.* A benevolent genie in Persian myth, used by Latino and Muslim families. **Aba, Abaan, Abanito.**

ABANU. *African, Ibo 'I have joined the family'.* Rhythmic, strong and buoyant.

♂ ABBA. *Hebrew, 'father'.* Double exposure: 1970s rock sensation *(Mamma Mia!)* and scholar/diplomat name in Israel.

ABBAS. *Hebrew, 'father'; Arabic, 'lion, stern'.* Not one of the five hundred names of Muhammad, but that of his uncle. **Abbah, Abban.**

♂ ABBOTT. *Hebrew, Aramaic, 'father'.* Neglected masculine surname with religious overtones; feminine nickname Abby could be a drawback. **Abbie, Abbot, Abby, Abot, Abott. International: Abboid** *(Gaelic),* **Abbé** *(French),* **Abad** *(Spanish),* **Abt** *(German).*

ABDALLAH. *Arabic, 'servant of Allah'.* A frequently used Arabic name. **Abdullah, Abdylla. International: Abdalla** *(Swahili).*

ABDIEL. *Hebrew, 'servant of God'.* More popular than you might think for a boy's name. **Abdel.**

ABDU. *Swahili, 'worshipper of God'.* The vowel ending energises this relative of Abdul.

ABDUL. *Arabic, 'servant of Allah'.* Widespread choice in the Muslim world. **Ab, Abdal, Abdall, Abdeel, Abdel, Abdoul, Abdu, Abdull.**

ABDULLAH. *Arabic, 'servant of Allah'.* Another Islamic favourite, the father of the Prophet Muhammad. **Abdalla, Abdallah, Abdulah, Abdulla.**

ABE. *Diminutive of* **ABRAHAM.** Old-time nickname that may follow in the fashionable footsteps of cronies Jake and Sam. **Abey, Abie.**

ABEEKU. *(ah-BAY-koo). Ghanan, 'born on Wednesday'.* Classic African day name, with rhythm and energy.

★**ABEL.** *Hebrew, 'breath'.* Name of Adam and Eve's unfortunate younger son, compensates with positive connotations: capable, competent, ready and willing. **Abell, Able, Avel.**

ABELARD. *German, 'noble, steadfast'.* Hero of medieval French romance, not neighbourhood-friendly. **Ab, Abalard, Abbey, Abby, Abelardo, Abelhard, Abilard, Adalard, Adelard.**

ABERDEEN. *Scottish place name.* Amiable, undiscovered geographic option.

ABI. *Turkish, 'older brother'.* Possibility for a first-born son.

♂ **ABIAH.** *Hebrew, 'God is my father'.* Gentle, rarely used Old Testament name. **Ab, Abia, Abisha, Aviyah. International: Abías** *(Spanish).*

ABIEL. *Hebrew, 'God is my father'.* Biblical name used by Puritans, sounds fusty today. **Abiell.**

♂ **ABIJAH.** *Hebrew, 'God is my father'.* Colonial era biblical favourite with energetic, modern aura; possible Elijah replacement.

♂ **ABILENE.** *English from Hebrew, 'grass'; place name.* New Testament, Texas and Kansas place name in the US; better for a girl. **Abalene, Abileen.**

ABIR. *Hebrew, 'strong, mighty, courageous'.* Place name of a settlement in Galilee in Israel. **Abeer, Abiri.**

★**ABNER.** *Hebrew, 'father of light'.* Neglected biblical name ready to flee Dogpatch. **Abnar, Abnor, Ebner, Ebnor. International: Ab, Avner** *(Israeli).*

ABRAHAM. *Hebrew, 'father of multitudes'.* The bearded Old Testament patriarch/ Lincolnesque image has kept this name lagging behind more popular biblical brothers: may be time to think about Baby Abie, or – even better – Baby Bram. **Abe, Abie, Abrahn, Braham, Bram, Ham. International: Abracham** *(Irish Gaelic),* **Abrahamo, Abramo** *(Italian),* **Aberhán, Abraán, Abrahán, Abrán, Avrán, Brancho, Ibrahim** *(Spanish),* **Abarran** *(Basque),* **Abrão** *(Portuguese),* **Abrasha, Avraam, Avram, Avramij** *(Russian),* **Avram** *(Greek),* **Aram** *(Armenian),* **Avraham, Avrom, Avron, Avrum** *(Hebrew),* **Avrumke** *(Yiddish),* **Ebrahim, Ibrahim** *(Arabic).*

ABRAM. *Hebrew, 'father of multitudes'.* Abraham's original name in the Bible; more user-friendly but with less substance.

♂ **ABRAXAS.** *Persian mythology dragon name.* A sci-fi name with earthly possibilities, but some playground peril. Fun fact: it evolved from abracadabra.

ABSALOM. *Hebrew, 'father of peace'.* Biblical (King David's beautiful, rebellious son) and literary (Chaucer, Faulkner) associations, solemn sound. **International: Absalon** *(French),* **Absalón** *(Spanish),* **Axel** *(Scandinavian),* **Avshalom** *(Hebrew).*

ACE. *Latin, 'one, unity'.* Jaunty nickname name starting to take flight among celeb parents.

ACHILLES. *Greek, 'thin-lipped'.* The name of great

Homeric hero with the vulnerable heel is widely used in European versions but rarely here. It makes a strong – probably too strong – statement. **International: Achille** *(French)*, **Achilleo** *(Italian)*, **Aquilles** *(Spanish and Portuguese)*, **Achill, Akhylle, Akilles** *(Eastern European and Russian)*, **Achilios, Achilleus** *(Greek)*.

ACKER, ACKERLY, ACKLEY. *English, 'meadow of oak trees'.* Three surnames lacking any sense of style or humour. **Accerly, Acklea, Acklee, Ackleigh, Ackerley.**

ACTAEON. *Latin, 'from Attica'.* A hyperkinetic name, might be more kid-friendly without the second *a*. **Acteon.**

ACTON. *English, 'village with oak trees'.* Very British, in a dated, monocled way – no action in view for Acton.

♂ **ADAIAH.** *Hebrew, 'God's witness'.* Rare Old Testament name with pleasing sound.

♂ **ADAIR.** *Scottish and Irish, 'oak tree ford'.* Adair has flair, the grace of a Fred Astaire. **Adaire, Adare, Adayre.**

ADAM. *Hebrew, 'son of the red earth'.* Revived in the 1960, this primal Old Testament name has been popular, only slipping out of the Top 25 in recent years. **International: Ádamh** *(Irish Gaelic)*, **Adamo** *(Italian)*, **Adamo, Adán, Addis, Adnon** *(Spanish)*, **Adão** *(Portuguese)*, **Aatami** *(Finnish)*, **Adamek, Adas, Adok** *(Polish)*, **Adi, Adrien** *(Hungarian)*, **Adamec, Adamek, Adamki, Adamok, Damek** *(Czech)*, **Adomas** *(Lithuanian)*, **Adamka, Adas** *(Russian)*, **Adem** *(Turkish)*, **Adi** *(Yiddish)*.

ADAN. *Spanish variation of* **ADAM.** Used most often in Hispanic cultures.

♂ **ADDISON.** *English, 'son of Adam'.* Cool guy name turned hot girl choice – the Madison of 2020. **Ad, Addisen, Addisson, Addysen, Addyson, Adisen, Adison, Adysen.**

ADELIO. *German, 'the father of the noble prince'.* Appealing, upbeat Spanish name.

ADEON. *Welsh.* This name of a legendary Welsh prince could serve as a more original

alternative to Adam or Aidan, though it does sound a bit chemical.

If You Like Adam,
You Might Love . . .

Abel

Abner

Addison

Asa

Caleb

Eli

Ethan

Gideon

Jacob

Jared

Jonah

Joseph

Josiah

Judah

Levi

Micah

Noah

Tobias

ADIL. *Arabic, 'just'.* Well used in the Arabic world, as is the related Aditya.

★ADLAI. *Hebrew, 'God's refuge'.* Old Testament name – he was the father of one of King David's herdsman – ripe for rediscovery. It can be pronounced either Ad-lie or Ad-lay. **Adlay, Adley.**

ADOLFO. *Latin form of* **ADOLPH.** One high-fashion brand that's actually a legitimate first name, though still linked to the tainted Adolph.

ADOLPH. *German, 'noble wolf'.* World War II stamped a permanent *verboten* on Adolph. **Ad, Dolf, Dolph, Dolphus. International: Adolphe** *(French),* **Adolfo** *(Italian),* **Adalfo, Adolfo, Dolfito, Dolfo, Fito** *(Spanish),* **Adolf** *(German, Swedish, Dutch, Danish),* **Adolphus** *(Swedish),* **Aatu** *(Finnish).*

ADOLPHUS. *Latin, 'noble wolf'.* More distinguished variation of Adolph – but still, *nein.*

ADONIS. *Greek, meaning unknown.* High-pressure name personifying masculine gorgeousness. **Addonis.**

♂ ADRIAN. *Latin, 'from the Adriatic'.* If you're not put off by the similarity to the feminine Adrienne, this long-term trendy name in England could be a winning choice. Adriano is a pleasing foreign version. **Ade, Adrean, Hadrian. International: Aidrian** *(Irish Gaelic),* **Adrien** *(French),* **Adriano** *(Italian),* **Adrián, Adrín** *(Spanish),* **Adrião** *(Portuguese),* **Arje** *(Dutch),* **Adorjan,** *(Hungarian).*

♂ ADRIEL. *Hebrew, 'God is my master'.* Biblical name getting some notice.

AEGIS, AEGEUS. *Greek, 'young goat'.* Often found as a brand name in the hi-tech and industrial worlds.

AENEAS. *Greek, 'the praised one'.* Legendary son of Venus and hero of Troy, but sounds vaguely biological in modern times. **Aineus, Ainneus, Eneas, Enneas.**

AESOP. *(EE-sop) Greek.* There once was a moralising fabulist who tried to make it as a baby name . . . and failed.

AGU. *Nigerian, 'leopard'.* More acronym than name.

AGUSTIN. *Latin, 'the exalted one'.* Popular in the Hispanic world, in honour of Saint Augustine.

AHAB. *Hebrew, 'uncle'.* Hard to think of this name without 'Captain' in front of it.

AHEARNE. *Celtic, 'owner of horses'.* Will not work and play well with most surnames. **Aherin, Ahern, Aherne, Hearn, Heris, Hern, Herne.**

AHMAD, AHMED. *Arabic, 'greatly praised'.* One of the five hundred plus variations on Muhammad, this is a favourite Muslim choice. **Achmad, Achmed, Achmet, Ahmet, Ahmod, Amad, Amadi, Amed, Emad.**

★♂ AIDAN. *Irish, 'little and fiery'.* An appealing Irish name that has been popular elsewhere in Britain too, though it has recently been descending in the Top 100 list.

Aidan and Aiden are both in Scotland's Top 25. **Adan, Aden, Aedan, Aedin, Edan. International: Aodhan** *(Irish Gaelic)*, **Aeddan, Aiden, Ayden, Edan** *(Welsh)*, **Ayden** *(Turkish)*.

♂ **AINSLEY.** *Scottish, 'one's own meadow'.* Suitable for a prospective butler. **Ainsleigh, Ainslie, Ainsly, Aynslee, Aynsley.**

♀ **AJA.** *Hindi, 'goat'.* Retro musical reference to classic Steely Dan rock album, but mostly for girls today.

AJAMU. *Nigerian, Yoruban, 'he fights for his desires'.* Rhythmic name sometimes associated with calypso singer King Ajamu.

AJANI. *Nigerian, Yoruban, 'the victor'.* An easily assimilated African name, a novel twist on Johnny.

AJAX. *Greek mythology name.* Be warned if you plan to move to the US: it would be too closely connected with a cleanser. To avoid teasing try the nickname Jax.

AKBAR. *Arabic, 'praised'.* Name of a great Indian Mogul king, a Matt Groening cartoon character and many Indian restaurants.

AKELLO. *Ugandan, 'I have brought forth'.* Energetic but mellow.

♂ **AKI.** *Japanese, 'born in the autumn'.* A name known in several cultures, also through animated book character Tiger Aki.

AKIM. *Russian, 'God will establish'.* Strong and commanding. **Kima.**

AKIRO. *Japanese, 'bright boy'.* Well used in Japan, the first name of famed director Kurosawa. **Aki, Akio, Akira.**

♂ **AKIVA.** *Hebrew, 'to protect, replace,' variant of* **YAAKOV.** Distinguished scholarly pedigree, but runs the risk of sounding feminine. **Akavya, Akeeva, Akiba, Akiv, Keeva, Keevah, Kiba, Kiva, Kivah, Kivi.**

ALADDIN. *Arabic, 'height of religion'.* Too tied to the magic lamp. **Aladian, Alladin.**

African Names

Akello
Asante
Banjul
Dabir
Dakarai
Jafari
Jelani
Kalif
Labaan
Luki
Mosi
Obi
Samori
Tau
Xola *(KOH-lah)*
Zuri

ALAMO. *Spanish, 'poplar tree'; also a San Antonio mission.* A name that would be remembered in the US, but for all the wrong reasons.

ALAN. *Irish, 'handsome, cheerful'.* In its three most popular spellings, this mid-century favourite has become a middle-aged grandpa name, given to very few of today's babies. Al, Alen, Alin Allan, Allayne, Allen, Alley, Alleyn, Allie, Allon, Alyn, Alynn. International: Ailin *(Irish)*, Ailean *(Scottish)*, Aland, Alleyne, Allyn, Alun *(Welsh)*, Alain *(French)*, Alano *(Italian and Spanish)*, Alao *(Portuguese)*.

♂ **ALANI.** *Hawaiian, 'orange tree'.* A name known in several cultures.

ALARD. *German, 'noble, steadfast'.* Stiff and square. **Alart, Allard, Ellard.**

ALARIC. *German, 'noble ruler'.* Ancient regal name that sounds modern enough to be considered. **Al, Alarick, Alarik, Aleric, Allaric, Allarick, Alric, Alrick, Ulrich, Ulrick, Ric, Rick.** International: Alarico, Rico *(Spanish)*, Adalrich, Alarich, Alrik, Aurick, Aurik, Ullric, Ullrich *(German)*, Alrik *(Swedish)*, Ulryk *(Polish)*.

ALASDAIR. *Scottish variation of* **ALEXANDER.** In this country, more recognisable with the Alistair spelling. **Alasdaire, Alasdare, Alisdair.**

ALASTAIR. *Irish variation of* **ALASDAIR.** *See* **ALISTAIR.** Al, Alasdair, Alastaire, Alastar, Alaster, Allastaire, Allaster, Allistir, Allystair.

ALBAN. *Latin, 'white, blond'.* One of the less appealing members of the army of names starting with *Al.* **Al, Albain, Alben, Albern, Albie, Albion, Alby.** International: Aubin *(French)*, Albino *(Italian, Spanish and Portuguese)*, Alva *(Spanish)*, Albek, Albinek, Binek *(Polish)*, Albin, Albinek, Binek *(Czech)*, Albins *(Latvian)*.

♂ **ALBANY.** *Place name.* An American place name possibility.

ALBEE. *Literary name.* For theatre-loving parents – an homage to one of the premiere twentieth-century playwrights.

ALBERT. *English, 'noble, bright'.* This name remained stylish for over eighty years, but with its serious, studious image (think Einstein, Schweitzer), it's far from fashionable today. Still, along with such stalwarts as Walter and George, it could now make an unusual yet classic choice. **Al, Albie, Alby, Bert,** Bertie, Berty, Burt, Elbert. International: Ailbhe *(Irish Gaelic)*, Adelbert, Ailbert *(Scottish)*, Aubert *(French)*, Alberto, Berto *(Italian, Spanish)*, Albrecht *(German)*, Albek, Bertek *(Polish)*, Alberik, Ales, Berco, Berti, Bertik *(Czech)*, Alberts *(Latvian)*, Albertko *(Slavic)*, Alvertos *(Greek)*.

♂ **ALCOTT.** *English, 'dweller at the old cottage'.* Shades of nineteenth-century New England, evoking memories of *Little Women* and *Little Men.* **Alcot, Allcott, Allkot.**

♂ **ALDEN.** *English, 'old, wise friend'.* A less than stylish surname name, but it might make a more distinctive alternative to such widely used but similar names as Aidan and Holden. **Aldin, Aldwin, Aldwyn, Elden, Eldin.**

ALDO. *Italian from German, 'old and wise'.* A spirited German name very popular in Italy and occasionally used elsewhere, Aldo could blend with an Anglo surname.

ALDOUS. *English from German, 'old and wise'.*

Somewhat stuffy, associated with author Huxley. **Aldas, Aldis, Aldus.**

ALDRICH. *English, 'old, wise ruler'.* Not bad surname name. **Al, Aldric, Aldrick, Aldridge, Alldric, Alldrich, Alldrick, Eldric, Rich, Rick.** International: **Audric** *(French).*

ALEC. *Diminutive of* **ALEXANDER.** Much fresher sounding than Alex. International: **Alick** *(Scottish),* **Alek** *(Russian).*

ALEEM. *Hindi, 'knowledgeable'.* Surname of a noted modern Urdu poet.

ALEJANDRO. *Spanish variation of* **ALEXANDER.** Softer and smoother than Alexander, the top boy's name in Spain could make a seamless transition to this culture. **Alehandro.**

ALEJO. *(ah-LAY-ho) Spanish, diminutive of* **ALEJANDRO.** Another appealing member of the Alexandrian clan.

★**ALESSANDRO.** *Italian variation of* **ALEXANDER.** Silky and sinuous take on

Alexander, a real winner. **Alessio, Sandro.**

ALESSIO. *Italian, diminutive of* **ALESSANDRO.** Used on its own in Italy, would be a welcome settler here.

♂ **ALEX.** *Diminutive of* **ALEXANDER, ALEXIS.** This independent form has become a classic in its own right. One of the truest unisex names, used almost equally for both sexes without sacrificing any of its masculinity. It's recently been slipping down the Top 100. **Aleks, Alik, Alix, Alleks, Allex, Allix, Lex.** International: **Olek** *(Polish),* **Alek** *(Russian).*

ALEXANDER. *Greek, 'defending warrior'.* Steady in the Top 25, the noble Alexander led to the popularity of so many spin-offs, such as Alex, Zander, Xan and Zan, that it almost feels as if the name world's been Alextrified out. **Al, Alec, Alecsander, Alex, Alexandar, Alexsander, Alexsandor, Alexxander, Alexzander, Alix, Alixander, Lex, Sandro, Sandy, Xan, Xander, Zan, Zander.** International: **Alastar** *(Irish Gaelic),* **Alasdair, Alistair** *(Scottish*

Gaelic), **Alexandre** *(French),* **Alessandro, Sandro** *(Italian),* **Alejandro** *(Spanish),* **Alexio** *(Portuguese),* **Sándor** *(Hungarian),* **Alexandru** *(Romanian),* **Olexa** *(Czech pet form),* **Aleksandr, Alexei, Alyosha, Sanya, Sasha, Shura** *(Russian),* **Alexandros, Alexios** *(Greek).*

♂ **ALEXIOS.** *Greek, 'defending warrior'.* Very popular on its native turf, foreign-sounding here. International: **Alessio, Alexius** *(Italian),* **Alejio** *(Spanish),* **Aleksy** *(Czech),* **Aleksei** *(Russian).*

♂ **ALEXIS.** *English variation of* **ALEXIOS.** Has definitely leapt into the female column. **Alexei, Alexes, Alexi, Lex.**

ALF. *Diminutive of* **ALFRED.** If Alfie is too formal for you.

ALFIE. *Diminutive of* **ALFRED.** In the Top 25 over here, where retro nickname names are ultratrendy, but it's less likely to happen elsewhere. **Alfey, Alfy, Alphey, Alphie, Alphy.**

ALFONSO. *Spanish, 'noble, ready'.* A royal name in España, snooty sounding here. **Alf, Alfie, Alfonz, Alfonzus, Fonz, Fonzie.**

Antiques Ready for Restoration

Alonzo

Amos

Atticus

Barnabas

Chester

Dexter

Dudley

Felix

Homer

Humphrey

Jasper

Josiah

Judah

Lemuel

Otto

Phineas

Thaddeus

Tobias

International: **Alphonsus** *(Irish),* **Alphonse** *(French),* **Alfonso** *(Italian, Swedish),* **Alfonzo, Alonso, Alonzo, Alphonso, Fonzi, Fonzo, Lonzo** *(Spanish),* **Affonso, Afonso** *(Portuguese),* **Alfons** *(German).*

ALFRED. *English, 'wise counselor'.* If you're looking for a path to Fred, we suggest going directly to Frederick. **Alf, Alfie, Alfryd, Fred, Freddie, Freddy, Fredo.** International: **Ailfrid** *(Irish Gaelic),* **Alfredo** *(Italian, Spanish),* **Alfreck, Alfrid** *(German).*

ALGER. *English, 'clever warrior'.* Harmless but charmless. **Algar, Allger.**

ALGERNON. *French, 'moustached man'.* Prissiness personified. **Algie, Algy.**

♂ **ALI.** *Arabic, 'supreme, exalted'.* This is one of the ninety-nine attributes of Allah, deemed by Muhammad to be a recommended name for a male child. In the US, it's been primarily associated with boxing immortal Muhammad Ali, known as 'the greatest'.

ALIJAH. *Spelling variation of* **ELIJAH.** This increasingly popular version changes the nickname from Eli to Ali.

ALISTAIR. *Scottish variation of* **ALEXANDER.** This sophisticated example could

and should be part of the next wave. **Alastair, Alisdair, Alister.**

ALLEN, ALLAN. *Celtic, 'handsome'.* Doubling the first consonant doesn't make Alan any more modern.

ALONSO. *See ALONZO.*

★**ALONZO.** *Spanish, diminutive of* **ALFONSO.** This friendly yet animated name could make a stylish choice outside the Hispanic community. **Alanzo, Alon, Alonso, Lon, Lonnie, Lonzo.**

ALOYSIUS. *Latin, 'famous warrior'.* Perfect name for a parrot. **Al, Aloisius.** International: **Alois** *(German).*

ALPHONSE. *German, 'noble, ready for battle'.* Rarely used and for good reason. Alonzo is a preferable choice. **Alf, Alonzo, Fonz, Fonzie.** International: **Alphonsus** *(Irish),* **Alfonso** *(Italian, Spanish),* **Affonso** *(Portuguese),* **Alfons** *(German),* **Alpheus** *(Greek).*

ALRIC. *German, 'ruler of all'.* Common in Sweden, problematic here. **Alrec, Alrick.**

ALTAIR. *Arabic, 'falcon'.* The eleventh brightest star in the sky has a celestial feel.

ALTO. *Latin, 'high'.* With its musical allusions, a harmonious possibility.

♂ **ALTON.** *English, 'dweller at the old town'.* The sort of formal surname name more popular in another era; Dalton's a more modern relation. **Allton, Alson, Alston, Alten, Altyn.**

ALUN. *Welsh spelling of* **ALAN***; river in Wales.* The vowel change makes the name slightly more modern.

♂ **ALVA.** *Hebrew, 'height, exalted one'.* Edison's middle name, too feminine for the modern male. **Alvah.**

ALVAR. *German, 'elf army'; Latin, 'fair, white'.* Hard to picture in a contemporary playground. **Al, Alvie, Alvy. International: Alvaro, Alverio** *(Spanish).*

ÁLVARO. *Spanish, 'elf army'.* The final *o* adds a good measure of attractiveness. **Albar, Albaro, Alvario, Alvarso, Alverio.**

ALVIN. *English, 'noble friend, friend of the elves'.* A little old-fashioned for a modern child. **Al, Alv, Alvan, Alven, Alvie, Alvis, Alvy, Alvyn. International: Aloin, Aluin** *(French),* **Alvino** *(Italian),* **Aluino** *(Spanish),* **Alwin** *(German).*

ALWYN. *Welsh river name.* Like Selwyn and Kelwyn, not on the current Richter scale of names.

AMADEO. *Italian, 'lover of God'.* See *AMEDEO.*

AMADEUS. *Latin, 'lover of God'.* Mozart's middle name makes an interesting pick for music-loving parents. Beats Wolfgang. **Amadayus, Amadeaus, Amadei.**

AMADO. *Spanish, 'loved'.* Romantic choice. **Amador.**

AMAHL. *Hebrew, 'hard labour'.* Known from the Menotti opera, subdued and gentle. **Amal, Amall.**

AMATO. *Italian, 'loved'.* Saint's name that emanates amore.

AMAZU. *Nigerian, Ibo, 'no one knows everything'.* Conveys a sense of amazement.

AMBROSE. *Latin, 'immortal one'.* An old favourite of British novelists, Ambrose has an air of blooming well-being and upper-class erudition. **International: Ambrós** *(Irish Gaelic),* **Emrys** *(Welsh),* **Ambroise** *(French),* **Ambrogio, Ambrosi** *(Italian),* **Broz, Brogio** *(Italian short form),* **Ambrosio** *(Spanish, Portuguese),* **Ambrosius** *(Dutch, German, Swedish),* **Ambrus** *(Hungarian).*

★**AMEDEO.** *Italian variation of* **AMADEUS.** This euphonious Italian name, often associated with the painter Modigliani, makes a recommended creative choice. **International: Amadeo, Amedée** *(French).*

♂ **AMERICA.** *Place name.* Hippy name when spelled Amerika, but difficult whatever shape it takes. **America, Americo, Americus, Amerika, Amerikah, Ameriko, Amerikus. International: Amerigo** *(Spanish).*

★**AMIAS.** *(um-EYE-us or AIM-ee-us) Latin, 'loved'.* Obscure name with an attractive sound and feel. **Ameus, Amyas.**

AMIEL. *Hebrew, 'God is with my people'.* Certain confusion with Emil. **Ammiel, Amyel.**

AMIN. *Arabic, 'faithful, trustworthy'.* Unfortunate association with Ugandan dictator Idi Amin.

AMIR. *Arabic, 'king, ruler'; Hebrew, 'treetop'.* A common Arabic name, the general title for an elevated official. **Ameer.**

AMON. *(Ā-mon) Hebrew, 'teacher, architect'.* Sounds confusingly like the Irish Eamon. Amun is the name of an ancient Egyptian god. **Amen, Amman, Ammon, Emmon.**

♂ **AMORY.** *German, 'industrious'.* The hero of an F. Scott Fitzgerald novel and the kind of executive-sounding surname name that became popular in the 1990s. **Emory.**

★**AMOS.** *Hebrew, 'to carry'.* Robust biblical name borne by one of the minor prophets of the Old Testament and ripe for revival by modern parents

looking for a choice that's both traditional and fresh.

AMPHION. *Greek mythology name.* Son of Zeus known for musical abilities, an edgy choice for music-minded families.

AMYAS. *Latin, 'loved'. See AMIAS.* **Ameus, Amias.**

ANASTASIOS. *Greek, 'resurrection'.* Greek name more familiar here in its feminine form, Anastasia. **Anstace, Stacy, Stassie, Stassy. International: Anastagio** *(Italian).*

ANATOLE. *Greek, 'from the east, rising sun'.* French name with exaggerated image sporting artist's beret, smock and pencil-thin moustache. **International: Anatolio** *(Italian),* **Anatoli, Anbatoly, Tolya** *(Russian),* **Anatol** *(Slavic),* **Anatolios** *(Greek).*

♂ **ANCHOR.** *Word name.* Plausible word name, denoting strength and stability. **Anka, Anker.**

ANDERS. *Scandinavian variation of* **ANDREW.** Friendly, unusual, but a

decidedly old-fashioned version of Andrew. **Ander, Anderson, Andirs, Andy.**

★**ANDERSON.** *Scandinavian, 'son of Anders'.* One of the most appealing of the new wave of surname names. **Andersen.**

ANDOR. *Hungarian variation of* **ANDREW.** Solemn.

ANDRÉ. *French variation of* **ANDREW.** French import that can be seen as pretentious and headwaiterish. **Andray, Andree Andrei.**

ANDREAS. *Original New Testament Greek variation of* **ANDREW.** A beautiful name, evocative of Old Master painters, but with a slightly feminine feel. **Andrius.**

ANDRÉS. *Spanish variation of* **ANDREW.** Has a nice flamenco flavour. **Antrez.**

★**ANDREW.** *Greek, 'strong and manly'.* Andrew, a Top 100 name, is among the most appealing of the classic boys' names, with more character and charm than James or John and a choice of nicknames: Andy makes it friendlier; Drew adds to its sophistication. **Andy, Drew. International: Aindréas andrias andriú** (Irish Gaelic), **Aindrea** (Scottish Gaelic), **Andras** (Welsh), **André** (French), **Andrea** (Italian), **Andrés** (Spanish) and**reu** (Catalan), **Andries** (Dutch), **Andreas** (German), **Anders** (Scandinavian), **Antero** (Finnish), **Ondrej** (Polish), **Andrei** (Russian), **Andras, Andreus, Andrian, Andros** (Greek).

ANDROCLES. Greek, 'glorious man'. Mythological name that's way too weighty for today's use.

ANDY. Diminutive of **ANDREW.** Most modern parents prefer Drew to the old Raggedy Andy.

ANEURIN. Welsh, 'honour'. A case where the jaunty nickname, Nye, is preferable to the original.

♂ **ANGEL.** Word name. Buffy the Vampire Slayer brought Angel into the Anglo-male camp, where it's now heard more frequently, though it still poses some gender confusion. **Angell, Angie. International: Aingeal**

(Irish Gaelic), **Ange** (French), **Angelo** (Italian), **Ángel** (Spanish), **Aniol** (Polish), **Angelov, Anzhel** (Eastern European), **Anshel** (Yiddish), **Angaros** (Persian).

ANGELO. Italian, 'angel, messenger'. Old-school Italian name falling from favour. **Anjelo.**

★**ANGUS.** Scottish, 'unique choice'. Rapidly moving from fuddy-duddy, kilt-wearing old Scotsman to hip young Brits; definitely a plausible choice, particularly for parents whose roots go back to Glasgow. **International: Aengus, Aonghus, Ennis, Gus, Oengus, Ungus.** (Irish).

ANSEL. German, 'with divine protection'. Associated with great western photographer Ansel Adams, this could make a creative artist-hero choice. **Ancell, Ansell.**

ANSELM. German, 'with divine protection'. More solemn than Ansel, but also possible. **International: Anselme** (French), **Anselmo** (Spanish, Portuguese), **Anshelm** (German), **Anzelm** (Polish).

ANSELMO. Italian from German, 'with divine protection'. Lighter Latin version of Anselm.

ANSON. English, 'son of Anne'. Dated matronymic: oxymoron?

Relaxed Names

Andy

Bailey

Barney

Ben

Boone

Brady

Cal

Casey

Charlie

Dugan

Eli

Fred

Harry

Jack

Jake

Mack

Moe

Ned

Rooney

Wylie

ANTHONY. *Latin, 'priceless one'.* This versatile, perennially popular name is comfortable anywhere; it's a safe choice – however it is starting to full from favour, recently slipping out of the Top 100. **Anfernee, Anthoney, Anthoni, Anthonie, Anthny, Antony, Tony.** International: **Antaine, Uaithne** *(Irish Gaelic),* **Antoine** *(French),* **Antonio** *(Spanish)* **Andone Andoni** *(Basque),* **Anton** *(German and Scandinavian),* **Toncse** *(Hungarian),* **Antoni, Tola, Tosia** *(Russian, Polish),* **Antal** *(Eastern European)* **Andonios, Antonios** *(Greek),* **Akoni** *(Hawaiian).*

ANTOINE. *French variation of* **ANTHONY.** Your friendly neighbourhood hairdresser. **Antawn, Antjuan, Antjwon, Antuan, Antuwain, Antwan, Antwain, Antwaine, Antwane, Antwann, Antwanne, Antwaun, Antwon, Antwone, Antwonne.**

ANTON. *German and Scandinavian variation of* **ANTHONY.** Cultured and cultivated.

ANTONIO. *Spanish and Italian variation of* **ANTHONY.**

Shakespearean and sexy. **Antone, Antonnio, Antonyo, Tonio, Tonito, Tony.**

ANWAR. *Arabic, 'brighter, clearer'.* Strongly identified with peace-accord-seeking Egyptian president Anwar el-Sadat.

AODH. *(OOH in Scotland or AY in Ireland) Gaelic, 'fire'.* Common in early Scotland, unworkable in modern Britain. Better to go with the modern Anglicisation: Hugh. **Aed.**

APOLLO. *Greek mythology name.* With mythological names rising, the handsome son of Zeus and god of medicine, music and poetry might offer an interesting, if high-pressure, option. **Apolo, Appollo, Appolo.**

APOLLINAIRE. *French literary name.* Uniquely poetic Gallic choice.

AQUILO. *(ah-KWIH-lo) Latin, 'eagle'.* Common Roman name mentioned in the Bible that has a crisply attractive sound. **Acquila, Acquilla, Aquilino, Aquilla.**

♂ **ARA.** *Arabic, 'rain-maker'; Armenian, 'handsome'.* One of the most melodious in the Armenian name pool. **Arra.**

♂ **ARABY.** *Place name.* Evocative but archaic silent-screen alternate name for Arabia. You might want to consider Barnaby instead.

ARAM. *Hebrew, 'height'.* Popular Armenian name with a pleasing sound that became known elsewhere through the books of William Saroyan, who named his son Aram.

ARAMIS. *French literary name.* One of Dumas' swashbuckling Three Musketeers, now better known as a men's cologne.

♂ **ARCHER.** *Occupational name.* Anglo-Saxon surname that feels more modern than most because of its on-target occupational associations. But it could also be associated with the fallen politician.

ARCHIBALD. *Teutonic, 'bold, noble'.* Although the full name might be tough to handle, the short form Archie is open and friendly – and very trendy here.

Arch, Archey, Archie, Archy. International: **Arhambault** *(French)*, **Archibald** *(Spanish)*.

ARCHIE. *Diminutive of* **ARCHIBALD.** An amiably retro nickname name, but be warned: zooming up the Top 50 at a fast pace. **Arch, Archey, Archy.**

♂ **ARDEN.** *English, 'valley of the eagle'.* Stronger when given to a girl. **Ardan, Ardin, Ardon.**

ARGENTO. *Latin, 'silvery'.* A more distinctive alternative to Angelo.

ARGO. *Greek mythology name.* The name of the ship sailed by Jason in his search for the Golden Fleece might now be confused with a popular retail store in this country.

ARGUS. *Greek, 'watchful guardian'.* In mythology, a creature with a hundred eyes, making it a better name for a camera than a baby.

ARGYLE. *Scottish, 'an Irishman, from the land of the Gaels'.* Nice Scottish sound, but too tied to jumpers and socks.

♂ **ARI.** *Hebrew, diminutive of* **ARIEL.** This short form of Ariel stands up better as a male name than its progenitor does. Also short for Aristotle, as in Onassis. **Arie, Arij, Aroe, Arri, Arye.**

ARIC. *Norse variation of* **ERIC.** This poor lad will spend his life saying, 'No, it's *Aric*, not *Eric!*' **Aaric, Arick, Arik Arric, Arrick.**

♂ **ARIEL.** *Hebrew, 'lion of God'.* Despite its distinguished pedigree and popularity in Israel, Disney's *Little Mermaid* feminised Ariel in this country forever. **Ari, Arial, Arie, Ariele, Arielle, Ariyel, Arriel.**

♂ **ARIES.** *Latin, 'a ram'.* Better than Capricorn or Cancer, not as usable as Leo.

ARISTEDES. *Greek, 'son of the best'.* This name of an early Greek Christian philosopher comes wearing a robe and a long white beard. **Ari, Aristede.**

ARISTOTLE. *Greek, 'superior'.* The great philosopher's name is commonly used in Greek families – and could work for exotically inclined British ones. **Ari.**

ARJUN. *(ar-JHOON) Hindi, 'one of the Pandavas'.* Popular in India and among the Indo-British, this name of the hero of a famous Hindu epic has an extremely pleasing sound. **Arjen, Arjin, Arju, Arjune.**

ARKADI, ARKADY. *Russian from Greek, 'Arcadia'.* Nice, bouncy three-syllable rhythm, à la Jeremy and Barnaby. **Arkadij.**

ARLEDGE. *English 'dweller at the rabbit lake'.* Stiff and formal surname. Try Roone instead.

♂ **ARLEN.** *Irish, 'pledge'.* A serviceable surname without much backbone. **Arlan, Arlin, Arlyn.**

♂ **ARLEY.** *English, 'from the rabbit meadow'.* Sounds a bit like Harley pronounced with a cockney accent. **Arleigh, Arlie, Arly.**

ARLO. *Spanish, 'berry tree'; English, 'fortified hill'.* Strongly associated with shaggy singer Arlo Guthrie, it has an animated and cheery feel, thanks to its upbeat *o* ending.

ARMAND. *French from German, 'soldier'; French variation of* **HERMAN.** Since the first production of *Camille* this has been considered one of the world's most romantic names, though it's rarely heard in this country. **Armande, Armond, Ormand, Ormond. International: Armando, Armano, Armani, Armino** *(Italian)*, **Armando, Armondo, Mando** *(Spanish)*, **Arek, Mandek** *(Polish)*, **Armands** *(Latvian)*, **Arman, Armen** *(Russian)*, **Arman, Armin, Armon, Armoni** *(Israeli)*.

ARMANDO. *Spanish from German, 'soldier'.* Another of the Latin names we expect to be seeing more of. **Armondo, Mando.**

♂ **ARMANI.** *Persian, 'desire, goal'; Italian surname.* Although this is catching on along with other brand names, we think it's better to use a personal family name than to appropriate Giorgio's.

ARMIN. *German, 'soldier, warrior'.* Armand might be a better choice. **Arman, Armen, Armon.**

ARMSTRONG. *English and Scottish surname, 'strong arms'.* Last name occasionally used as a first, can be seen as a Lance Armstrong athlete-hero name.

ARNAU. *Catalan variation of*

ARNOLD. A name sometimes used by Latino parents, considerably more muscular than the Anglo version.

ARNE. *Dutch and Scandinavian variation of* **ARNOLD.** Works better as a full name than Arnie does as a nickname.

ARNO. *German, 'eagle'.* Subtract the last two letters of Arnold and you're left with a much more modern-sounding name. **International: Arnou, Arnoux** *(French)*.

ARNOLD. *English from German, 'ruler, strong as an eagle'.* A name that, despite strongman Schwarzenegger, does not have much muscle. **Arnie, Arnald, Arnoll. International: Ardál** *(Irish Gaelic)*, **Arnaud, Arnauld, Arnaut** *(French)*, **Arnoldo,** *(Italian)*, **Arnaldo** *(Spanish and Portuguese)*, **Arnau** *(Catalan)*, **Arend, Arne** *(Dutch)*, **Arnd, Arno** *(German)*, **Arne** *(Scandinavian)*, **Arneld, Arnljot** *(Norwegian)*, **Arni** *(Icelandic)*.

ARON. *Hebrew and Spanish variation of* **AARON.** This shortened variation of Aaron – it was Elvis's middle name – is popular in the US. **Aaron, Arron, Arun.**

AROON. *Thai, 'dawn'.* Unrelated, but a dramatic twist on the quiet Aaron.

ARRIGO. *Italian variation of* **HENRY** *and* **HARRY**. Think Harry with a go-getter ending.

ARRIO. *Spanish, 'war-like'.* Less substantial than many other Latin choices.

♂ **ARROW.** *Word name.* Implications of being straight and swift lend this word great potential as a name.

ARSENIO. *Spanish from Greek, 'virile, strong'.* A name that is now ready to be adopted elsewhere. **Arsen, Arsenios, Arsenius, Arseny, Arsinio, Senio.** International: **Arséne** *(French)*, **Arsanio, Arsemio, Eresenio** *(Spanish)*, **Arseni** *(Russian)*.

ART. *English, diminutive of* **ARTHUR**. Its meaning may be creative; its abbreviated sound is not. **Artigan, Artin.**

ARTEMAS. *Greek, 'gift of Artemis, goddess of the hunt'.*

This name has a nice mythological, historical, Three Musketeers-ish ring. **Aerimus, Artemis, Artemus. International: Artemio** *(Spanish)*.

ARTHUR. *Celtic, 'noble one, bear man'.* Once the shining head of the Knights of the Round Table, Arthur's image has long since dulled. But some stylish parents are restoring it as a neglected classic. **Art, Arte, Arther, Arthor, Artie, Arty, Authur. International: Artur** *(Irish)*, **Artair** *(Scottish Gaelic)*, **Artus** *(French)*, **Arturo** *(Spanish, Italian)*, **Artek, Arto** *(Finnish)*, **Arturek** *(Polish)*, **Artis** *(Czech)*, **Anthanasios, Thanos** *(Greek)*.

ARVID. *Norwegian, 'eagle-tree'.* Scholarly, bespectacled image. **Arv, Arvad, Arve, Arvie.**

ARVIN. *German, 'friend of the people'.* An anorak name – it won't be a friend to the growing lad. **Arv, Arven, Arvind, Arvy.**

ARYAN. *Indo-Iranian, 'warrior, honourable'.* Very popular Iranian name catching on elsewhere; Arian or Arya spelling would avert hot potato racist connotations. **Arian, Arya.**

ARYE. *Hebrew, 'lion'.* Usually shortened into the Ary or Ari form. **Ari, Ary, Aryeh.**

♂ **ASA.** *Hebrew, 'doctor, healer'; Japanese, 'born in the morning'.* Short but strong biblical name with multicultural appeal. **Aza.**

♂ **ASH.** *Nature name; also diminutive of* **ASHER**. Has arboreal-nature appeal. And your little boy will prize it as the name of the hero of the Pokémon cartoons. **Ashe.**

★**ASHER.** *Hebrew, 'fortunate, blessed, happy one'.* Excellent Old Testament choice, less overused than Adam and Aaron. **Ash, Ashor, Ashur, Asser, Osher.**

♂ **ASHLEY.** *English, 'ash tree meadow'.* Popular name for both the girls and boys, although it's recently slipped out of the boys Top 100. **Ash, Asheley, Ashelie, Ashely, Ashlie.**

ASHTON. *English, 'ash trees place'.* The recent ascent of this English surname could be due to the megapopular *Ash* beginning. It has just entered the Top 100. **Ashten, Ashtin, Ashtyn.**

ASMUND. *Scandinavian, 'God is protector'.* Only occasionally heard in this country.

♂ **ASPEN.** *Nature and place name.* As trendy as the chic Colorado ski resort in the US and film festival, but Aspen is fast becoming cooler for girls than for boys. **Aspin, Aspyn.**

ASTON. *English, 'eastern settlement'.* Has an upscale aura, perhaps due to the luxury James Bond Aston Martin car. **Asten, Astin.**

ATLAS. *Greek, 'bearing the world'.* Would you really want your baby boy to carry the weight of the world on his shoulders?

★**ATTICUS.** *Latin, 'from Athens'.* Trendy Roman feel combined with the upstanding, noble image of Atticus Finch in *To Kill a Mockingbird* make this a potential winner. **Aticus, Attikus.**

ATTILA. *German, 'little father'.* Stun-gunned by the fifth-century Hun. **Atila, Atilo, Attilla.**

ATU. *Ghanan, 'born on Saturday'.* Typical African day-of-the-week name.

AUBERON. *English from German, 'noble, bear-like'.* More commonly used in the Oberon version, but this form has a gentler autumnal feel. **Auberron, Oberon, Oberron.**

♂ **AUBREY.** *English from French, 'elf ruler'.* Upscale British name being used more for girls. . . . and less for boys. **Aubry, Aubury.**

♂ **AUBURN.** *Colour name.* Most of the colour names are reserved for the girls, but here's a perfect one for a boy.

★♂ **AUDEN.** *English, 'old friend,' literary name.* The surname of the distinguished modern poet W. H. has recently started to be seen as a first name option, used for both sexes; appreciated for its pleasing sound as well as its poetic link. **Audon, Audun.**

AUDIO. *Word name.* When a Hollywood semi-celebrity dubbed her son Audio Science, we saw it as a bid for attention. We don't recommend Audio or Video for even the most intrepid baby namer.

★♂ **AUGUST.** *Latin, 'majestic venerable'; month name.* Heating up in Hollywood (Garth Brooks even used it for his daughter), this German and Scandinavian classic is a good choice for a baby born in the month. **Augie, Gus, Gussie. International: Agaistin, Aguistin** *(Irish),* **Août, Auguste, Augustin** *(French),* **Agosto** *(Italian),* **Augusto, Agostino, Agustin, Agusto** *(Spanish),* **Agoston, Agusztav** *(Hungarian),* **Avgust** *(Russian),* **Augustin, Augustinos** *(Greek).*

AUGUSTEN. *German variation of* AUGUSTUS, AUGUSTINE. Confessional memoirist Augusten Burroughs is the first literary notable in this family of names since the confessional saint.

AUGUSTINE. *English variation of* AUGUSTUS. More substantial (and saintly) than August, Augustine, along with its nickname Gus, is definitely a viable choice. **International: Agaistin** *(Irish*

Gaelic), **Agostino** *(Italian),* **Augustín** *(Spanish and French),* **Augustus** *(Slavic),* **Augustinos** *(Greek).*

AUGUSTUS. *Latin, 'the exalted one'.* Parents are beginning to look at imposing but fusty-sounding names like this one with fresh eyes: they definitely make a strong statement. **Augie, Gus.**

AURELIO. *Italian variation of* **AURELIUS.** Exotic and energetic.

AURELIUS. *Latin, 'the golden one'.* Given the supermodel seal of approval by Elle Macpherson, this is another of the Roman emperor names now in the realm of possibility. **International: Auryn** *(Welsh),* **Aurel, Aurelien, Aurelian** *(French),* **Aurelio** *(Italian),* **Aureline** *(Basque),* **Aurek** *(Polish),* **Aranyu** *(Hungarian),* **Avreliy** *(Russian).*

♂ **AUSTEN.** *Shortened form of* **AUGUSTINE,** *literary surname.* Parents who love the great English novelist Jane Austen may choose this spelling of the popular name to honour the

author of *Emma* and *Pride and Prejudice.*

AUSTIN. *English, shortened form of* **AUGUSTINE.** After reaching the peak of its popularity in the 1990s, this attractive American place name has been gradually losing favour in the US; perhaps done in by the smarmy Austin Powers. **Astin, Austen, Auston, Austyn.**

♂ **AUTRY.** *French, 'ancient power'.* Loose, lean and lanky cowboy name.

♂ **AVERILL.** *English from French, 'April'.* A distinguished name. **Averel, Averell, Averil, Averyl. International: Abril** *(Spanish, Portuguese and Arabic).*

♂ **AVERY.** *English, 'ruler of the elves'.* A last-name-first-name being used increasingly for girls, perhaps because of its similarity to Ava and Ivory. **Avary, Averey, Avry, Avory.**

AVI. *Hebrew, 'father'.* This short form of many Hebrew names *(see below)* is often used on its own in Israel. **Aviav, Avidan, Avidor, Aviel, Aviram, Avniel.**

AVIV. *Hebrew, 'springtime, freshness, youth'.* Strongly associated with the city of Tel Aviv. **Avivi.**

US Place Names

Albany
Atlanta
Augusta
Austin
Boston
Cheyenne
Columbia
Denver
Dover
Helena
Jackson
Juneau
Lincoln
Madison
Olympia
Phoenix
Pierre
Raleigh
Salem
Trenton

Stellar Starbabies Beginning with A

Ace	Natalie Appleton
Adam	Des O'Connor
Adrian	Edie Brickell & Paul Simon
Alastair	Rod Stewart, Andrew Lloyd Webber
Alimayu Moa-T	Wesley Snipes
Amedeo	John Turturro
Anderson	Edie Falco
Andres	Andy Garcia
Anton	Beverly D'Angelo & Al Pacino
Antonio Carlos	Anthony Field *(Blue Wiggle)*
Arthur Elwood	Jasmine Guinness
Augustin James	Linda Evangelista
Aurelius	Elle MacPherson

AXEL. *German, 'father of peace'; Scandinavian variation of* **ABSALOM.** The perfect heavy metal rock name. **Aksel, Ax, Axe, Axell, Axil, Axill, Axl, Axyl. International: Aksel** *(Norwegian),* **Akseli** *(Finnish).*

AXTON. *English, 'sword stone'.* Macho.

AYDAN. *Spelling variation of* **AIDAN.** Becoming increasingly popular as one of the many alternate spellings of Aidan.

AYDIN. *Turkish, 'intelligent'.* As a homophone of Aidan, assured of a smooth path to assimilation.

AYU. *African, Yoruban, 'joy'.* Rhythmic and exotic.

♂ **AZA.** *Arabic, 'comfort'.* Similarity to the biblical name Asa makes it ripe for adaptation.

★**AZARIAH.** *(az-ah-RI-ah) Hebrew, 'helped by God'.* A rare biblical name that moves way beyond Adam and Abraham; its pleasant sound makes it one to watch. **Azael, Azaia, Azaryah, Azria, Azriah, Azuriah. International: Azarius** *(Greek).*

♂ **AZIEL.** *Hebrew, 'God is my strength'.* Rarely used name that connotes zeal. **Azeel.**

AZIZI. *Swahili, 'precious treasure'.* Two *z*'s equal double pizzazz. **Aziz.**

AZRIEL. *Hebrew, 'God is my help'.* More masculine than Ariel, more unusual than Israel. **Azreal.**

AZZAM. *Arabic, 'determined'.* Might be open to some 'shazam!' teasing.

B boys

BABSON. *English, 'son of Barbara'.* Only if he actually is. **Babsen, Babsson.**

BACCHUS. *Greek mythology name.* Only if you're hoping for your son to become a wine-besotted poet.

BACH. *German, 'dweller near the brook'.* Although there are plenty of Bachs in the world besides Johann Sebastian, everyone will assume you're honouring the great composer – and why not?

BACHELOR. *French, 'unmarried man'.* Melodic word that nonetheless feels more like a prediction than a name. **Bachellor, Batcheler, Batcheller, Batchellor, Batchelor.**

BADAR. *Arabic and Hindi, 'full moon'.* Strong name, romantic image.

BADEN. *German, 'son of Bade'.* If Braden and Caden, why not Baden? **Badan, Badin, Badon, Badyn, Baeden, Bayden, Baydin, Baydon.**

BADER. *German occupational name, 'barber, surgeon'.* This may be an interesting way to honour a loved one who is a doctor. . . . or a hairdresser.

BAER. *German, 'bearlike, dweller at the sign of the bear'.* Reversed vowels make it seem less fierce.

♂ **BAEZ.** *Spanish surname.* The last name of folksinger Joan is melodic in its own right.

BAGGIO. *Italian, 'toad'.* Too much like baggage.

BAHRAM. *Iranian, 'good-natured, nice'.* Interesting name with affable meaning.

♂ **BAILEY.** *English occupational name, 'law enforcer, bailiff'.* Extremely amiable, open-sounding surname that's in the Top 100, but also well-used for girls. **Bail, Baileigh, Baily, Baley, Bay, Baylee, Bayley, Bayly.**

BAIN. *Gaelic, 'white, fair'.* Not a very desirable pick – you wouldn't want your child to be the Bain/bane of your existence.

BAINBRIDGE. *British, 'bridge over the river Bain'.* We'll have our sherry in the parlour, please, Bainbridge. **Bain, Banebridge, Baynbridge, Bayne, Baynebridge.**

BAIRD. *Scottish occupational name, 'minstrel, poet, balladeer'.* Original choice with poetic and melodic undertones. **Bar, Bard, Barde, Barr, Bayerd, Bayrd, Bay.**

BAKER. *English occupational surname.* One of the best of the newly hip occupational names.

BAKU. *Place name, capital of Azerbaijan.* Why settle for Boston when you can name your child for someplace so much more exotic?

BALBO. *Latin, 'mutterer'.* More appropriate for a chimp than a human child. **Bailby, Balbi, Balbino, Ballbo.**

BALDEMAR. *German, 'bold and renowned'.* The name of a monk who is the patron saint of blacksmiths – not a twentieth-century occupation or baby name. **Baldomar, Baldomero, Baumar, Baumer.**

♂ **BALDWIN.** *German, 'brave friend'.* One 'bald' name we can get behind, thanks to pioneering African-American author James Baldwin. **Bald, Baldewin, Baldwinn, Baldwyn, Baldwynn, Baudwin. International: Baudoin, Baudouin** *(French).*

BALFOUR. *Scottish, 'the village by the pasture'.* Historically interesting via the 1917 Balfour Declaration, which supported the creation of a Jewish state in Palestine. **Balfer, Balfor, Balfore.**

BALIN. *Hindi, 'mighty sword'.* Unusual Asian option and also the name of the Dwarf Lord from *Lord of the Rings.*

BALLIOL. *Scottish, 'wall, fortification'.* Fun to say (try it) and a melodic middle name possibility.

♂ **BALLOU.** *French, 'from Bellou'.* Maybe it's the sexy screen image of Cat Ballou that keeps us from seeing this for a boy.

BALTHASAR. *Greek, 'God protects the king'.* One of the biblical Three Kings who visited the infant Jesus, also used by

Shakespeare and in the oil-rich Getty family; offbeat and intriguing. **International: Balthazar, Baltasaru** *(French),* **Baldassare** *(Italian),* **Baltasar** *(Spanish),* **Balthazar, Belshazzar** *(Hebrew).*

BALTIMORE. *Place name.* Place names are extending their range, but this American city is a bit stiff.

BALTON. *Modern invented name.* Dalton with a *B.* The original is better.

BALZAC. *Literary name.* Dashing middle name choice for admirers of the French author.

♂ **BANAN.** *Irish, 'white'.* Unusual and attractive entry to the growing Irish name canon. **Bannan, Bannon.**

BANCROFT. *English, 'field of beans, dweller near the bean farm'.* An upper-crusty-sounding name with humble origins. **Bancrofft, Banfield, Bank, Banky.**

BANGKOK. *Place name.* This is one place name we'd put off-limits, for obvious reasons.

♂ **BANJO.** *Word name.* When actress Rachel Griffiths chose this highly unusual name for her son, many assumed it was a bizarre invention. But a noted Australian poet (Griffiths is an Aussie) is known by this name.

BANNER. *English occupational surname, 'flag bearer'.* Tanner with a *B,* but a choice with enough charm and heft to transcend its trendy roots.

BANNING. *Irish, 'small, fair one'.* If you like the Irish surname feel, there are loads of more congenial options.

BANYAN. *Indian, 'the God tree'.* This evocative name of a dramatic tropical Indian fig tree is ready to move west.

BAPTISTE. *French, 'baptist,' from Greek, 'to dip'.* Traditionally used by the ultra-religious. **International: Battista, Battiste, Bautiste** *(Italian),* **Baptista, Bautista** *(Spanish).*

BARABBAS. *Aramaic, 'son of the father'.* Barabbas was a murderer Pontius Pilate freed while condemning Jesus to die.

Not the nicest biblical namesake, to say the least.

BARAK. *Hebrew, 'lightning'.* An Old Testament warrior whose name still sounds tough. **Baraq.**

BARAM. *Israeli, 'son of a nation'.* This is one of hundreds of modern Israeli names that are unknown here but could translate to our culture.

♂ BARBEAU. *French occupational name, 'fisherman'.* Too feminine via resemblance to both Barbara and Bardot.

BARBER. *French occupational name, 'beard'.* This name's all-male occupational roots help it break the Barbara bonds, but still not the most inspiring surname choice. **Barbar, Barbour.**

BARBOSSA. *Film character name.* The captain of the *Black Pearl* in the movie *Pirates of the Caribbean* is not much of a namesake inspiration.

BARCLAY. *English and Scottish, 'where birches grow'.* In the UK, Barclay would not escape association with one of the largest banks. Of course, Barclay is the phonetic spelling of Berkley – both sound like old-fashioned butler names. **Bar, Bardey, Barklay, Barkley, Barklie, Barrclay, Berk, Berkeley, Berkie, Berkley, Berklie, Berky.**

BARD. *Irish variation of* **BAIRD.** Great middle name choice for Shakespeare lovers. **Bar, Barde, Bardo, Barr.**

BARDEN. *English 'barley valley'.* Rarely heard last-name-first choice with nice garden-like feel. **Bardon, Borden, Bordon.**

BARDO. *Scandinavian saint name; also Aboriginal, 'water'.* Poetic beginning and upbeat ending.

BARDOLF. *English, 'axe-wolf'.* Shakespeare's classic drunken fool. **Bardolph, Bardon, Bardoul, Bardulf, Bardulph.**

BARDRICK. *Teutonic, 'axe-ruler'.* Sounds like . . . a Teutonic axe-ruler. **Bardric, Bardrich.**

BARKER. *English occupational name, 'shepherd' or 'tanner'.* Either Shepherd or Tanner is more appealing than this somewhat harsh cognate.

♂ BARLEY. *English, 'grower or seller of barley'.* Rhymes with the posh Harley Street, known for its elite doctors, as well as being the name of a grain.

BARLOW. *English, 'bare hillside'.* You'd definitely get a lot of 'huh?'s with this name, but it does have some appeal. **Barlo, Barlowe, Barrlowe.**

BARNABAS. *Aramaic, 'son of comfort'.* Attractive but a bit old-fashioned; we prefer the update Barnaby. **Barnabus, Barnebas, Barnebus.**

★BARNABY. *English variation of* **BARNABAS.** Genial and energetic with an Irish-sounding three-syllable lilt, Barnaby is an ancient name that manages to be both unusual and highly attractive. A real winner. **Barn, Barnabee, Barnabey, Barney, Barni, Barnie, Barno, Barny, Bernabi, Burnaby. International: Barnaib** *(Irish),* **Barnabé** *(French),* **Barnaba, Bernaba** *(Italian),* **Barnebas, Barnabe** *(Spanish),* **Barna** *(Hungarian).*

BARNES. *English, 'someone who lives or works near the barn'.* A fairly charmless family name. **Barns.**

BARNETT. *English, 'place cleared by burning'.* Has some creative credibility via abstract painter Barnett Newman, but we'd prefer his nickname, Barney. **Barnet, Barney, Barnie, Baronet, Baronett, Barren, Barrie, Barry.**

BARNEY. *Variation of* **BARNABUS.** A hot name among hip Londoners – but be careful it's not associated with the purple dinosaur. **Barny, Barnie.**

BARNUM. *English contraction of 'baron's home'.* Inevitable circus association. **Barnham.**

BARON. *English word name.* If you're going to choose a noble word name, why not aim higher and pick Duke, Prince . . . or King? The Donald Trumps picked the Barron spelling for their little princeling. **Baran, Barren, Barron.**

BARR. *Irish diminutive of* FINBAR. We like a cool bar as much as the next fun-loving adult . . . but not as a baby's name.

♂ **BARRETT.** *German, 'bear strength'.* Pleasing sound and pleasing association with poet Elizabeth Barrett Browning. **Barat, Baret, Barrat, Barratt, Barret, Barrey.** International: **Barraud** *(French).*

BARRIC. *English, 'grain farm'.* Perfect choice if your baby has grandpas named Barry and Eric, but also a bit military. **Barrick, Beric.**

BARRON. *See BARON.*

BARRY. *Irish, 'spear'.* This Anglicised form of Bearach or short form of Finbarr predates the Gary-Cary tight black pants/white socks era and shows no signs of revival. **Bar, Baris, Barra, Barree, Barrey, Barrie.**

BART. *Diminutive of* **BARTHOLOMEW.** Permanent property of that devilish little Simpson kid.

BARTHOLOMEW. *Hebrew, 'farmer' or 'son of the earth'.* An apostle's name that's been out of favour for centuries but might appeal again to the parent in search of an old but rare choice. Problems: the natural short form Bart and that final *mew* sound. **Bart, Bartelby, Bartho, Barthol, Barthold, Bartholomeus, Bartlet, Bartlett, Bartow, Bartt, Bat.** International: **Bairtliméad** *(Irish Gaelic)*, **Parthalan, Partholon** *(Irish)*, **Parlan** *(Scottish Gaelic)*, **Barthélemy, Bartholome, Bartholmieu** *(French)*, **Bartolomeo, Meo** *(Italian)*, **Balta, Bario, Barolo, Bartoleme, Bartoli, Bartolomeo, Toli** *(Spanish)*, **Bartel** *(Dutch and German)*, **Barthel, Bartol, Bertel** *(German)*, **Bardo** *(Danish)*, **Barthelemy** *(Swedish)*, **Perttu** *(Finnish)*, **Bartek, Bartos** *(Polish)*, **Barta, Bartalan, Bertalan, Berti** *(Hungarian)*, **Bartek, Barto, Bartosz, Bartz** *(Czech)*, **Varfolomei** *(Russian)*.

BARTLEBY. *Literary name.* Bartleby (that's his last name) the Scrivener is a famous Herman Melville character whose surprisingly powerful refrain was, 'I would prefer not to'. Or, in the immortal words of any two-year-old: No!

BARTLETT. *Diminutive of* **BARTHOLOMEW**. Either you're going to have yourself a Bart . . . or an anorak who's constantly citing quotations. **Bartlet, Bartlitt.**

BARTON. *English, 'from the barley settlement'.* More user-friendly, though less substantial, than Bartholomew. **Bart, Bartan, Barten, Bartin, Bartyn.**

BARTRAM. *Scandinavian, 'glorious raven'.* The raven was a holy bird in Norse mythology, giving this choice some resonance beyond other Bart variations. **Bertram, Barthram.**

BARUCH. *Hebrew, 'blessed'.* Think of this as the Hebrew equivalent of Benedict or Benito; best for observant Jews. **Barruch, Barrush, Baruchi, Barukh, Boruch.** International: **Barrucio** *(Italian)*, **Berakhiah** *(Hebrew)*.

★**BAS.** *Dutch, diminutive of* **BASTIAAN** *and* **SEBASTIAAN**. A fashionable name in its own right in the

Netherlands, where it's in the Top 10. Used throughout the Continent, it may have a future here as a straightforward-but-charming nickname name. Baz is another similar possibility.

BASIL. *Greek, 'regal'.* It's an herb, it's an early Christian name and it's got possibilities here, though a bit effete, à la Basil Rathbone. **Bas, Baz.** International: **Breasal** *(Irish)*, **Bale, Basile, Basle** *(French)*, **Basilio** *(Italian and Spanish)*, **Basle** *(German)*, **Basilius, Basle** *(Swedish)*, **Basek** *(Polish)*, **Bazel, Vazul** *(Hungarian)*, **Vasile** *(Romanian)*, **Bazil, Vasil** *(Czech)*, **Vas, Vaslek, Vasili, Vasily, Vassily, Vasya, Wassily** *(Russian)*, **Bazel, Bazyli** *(Slavic)*, **Basul** *(Arabic)*.

BASSETT. *English, originally a nickname for a short person.* Nothing but a hound dog. **Basett, Basset.**

BASTIEN. *Latin, diminutive of* **SEBASTIEN**. In this form, as Sebastian or as Bas, a fashionable continental name with a possible future here. International: **Bastiaan** *(Dutch)*.

BATES. *English, 'son of Bate (Bartholomew)'.* Hard to discount the creepy Norman B.

BAUER. *German, 'farmer, tiller of the soil'.* A surname name with an occupational background . . . and newfound possibilities. **Bower, Bowers.**

BAXLEY. *English, 'baker's meadow'.* A more unusual, if slightly snooty, masculine Bailey alternative. **Baxlea, Baxlee, Baxlie, Baxly.**

BAXTER. *English occupational name, 'baker'.* An *x* makes any name cooler. **Bax, Baxley.**

♂ **BAY.** *Vietnamese, 'seventh child'; nature name.* Like River and Lake, a cool, refreshing modern water-related choice. **Bai.**

BAYARD. *(BYE-yard) English, 'russet-haired'.* An old English redhead name – one of the few that doesn't begin with the letter *r* – with references both to a famous French knight and a magical horse. **Bay, Bayerd, Bayrd.**

BAYLESS. *French occupational name, 'bailiff'.* Offers much less than Bay. **Bayliss.**

♂ **BAYOU.** *(bye-you) Nature name.* A slow and sultry choice that's definitely cool for babies of either gender.

BAZ. *See BAS.*

BEACAN. *Irish, 'tiny one'.* An attractive ancient Irish saint's name that conjures up a beacon of light. **Beag, Beagan, Bec, Becan, Beccan.**

♂ **BEACH.** *Nature name.* With the tide coming in on a new wave of word names, this one is sure to catch on, especially for parents who relish sun, sand and surf. Forest lovers can spell it Beech, like the tree.

BEACON. *English, 'signal light'.* A word name with an appealing and illuminating meaning.

BEAL. *English from French, 'fair, handsome'.* Could be a possible and more modern, namesake for Uncle Neal. **Beale, Beall, Bealle, Beals, Beel, Beele, Beell, Beil, Beile, Beill.**

BEAMAN. *English occupational name, 'beekeeper'.* This occupational choice is less appealing than such brethren as Baker and Baxter. **Beamann, Beamen, Beamon, Beeman, Beemon.**

BEAMER. *English, 'trumpet player'.* Might make a good middle name for the child of a musician, though people could think you were honouring your BMW. **Beemer.**

BEAR. *Animal name.* Nature names – animals, birds, fish, trees, plants – are hot, though Bear may seem a little aggressive.

BEARCHÁN. *(BAR-uh-hawn) Irish, 'little spear'.* This was a common name in early Ireland, borne by numerous saints, but pronunciation problems would make it prohibitive here. **Bercan.**

★**BEAU.** *French, 'handsome'.* Suggests someone devilishly handsome, with a large measure of charm – a nice image to bestow on your boy. **Beal, Beale, Beauregard, Bo, Boe.**

BEAUCHAMP. *French, 'the beautiful field'.* Pronounced

Beecham, but still too fancy and fey. Likewise **Beaufort** (beautiful fort), **Beaufoy** (beautiful beech tree) and **Beaumont** (beautiful mountain). **Beecham.**

BEAUREGARD. *French, 'beautiful gaze'.* Better suited to a beagle than a boy. **Beau, Bo.**

♂ **BECAN.** *Irish, 'little man'.* More user-friendly Anglicised form of Beacan, could profit from kinship with the popular Beckett.

♂ **BECK.** *English, 'home near the brook', short form of* **REBECCA.** The popular single-named alternative singer (born Bek) has moved this one-time shortening of Becky into male territory. **Becker, Beckman.**

★♂ **BECKETT.** *English and Irish, 'home near the brook'.* A handsome name rich in literary associations with major Irish playwright Samuel Beckett that has recently become hot among celebs – including Conan O'Brien, Melissa Etheridge and Malcolm McDowell. **Becket, Beckitt.**

BECKHAM. *English, 'home near the brook'.* For football fans wishing for a son who can bend it like Beckham.

BEDE. *English, 'prayer'.* A famous seventh-century saint and church historian whose name has not survived as well as his works.

BEELZEBUB. *Hebrew, 'lord of the flies'.* The name of the devil. Enough said. **Baalzebub.**

BEHAN. *Irish, 'bee'.* An Anglicised derivative of the Gaelic name Beatha, meaning 'life,' best known as the surname of Irish playwright Brendan Behan. **Beachán, Beathán.**

♂ **BEIGE.** *Colour name.* Bland and better for a girl besides.

♂ **BELA.** *(BAY-la) Czech, 'white'.* With Bella so popular for girls, we discourage you from naming your son after *Dracula* actor Bela Lugosi – or even composer Béla Bartók.

BELCHER. *English from French, 'pretty face'.* Try telling the kids it *really* means 'pretty face' and not 'burper'.

BELDEN. *English from French, 'pretty valley'.* A charmless surname name. **Beldene, Beldon, Bellden, Belldene, Belldon.**

BELISARIO. *Spanish from Greek, 'swordsman'.* Romantic, dashing, but a bit too elaborate.

♂ **BELL.** *English and Scottish occupational name, 'ringer of the bell'.* Simplicity and pleasant associations give this word real possibility as a first name – but somehow it seems better for a girl, à la Belle.

♂ **BELLAMY.** *English and Irish from French, 'fine friend'.* Undiscovered surname with an admirable meaning and upbeat rhythm. **Belamy, Bell, Bellamey, Bellamie, Bellemy.**

BELLO. *Italian, 'handsome, beautiful'.* Too close to both Bella and belly to make it as a first name, despite its enticing meaning.

BELLOW. *English occupational name, 'bellows maker'.* Might be an honour towards novelist Saul Bellow, although bellowing is not the gentlest of sounds. Consider Saul instead. **Beli, Bellewn.**

BELVEDERE. *Italian, 'beautiful view'.* What the spoilt child in a Victorian novel might be

named. **Bellveder, Bellvedere, Bellvidere, Belvider, Belvidere.**

BEN. *Hebrew, 'son of'.* This diminutive of, most commonly, Benjamin or Benedict, can easily stand on its own as a simple, strong, nice-guy choice, though it's somewhat attenuated. It's in the Top 50. **Benjie, Benn, Bennie, Benno, Benny.**

BENAIAH. *Biblical, 'son of the Lord'.* An unusual biblical choice that can get you to Ben.

BENEDETTO. *Italian, 'blessed'.* This Italian form of Benedict sidesteps the Benedict Arnold association that still clouds the English version.

BENEDICT. *Latin, 'blessed'.* Parents who like Ben and Benjamin but find those forms too popular sometimes consider Benedict – now sanctioned as the name of the current pope – as a more distinctive choice, despite its lasting link to the traitor Benedict Arnold. **Ben, Bendick, Bendict, Benedikte, Benedykt, Bennedict, Bennedikt, Bennet, Bennett, Bennie, Bennito, Bennt, Benny, Betto,**

Dick, Dix. International: **Benen** *(Irish)*, **Benneit** *(Scottish Gaelic)*, **Benôit** *(French)*, **Benedetto** *(Italian)*, **Benicio, Benedicto, Benito** *(Spanish and Portuguese)*, **Benet** *(Catalan)*, **Benedick, Benedikt, Bendix** *(Dutch)*, **Bendt** *(Danish)*, **Beng** *(Swedish)*, **Bendik** *(Norwegian)*, **Pentti** *(Finnish)*, **Bence, Bendek** *(Hungarian)*, **Benes** *(Czech and Slavic)*, **Benedek, Benedik, Benke** *(Eastern European)*, **Benedikt, Venedict, Venedikt, Venka, Venya** *(Russian)*, **Venedict** *(Greek)*, **Benoit** *(Yiddish)*.

BENEN. *Irish, 'mild'.* This name of an ancient Irish saint – a favourite disciple of Saint Patrick – could be an option for parents in search of a more distinctive alternative to Brendan or Aidan.

♂ **BENEVOLENT.** *Word name.* One of the new generation of virtue names, with Peace and Justice taking over from the Puritans' Absolution and Forgiveness, but this one is still a bit heavy to carry.

BENICIO. *(ben-EE-see-ō) Spanish, 'blessed'.* Smouldering

Spanish actor Benicio Del Toro made this version a possibility elsewhere.

BENIGNO. *(ben-NEEN-yo) Latin, 'kind, wellborn'.* From the root that gives us 'benign', not as accessible as such names as Bruno and Benicio.

BENJAMIN. *Hebrew, 'son of the right hand'.* Sensitive Old Testament name of the son of Jacob and Rachel, associated with many other distinguished figures, including Benjamin Franklin, which has enjoyed widespread favour for decades – and is attractive and strong enough to hold its place in the Top 25. **Benejamen, Beni, Benjaman, Benjamen, Benjamon, Benjee, Benjey, Benji, Benjie, Benjiman, Benjimen, Benjy, Benn, Bennie, Benno, Benny, Benyamin, Benyanrino, Binyamino. International: Bannerjee** *(Gaelic),* **Beniamino, Benjamino** *(Italian),* **Beniamín, Benja, Benjamé, Benjammén, Benjemín, Chelín, Min, Mincho, Mino, Venjamín** *(Spanish),* **Benkamin** *(Basque),* **Benjaminho** *(Portuguese),* **Beniamin** *(Slavic),* **Veniamin**

(Greek), **Binyamin** *(Israeli),* **Beinish** *(Yiddish),* **Peni'amina Peni** *(Hawaiian).*

BENNETT. *English, 'blessed'.* Ben with a bow tie. **Benedict, Benet, Benett, Bennet.**

♂ **BENNING.** *German, 'son of Bernhard'.* Delete an *n* and you could pay tribute to Warren Beatty's wife Annette Bening.

BENNO. *German, tenth-century saint.* A cool name in its own right but more likely to be used as a nickname for Benjamin. **Beno.**

BENOÎT. *(Ben-wa) French variation of* **BENEDICT.** Once you get past the pronunciation hurdle, an elegant, sexy choice.

BENONI. *Hebrew, 'son of my sorrow'.* What the Old Testament Rachel originally named Benjamin, before his father changed it; rarely heard today.

BENSON. *English, 'son of Ben'.* **Bensen, Benssen, Bensson.**

BENTLEY. *English, 'meadow with coarse grass'.* Or, an incredibly expensive English car.

Ben, Bentlea, Bentley, Bentlie, Bently, Lee.

BENVENUTO. *Italian, 'welcome'.* In Italy, often refers to the joy at the birth of a long-awaited child. **International: Bienvenido** *(Spanish).*

BENYAMIN. *Hebrew, 'son of the right hand'.* Benjamin for purists. *See* **BENJAMIN.**

BERED. *Hebrew, 'hail'.* Mentioned in the Old Testament as both a place name and a grandson of Ephraim, this would make a fairly obscure biblical choice.

BERENGER. *German, 'warrior fighting with a spear'.* Last-name-first-name with a romantic but dangerous edge.

BERESFORD. *English, 'ford where barley grows'.* Upper-crusty hotelish surname.

BERG. *German, 'mountain, hill'.* Earthbound surname that few would make as first choice. **Berger, Bergh, Burg, Burgh.**

BERGEN. *Scandinavian, 'lives on a hill'.* Norwegian city name heard much more often as a last name than a first. **Bergin, Birgin.**

BERGER. *German, Dutch and Swedish, 'lives on a hill'.* No kid would want to be open to all those burger jokes. **Bergeron.**

♂ **BERIAH.** *Hebrew, 'in fellowship' or 'in envy'.* Unusual biblical name that may be too close in sound to the feminine Mariah. **Beri.**

BERILO. *(bay-REE-low) Spanish from Greek, 'beryl, pale green gemstone'.* A Latin name with a lot of tango flair. **Barilio, Berillo.**

♂ **BERIN.** *Latin, 'fair-haired'.* Fresh choice, but with feminine lilt. **Birin, Birinus.**

BERKELEY. *English, 'where birches grow'.* A pretentious name that firmly belongs to another era. **Barcley, Barklay, Barkley, Barklie, Berk, Berkie, Berklee, Berkley, Berky, Birkeley, Birkley.**

♂ **BERLIN.** *German, 'borderline'.* Edgy German capital with definite possibilities as a baby name. **Berlyn.**

BERN. *German, 'bear'.* Hip short form of Bernard; also Swiss place name. **Berne, Bernie, Berny.**

BERNARD. *German, 'strong, brave as a bear'.* Though the patron saint of mountain climbers, still an unathletic, outdated name with a highly intellectual image. **Barnard, Barney, Barnhard, Barnie, Barny, Bear, Bearard, Bern, Bernarr, Bernie, Bernis, Burnard. International: Bearnard** *(Gaelic),* **Bernal, Bernardin, Bernon, Bernot** *(French),* **Bernadino** *(Italian),* **Bernal, Bernardel, Bernardino, Bernardito, Bernardo, Nardo** *(Spanish),* **Benat** *(Basque),* **Bernat** *(Catalan),* **Beno, Berend, Bernhard, Bernhardt, Bernhart** *(German),* **Bernt** *(Scandinavian),* **Benek, Bernardyn** *(Polish),* **Bernek, Berno** *(Czech),* **Berngards** *(Russian),* **Vernados** *(Greek).*

BEROLD. *English, 'bear rule'.* Too close to Beryl for a boy. **Berholt.**

BERQUIST. *Swedish, 'mountain twig'.* Few Scandinavian names make the journey elsewhere . . . and this one shows you why. **Bergquist.**

♂ **BERRY.** *Nature name.* If not for Motown founder Berry Gordy, this name would now be totally in the girl group.

BERT, BERTIE. *English, diminutive variation of* **ALBERT** *and* **BERTRAM**. A once-popular nickname for Albert and Bertram now being polished up by hip Brits, but still hibernating elsewhere. **Bertie, Berty, Burt, Burty, Butch.**

BERTHOLD. *German, 'bright strength'.* One bright spot: famous namesake *Threepenny Opera* playwright Berthold (later known as Bertolt) Brecht. **Bertell, Bertil, Berthoud, Bertol, Bertold, Bertolde, Bertoll.**

BERTON. *English, 'fortified town'.* Prissy. **Bert, Bertie, Bertin, Burt, Burton.**

BERTRAM. *German, 'bright raven'.* Old Norman name last current in the 1930s. **Bart, Bartram, Bert, Bertie, Berton,**

Bertran, Bertrando, Bertranno. International: Bertrand *(French)*, Beltrán, Beltrano *(Spanish)*.

BERTRAND. *French and English variation of* **BERTRAM.** This name of famed philosopher Bertrand Russell becomes slightly more plausible with the French pronunciation, *bare-TRAHN.*

BERWIN. *English, 'bright friend'.* One step up from Irwin and that's not nearly enough. **Bervin, Bervyn, Berwinn, Berwyn, Berwynn, Berwynne.**

♂ **BEVAN.** *Welsh, 'son of Evan'.* This Welsh surname might be an interesting alternative to the popular Evan, though that *Bev* beginning conjures up a fifty-five-year-old woman named Beverly. **Beavan, Beaven, Bev, Beven, Bevin, Bevon, Bevvin, Bewan, Bewon, Bivian.**

BEVIS. *French, 'from Beauvais'; Welsh, 'son of Evan'.* Well, it's better than Butthead. **Beauvais, Beavess, Beavis, Beviss.**

BEZAI. *Hebrew, 'eggs'.* Biblical family with 323 children. That's a lot of eggs.

BICKFORD. *English, 'axe man's ford'.* Surname doomed to remain a surname.

BIFF. *American nickname.* The quintessential mid-century nickname, famously found in Arthur Miller's play *Death of a Salesman.*

BILL. *English, diminutive of* **WILLIAM.** Most Bills today are dads . . . or grandpas. The younger Williams are usually nicknamed Will, or called by their full names. **Bil, Billie, Billy, Byll.**

BILLY. *English, diminutive of* **WILLIAM.** Cute kid with freckles, bouncing along in the Top 100 list. Cool couple Helena Bonham Carter and Tim Burton put the name Billy Burton on their son's birth certificate. **Billie.**

♂ **BIMINI.** *place name.* Name of a tiny Bahamian island that's better suited to a girl.

BING. *German, 'kettle-shaped hollow'.* There was only one, nicknamed Der Bingle – and he was really Harry.

BINGO. *Word name.* A name best for pets.

★**BIRCH.** *Nature name.* Lovely image of the tall, strong but graceful white-barked tree. **Birk, Burch.**

BIRKETT. *English, 'birch coastland'.* Birch or even Burke is better. **Birket, Birkit, Birkitt, Birky, Burket, Burkett, Burkitt.**

BIRLEY. *English, 'meadow with the cow shed'.* Girly. **Birlie, Birly, Burleigh, Burley.**

BIRNEY. *English surname, 'island with the brook'.* Bernie, with airs. **Birnie, Birny, Burney, Burnie.**

BIRTLE. *English, 'hill of birds'.* Brittle. **Bertie, Birt, Birtie.**

BISHOP. *English occupational name.* Reese Witherspoon's Deacon has opened this churchy direction for occupational names. **Bishopp.**

BIX. *Modern nickname.* Biff's cooler brother, thanks to that final *x*; could be a hero name for jazz lovers, via the great Bix (born Leon) Beiderbecke.

Tree Names

Apple
Ash
Aspen
Banyan
Beech
Birch
Branch
Cedar
Elm
Forrest
Grove
Hazel
Ilara
Juniper
Kamilah
Laurel
Leaf
Linden
Oak
Olive
Park
Pine
Sequoyah
Spruce
Sylvan
Willow

BJORN. *Swedish, 'bear'.* One of the best-known Scandinavian names, thanks to tennis great Björn Borg. **Bernard, Bjame, Bjarn, Bjarne, Bjorne.**

BJORNSON. *Scandinavian, 'son of Bjorn'.* Leave it at Bjorn. **Bjornsen.**

BLACK. *Colour name.* Unlike Rose and Blue, this colour name is not ready for prime time.

BLACKBURN. *English, 'black brook'.* Somewhat dashing surname, but with serious teasing potential. **Blackburne.**

BLACKWELL. *English, 'black well or stream'.* Dark.

BLADE. *Word name.* One of the new crop of boys' names that manage to be unconventional and macho at the same time – though Blade verges on the threatening.

♂ **BLAINE.** *Irish, 'slender, angular'.* Attractive surname name of a seventh-century Scottish saint, but it can sound a bit feminine. **Blain, Blane, Blayne.**

♂ **BLAIR.** *Scottish, 'dweller on the plain'.* One of the first generation of cool surname names, now largely gone to the girls. **Blaire, Blayr, Blayre.**

♂ **BLAISE.** *French, 'one who stutters'.* An ancient Christian martyr name, also Merlin the Magician's tutor; its relation to Blaze gives it a fiery feel. **Blayse, Blayze, Blaze. International: Blaisot, Blaise** *(French),* **Biagio** *(Italian),* **Blas** *(Spanish),* **Braz** *(Portuguese),* **Blasi, Blasius** *(German),* **Blazek** *(Polish),* **Balas, Balasz, Ballas** *(Hungarian),* **Vlas** *(Russian).*

♂ **BLAKE.** *English, means both 'black, dark-haired' and 'fair-haired'.* Early unisex option, it still a sophisticated choice for a boy.

♂ **BLAKELY.** *English, 'dark woodland clearing'.* Takes things one syllable too far. **Blakelee, Blakeleigh, Blakeley, Blakelie.**

BLANCO. *Spanish, 'fair, white'.* Unlike the feminine Blanca, this name for some reason seems to put more emphasis on the 'blank' aspect. **Bianco.**

BLANFORD. *English, 'grey man's ford'.* Comes with a monocle. **Blandford.**

♂ **BLAZE.** *Latin, 'one who stutters'.* Originally a form of Blaise, though now more likely to be a hot word name; used for both sexes. **Blaise, Blaise, Blase, Blayze.**

BLEDDYN. *(BLETH-in) Welsh, 'wolf's cub'.* Unusual two-syllable choice with a real pronunciation challenge.

BLIGH. *English variation of* BLYTHE. Too tightly associated with the real-life villainous Captain Bligh of *The Mutiny on the Bounty.*

♂ **BLISS.** *English word name, 'intense happiness'.* If you use this for a boy, it had better be a family name, hidden away in the middle.

♂ **BLUE.** *Colour name.* Among the coolest of the cool colour names, particularly popular with celebs as a unisex middle name. **Bleu, Blu.**

♂ **BO.** *Norse nickname, 'to live'.* A popular name in Denmark, in this country Beau would have more substance. **Beau, Boe, Bow.**

★**BOAZ.** *Hebrew, 'swiftness'.* Now that such Old Testament patriarchs as Elijah and Moses fill the playground, Boaz seems downright baby-friendly, having more pizzazz than many of the others. **Bo, Boas, Boase.**

BOB. *English, diminutive of* ROBERT. Kids love Bob the Builder, but do they want to *be* Bob the Builder? **Bobbee, Bobbey, Bobbie, Bobby, Bobo.**

BODI. *Hungarian, 'God protect the king'.* An affectionate-seeming name from a Slavic culture.

BODHI. *Sanskrit, 'awakening'.* The Buddhist concept of Bodhi is spiritual awakening and freedom from the cycle of birth, karma and death. An unusual name for a son.

BOGART. *Gaelic, 'marshlands'; German, 'small bowl'.* What it really means: you're a *Casablanca* fan. **Bogie, Bogy.**

Cool Biblical Names

Abel
Abner
Amos
Asa
Asher
Boaz
Elijah
Ezekiel
Ezra
Gideon
Isaac
Isaiah
Jabez
Jethro
Josiah
Jude
Levi
Malachi
Micah
Moses
Obadiah
Phineas
Samson
Simeon
Tobiah
Zebedee

BOGDAN. *Russian, 'gift from God'.* Funny, you don't sound Russian. **Bogdasha.**

BOHDAN. *Ukrainian variation of* **DONALD.** Cooler than Donald. But then again, what isn't? **International: Bogdan, Bogdashka, Danya** *(Russian).*

BOLAN. *Irish, 'little poet'.* An Irish surname name with a combination of boldness and élan. Some might connect it to the founder of the group T. Rex – Marc Bolan.

BOLIVAR. *Basque, 'mill at the riverbank'.* Revolutionary choice. **Bolevar, Bollivar.**

♂ **BOLIVIA.** *place name.* A wonderful geographic option, if only the final *a* didn't feminise it.

BOLTON. *English, 'dwelling in an enclosure'.* Severe surname choice. **Bollton, Boltan, Boltin.**

♂ **BOMBAY.** *Indian place name.* The real city is now known as Mumbai, but the original name is far more evocative.

♂ **BONANZA.** *Word name.* Wildly optimistic – and unrealistic – choice.

BONAVENTURE, BONAVENTURA. *Latin, 'good fortune'.* The kind of middle name you confess only at gunpoint.

BOND. *English, 'peasant farmer'.* For 007 fans, a great middle name choice – or even a first.

BONIFACE. *Latin, 'fortunate, of good fate'.* A name only a pope could carry. **International: Bonifacio** *(Italian, Spanish and Portuguese),* **Bonifaz** *(German).*

★**BOOKER.** *English occupational name, 'scribe'.* A very cool name, for writers, R & B fans and those wanting to pay tribute to Booker T. Washington.

★**BOONE.** *English from French, 'a blessing'.* Appealing surname with a laid-back, backwoods feel. **Boon.**

BOOTH. *English and Scottish, 'small dwelling place, shed'.* Short but not particularly sweet surname. **Boot, Boote, Boothe, Booths, Both.**

BORDEN. *English, 'den of the boar'.* **Bordin.**

BORIS. *Slavic, 'to fight'.* One of the old Russian names being revived by chic Europeans. Are you cool enough to call your kid Boris, like the popular tennis player? More to the point, will your son be cool enough to live with such a potentially clunky name? **Boriss, Borris, Borys.**

BORROMEO. *Italian saint name.* A rarely heard saint's name – Saint Charles Borromeo is the patron of apple orchards and stomach diseases. Romeo would be better.

BOSCO. *Italian saint name.* Not likely to be a popular choice in the modern world.

BOSLEY. *English, 'meadow near the woods'.* Another servile surname, this one connected to the go-between character in *Charlie's Angels.* **Boslea, Boslee, Bosleigh, Bosly.**

♂ BOSTON. *Place name.* With the popularity of place names from Brooklyn to Brazil, the attractive and distinctive Boston is surely about to rise.

BOSWELL. *English, 'well near the woods'.* Well known in literature for Boswell's *Life of Johnson.*

BOTAN. *Japanese, 'peony'.* One Japanese name that feels Western, though not quite British.

BOTHAM. *English, 'he who lives in a broad valley'.* Hitting bottom.

BOURBON. *Word name.* Not even for Brandy's twin brother. **Borbon.**

BOURNE. *English, 'one who lives near a stream'.* A surname with more force than most. **Born, Borne, Bourn, Burn, Burne, Byrn.**

♂ BOUVIER. *French occupational name, 'herdsman'.* So tied to being Jacqueline Kennedy's maiden name that it's best saved for a girl.

BOWEN. *Welsh, 'son of Owen'.* Good choice if you're looking for an alternative to Owen. **Bow, Bowie, Bowin.**

BOWIE. *Scottish, 'blond'.* David Bowie dyed it blond and gave it rhythm. **Bow, Bowen.**

BOYCE. *Scottish, from French, 'lives by the woods'.* CEO name. **Boice, Boise.**

BOYD. *Scottish, 'blond'.* Has a bit of a hayseed image and that *oy* sound is tough to work with.

BOYER. *English and French, 'bow-maker, cattle herder'.* Two completely different images come from its national pronunciations – *BOY-err* or *boy-AY* – the latter giving it an effete French accent.

BOYNE. *Irish, 'white cow'.* The famous Battle of the Boyne, in Ireland, vanquished the Catholic king. **Boine, Boyn.**

BOYNTON. *Irish and English, 'town near the Boyne'.* Oy! That sound again!

BOZRAH. *Biblical place name.* A city in southern Jordan that some believe will be the site of the Second Coming.

BRAD. *Diminutive of* **BRADLEY.** Pitt is the prototypical blond Brad. **Bradd.**

BRADAN. *Irish, 'salmon'.* This now-popular name has spawned several different spellings. Many parents choose it solely for its style and sound, but we like the history behind this version: the bradan feasa is the 'Salmon of Knowledge' in the legend of Finn McCool. **Braddan, Bradden, Braden, Bradeon, Bradin, Bradun, Braedan, Braeden, Braedin, Braedon, Brayden, Braydon.**

BRADBURY. *English, 'dweller near the wood fort'.* Possibility for fans of science fiction writer Ray. **Bradberry, BradbURRY.**

BRADEN. *English, 'wide valley'.* One of the trendiest of the new two-syllable boys' names that have appeared in the past few years, including the rhyming Aidan, Caden, Kaden and Jaden.

Bradan, Bradin, Bradon, Braiden, Braidin, Brayden, Braydon.

BRADFORD. *English, 'wide river crossing'.* Brad in a Brooks Brothers suit. **Braddford, Bradman.**

♂ **BRADLEY.** *English, 'wide meadow'.* Brad in a BHS suit. Sounds fresher for a girl. **Brad, Bradd, Bradlea, Bradleigh, Bradlie, Bradly, Bradman, Bradney, Lee.**

BRADSHAW. *English, 'broad forest'.* Another attractive last name as first.

♂ **BRADY.** *Irish, 'broad meadow,' 'one with broad eyes'.* The name is friendly and energetic and a popular choice – it's currently in the Top 50.

BRAHAM. *English, 'flood plain'.* Rarely heard name that could be a subsitute for Graham. **Braheim, Brahiem, Brahima, Brahm.**

♂ **BRAHMS.** *German surname.* A melodic choice for lullaby-lovers. **Brahms.**

BRAINARD. *English, 'courageous raven'.* We can hear the kids teasing him from here. **Brainerd, Braynard.**

★**BRAM.** *Dutch variation of* **ABRAHAM.** Has an unusual measure of character and charm for a one-syllable name; it started as a hipper-than-Abe diminutive of the biblical Abraham, but it's also an independent Irish and Dutch name made famous by *Dracula* creator Bram Stoker. **Bramm, Bran, Brann.**

BRAMWELL. *English, 'well where the gorse grows'.* The only boy in the Brontë family; the name has a lonely *Wuthering Heights/Jane Eyre* feel. **Bramwel, Braimvyll, Branunell, Branwell, Branwill, Branwyll.**

♂ **BRANAGAN.** *Irish, 'little raven'.* Bold Irish surname, full of energy and cheer. **Branigan, Brannigan.**

★♂ **BRANCH.** *Word name.* Attractive name with associations both with trees and with branching out into new worlds. Combination of nature and a positive spiritual feel makes it a winner.

BRAND. *English, 'firebrand, sword'.* Rugged and straightforward brand-new name, though you might not like the idea of branding your son. **Brander, Brant, Brantley, Brantlie, Brantly.**

BRANDEIS. *Place name from Czech town of Brandýs.* A name that hasn't made it in the popularity lists elsewhere.

BRANDON. *English, 'broom-covered hill'.* A forebear of the Braden-Caden pack, Brandon had a great run of popularity, but it has recently slipped out of the Top 50. **Brand, Branden, Brandin, Brandyn, Brannon, Branton.**

BRANDT. *German, 'dweller on burnt land'.* Less commercial-sounding than Brand.

♂ **BRANLEY.** *English, 'raven meadow'.* Rather than being manly, the *-ley* ending is feminine, à la Ashley. **Branlea, Branlee, Branlie, Branly.**

♂ **BRANNON.** *Irish variation of* **BRENNAN.** Occasionally used as an alternative to

Brandon or Brennan. **Brahnen, Brannan, Brannin.**

BRANSON. *English, 'son of the raven'.* Virgin Airlines entrepreneur Richard spotlighted this name – however it is also reminiscent of the pickled onions, making it unlikely to be a popular choice here.

BRANT. *German, 'sword'.* Brisk. **Brandt, Brannt, Brantt.**

BRANTON. *Gaelic and English, 'farmstead overgrown with broom'.* Sounds like an attempt to make Brandon more 'original'. **Brannton, Branten, Brantin.**

♂ **BRAQUE.** *Artist name.* A strikingly creative and unique surname name well worth considering, recalling the great cubist paintings of Georges Braque.

BRASON. *Modern invented name.* Jason with a *Br.*

BRÁULIO. *Spanish from German, 'glowing'.* Bráulio was a medieval bishop and saint whose name has an energetic, modern quality. **Bravilio, Bravlio.**

BRAUN. *German, 'brown'.* Has some highly unfortunate World War II associations.

BRAVO. *Italian word name.* One way to encourage some cheers for your little one, but not recommended. **Brahvo, Brawo.**

BRAWLEY. *English, 'meadow at the slope of the hill'.* A rowdy name nobody ever heard of, till Nick Nolte gave it to his son. **Brauleigh, Braulie, Brauly, Brawlea, Brawleigh, Brawly.**

BRAXON. *Modern invented name.* Jaxon with a twist. *Another* twist.

♂ **BRAXTON.** *English, 'Brock's settlement'.* Might appeal to fans of singer Toni.

BRAY. *Irish place name, from French, 'marsh'.* Can't help thinking of a donkey. **Brae.**

BRAZIER. *Occupational name, 'worker with brass'.* Would be an obscure but winning entry in this category, except for its similarity to the word *brassiere,* which would certainly arouse unwanted attention in secondary school. **Braiser, Braser, Brasier, Braiser, Brazer.**

♂ **BRAZIL.** *Place name.* A geographical name that does the samba . . . and was also borne by a Celtic saint: a winning combination. **Brasil, Brasilia.**

BRECCAN. *Irish, 'freckled, speckled'.* This name of a saint from the Isle of Aran also appears in myth and fantasy fiction, giving it an intriguing, mystical air. **Breck, Brecon. International: Breácan** *(Irish).*

♂ **BRECK.** *Scottish, 'speckled'.* Sudsy name that could be a new character on *Coronation Street.*

BRENDAN. *Irish, 'prince'.* According to Irish legend, Saint Brendan the Voyager was the first European to touch American soil, lending the name an adventurous lilt. **Brendano, Brendin, Brendon, Brendyn.**

Cool Saints' Names

Adrian

Amias

Austin

Blane

Breccan

Bruno

Cassian

Cloud

Conan

Elias

Fabian

Finnian

Isaac

Jonah

Julian

Kieran

Lorcan

Oliver

Quentin

Romeo

Rufus

Rupert

Zeno

★ ♂ **BRENNAN.** *Irish, 'descendent of the sad one'.* Winning Irish surname name, more modern than Brian or Brendan, more unusual than Conor and Aidan. **Brenan, Brennen, Brennin, Brennon, Brenyn.**

BRENNER. *English, 'charcoal burner'.* That *er* ending definitely adds to its stylishness.

BRENT. *English, 'dweller near the burnt land'.* One of several blunt *B* names just this side of the gender divide. **Brennt, Brentan, Brenten, Brentin, Brenton, Brentt.**

♂ **BRETT.** *Celtic, 'from Brittany'.* An unusual name that could suit a boy with a celtic background. **Bret, Brette, Bretton, Brit, Briton, Britt, Britte.**

♂ **BRETTON.** *French, 'from Brittany'.* Veering towards Brittany. **Breton.**

BREVIN. *Modern invented name.* If you're tired of Kevin and Devin, you might consider the newly coined Brevin.

BREWSTER. *English occupational name, 'brewer'.* With its slightly cocky feel, this well-used surname is not often heard as a first. **Brewer.**

BRIAN. *Irish, 'strong, virtuous and honourable'.* Long among the most popular of the Irish imports, Brian, like Ryan, is gradually being replaced by such upstart brothers as Aidan and Conor. Brian Boru was the most famous of all Irish warrior-kings. **Briano, Briant, Brien, Brion, Bryan, Bryant, Bryen, Bryent, Bryon.**

♂ **BRICE.** *Celtic, 'bright strength'; Welsh, 'speckled, freckled'.* Old saint's name that now has a sleek and sophisticated image; it's elegant and efficient almost to the point of cliché. **Bryce. International: Brychan** *(Welsh).*

BRICK. *Anglicised form of various names; Irish Gaelic, Ó Bruic; German, Brück or Breck, meaning 'swamp' or 'wood'; Jewish (Ashkenazic), Brik 'bridge'; Slovenian, Bric, 'dweller from a hilly place'.* Gosh and we thought it was just a macho word name. **Bric, Brik, Bryck, Bryk.**

♂ **BRIDGE.** *Word name.* A new name with the potential for spanning across a far-reaching future.

BRIDGER. *English, 'lives near the bridge'.* A trendy two-syllable name with the fashionable *er* ending, Bridger connotes a person who makes connections and spans disjointed places. A good choice for a child with a cross-cultural background.

BRIGGS. *English variation of Bridges.* Priggish.

BRIGHAM. *English, 'little village near the bridge'.* Mormon leader Brigham Young may inspire some namesakes. **Brigg, Briggham, Briggs.**

♂ **BRILEY.** *Modern invented name.* Brian meets Riley. **Brilie, Brily, Bryley, Bryly.**

♂ **BRINLEY.** *English, 'burnt meadow'.* Surname name with feminine final *ley.* The Welsh name Bryn, though also unisex and veering towards the girl world, is far more attractive.

Brindley, Brindly, Brinlee, Brinleigh, Brinly, Brinsley, Brynly.

♂ **BRIO.** *Italian, 'vivacity, zest'.* Zesty.

BRISTOL. *British place name.* This name of a busy UK city has a brisk and bustling air about it – but it also has negative slavery connections. **Bristow.**

♂ **BRITAIN.** *Place name.* The popularity of all forms of Brittany for girls knocks this somewhat out of consideration, but not completely.

♂ **BRITTON.** *English, 'from Britain'.* One case where a spelling variation improves the name. **Bretton, Brit, Briton, Britt.**

BROCK. *English, 'badger'.* Strong name for a boy, rising in Oz. **Broc, Brocke, Brok.**

BROCKTON. *English, 'badger settlement'.* Brock plus. **Brockten, Brocktin, Brocton.**

BRODER. *Scandinavian, 'brother'.* One of the more

unfamiliar – and unappealing – Nordic choices.

BRODERICK. *Norse, 'brother'; variation of RODERICK.* Despite its brotherly meaning, sounds rather formal and cold. **Brod, Broddy, Broder, Broderic, Brodric, Brodrick, Ric, Rick, Rickey, Rickie, Ricky.**

BRODNY. *Slavic, 'one who lives near a stream'.* Off-putting cousin of Bradley and Rodney.

★**BRODY.** *Scottish, 'muddy place, ditch'.* When bad meanings happen to good names. Brody is slightly less common than Brady, making it a more distinctive choice. **Brodee, Brodey, Brodie, Broedy.**

BROGAN. *Irish, 'small shoe'.* May follow Logan into the limelight, bringing its own Irish brogue along with it. **Broggan.**

BROM. *English, diminutive of* **BROMLEY.** Attached to one of the heroes of Christopher Paolini's megapopular fantasy novel *Eragon,* this name sounds strong yet sensitive.

BROMLEY. *English, 'meadow where broom grows'.* Stiff surname choice. **Brom, Bromlea, Bromlee, Bromleigh, Broomlie.**

BRON. *Polish diminutive of Bronislaw.* Crisply appealing.

BRONCO. *Spanish, 'rough, unbroken horse'.* For the parent who might also have Buck and Ryder on his list.

BRONE. *Irish, 'sorrow'.* An old saint's name that, even with the post-Aidan wave of Irish names, is a bit too close to crone. **Bron.**

BRONISLAW. *Polish, 'weapon of glory'.* Fine to honour a family tradition, as long as you promise to call him Bron.

BRONSON. *English, 'son of brown-haired one'.* An old-fashioned name that has some contemporary appeal. **Bron, Bronnson, Bronsen, Bronsin, Bronsonn, Bronsson.**

♂ **BROOK.** *Nature name.* Gone to the girls. **Brooke, Brooker, Brookes, Brookie, Brooks.**

♂ **BROOKLYN.** *Place name.* Posh Spice and David Beckham's little boy notwithstanding, this name is popular mainly for girls, with a whole raft of new feminine spellings taking it away from the New York borough.

BROOKS. *English, 'of the brook'.* Surname name, with more masculine heft than Brook or Brooklyn.

BROSNAN. *Irish, 'dweller near the Brosna River'.* Actor Pierce made both his first and last name sexier.

♂ **BROWN.** *Colour name.* As rich and warm as the tone it denotes, but the Italian version Bruno has more spark and substance.

BRUCE. *Scottish and English from French, 'from the brushwood thicket'.* Norman place name made famous by the Scottish king Robert the Bruce, who won Scotland's independence from England in 1327; it's perennially popular in Scotland, but rarely used for babies here and now. **Brucey, Brucie.**

★**BRUNO.** *German, 'brown'.* A popular name throughout Europe that deserves more fashion status here. Stylish cookbook writer Nigella Lawson has a son named Bruno. **Bruin, Bruino, Brun.**

BRUTUS. *Latin, 'heavy'.* The quintessential brute: any child with this name would spend much of his life hearing 'Et tu . . .'. **Bruto.**

BRYAN. *Variation of* **BRIAN.** *See* **BRIAN.** **Bryen.**

BRYANT. *Variation of* **BRIAN.** Brian with attitude.

♂ **BRYCE.** *Variation of* **BRICE,** *also place name.* Using a *y* where an *i* will serve complicates matters unnecessarily. **Brice, Brycen, Bryson.**

♂ **BRYN.** *Welsh, 'hill'.* Nice name, well used in Wales, but feminine elsewhere. **Brin, Brinn, Brynmor, Brynmore.**

BRYSON. *English, 'son of Brice'.* A surname name that can transition to first. **Brysen, Brysin.**

BUCHANAN. *Scottish, 'place of the cannon'.* If you're looking for an American presidential name, Truman and Jackson are better options.

BUCK. *English, 'male deer'.* Comedian Roseanne Barr chose this for her son . . . which seems in character. **Buckey, Buckie, Bucky.**

BUCKLEY. *English, 'meadow of the deer'.* Mummy's boy.

BUCKMINSTER. *English, 'monastery where deer dwell'.* Innovative architect, inventor and thinker Buckminster (universally known as Bucky) Fuller makes this vaguely possible.

BUD. *English nickname.* This is a name you get stuck with, not (we hope) one your parents choose for you. **Budd, Buddey, Buddie, Buddy.**

BUELL. *Welsh, 'dwelling'; also Dutch occupational name for a hangman.* The Dutch definition is enough to keep most people away. **Buel, Bueller, Buhl, Buhler.**

BUFF. *Modern nickname, also colour name.* Has too many slangy connotations to be considered.

BUNYAN. *English from French, 'swelling'.* Mythic lumberjack Paul may inspire some namesakes despite its relationship to a similarly pronounced foot problem.

BURBANK. *English, 'riverbank where burrs grow'.* About as glamourous a place name as Liverpool or Birmingham.

BURFORD. *English, 'ford near the castle'.* Stuffy. **Bufford, Buford.**

BURGESS. *English, 'inhabitant of a fortified town'.* Related to the word *bourgeois;* actor Burgess Meredith put this surname in first place. **Burges, Burgiss.**

♂ **BURGUNDY.** *French place name; also colour name.* Ron Burgundy was Will Ferrell's fictional helmet-haired newsman, but this colour name is much more suited to a girl.

BURKE. *French, 'from the fortress'.* Simple, usable surname choice. **Berk, Berke, Birk, Birke, Bourke, Burk.**

BURL. *English, 'knotty wood,' 'butler'.* Has a nicely fragrant woodsy feel. **Burle.**

BURLEIGH. *English, 'meadow belonging to a manor'.* Let's hope he's 'burly'. **Burley, Burli, Burlie, Burly, Byrleigh, Byrley.**

♂ **BURMA.** *Place name.* One place name that's far off the beaten track and better for girls, despite the connection with the dated Irma.

♂ **BURNE.** *English, 'the brook'.* Has a certain fiery charm. **Beirne, Bourn, Bourne, Burn, Byrn, Byrne, Byrnes.**

♂ **BURNET.** *English from French, 'brown'.* We don't see this one making it unless you have a compelling family reason. **Bernet, Bernett, Burnett.**

BURNEY. *English, 'island of the brook'.* Though they sound exactly alike, this spelling makes it much more elegant than Bernie. **Beirney, Beirnie, Burnie.**

Stellar Starbabies Beginning with *B*

Bamboo	Big Boi *(Outkast)*
Banjo	Rachel Griffiths
Barron	Melania & Donald Trump
Bay	Kristie Allsopp
Beau	Art Garfunkel, Tanya Tucker
Beckett	Conan O'Brien, Melissa Etheridge, Malcolm McDowell
Benjamin	Annette Bening & Warren Beatty
Billy	Helena Bonham Carter & Tim Burton
Blake	Rosie O'Donnell
Boman	Matthew Modine
Braison	Billy Ray Cyrus
Brandon	Pamela Anderson & Tommy Lee
Brooklyn	Victoria & David Beckham
Bruno	Nigella Lawson
Buck	Roseanne Barr

BURNS. *Scottish and English, 'from the burnt house'.* The final *s* turns this name into a manservant.

BURR. *English, 'bristle'.* Ruggedly appealing word name in the Thorn/Rider/Storm school of boys' names.

BURROUGHS. *English, 'dwelling place'.* Most parents attracted to this name will be devotees of the author William and would be better off using it in the middle. **Burr, Burrows.**

BURTON. *English, 'fortified enclosure'.* Prissy, no matter how you spell it. **Bert, Berton, Burt, Burtt.**

BUSBY. *English, 'shrub farm'.* A busby is the tall fur hat palace guards wear in England; also the unique first name of iconic movie choreographer Busby Berkeley. **Busbee, Busbey, Busbie, Bussby.**

BUSCH. *German, 'dweller near the bush'.* **Busche, Bush.**

BUSTER. *Modern nickname.* Another old-fashioned nickname in the Bud/Buzz/Biff mould; this one's a bit belligerent. **Busta.**

BUTCHER. *English occupational name.* One occupational name unlikely to find a single taker. **Butch.**

BUTLER. *English occupational name.* We don't see that bright a future for this one either. **Buttler.**

BUXTON. *English, 'boulders that rock at a touch'.* Sounds too much like buxom.

BUZZ. *Modern nickname.* Brother for Biff and Bud.

♂ BYATT. *English, 'by the enclosure'.* For fans of the (female) author A.S.; makes an interesting alternative to Wyatt or the hotelish Hyatt.

BYRAM. *English variation of* **BYRON.** Why not stick with the original?

★BYRON. *English, 'barn for cows'.* This name has always had a romantic, windswept image thanks to the poet Lord Byron. **Beyren, Beyron, Biren, Biron, Buiron, Byram, Byran, Byrom.**

C *boys*

CABLE. *French, 'rope'.* Drop the C and arrive at an established biblical name. **Cabel, Cabell.**

♂ CABOT. *French, 'to sail'.* Attractive English surname associated with the daring early Italian-born British explorer. **Cabbot, Cabbott.**

CADAO. *(kah-DAH-oh) Vietnamese, 'song'.* Rhythmic and exotic.

CADDOCK. *Welsh, 'eagerness for war'. See CADOC.* **Cadog.**

CADE. *English, 'round' or 'barrel'.* Strong, ultramasculine and modern, Cade is becoming a popular choice, along with cousins Caden and Cale. **Caden, Caide, Cayde, Kade, Kaden, Kayden.**

CADELL. *Welsh, 'battle'.* A surname that is unlikely to win many supporters. **Caddell, Cadel.**

♂ CADEN. *Modern invented name.* A key member of the rhyming contingent that dates all the similar sounding Cadens, Jadens, Braedons and Aidans as part of a millennial megatrend. **Cadan, Cadin, Cadon, Cadyn, Caiden, Caedon, Cayden, Kaden, Kaiden, Kayden.**

CADMAN. *Anglo-Saxon, 'warrior'.* Caedmon is considered the first English poet – a nice literary tie-in to the streamlined version. **Cadmon, Caedmon.**

CADMUS. *Greek, 'from the east' or 'one who excels'.* A dragon-slaying hero of Greek

mythology who also invented the alphabet, but the caddish opening and musty *mus* ending could be negatives. **Cadmos, Cadwallader.**

CADOC. *Welsh, 'battle'.* This Welsh saint's name has an industrial edge.

CADOGAN. *(kah-DUG-gan) Welsh, 'honour in battle'.* This surname borne by several early Welsh leaders has a lot of energy.

♂ **CAELAN**. *Scottish variation of* **NICHOLAS**. One of the rarer, more appealing forms of this family of names. **Cael, Caelon, Cailan, Calen, Calin, Callan, Callon, Calyn, Caylan.**

CAESAR. *Latin, 'long-haired'; also clan name.* The name of the greatest Roman of them all is rarely used outside Latino families, where the César spelling is preferred. **Caeser, Caezar, Seasar, Sezar. International: Césaire, César, Chesare** *(French)*, **Ceasario, Cesare, Cesareo** *(Italian)*, **Cecha, César, Cesareo, Cesario, Cesaro, Carito** *(Spanish)*, **Kesar** *(Basque)*, **Kaiser** *(German)*, **Arek, Cezar, Cezary, Cezek** *((Polish)*, **Casar, Cezar, Kaiser** *(Bulgarian)*, **Kesar** *(Russian)*.

♂ **CAGNEY**. *Irish, 'tribute'.* Synonymous with spunk. **Cagny.**

♂ **CAIDEN**. *See* **CADEN**. An increasingly well-used spelling of Caden/Kaden.

♂ **CAILEAN**. *(KAH-lun) Irish, 'pup, cub'.* This is the original Gaelic spelling of the Anglicised Colin – more authentic, yes, but could make your child's life unnecessarily complicated. **Caelan, Cailen, Cailin, Caillen, Calan, Caley, Colin, Kaelan, Kaelin, Kalan, Kalen, Kalin.**

CAIN. *Hebrew, 'spear,' 'possessed'.* Cain, the name of the first murderer, was until recently seldom heard outside of the Old Testament and soap operas. Vary the spelling to sidestep the negative biblical connection. **Caine, Cainen, Cane, Cayne, Kane, Kain, Kayne, Kean, Keane.**

♂ **CAIRN**. *Scottish, 'mound of rocks'.* In Scotland, a cairn is a heap of stones placed on a grave – not the most appealing association. **Cairne.**

♂ **CAIRO**. *place name.* Exotic place name possibility with upbeat *o* ending. **Cai, Kyro.**

CAIUS. *Latin, 'rejoice'; variation of* **GAIUS**. Classical and serious. **Cai, Caio, Kay, Kaye, Keye, Keyes, Keys.**

CAL. *Diminutive of* **CALVIN**. A homey sitting-by-the fire-type nickname name. **Kal.**

CALBERT. *English, 'calf-herder'.* Putting a *C* before Albert doesn't make this old occupational name any more contemporary. **Calburt, Colbert.**

♂ **CALDER**. *English, 'rocky water'.* Artistic associations with the sculptor who invented the mobile make this one of the more creative surname choices.

CALE. *Diminutive of* **CALEB**. This up-and-coming single-syllable name has one drawback: it sounds like the green, leafy vegetable. **Cael, Caile, Cayle, Kale.**

★**CALEB**. *Hebrew, 'bold, intrepid'.* This attractive Old Testament name, belonging to one of only two young people to enter the Promised Land, is in hot pursuit of Jacob as the leading biblical boy's name. **Cal, Cale, Caley, Calub, Calyb, Cayleb, Caylyb, Kale, Kaleb, Kalyb, Kayleb, Kaylob, Kaylyb.**

♂ **CALEN**. *Modern invented name.* A recently created

member of the Cale family, with a trendy unisex aura. **Caelen, Cailen, Calin, Kaelen, Kalen, Kalin.**

♂ **CALENDAR.** *Word name.* If you don't want to limit yourself to one month of the year, this unique possibility offers the plus of the friendly nickname, Cal.

♂ **CALHOUN.** *Irish, 'from the narrow forest'.* A beaming, friendly Irish last-name-first-name waiting to be discovered. **Calhoon, Calhoun, Calhoune, Callhoun.**

♂ **CALIFORNIA.** *Place name.* The sidekick in a John Wayne western.

★♂ **CALIXTO.** *(cah-LEEKS-toe) Greek, 'beautiful'.* Known in Spain as the name of a pope and martyr, this has a lot of energy and futuristic spirit, thanks in part to the attention-grabbing *x*. **Cal, Calesto, Calexto, Cali, Calistaro, Caliste, Calisto, Calistu, Calix, Calixte, Calliste, Callixte, Callixto, Kalixto.**

♂ **CALLAGHAN.** *(CAL-a-han) Irish, 'lover of churches'.* A classic Irish 'top-o'-the-mornin' surname with a lot of rhythm and pizzazz. **Calahan, Calihan, Callahan, Ceallach, Cellachan, Kellach.**

♂ **CALLISTER.** *Variation of Irish surname MacCallister, 'son of Alister'.* Can be used either with or without the addition of *Mac*.

★♂ **CALLOWAY, CALLAWAY.** *Irish from Latin, 'pebbly place'.* Another animated Irish surname, this one with jazzy ties to the immortal 'Dean of American Jive,' Cab Calloway.

★**CALLUM, CALUM.** *Scottish variation of* **COLOMBIA.** This charming name has been in the Top 25 consistently in recent years. In this country, it's a more popular alternative to Colin and Caleb. **Cal, Colm, Colum.**

♂ **CALM.** *Word name.* A modern virtue name, particularly desirable in this pressure-cooker world.

CALTON. *Latin, 'calf farm'.* The kind of hybrid name – it sounds like a blend of the

Jazz Names

Bechet
Basie
Bessie
Billie
Bix
Calloway
Cassandra
Coleman
Coltrane
Dinah
Django
Ella
Ellington
Etta
Jarrett
Jaz/Jazz
Joplin
Kenton
Lionel
Louis
Mercer
Miles
Mingus
Parker
Quincy
Thelonius
Tyree

boys' names

popular Caleb and Colton – that could catch on despite its lack of pedigree.

★CALVIN. *Latin, 'bald, hairless'.* A slightly quirky but cozy name that has a fashion edge thanks to Calvin Klein. **Cal, Kal, Kalvin, Vin, Vinnie. International: Calvino** *(Italian).*

♂ CALYPSO. *Greek, 'she who hides'.* Rhythmic route to the nickname Cal, but it would take a mighty strong persona to cope with the playground problems.

♂ CAMDEN. *Scottish, 'winding valley'; British place name.* London Boy name. This is a case where the name is as attractive as the place that inspired it. The same couldn't be said about the American city in New Jersey – although the name is popular in the US. **Camdan, Camdin, Camdon, Camdyn, Kamdan, Kamden, Kamdin, Kamdon, Kamdyn.**

♂ CAMERON. *Scottish, 'crooked nose'.* Popular both in Scotland and Hollywood, for both boys and now girls (thanks to Cameron Diaz), this Top 50 name, with its good-looking, sensitive aura, has generated a deluge of variant spellings, the most prominent of which is Camron. **Cam, Camaeron, Camaron, Cameran, Camerin, Camerron, Camey, Cammeron, Camren, Camron, Camryn, Kam, Kameron, Kamren, Kamron, Kamryn.**

♂ CAMPBELL. *Scottish, 'crooked mouth'.* The seventh most common surname in Scotland is now being considered as a last-name-first choice, accessible but unusual. **Cambell.**

CAMRON. *See CAMERON.*

CÁNDIDO. *Latin, 'pure, white'.* Projects a feeling of openness and candor. **International: Candide** *(French).*

♂ CANNON. *Word name.* Unusual but trendy two-syllable boys' name. **Canaan, Cannan, Cannen, Canon, Kanaan, Kanon.**

♂ CANTON. *Place name.* Not nearly as exotic as some of the more distant names in the atlas, Canton fits into the category of the no-nonsense, new-sounding boys' names many parents are looking at.

CANUTE. *Scandinavian, 'knot'.* More familiar in its *K* forms, that may prove rough for a modern boy. **Cnut, Knut, Knute.**

♂ CANYON. *Spanish word name.* Evocative of natural splendour; an intriguing new possibility.

♂ CAOLÁN. *(KAIL-aun) Irish Gaelic, 'slender lad'.* Gaelic spellings can complicate even potentially attractive names. **Kalen, Kealan, Keelin.**

CARADOC. *Welsh, 'amiable, beloved'.* An ancient Celtic name too difficult for any preschool elsewhere. **Caradawg, Caradog.**

♂ CARBRY, CARBERY. *Irish, 'charioteer'.* A name scattered throughout Irish mythology, with an intriguing if feminised sound. **Carbury, Carrbry.**

♂ CARDEN. *English occupational name, 'wool carder'.*

Highly unusual but stylish-sounding occupational name, with a pleasant association with gardens. **Card, Cardan, Cardin, Cardon.**

CAREW. *Welsh, 'fort near a slope'.* Noted bearers of this surname include a metaphysical poet and a Nobel Prize winner, so there's some hero-name inspiration. **Carewe, Carrew, Crew, Crewe.**

♂ **CAREY.** *Irish, 'dark, black'.* All forms of this name have slipped out of the boys' territory, having been feminised in the 1960s and 70s. **Carrey, Cary, Karey, Kary.**

CARL. *German variation of* **CHARLES.** This no-nonsense German variation of Charles is strong and still well used, but lacks much sensitivity or subtlety; the Latin forms have far more energy. **International: Carlus, Cathal** *(Irish),* **Carlino, Carlo, Carolo** *(Italian),* **Carlito, Carlo, Carlos** *(Spanish),* **Carel, Carolu, Karel** *(Dutch),* **Karl** *(German and Scandinavian),* **Kalman** *(German),* **Kalle** *(Finnish),* **Karol, Karolek** *(Polish),* **Karcsi, Kari, Károly** *(Hungarian),* **Karel, Karlik, Karol** *(Czech),* **Karlen, Karlin** *(Russian),* **Carolos** *(Greek),* **Kale** *(Hawaiian).*

CARLETON. *English, 'settlement of free men'.* An upscale name almost to the point of caricature. **Carl, Carletun, Carlton, Charleston, Charleton, Charlton.**

♂ **CARLIN.** *Irish, 'little champion'.* Although an authentic Irish male name, the *lin* ending seems more appropriate for a girl. **Carling, Carlyn, Karlin, Karlyn. International: Ceabhallan** *(Irish).*

♂ **CARLISLE.** *English, 'from the walled city'.* Sounds more like a hotel than a person. **Carlyle.**

CARLO. *Italian variation of* **CHARLES.** Energetic Italian classic that would blend with a surname of any ethnicity.

CARLOS. *Spanish variation of* **CHARLES.** A name with huge popularity in the Hispanic community. **Carlito, Carlitos,** Carlo, Carrlos, Lito, Litos.

♂ **CARLOW.** *Irish place name, 'four-part lake'.* Gives Carlo a place name/surname spin. **Carlowe.**

CARLSEN. *Scandinavian, 'Carl's son'.* Good way to honour Scandinavian roots, or an ancestor named Carl or Charles. **Carlson, Carlssen, Carlsson, Karlsen, Karlson, Karlssen, Karlsson.**

CARLTON. *See CARLETON.*

CARLYLE. *See CARLISLE.*

♂ **CARMEN.** *Spanish variation of* **CARMEL.** Much more often heard as a girl's name in this country.

CARMICHAEL. *Scottish, 'fort of Michael'.* Most parents would prefer to leave the *car* part parked in the garage.

♂ **CARMINE.** *Latin, 'vivid red'.* This traditional Italian name could have a whole new life when viewed as a colour name. **Carman, Carmen, Carmin, Carmino, Karman, Karmen.**

TV Guide
Names

Alan
Ant
David
Dec
Dermot
Gary
Frank
George
Gordon
Graham
Jamie
Jonathan
Jeremy
Martin
Michael
Neil
Noel
Simon

CARNEY. *Irish, 'victory'.* It has the boisterous carnival connection, and it sounds like there's a link with meat-eaters. Perhaps a name worth skipping over. **Carny, Kearney.**

♂ **CARO.** *Italian, 'dear'.* The meaning is endearing, but it also feels uncomfortably like a short form for Caroline.

♂ **CARROLL.** *Anglicised variation of Irish* **CEARBHALL,** *'hacking with a weapon'.* Carol is rarely heard as a girl's name anymore, Carroll even less so for a boy. **Carol, Caroll, Carolus, Carrol, Cary, Caryl, Caryll.**

♂ **CARSON.** *Irish and Scottish, 'son of the marsh-dwellers'.* An androgynous executive-type name, with a dash of the Wild West via Kit Carson, that's moving up the boys' popularity ladder and down the girls'. **Carrson, Carsan, Carsen, Karson.**

CARSTEN. *German variation of* **CHRISTIAN.** A little bit Carson, a little bit Austin, a little bit muddled. **Carston, Karsten.**

♂ **CARTER.** *English occupational name, 'cart-maker or driver'.* The ultimate trendy Yuppie name, popular for almost two decades, gets a fresh boost when seen as a trendy occupational name. **Cartier.**

CARUSO. *Italian surname.* Operatic.

♂ **CARVER.** *English, 'sculptor'.* Both a creative name because of its link with the arts and a possible hero name via the American George Washington Carver.

♂ **CARY.** *Latin, 'pleasant stream'.* Cary Grant's debonair, masculine image hasn't stood up to the large number of female Carries. **Carey, Kary, Kerry.**

♂ **CASE.** *Word name.* Brisk and unconventional name that could be a style stand-in for confederates Casey, Chase, Cale and Cade.

♂ **CASEY.** *Irish, 'brave in battle'.* A name with a big wide grin, Irish, friendly, open and suited to both sexes. Not as popular as it once was. **Cace, Cacey, Cayce, Caycey, Kacey, Kacy, Kasen, Kasey.**

CASH. *Word name; also diminutive of* **CASSIUS.** A tad mercenary, but a little laid-back Johnny Cash-like too.

♂ **CASHEL.** *Irish, 'castle, stone fort'.* Often spelled Caislin or Cashlin in Ireland, this unusual Gaelic name was chosen by actor Daniel Day-Lewis and his writer-director wife Rebecca Miller for their son.

CASIMIR. *Polish, 'announcing peace'.* This traditional name of Polish kings would have problems assimilating here. **Casmir, Kasimer, Kazmer. International: Casimiro** *(Spanish)*, **Kasimir** *(German)*, **Kazimir** *(Czech)*.

♂ **CASON.** *Modern invented name.* Rhymes with the popular Jason, Mason and Brayson. **Casen, Caysen, Cayson, Kasen, Kason, Kayson.**

CASPAR, CASPER. *Persian, 'keeper of the treasure'; German, 'imperial'.* After half a century, this otherwise feasible name is still linked to the friendly ghost, which didn't scare model Claudia Schiffer, who chose it for her son. **Cass. International: Gaspard, Jasper** *(French)*, **Gasparo** *(Italian)*, **Casparo, Gaspar, Gazpar** *(Spanish)*, **Kaspar** *(German)*, **Casper, Kaspar** *(Scandinavian)*, **Jesper** *(Danish)*, **Kasper** *(Polish)*, **Gaspar, Gazsi** *(Hungarian)*.

★ ♂ **CASPIAN.** *Place name.* If you're looking for a truly unusual geographical name, consider this salty sea between Asia and Europe; also a prince in the *Narnia* books.

♂ **CASS.** *Diminutive of* CASPER *etc.* A lighter if more feminine variation of any of the weightier names beginning with *Cas*; once associated with singer Mama Cass. **Kass.**

★ ♂ **CASSIAN.** *Latin, 'fair, just'.* A saint and Latin clan name that is virtually unused and waiting to be discovered. **International: Casiano, Cassio** *(Italian)*.

♂ **CASSIDY.** *Irish, 'curly-headed'.* A lean and lanky Irish cowboy name (Butch Cassidy) that has been lassoed by the females of the species. **Casidy, Cassady, Cassedy, Cassidey, Kasidy, Kassidy.**

♂ **CASSIEL.** *Latin, 'angel of Saturday'.* This name of the archangel who protects those born under the sign of Capricorn might make a distinctive choice for a child with a December-January birthday.

CASSIUS. *(CASH-us) Latin, 'hollow'.* Cassius Clay was an abolitionist and the birth name of Muhammad Ali; also a Shakespearean name with the feel of antiquity that is coming into fashion. **Casius, Casseus, Casshus, Cassio.**

CASTOR. *Greek, 'beaver'; Latin, 'pious one'.* Forget the oil. It's one of the twins that make up the constellation Gemini and a mythological name on the cutting-edge of fashion; used by Metallica's James Hetfield. **Caster, Castorio, Kastor.**

CATO. *Latin, 'all-knowing'.* Conjures up images of ancient Roman statesmen and southern antebellum retainers. **Catoe, Cayto, Kaeto, Kato. International: Caton** *(French)*.

CATULLUS. *Latin, meaning unknown.* Bearded, fusty name of great old Roman lyric poet; just what the bold vanguard baby namer might be looking for.

CAVANAGH *Irish, 'son of the monk'.* Pleasant Irish last name that could be a more masculine alternative to the overused Cassidy. **Cavanaugh, Kavanagh, Kavanaugh.**

♂ **CAYDEN.** *Modern invented name.* A popular substitute spelling for Kaden, Cayden itself is gaining in popularity. **Caden, Cadin, Cadon, Cadyn, Caeden, Caedin, Caedyn, Kaden, Kadin, Kadon, Kadyn.**

CAYMAN. *Place name.* Connection to the Caribbean Cayman Islands gives this a nice resortish feel.

♂ **CAYO.** *Latin, 'the happy ones'.* Rare and rhythmic.

CECIL. *Latin, 'blind'.* Once a powerful Roman clan name, Cecil has lost much of its potency over the years. It now has a prissy feel, though it retains a strong presence in the sports and jazz worlds. **Cecill, Siseal. International: Cecilio** (*Italian*).

♂ **CEDAR.** *Word name.* Like Oak, Pine and Mahogany, one of the new tree/wood names that parents are starting to consider; this one's particularly aromatic.

CEDRIC. *Celtic, 'model of generosity'.* Invented by Sir Walter Scott for an *Ivanhoe* character, then sissified as Little Lord Fauntleroy, a stereotype ready to be broken. **Caddaric, Ced, Cederic, Cedrec, Cedrick, Cedro, Rick, Sedric, Sedrick, Sedrik.**

♂ **CELADON.** *Colour name.* Like Cerulean, one of the new and unusual colour names – it's a soft greyish-green – suitable for a boy.

CELESTINO. *Latin, 'belonging to heaven'.* Classic Italian name with celestial vibes. **Alestino, Calestino, Celestín, Selestino, Selistino.**

CELIO. *(SAY-leo) Latin, 'belonging to heaven'.* A welcoming name that seems to say 'hello'. **Celín, Chelo, Lino.**

CELLINI. *(chell-EE-nee) Italian surname.* Benvenuto Cellini, the great Italian sculptor and writer – a true Renaissance man – could inspire this creative choice.

CELLO. *Word name.* If Viola is a credible girl's name, why not the mellow Cello for a boy?

♂ **CERULEAN.** *Colour name.* Just beginning to be heard as a name. Though it works for both genders, the fact that it's a majestic light blue makes it particularly appropriate for a boy.

CÉSAR. *Latin, 'long-haired'.* The preferred spelling of Caesar for the many Hispanic families who have made it popular in their community. **Ceasar, Cesare, Cezar.**

CHAD. *English, 'battle warrior,' from surname* **CHADWICK.** This is a saint's name, but it is also remnant of the Brad-Tad era and still holds some surfer-boy appeal for a number of modern parents. **Chaad, Chadd.**

CHADWICK. *English, 'warrior' or 'dairy farm'.* A snooty-sounding pathway to the cooler short form, Chad.

CHAIM. *Hebrew, 'life'.* Despite its affirmative meaning, Chaim barely survived early Jewish immigration, being watered down to Hyman and Hymie. Now, the original is experiencing a revival. **Chai, Chayim, Chayyim, Chayym, Haim, Hayim, Hayvim Hayyim, Hy, Hyman, Hymen, Hymie, Khaim.**

CHALIL. *Hebrew, 'flute'.* Rarely heard in this country. **Halil, Hallil.**

♂ **CHANCE.** *French variation of* **CHAUNCEY.** Once a cavalier gambler-type name, Chance has entered the mainstream and is rising rapidly; endorsed by such celebrity dads as Paul Hogan.

CHANCELLOR. *English, 'chief secretary'.* Most modern parents would prefer the more manageable Chance. **Chance, Chancelor, Chansellor, Chaunce.**

♂ **CHANDLER.** *French occupational name, 'candle-maker'.* With TV's *Friends* having vanished into rerun land, this prime-time name of one of its characters has begun to cool.

♂ **CHANEY.** *French, 'oak tree'.* A variant spelling that will avoid – at least on paper – any unwanted reference to American Republican politics. **Chainey, Chany, Cheney, Cheyne, Cheyney.**

CHANG. *Chinese, 'smooth, free, unhindered'.* An Asian favourite.

CHANIEL. *Hebrew, 'the grace of God'.* Highly unusual; conceivable alternative to Daniel. **Channiel, Haniel, Hanniel.**

CHANNING. *Latin, 'canal'.* Future CEO. **Canning, Cannon, Canon, Chan, Chann, Channe, Channon.**

CHAPIN. *(CHAY-pin) French, 'clergyman'.* An undiscovered last-name-first option.

CHAPLIN. *English, 'clergyman of a chapel'.* Two conflicting images: the beloved Little Tramp and a minister, often to the military. **Chaplain.**

♂ **CHARAKA.** *Hindi, 'wanderer'.* The name of the visionary second-century BC Indian physician, a definer of diseases and believer in a sound mind and body: a worthy inspiration.

CHARLES. *French from German, 'free man'.* If a classic can be called an up-and-comer, then Charles is it. This long-time traditional favourite has recently slipped from the Top 50, but it may be resuscitated by many celeb parents, from Jodie Foster to Russell Crowe, honouring a distinguished history dating back to Charlemagne – the original Charles the Great. **Carl, Carroll, Cary, Chad, Charley, Charlie, Charlot, Charls, Charlton, Charly, Chas, Chay, Chaz, Chazz, Chick, Chip, Cholly, Chuck. International: Tearlach** *(Gaelic),* **Séarlas** *(Irish Gaelic),* **Carlus** *(Irish),* **Siarl** *(Welsh),* **Charlot** *(French),* **Carlo** *(Italian),* **Carlos** *(Spanish),* **Xarles** *(Basque),* **Karel** *(Dutch),* **Karl** *(German),* **Kaarle** *(Finnish),* **Carel, Karol** *(Polish),* **Károly** *(Hungarian).*

★**CHARLIE.** *English, diminutive of* **CHARLES.** Good-time Charlie is back and in the Top 10. More parents these days are opting to put this friendly, genial nickname on the birth certificate – though we'd recommend you use it as a pet form of the more serious Charles. **Charley, Charly.**

♂ **CHARLOT.** *(shar-low) French nickname for* CHARLES. The way the French allude to Charlie Chaplin could make a charming name on its own, or a hip nickname alternate to Charlie or Chuck. **Charlo, Sharlo, Sharlot.**

CHARLTON. *English, 'settlement of free men'.* An upper-crust, out-of-style surname name associated with actor Heston. **Carleton, Carlton, Charleston, Charleton.**

♂ **CHASE.** *French, 'to hunt'.* Sleek and ultraprosperous sounding name redolent of the worlds of high finance and international banking that's been well used during the last decade. **Chace, Chasen, Chason, Chayace, Chayce, Chayse, Chaysn.**

CHASIN, CHASON. *(CHAH-sohn) Hebrew, 'strong, mighty'.* Old-fashioned Jewish name that could be seen as modern. **Hasin, Hason, Hassin.**

CHAUCER. *English, 'maker of breeches'.* One of the most distinguished names in literature could become a hero name in a family of poetry-lovers – or be seen as a trendy new occupational name.

CHAUNCEY, CHAUNCY. *Latin, 'chancellor'.* A name halfway between its old milquetoast image and a more jovial Irish-sounding contemporary one. **Chance, Chancey, Chaunce, Chaune, Chaunsey, Chaunsy, Chawncey, Choncey.**

CHAVEZ. *Spanish place name.* The perfect Latin-accented hero name to honour labour activist César Chavez. **Chavaz, Chevez.**

CHAVIV. *Hebrew, 'loved one'.* Lively sounding Hebrew choice. **Habib, Haviv.**

CHAZ. *Diminutive of* **CHARLES.** The jazziest nickname for Charles. **Chas, Chazz.**

CHAZON. *(Chah-zohn) Hebrew, 'prophecy, revelation'; also a place name in Galilee.* This is one of several Hebrew names with the beginning syllable *Chaz.* **Chazaiah, Chazaya, Chaziel, Chezyon, Hazon.**

CHÉ. *Spanish, diminutive of* **JOSÉ.** Strongly associated with Cuban revolutionary Guevara. **Chay.**

★**CHEEVER.** *English, 'female goat'.* Nice, cheery sound, literary tie to writer John Cheever and subliminal association with the desirable word *achiever:* all strong pluses.

CHEN. *Chinese, 'great, tremendous'.* Asian name with positive meaning.

♂ **CHENEY.** *French spelling variation of* **CHANEY.** Strong, solid surname name; might be seen to reflect your political leanings if in the US.

★CHESTER. *Latin, 'fortress, walled town'; place name.* Comfortable, little-used teddy bear of a name that suddenly sounds both quirky and cuddly; chosen by Tom Hanks and Rita Wilson for their son. **Caster, Castor, Chesleigh, Chesley, Chess, Cheston, Chet.**

CHEVY. *French, diminutive of* **CHEVALIER,** *'horseman, knight'.* Eternally tied to the second name Chase, via first the old English battle and ballad and the goofy American comedian (who was born Cornelius). **Chevey, Chevie, Chevvy.**

♂ **CHEYENNE.** *Sioux, 'people of a different language'.* Started as a western male name, but has been lassoed into cowgirl territory.

CHICO. *Spanish, 'boy'; also diminutive of* **FRANCISCO.** Friendly but flimsy.

♂ **CHILI.** *Word name.* Spicy but insubstantial nickname name.

CHIP. *Pet name for* **CHARLES.** Only if you're madly nostalgic for 1960s TV.

CHIRICO. *(KEER-ee-ko) Italian surname.* Surrealist artist-inspired creative choice.

♂ **CHRIS.** *English nickname for* **CHRISTIAN, CHRISTOPHER and CHRISTINE.** Long-running nickname used almost equally for boys and girls. **Chriss, Cris, Criss, Crys, Cryss, Kris, Krys.**

♂ **CHRISTIAN.** *Greek, 'anointed one'; English from Latin, 'follower of Christ'.* A popular name in recent decades, Christian is threatening to overtake Christopher. Once considered overly pious, it's now seen as making a bold statement of faith by some. It also has secular appeal for others; Cristian is a popular spelling. **Chris, Christer, Christie, Christino, Christo, Christy, Cristino, Cristy, Kit, Kris, Krister, Kristo, Krystian, Krystiano. International: Chréstien, Chrétien, Cretien** *(French),* **Cristian, Cristiano** *(Spanish),* **Kerstan, Christiaan, Cristiaan** *(Dutch),* **Carsten, Karsten, Krischan** *(German),* **Kristian** *(Scandinavian),* **Christiansen** *(Danish),* **Krist** *(Swedish),* **Christiano, Christion, Christos** *(Greek).*

♂ **CHRISTMAS.** *English word name.* Very occasionally given to boys born on that day; Noel is a more common choice.

CHRISTO. *Slavic, diminutive of* **CHRISTOPHER.** Jauntier than Chris, associated with the installation artist (who wrapped up the Reichstag in Berlin) of that name.

CHRISTOPHER. *Greek and Latin, 'one who carries Christ'.* Fashionable classic, thanks to a strong, sincere, straightforward image, combined with a softer, more modern sound than, say, Robert or Richard. But it's rapidly slipping down the Top 100. **Chris, Christo, Christobel, Christof, Christoff, Christoffel, Christofor, Christy, Cris, Cristofer, Cristopher, Cristovano, Kip, Kit, Kitt, Kris, Kristo, Kristofel, Kristoff, Kristofor, Kristoforos, Kristopher, Kristos, Krys, Krystofer, Krystopher, Tofer, Topher.**

CHRISTOS. *Greek, diminutive of* **CHRISTOPHER.** A Greek classic. **Cristos, Khristos, Kristos.**

Christopher's International Variations

Irish Gaelic	Críostóir
Gaelic	Crisdean
Irish	Criostal, Criostoir
Scottish	Christie, Kester
Welsh	Crist
French	Christophe
Italian	Cristoforo
Spanish	Christos, Cristóbal
Portuguese	Cristovão
Dutch	Christofel
German	Christoforus, Christoph, Stoffel
Scandinavian	Kristof, Kristoffer
Danish	Christoffer, Christofferson
Swedish	Kristoffer
Finnish	Risto
Polish	Krzysztof
Romanian	Cristofor
Czech	Krystof
Russian	Christoffer, Khristofor
Ukrainian	Khrystofor
Greek	Christophoros, Khristos, Kristo
Armenian	Kristapor
Hawaiian	Kilikikopa

♂ **CHRISTY.** *Greek, diminutive of* **CHRISTOPHER.** Common nickname for Christopher in Ireland, too feminine for use elsewhere.

CHUCK. *Diminutive of* **CHARLES.** So far out it's almost ready to be let back in. **Chuckie, Chucky.**

CHURCHILL. *English, 'hill of the church'.* Distinguished though it is, it will never shake its portly cigar-smoking image. **Churchil.**

CIAN. *(KEE-an) Irish, 'ancient'.* A handsome Irish name, very popular in that country, but here better spelled Kean – or even Keen. **Kean, Keandre, Keane, Keen, Keenan, Keene, Keondre, Kian.**

CIANÁN. *(KEE-nahn) Irish, diminutive of* **CIAN.** Sticklers for authenticity might opt for this original spelling, but most others will go for one of the phonetic versions. **Keanan, Keenan, Keenon, Kenan, Keyan, Keyon, Kienan.**

CIAR. *(KEER) Irish, 'dark'.* See *KEIR.*

CIARÁN. *(KEER-aun) Gaelic, 'little black-haired one'.* See *KIERAN.* Ciaren, Kearn, Kern, Kerne, Kiaran, Kieran, Kieron, Kyran.

CICERO. *Latin, 'chickpea'.* Roman statesman's name once used for slaves by owners trying to show off their classical education – and rarely heard since. A bold baby namer could try to bring it into modern life.

CIELO. *(chee-EL-oh) Italian, 'sky'.* Expansive, sunny Italian word name.

CILLIAN. *(KIL-yan) Irish, 'war, strife'.* See *KILLIAN.* Cillín, Kilian, Killian.

CIPRIANO. *(see-pree-AH-no) Latin, 'from Cyprus'.* A saint and surname often heard in Italy. Ciprien, Cyprian, Cyprien, Siprian, Siprien, Sipran. International: Cebrián *(Spanish)*, Cebrià *(Catalan)*.

CIRO. *(SEE-ro) Italian variation of CYRUS.* This name of an old Hollywood nightclub still retains a spark of glamour.

♂ **CLAIBORNE.** *French and German, 'boundary with clover'.* Women's designer name, a bit femme for a baby boy. Claiborn, Claibourn, Claibourne, Clay, Clayborn, Clayborne, Clayborney, Claybourn, Claybourne, Clayburn, Klaiborn, Klaibourne.

♂ **CLANCY.** *Irish, 'red-haired warrior'.* One of the original Irish surname names, as energetic as ever. Clancey, Clancie.

♂ **CLARE.** *Diminutive of CLARENCE.* Has been used strictly for girls for many decades.

CLARENCE. *Latin, 'bright'.* The name of the guardian angel in *It's a Wonderful Life* is rarely heard the rest of the year because of its studious, near-nerdy image. Clair, Claire, Claran, Clarance, Clare, Clarens, Claron, Clarons, Claronz, Clarrance, Clarrence, Klarance, Klarenz, Sinclair.

CLARK. *English, 'clerk'.* Has lost its Superman superpowers. Clarke, Clerc, Clerk.

♂ **CLAUDE.** *French from Latin, 'lame'.* Soft-spoken French name that conjures up the pastel colours of Monet and harmonies of Debussy. International: Claud, Claudian, Claudien, Claudiu, *(French)*, Claudio *(Italian, Portuguese)*, Cladio, Claudio, Claudicio, Claudios, Clavio, Glaudio *(Spanish)*, Claudius *(German)*, Claudios *(Greek)*, Klaudiusz *(Polish)*, Kolos *(Hungarian)*, Klavdii *(Russian)*.

★**CLAUDIO.** *Italian from Latin, 'lame'.* This very appealing Italian name is featured in not one, but two Shakespearean plays. Claudius.

CLAUS. *Scandinavian and German variation of NICOLAS.* And how is Mrs Claus? Claes, Class, Klaas, Klasse, Klaus *(Dutch)*, Clause, Klaus *(German)*, Launo *(Finnish)*.

CLAY. *English word name; diminutive of CLAYTON.* Rich one-syllable name with a handsome-rogue image. Klay, Klee.

CLAYTON. *English, 'place with good clay'.* Almost fits into the

These names – many traditionally starting with the letter C – are now being spelled with either C or K as their first initial.

Cade or Kade
Caden or Kaden
Caelean or Kaelan
Cai or Kai
Cale or Kale
Caleb or Kaleb
Callen or Kallen
Camden or Kamden
Cameron or Kameron
Carl or Karl
Carlsen or Karlsen
Carson or Karson
Carsten or Karsten
Casey or Kasey
Caspar or Kaspar
Cato or Kato
Christian or Kristian
Christopher or Kristofer
Cian or Kian
Clay or Klay
Clayton or Klayton
Clement or Klement
Coby or Koby
Cody or Kody
Cordell or Kordell

wildly popular Jaden-Caden-Braden family – but not quite; a possibility for parents who want a similar but more traditional name. Clay, Clayten, Klayton.

CLEANTH. *Greek, 'clean, pure'.* Pastoral poetry name, associated with shepherds and nymphs. **Cleante, Cleanthe, Cleneth, Clianth, Clianthes, Kleanth, Kleanthes. International: Cleandro, Cleanto** *(Spanish).*

♂ **CLEARY.** *Irish, 'scholar'.* Irish surname with several unpleasant rhymes – teary, weary, leery. **Cleery.**

CLEAVON. *English, 'of the cliff'.* Deservedly obscure. **Cleevon.**

CLEM, *English, diminutive of* **CLEMENT.** Laid-back and humble, with a distinctive down-home charm.

CLEMENT. *Latin, 'mild, merciful'.* This name of fourteen popes and several saints has a mild, positive, slightly antiquated feel, like the phrase 'clement weather'. **Clem, Clemense, Clements, Clemmie, Clemmons, Clemmy.**

International: **Cléimeans** *(Irish Gaelic),* **Cliamain** *(Scottish Gaelic),* **Clémence, Clément** *(French),* **Clemente** *(Italian, Spanish),* **Klemens** *(German, Danish, Swedish),* **Clemens** *(Danish),* **Kelemen** *(Hungarian),* **Klema, Klement, Klemo** *(Czech),* **Kliment** *(Russian, Czech, Bulgarian),* **Clementius** *(Latin).*

CLEON. *Greek, 'glorious, renowned'.* Rare and distinctive name with intimations of antiquity, also a Shakespearean character. **Kleon.**

CLETE. *Greek, diminutive of* **CLETUS.** Heavy-footed.

CLETUS. *Greek, 'called forth'.* Sounds a bit anatomical. **Cleatus, Clete, Cletis.**

CLEVE. *Diminutive of* **CLEVELAND.** Appealing short form of the stuffy Cleveland, occasionally used on its own.

CLEVELAND. *English, ' hilly land, from the cliff'.* A presidential and place name that's not a stand-out in either category. **Cleaveland, Cleavland, Cleavon, Cleon, Cleve, Clevon.**

CLIFFORD. *English, 'lives near the ford by the cliff'.* Beginning to overcome a slightly stodgy intellectual image and showing signs of possible revival. Kids might or might not like the association with the big red dog. **Cliff, Clift, Clyfford, Clyford.**

CLIFTON. *English, 'place on a cliff'.* A less-used cross between Clifford and Clinton. **Cliff, Cliftun, Clyff, Clyfford, Clyffton, Clyftun.**

CLINT. *English, diminutive of* **CLINTON.** As flinty and steely as Mr Eastwood.

CLINTON. *English, 'hilltop town'.* After its high-profile presidential term, dropped out with Bill. **Clint, Clintt, Clinttun, Clynton, Klint, Klinton.**

CLIVE. *English, 'lives near a high cliff'.* Clipped name in a pith helmet and pencil-thin moustache. **Cleve, Clyve.**

♂ **CLOUD.** *Nature name.* Like Sky and Sunshine, this fluffy name from the hippy 1970s has floated back onto the naming radar.

CLOVIS. *Teutonic, French, early form of* **LUDWIG** *or* **LOUIS.** An aromatic, unconventional name. **Clove, Clovus, Klove, Klovis.**

♂ **CLUNY.** *Irish, 'from the meadow'.* Likable Irish surname name, but bound to be confused with Clooney. **Clooney, Cloony, Clunainach.**

★**CLYDE.** *Scottish river name.* In the past, it may have been an outlaw (with Bonnie) and somewhat anorak, but Clyde has always had an element of jazzy cool that could overcome all the rest. **Clide, Clydell, Klyde.**

COAL. *Word name.* This recently coined respelling of Cole darkens its image. **Coale, Koal.**

♂ **COBY.** *English, diminutive of* **COBURN** *or* **JACOB.** The new Cody. **Cobey, Cobi, Cobie, Kobe, Kobey, Kobi, Kobie, Koby.**

♂ **CODY.** *English, 'helpful, pillow'.* Riding off into the sunset. **Codey, Codi, Codie, Kodee, Kodey, Kodie, Kody.**

♂ **COLBY.** *English, 'coal town'.* Could this become a red hot name? **Colbee, Colbey, Colbie, Collby.**

★COLE. *English, 'coal, dark';
also diminutive of* **NICHOLAS.**
A short name that embodies a
lot of richness and depth,
rapidly rising in popularity.
**Coal, Colby, Coleman, Colis,
Collier, Collyer, Kohl, Kole.**

COLEMAN. *English, 'servant
of Nicholas'.* Name of three
hundred saints, a mustard and
your own baby boy? **Colman,
Kohlman, Kolman.**
International: Colombain
(French), **Columbano** *(Italian),*
Kálmán *(Hungarian).*

COLERIDGE. *English, 'ridge
where charcoal is burnt'.* Name
of a poet, but not particularly
poetic. **Colerige, Colridge,
Colrige.**

♂ **COLIN.** *Scottish, 'pup or
cub'; also diminutive of*
NICHOLAS. Thanks to its
dashing image and *c*-initialed
two-syllable sound, Colin/Collin
is definitely headed for
superstardom. **Colan, Cole,
Collan, Collen, Collin, Collon,
Collyn, Colyn, Kolin.**
International: Cóilean *(Irish
Gaelic),* **Coilin** *(Irish),* **Cailean**
(Scottish Gaelic).

COLLIER. *English occupational
name, 'coal miner'.* Dated
occupational surname. **Colier,
Colis, Collayer, Collis, Collyer,
Colyer.**

COLLIN. *Scottish variation of*
COLIN *and* **COLLINS.** *See*
COLIN.

COLM. *Irish variation of Latin*
COLUMBA, *'dove'.* Popular
name in Ireland that could
immigrate. Just don't forget to
pronounce the *l.* **Calum, Callum,
Colom, Colum, Columb.**

COLMAN. *See* **COLEMAN.**

♂ **COLORADO.** *Place name.*
More distinctive and masculine
than two other American place
names – Dakota or Sierra.

COLT. *Word name.* The kind of
unconventionally macho name
trendy now, associated with
horses and guns.

COLTEN. *See* **COLTON.**

COLTER. *English, 'colt herder'.* A
variation on the popular Colton.

COLTON. *English, 'from the
coal or dark town'.* Trendy two-

syllable choice, with a host of
spellings. **Coalten, Coalton,
Coleton, Collton, Colston, Colt,
Coltan, Colten, Coltin, Colton,
Coltyn, Koltan, Kolten, Koltin,
Kolton, Koltyn.**

♂ **COLTRANE.** *Irish surname.*
The great sax player John
Coltrane could be a cool
naming inspiration for a
jazz fan.

COLUM. *Latin, 'dove'.* This
Irish name rarely heard
elsewhere makes an interesting
alternative to Colin. **Calum,
Callum, Colm, Kolm, Kolum.**

COLUMBO. *Latin, 'dove'.*
Grandmas will remember the
old TV detective show;
playmates won't. **International:
Colum** *(Irish),* **Colombo**
(Spanish).

COLUMBUS. *Variation of*
COLUMBO. Probably best to
stick with Christopher.
Colombe, Colombo.

COMO. *Italian place name.*
Singer Perry is long gone, but
the beautiful northern Italian
lake conjures up a clear and
tranquil image.

CONAIRE. *(KON-er-ee) Irish, uncertain meaning.* Despite the pronunciation, it looks a bit like an airline. **Connery, Connory, Connorry.**

CONAL, CONALL. *Irish, 'strong as a wolf'.* Are there too many Connors in your neighbourhood? This name is equally authentic and much more unusual. **Comhnall, Conel, Conell, Connal, Connally, Connaly, Connel, Connell, Connelly.**

★**CONAN.** *Irish, 'little wolf'.* The fierce image of the Barbarian has been replaced by the amiable O'Brien, making Conan one of the new, desirable Irish choices; a perfect alternative to Conor. **Con, Conant, Conn, Connie.**

CONCORD. *Word name.* With its harmonious meaning, this could be a modern virtue name – and your boy might like the link to the super-fast jet.

CONLAN. *Irish, 'hero'.* Undiscovered Irish surname. **Con, Conn, Conlen, Conley, Conlin, Conlon, Connlyn.**

♂ **CONNELLY.** *Irish, 'love, friendship'.* An open, inviting and rarely used Irish surname. **Con, Conelly, Conn, Connally, Connaly, Connely.**

CONNER. *See CONNOR.*

♂ **CONNERY.** *Irish, 'warrior-lord'.* This name of a mythical king of Tara is strongly associated with actor Sean. **Conaire, Conery, Connary.**

♂ **CONNOR, CONOR.** *Irish, 'lover of hounds'.* An appealing name of a featured player in Irish mythology that is rapidly catching up elsewhere with the popularity it has long enjoyed in the Emerald Isle: it's currently in the Top 50. **Cahner, Con, Conn, Conner, Connory, Konnor. International: Concobhar** *(Irish Gaelic).*

CONRAD. *German, 'bold advisor'.* Intellectual and masculine? Or an anorak and old-fashioned? Your call. **Con, Connie, Conrade, Cort, Curt, Duno, Koen. International: Corrado** *(Italian),* **Conrado** *(Spanish),* **Conrao** *(Portuguese),* **Koenraad, Kort** *(Dutch),* **Konrad,**

Irish Surnames

Branigan
Brody
Calhoun
Callahan
Connolly
Delaney
Donahue
Donovan
Finn
Finnegan
Fitzgerald
Flannery
Gallagher
Kennedy
Maclean
Madigan
Maguire
Malloy
Murphy
Nolan
O'Brien
O'Hara
Phelan
Quinn
Rafferty
Tierney

boys' names

Kurt *(German)*, Konrad *(Swedish, Polish)*.

CONROY. *Irish, 'wise'.* One *Con* name that sounds very out of date.

♂ CONSTANT. *French from Latin, 'steadfast'.* A traditional French male name that could, with English pronunciation, become an admirable word name.

CONSTANTIN, CONSTANTINE. *Latin, 'steadfast'.* Rather bulky and unwieldy name for a modern child, despite – or because of – heavy historical associations with the first Christian head of the Roman Empire. Con, Connie, Stan, Tino. International: Còiseam *(Scottish Gaelic)*, Constant, Constantin *(French)*, Constanzo, *(Italian)*, Constantino *(Spanish)*, Konstantin *(Czech, Hungarian, Scandinavian, German)*, Konstancji, Konstanty, Konstantyn *(Polish)*, Konstantin, Kostya *(Russian)*, Constantinos, Costa, Kastas, Konstantinos, Kostas, Kostis *(Greek)*.

CONWAY. *Irish, 'hound of the plain'.* Once the exclusive property of country signer Conway Twitty, but now might join the in-crowd Connor/Colton/Corbin contingent.

★COOPER. *English occupational name, 'barrel-maker'.* This genial yet upscale surname was one of the first occupational last names to catch on and it's still continuing its rise, especially popular in Australia. Coop.

♂ CORBIN. *Latin, 'raven'.* This is the name of the castle where the Holy Grail was said to be hidden. Its use is only now escalating as part of the mania for two-syllable names starting with *c* or *k*. Corben, Corbet, Corbett, Corbie, Corbit, Corbitt, Corby, Corbyn, Corvin, Cory, Korbin, Korbyn.

♂ CORBY. *English, diminutive of* CORBIN. A casual take on Corbin.

♂ CORCORAN. *Irish, 'ruddy-faced'.* Corky was a moniker of the 1950s, Corcoran a better fit for these times. Cochran, Cork, Corkie, Corky, Korcoran, Korky.

CORD. *Diminutive of* CORDELL. A severe and brawny word name without much soul.

♂ CORDELL. *English occupational name, 'maker or seller of rope or cord'.* An aristocratic occupational name, though the *-ell* ending brings it down-market. Cord, Cordale, Cordas, Corday, Cordelle, Kord, Kordale, Kordell, Kordelle.

CORDOVAN. *Spanish, 'native of Cordova'.* Leathery, masculine image, complete with user-friendly short form. Cord.

CORENTIN. *(kor-en-TAN) French, Breton, 'tempest, hurricane'.* An intriguing saint's name fashionable in France but virtually unknown here – which you may consider a big plus. Corentino, Corey, Corien, Cory, Curi, Kaou, Tin.

♂ COREY. *Irish, 'from the hollow'.* It briefly appeared in the Top 100 recently, but it's more of a middle-aged name. **Correy, Corrie, Corry, Cory, Currie, Curry.**

♂ **CORIN.** *Latin, 'spear'.* Used by Shakespeare in *As You Like It*, this unusual name could make a more distinctive alternative to Corey or Colin. **Coren, Corrin, Cory, Cyran, Koren, Korin, Korrin.**

CORK. *Irish, 'swamp, marsh'.* Buoyant but lightweight. **Corky.**

★**CORMAC.** *Irish, 'charioteer'; Greek, 'tree trunk'.* Offbeat and upbeat, this evocative Irish name that runs through Celtic mythology is known elsewhere via novelist Cormac McCarthy. **Cormack, Cormag, Cormic, Cormick, Mac, Mack.**

CORNEL, CORNELL. *Medieval form of* **CORNELIUS.** Better known now as an American university than as a name. **Cor, Cornall, Corney, Corny. International: Corneille** *(French),* **Kornelis, Kees, Cees** *(Dutch),* **Kornel** *(Czech, Polish).*

CORNELIUS. *Latin, 'horn'.* As soon as the word *corny* entered our slanguage, this name was in

trouble. **Cornall, Cornel, Cornell, Corny, Neil, Niels. International: Corneille** *(French),* **Cornelio** *(Spanish),* **Krelis, Cornelis, Kees** *(Dutch),* **Korneliusz** *(Polish),* **Kornel** *(Czech).*

CORRADO. *Italian variation of* **CONRAD.** A Latinate name with a lot of dash and bravado.

CORT. *German, 'brave'.* Short and curt. **Corty, Court, Kort.**

★**CORTEZ.** *Spanish surname, 'courteous'.* The current craze for surname names is now moving beyond the English and Irish surnames to include exotic Spanish names like this historic one. **Cortes, Kortes, Kortez.**

CORY. *Irish, 'from the hollow'.* See *COREY.*

COSIMO. *Italian variation of* **COSMO.** Dramatic, worldly and exotic and chosen by singer Beck and his wife, Marissa Ribisi, for their son.

★**COSMO.** *Greek, 'universe'.* Some pioneering parents have been considereing if this expansive Greek name that

seems to embrace the whole cosmos could make a creative and cool choice for their newborn son. **Cos, Coz, Kos, Kosmo, Koz. International: Cosimo** *(Italian),* **Cosme** *(Spanish).*

♂ **COTTON.** *Word name.* A name heard in Puritan times, however it would make a too-soft choice today for today's boys. **Cotten.**

♂ **COTY.** *French surname.* Cosmetic reinvention of Cody. **Cotey, Koty.**

COUNT. *Word name.* Nobility names like Duke and Count seem to be forming a minitrend: with Prince and King also in the mix. But not the classiest choices.

♂ **COURTNEY.** *French, 'courteous, from the court'; also Old French nickname, 'short nose'.* Since this courtly old name has been used mostly for girls for decades, it's now out-of-bounds for boys. **Cortland, Courtenay, Courtland, Courtnay.**

♂ COVE. *Nature name.* A new word name possibility with a safe, protected feel.

CRAIG. *Scottish, 'from the rocks'.* Single-syllable baby-boomer name, still common in its native Scotland, but most modern parents would prefer something like Kyle. **Kraig.**

CRANE. *English nickname for tall man with long, thin legs; nature name.* This elegant last name has great potential to turn into a first name. **Crain, Craine, Crandall, Crandell, Crayn, Crayne, Krane. International: Grue** *(French)*, **Gru** *(Italian, Spanish)*, **Kran** *(Scandinavian, German, Polish and Russian)*, **Daru** *(Hungarian)*, **Yeranos** *(Greek)*, **Yashtahi** *(Arabic)*.

CRANSTON, CRANDALL, CRANLEY. *English, 'the crane town'.* Three retired members of the Board.

CRAVEN. *English, 'garlic place'.* Since this is a word that pertains to cowardice, not a wise choice.

CRAWFORD. *English, 'ford where crows gather'.* A common surname in Scotland, but a starchy first name choice. **Crawfard, Crawferd, Crawfurd.**

CREIGHTON. *(CRAY-ton) English and Scottish, 'hilltop town, rocky place'.* Here is one instance where a phonetic spelling might be better. **Crayton, Crichton.**

CREW. *English word name.* Yet another word name that has been added to the baby name lexicon.

CRICHTON. *(KRY-ton) Welsh, 'from the hilltop town'.* Nineteenth-century butler name with pronunciation challenge. **Creighton, Crighton.**

★CRISPIN. *Latin, 'curly-haired'.* Saint's name that has as an image much like its first syllable: crisp, autumnal and colourful. **Cris, Crispanius, Crispen, Crispian, Crispus, Crisspin. International: Crepin** *(French)*, **Crispino** *(Italian)*, **Crispo** *(Spanish)*, **Krispin** *(German, Hungarian, Czech)*.

CRISPUS. *Latin variation of* **CRISPIN.** Ancient Roman names have definite style value, but the Crispin version feels better suited to a modern boy.

CRISTÓBAL. *Spanish variation of* **CHRISTOPHER.** Frequently used in the Spanish-speaking community; Christopher Columbus was born Cristóbal Colón.

CROCKETT. *English, 'large curl'.* Though Davy Crockett is an American childhood hero, most kids would not like to have a name starting with the teasable *crock*. **Crock, Crocket, Croquet, Croquett, Krock.**

♂ CROIX. *French, 'cross'.* Pronounced *croy*, this is an unusual name.

CRONAN, CRONIN. *Irish, 'dark one'.* A distinctive alternative to Conan. **Cronon, Cronyn.**

CRONUS. *Greek mythology name.* A Titan in Greek mythology, would not work in the modern world.

♂ CROSBY. *Irish, 'village with crosses'.* Attractively laid-back Irish surname with retro musical associations to Bing and Crosby, Stills and Nash. **Crosbey, Crosbie.**

★♂ **CRUZ.** *Spanish, 'cross'.* For a single-syllable Latino surname, this new popular kid on the block – its popularity is up 245 percent – packs a lot of energy and charm. Victoria and David Beckham named their third son Cruz – following Brooklyn and Romeo. Other parents may prize its Christian associations.

CUARTO. *Spanish, 'a fourth, a quarter'.* A possibility for a fourth-born child.

♂ **CUBA.** *(Coo-ba) place name.* Actor Cuba Gooding Jr brought this spirited geographic name to the fore. **Cubah, Kuba.**

♂ **CULLEY.** *Irish, 'the meadow'.* Cheerful and distinctive. **Cully.**

♂ **CULLEN.** *Irish, 'puppy, cub'.* An Irish surname that presents another twist on Colin – though it could be confused with it. **Cullan, Cullin, Cullinan.**

CULVER. *English variation of* **COLUMBA**. In the currently

Stellar Starbabies Beginning with *C*

Caleb	Julianne Moore
Cameron	Louise Brown
Cannon	Larry King
Cash	Saul 'Slash' *(Guns N' Roses)* Hudson
Cashel	Rebecca Miller & Daniel Day-Lewis
Caspar	Claudia Schiffer
Castor	James *(Metallica)* Hetfield
Chance	Paul Hogan
Charles	Jodie Foster, Chris O'Donnell, Danielle Spencer & Russell Crowe
Charlie	Peter Kay, Louise & Jamie Redknapp
Chester	Rita Wilson & Tom Hanks, Davina McCall
Clyde	Catherine Keener & Dermot Mulroney
Connor	Nicole Kidman & Tom Cruise
Cody	Robin Willimas
Colin	Paul *(Kiss)* Stanley
Cooper	Bill Murray, Tim Matheson, Philip Seymour Hoffman
Cosimo	Marissa Ribisi & Beck
Cruz	Victoria & David Beckham

popular solid, serious, two-syllable mould. **Colver, Cully.**

CURRAN. *Irish, 'hero, champion'.* Unusual and savoury, calling to mind curry and currants. **Curren, Currey, Currie, Currin, Curry.**

CURRIER. *English occupational surname, 'person who dressed leather after it was tanned'.* Has a fresh occupational name feel, combined with old-fashioned Currier & Ives charm.

♂ **CURRY.** *Word name.* Spicy but a touch girlish. **Currey, Currie, Currier.**

CURT. *Diminutive of* **CURTIS.** Short and to the point, muscular and strong. **Cort, Kurt.**

♂ **CURTIS.** *French, 'courteous, polite'.* An attractive if shopworn name that has been borne by several significant musicians and athletes. **Cort, Court, Curt, Curtel, Curtice, Curtiss. International: Curcio** *(Spanish),* **Kurt, Kurtis** *(German).*

CUTHBERT. *English, 'famous, brilliant'.* Playground poison.

CUTLER. *English occupational name, 'knife maker'.* Cooper would be a more engaging *C*-starting occupational choice.

CY. *Diminutive of* **CYRUS.** Where Sam, Max and Gus may be leading us. **Si, Sy.**

♂ **CYAN.** *English, 'greenish blue colour'.* A highly unusual colour name, a classmate of Celadon and Cerulean.

CYPRIAN. *Greek, 'from Cyprus'.* With a long and noble history – Cyprian was one of the great Christian Latin writers – this could make a highly unusual but meaningful choice. **Ciprian, Ciprien. International: Cyprien** *(French),* **Cipriano** *(Italian).*

♂ **CYPRUS.** *Place name.* This Mediterranean island name would be a plausible choice for parents with a Greek or Turkish heritage.

CYRANO. *Greek, 'from Cyrene'.* Like Pinocchio, unlikely to recover from its long-nosed reputation.

CYRIL. *Greek, 'lordly'.* A name with a monocle in one eye and an ascot in place of a tie. **Ciril, Cyrill. International: Coireall** *(Irish Gaelic),* **Cyrille** *(French),* **Cirillo, Ciro** *(Italian),* **Cirilo, Ciro** *(Spanish and Italian),* **Kiril** *(Bulgarian),* **Cyrillio, Cyrek, Cyryl** *(Eastern European),* **Kirill, Kiryl** *(Russian).*

CYRUS. *Persian, 'sun' or 'throne'.* Very popular in the Iranian community, this name of the founder of the Persian Empire has a more relaxed image for most British people. **Cy, Cyress, Cyrie, Cyris, Cyriss, Cyro, Syris, Syrus.**

D boys

DAAN. *Scandinavian variation of* **DANIEL.** Dan with a little something extra.

♂ **DABNEY.** *French, 'from Aubigny'.* Dapper-sounding choice with old roots that has definite teasability potential in the playground. **Dabnee, Dabnie, Dabny.**

♂ DACEY. *Irish, 'from the south'.* Too lacy for a boy. **Dace, Dacian, Dacrius, Dacy, Daicey, Daicy.**

DACIAN. *Modern invented name.* If it looks like a name and sounds like a name . . .

DAEDALUS. *Greek, 'craftsman'.* Name of a tragic mythological hero, used as a surname in the works of James Joyce; heavy and ponderous for a British boy – and the *dead* beginning doesn't help either. **Daidalos, Dedalus.**

DAFYDD. *(DAY-vith) Welsh variation of* **DAVID.** Extremely common in Wales, but bewildering elsewhere. **Daffy, Dafi, Dai, Dei, Deian, Deicÿn, Deio.**

DAG. *Scandinavian, 'daylight'.* Norse god who's the son of light plus historic diplomat Dag Hammarskjöld combine to boost its appeal – though it might be too close to *dog*. **Dagget, Daggett, Dagny.**

DAGWOOD. *English, 'shining forest'.* One place name/surname unlikely to be revived.

DAHY. *(DAY-hee) Irish, 'quick-footed'.* A long shot, but it could join the crop of dashing Irish surname names. **Dahey.** **International: Daithi** *(Irish Gaelic).*

♂ DAI. *Welsh, 'to shine'; Japanese, 'great'.* A cross-cultural name that can be a nickname for David and can be pronounced *Day* (preferable to *die*), but is also the name of a vicious Asian villain. **Day, Dei.**

♂ DAKOTA. *Native American, Sioux, 'friendly one'.* An early and popular unisex American place name, Dakota is starting to fall out of fashion. **Daccota, Dakoda, Dakodah, Dakoeta, Dakotah, Dekota, Dekohta, Dekowta.**

♂ DALE. *English, 'valley'.* Has lost virtually all its masculine punch. **Daile, Daley, Dalian, Dalle, Dallin, Dayle.**

♂ DALEY. *Irish, 'assembly, gathering'.* Much stronger than Dale for a boy. **Dailey, Daily, Daley, Daly, Dawley.** **International: Dalaigh** *(Irish Gaelic).*

Names That Mean Friend or Friendly

Alden
Alvin
Amica
Amity
Amy
Arden
Auden
Bellamy
Dakota
Darwin
Edwin/Edwina
Elvin
Farquahar
Irvin/Irving
Kahlil/Khalil
Nakotah
Rafiq

DALFON. *Hebrew, 'raindrop'.* Definitely a name you won't hear in every playground, partially because of its synthetic-fabric sound. **Dalphon.**

♂ DALLAS. *Irish, 'skilled'; place-name in Scotland and Texas.* Relaxed, laid-back name with broad appeal, although none of the American place names packs the same style power they did a few years ago. **Dal, Dalles, Dallis, Dallous.**

♂ **DALLIN.** *English, 'from the valley'.* A Dale relative with a bit (a tiny bit) more masculine heft. **Daian, Dallen, Dallon, Dallyn.**

DALMAZIO. *Latin, 'from Dalmatia'.* Ancient Italian martyr's name that's a rarity here and now. **International: Dalmatius** *(Latin)*, **Dalmacio** *(Spanish).*

♂ **DALTON.** *English, 'the settlement in the valley'.* There used to be only one Dalton – screenwriter Dalton Trumbo – but now there are many more, inspired by the name's resemblance to two-syllable unisex favourites: Colton, Holden and cousins. **Daleton, Dallton, Daltan, Dalten, Daltun.**

DALY. *See* **DALEY.**

DALZIEL. *Scottish, 'the small field'.* If you want a truly unusual name with authentic roots, this one certainly fits on both counts.

DAMARIO. *Spanish from Greek, 'to tame'.* Dark and handsome. **Damarios, Damaris, Damarius, Damaro, Damero.**

DAMASO. *Spanish from Greek, 'to tame'.* A Damian relative and the name of an ancient Spanish pope with modern possibilities. **Damase, Damasiano, Damasu, Damasus, Dámazo, Damisio, Domasio, Dómaso.**

DAMEK. *Slavic variation of* **ADAM.** Adam with a Slavic accent. **Adamec, Adamek, Adamik, Adamok, Adham, Danuck, Damicke.**

DAMIAN. *Greek, 'to tame, subdue'.* Damian has sidestepped its demonic horror film overtones, leaving a basically friendly and charming Irish image. A well-used upper-class name in England, it is growing in popularity elsewhere. **Daemon, Daimen, Damen, Dameon, Damiane, Damianos, Damianus, Damion, Damon, Damyen, Dayman, Daymian, Daymen. International: Daman** *(Irish)*, **Dyfan** *(Welsh)*, **Damiano** *(Italian)*, **Damián** *(Spanish)*, **Damião** *(Portuguese)*, **Damek, Damjan** *(Hungarian)*, **Damien, Damyan, Damyon, Dema, Demyan** *(Russian).*

DAMON. *English variation of* **DAMIAN.** In a classic myth, Damon and Pythias were symbols of true friendship and this name does project a friendly, strong, positive aura, much like the persona of actor Matt. **Daman, Damen, Damin, Daymon. International: Damone** *(Italian)*, **Daimon** *(Greek).*

DAN. *Hebrew, 'God is my judge'; diminutive of* **DANIEL.** Often stands alone in Israel, but rarely here.

♂ **DANA.** *English, 'from Denmark'.* Not often heard as a male name these days.

♂ **DANAR.** *Modern invented name.* In *Star Trek's* twenty-fourth-century scenario, the perfect human, but it's not the perfect twenty-first-century name.

♂ **DANCER.** *English word name.* Danger of other kids relating it to Santa's reindeer.

♂ **DANE.** *English, 'from Denmark'.* More masculine Dana alternative, with added style edge. **Dain, Daine, Dayn, Dayne. International: Danek** *(German).*

♀ **DANI.** *(DAH-nee) Diminutive of* **DANIEL.** Sounds like Donny, looks like Danny and feels like a girls' name.

DANIEL. *Hebrew, 'God is my judge'.* A perennial favourite – still in the Top 10 – Daniel is one of only a handful of male names that sounds both classic and modern, strong yet approachable and popular but not clichéd, with a strong Old Testament pedigree. The only real downside: there are a lot of Daniels named each year. **Dan, Danal, Dane, Daneal, Dannie, Danny, Danyal, Danyel, Danylo. International: Dainéal, Dainial** *(Irish Gaelic),* **Deiniol** *(Welsh),* **Danial, Dannel** *(French),* **Daniele** *(Italian),* **Danialo, Danilo, Donelo, Nelo, Nilo** *(Spanish),* **Danele** *(Basque),* **Dannel** *(Swiss),* **Daneel** *(Dutch),* **Taneli** *(Finnish),* **Danek** *(Polish),* **Dacso, Daniil, Dani** *(Hungarian),* **Danek, Danko, Dano** *(Czech),* **Daneil** *(Eastern European),* **Danil** *(Bulgarian),* **Daniels** *(Latvian),* **Daniell, Daniil, Danil, Danila, Danilka, Danya, Danylo** *(Russian),* **Danilo** *(Ukranian),* **Dani, Daniyel** *(Israeli).*

DANNER. *German, 'dweller near the fig tree'.* The authentic pronunciation brings it perilously close to Donna.

DANO. *Czech variation of* **DANIEL.** Groovier than Daniel, with an engaging, upbeat energy.

DANTE. *(DON-tay) Latin diminutive of* **DURANTE.** The great medieval poet's name is widely used in Italian communities – and beyond. **Danté, Dantae, Dantay, Dontae, Dontay, Donte. International: Duran, Durante** *(Italian).*

DANTON. *French variation of* **DANTE.** Has the two-syllable sound so popular for boys, though adding an apostrophe – and turning it into D'Anton – changes the name entirely. **Danten, D'Anton, Dantun, Dantyn.**

♂ **DANUBE.** *River name.* Some parents are turning to rivers and other bodies of water in the search for undiscovered place names and this has the feel of a Viennese waltz. **Donau.**

♀ **DANYA.** *Russian variation of* **DANIEL.** Appealing Daniel diminutive, though its similarity to the feminine Tanya is a problem.

DAOUD. *(dah-ood) Arabic variation of* **DAVID.** Intriguing David alternative, though British tongues will have trouble wrapping themselves around three vowels in a row.

DAPHNIS. *Greek, 'laurel'.* Mythological shepherd in love with Chloe, whose name, though the *s* is pronounced, is still too close to the thoroughly feminine Daphne.

DAQUAN. *Invented name.* One of several similar names used almost exclusively by African-Caribbean parents. **Daquanne, Dekwan, Dekwohn, Dekwohnne, Dequan, Dequanne.**

♂ DARBY. *Irish, 'free one' or 'free from envy'; Norse, 'from the deer estate'.* Lighthearted, spirited Irish-accented name. Works particularly well with an *O'* surname, as in *Darby O'Gill and the Little People*. **Darbey, Darbie, Derby.**

♂ DARCY. *Irish, 'dark one'; French, 'from Arcy' or 'from the fortress'.* The ultimate Jane Austen hero name, a bit feminine though zooming up the Australian popularity list. **Darcey, D'Arcy, Darsey, Darsy.**

♂ DARIAN. *Variation of* DARIUS. Darren wannabe that peaked in the 1990s. **Darien, Darion, Darrian, Darrien, Darrion, Darryan, Darryen, Darryon, Daryan, Daryen, Daryon.**

DARIO. *Italian variation of* DARIUS. More creative and classier than Mario.

DARIUS. *Greek, 'rich, kingly'.* Emperor Darius the Great was a key figure in ancient Persian history; his name today has an appealingly artistic image, which might well be found on a concert program or gallery announcement. **Darias, Dariess, Darious, Darrius, Derrius. International: Dario** *(Italian),* **Dariusz** *(Slavic).*

♂ DARL. *Literary name.* This name of a character in Faulkner's *As I Lay Dying* sounds as though it was cut off at the middle.

DARNELL. *English, 'the hidden spot'.* Doo-wop name. **Darnall, Darnel, Darnley.**

DAROLD. *Modern invented name.* You can dress up Harold, but you still can't take him out.

♂ DARRELL. *French, 'dear one, beloved'.* Beach boy name of the 1960s, dad or grandpa name today. **Darral, Darrell, Darrill, Darrol, Darroll, Darryl, Darryll, Darty, Daryl, Derrel, Derrell, Derril, Derrill, Deryl, Deryll.**

♂ DARREN. *Irish, 'little great one'.* Darren and wife Sharon shop for 1950s memorabilia on eBay. Darien might offer an update. **Daeron, Daren, Darin, Daron, Darran, Darrin, Darring, Darron, Daryn, Derrin, Derron.**

DARROW. *English, 'spear'.* This is a little too soft sounding to make a suitable boy's name. **Darro.**

DARSHAN. *Sanskrit, 'perceptive one'.* This name is widely used in India.

DART. *English place and word name.* This British river name sounds sleek and strong but perhaps a bit too energetic.

D'ARTAGNAN. *French, 'from Artagnan'.* The least usable of the *Three Musketeers* names.

DARTON. *English, 'deer town'.* Obscure, though legitimate, name that could be used to honour a relative named Barton or Martin. **Dartan, Darten, Dartin.**

DARWIN. *English, 'dear friend'.* Enough parents have found naturalist Darwin a worthy hero to keep his name popular for several years – unless they just liked its trendy two-syllable sound. **Darwon, Darwyn, Derwin, Derwynn.**

DASAN. *(DAY-sun) Native American, 'son of bird clan leader'.* Name from legend that might be an interesting Jason alternative.

♂ **DASH.** *Diminutive of* **DASHIELL.** A nickname that can stand on its own and sounds, well, dashing.

★**DASHIELL.** *Scottish surname, meaning unknown.* Though missing from most other name books, Dashiell is among the hottest new names. Chosen by celebs like Cate Blanchett and author Helen (*Bridget Jones*) Fielding; with its great dash and panache, it's associated with detective writer Dashiell Hammett (born Sam, as in Sam Spade), Dashiell being his mother's maiden name.

DATHAN. *Hebrew, 'fountain'.* Obscure Old Testament name that rhymes with (and might be a substitute for) Nathan.

DAUMIER. *French artist name.* If you're seeking a French artist name that goes beyond Monet and Manet, Daumier – known for his revealing caricatures –

makes a rich, sophisticated choice.

DAVENPORT. *English word name.* This old-time name for a desk would not be comfortable as a baby name.

DAVIAN. *Modern invented name.* David plus Damian equals hybrid name beginning to rise. **Daivian, Daivyan, Davien, Davion, Davyan, Davyen, Davyon.**

DAVID. *Hebrew, 'beloved'.* Serious yet simpatico, with deep biblical roots as the name of the Old Testament hero who triumphed over the mighty Goliath and inspired one of Michelangelo's finest sculptures, David is an enduring classic, but it's slipping down the Top 100. A royal name well used in many cultures, it is still a safe and timeless choice. **Daffy, Dave, Davey, Davidde, Davie, Davies, Davin, Davis, Davon, Davy, Davyd, Davydd. International: Dáivi** (*Irish*), **Dàibhidh** (*Scottish*), **Daffydd, Dai, Dewi, Taffy** (*Welsh*), **Davide** (*French*), **Devi** (*Breton*), **Dabid** (*Basque*), **Daoud, Daved, Daven** (*Scandinavian*), **Taavi**

(*Finnish*), **Dawid** (*Polish*), **Davi** (*Israeli*), **Tevel** (*Yiddish*), **Daoud** (*Arabic*).

DAVIDSON. *English, 'David's son'.* Can be used as a middle name to honour Dad or Grandpa David.

━━━⎯⊸⊘⊶⎯━━━

Names All Your Friends Will Think Are Cool

Ash

Beckett

Cormac

Cruz

Dashiell

Donovan

Elvis

Finn

Gus

Hudson

Jackson

Jude

Matteo

Miles

Nico

Rowan

DAVIES, DAVIS. *Welsh, 'son of David'.* Both fresher and cooler spins on David. **Dave, Davidson, Davies, Davison, Daviss, Davy, Daw, Dawe, Dawes, Dawson.**

DAWSON. *Welsh, 'son of David'.* This is one of the more modern-sounding Welsh names, making it worthy of consideration for a son. **Dawsen.**

DAX. *French place name.* A Dax on *Star Trek* prompted a brief blip in popularity, as did its appealingly energetic sound.

DAXON. *Modern invented name.* May tagalong after fast-rising cousin Jaxon.

DAXTER. *Modern invented name.* Video-game name. Enough said.

♂ **DAY.** *Word name.* Many African tribes have a tradition of naming children for the day or time they were born – Friday, Afternoon – a practice finding new life in the Western world as word names become more popular. **Daye.**

♂ **DAYTON.** *English, variation of* **DEIGHTON,** *'place with a dike'.* If Dayton is finding favour with parents, it's because of its popular two-syllable surname feel and *on*-ending. **Datan, Daten, Datin, Daton, Datun, Daytan, Dayten.**

DEACON. *Greek, 'messenger, servant'.* This name was transposed from the word for a church officer to a baby name when American actor Reese Witherspoon and Ryan Phillippe chose it for their son, and ex-*Miami Vice* star Don Johnson followed suit. **Deakin, Deecon, Deekon.**

♂ **DEAN.** *English, 'lives in a valley' or 'church official'.* Surfer boy, now beached out. Diane Keaton used it as her *daughter*'s middle name. **Deane, Deen, Dene, Deyn, Dino.**

DeANDRE. *Modern invented name.* Obviously, Andre with the prefix *De-*, which denotes 'son of'. **D'Andre, DeAndrae, DeAndray, Diandray, Diondrae, Diondray.**

♂ **DECCAN.** *place name.* The vast plateau in central India makes an intriguing first name, similar to the better-known Irish Declan.

♂ **DECEMBER.** *Word name.* Like most month names, this works better for girls.

DECIMUS. *Latin, 'tenth'.* Might see some new life thanks to cutting-edge fashion for ancient Roman names. **Decio.**

DECKER. *German occupational name, 'roofer'.* Brawny name chosen for his son by rocker Nikki Sixx of Mötley Crüe.

★**DECLAN.** *Irish, meaning unknown.* The amiable and appealing name of an Irish saint (and the real first name of singer Elvis Costello), Declan is very popular in the Emerald Isle. Here, it's only recently left the Top 100 but its star is dimming. **Declyn.**

♂ **DECLARE.** *Word name.* A word name in the Puritan vein, à la Remember or Experience, which a few daring namers are beginning to consider.

DEEPAK. *Sanskrit, 'lamp, light'.* Spiritual author Deepak Chopra made this familiar, if not particularly accessible, outside the Indian community. **Deepack, Dipak.**

DeFOREST. *English, 'living near the forest'.* Just Forest will do. **DeForrest.**

DEI. *Welsh, diminutive of* **DAFYDD/DAVID.** Simplify things and spell it Dai, or even Day.

DEION. *Modern invented name.* Elaboration of Dion – it would be easier to stick with the original, especially when it comes to spelling the name. **Dion.**

DEL. *English, diminutive, 'small valley'.* The kind of name was last found in the 1950s, and even then it was probably a nickname for Delbert. **Dell.**

♂ **DELANEY.** *Irish, 'dark challenger'.* One Irish family name that the girls have definitely captured as their own. **Delaine, Delainey, Delainy, Delane, Delany.**

DELANO. *French surname, 'from the forest of nut trees'.* Popular President Franklin Delano Roosevelt inspired a brief fashion for this as a first name in the US in the 1940s; almost never heard today.

DELBERT. *English, 'day-bright'.* Problematic, even if not for Dilbert. **Bert, Bertie, Dalbert, Dilbert.**

DELGADO. *Portuguese and Spanish, 'slender, thin'.* This originated as a nickname for a skinny person; could make a rhythmic first name as well.

DELIAS. *Greek, 'from Delos'.* Delos was a sacred island to the ancient Greeks and its namesake is rarely used. A more interesting and musical choice might be Delius, after the British-born composer of lush rhapsodies. **Deli, Delos, Deltas.**

DELMAR. *Spanish, 'of the sea'.* Could be considered by a family with sailing interests. **Delmer, Delmore.**

DELMORE. *French, 'of the sea'.* Even passionate admirers of

poet Delmore Schwartz would probably look elsewhere for their son's name. **Delmar, Delmer, Delmor.**

DELROY. *French, 'servant of the king'.* Gone, along with Elroy and Leroy. **Delroi.**

DEMETRIUS. *Greek, 'follower of Demeter'.* Classic Greek name that is hard to think of without following it with '. . . and the Gladiators'. Dimitri would be far cooler. **Dametrius, Demetrice, Demetrien, Demetris, Demitrio, Demitrios, Dimetre, Dimitrios, Dimitrious, Dimitry, Dmitrios, Dmitry. International: Demetre** *(French),* **Demetrio** *(Italian, Spanish),* **Demeter, Dometer, Domotor, Dymitr** *(Polish),* **Dimitr** *(Bulgarian),* **Dima, Dimitri, Dmitri, Dmitrik, Mitya** *(Russian),* **Demetri, Demetrios, Demitrius, Dhimitrios, Dimitros, Dimos, Mimis, Mitros, Mitsos, Takis** *(Greek).*

♂ **DEMOCRACY.** *Word name.* Righteous brother of Peace and Justice – all of whom might have a hard time during playground recess.

Two-Syllable Standouts

August

Calvin

Dermot

Forrest

Garrett

Griffin

Harry

Homer

Hudson

Ian

Isaac

Jasper

Joaquin

Jonah

Joseph

Levi

Lucas

Moses

Noah

Owen

Patrick

Theo

Thomas

Wyatt

DEMOS. *Diminutive of Greek* **DEMOSTHENES,** *'the people'.* Related to the word democracy and easier as a name. **Detnas.**

DEMPSEY. *Irish, 'proud, haughty'.* Spunky Irish surname that still has a pugnacious feel from its lingering association with one of boxing's greatest champs, Jack Dempsey. **Dempster, Dempsy.**

♂ **DENALI.** *Place name.* Alaska's Denali National Park is the home of Mount McKinley, endowing the name with a lofty feel.

DENHAM. *English, 'village in a valley'.* Legitimises the newly coined Denim, as does the Scottish place name Denholm (both pronounced *DEN-um*). **Denholm.**

♂ **DENIM.** *Word name.* Singer Toni Braxton chose to give her son this fabric name; better just to dress your kid in jeans. **Denham, Denym.**

DENIZ. *Turkish, 'sea, waves'.* Jazzy Dennis.

DENNIS. *French from Greek, vernacular form of* **DIONYSIUS.** The Irish-sounding name of the patron saint of France was popular in the 1940s and 50s but has been slipping ever since. **Den, Deni, Denies, Denis, Dennet, Denney, Dennie, Dennison, Denny, Dennys, Deon, Dionisio, Dionysius, Dionysus. International: Denes, Denijs, Denis, Deniss, Denney, Denys, Dion, Dione** *(French),* **Dunixi** *(Basque),* **Dinis** *(Portuguese),* **Dionizy** *(Polish),* **Dénes** *(Hungarian),* **Dennes** *(Eastern European),* **Deniskov, Denka, Denya** *(Russian).*

DENNISON. *English, 'son of Dennis'.* The son is now more attractive than the father. **Den, Denison, Denisson, Dennyson, Tennyson.**

♂ **DENNY.** *Diminutive of* **DENNIS.** Has more of a ring for a girl than a boy. **Den, Deni, Dennie.**

♂ **DENVER.** *Place name, 'green valley'.* American place name, oddly more popular there in the

1920s; Aspen is a more
fashionable choice today.

DENZEL. *Cornish, 'from the
high stronghold'*. This old
Cornish name took on a whole
new identity via American actor
Denzel Washington, who has
inspired many namesakes.
The actor was named after
his father, who was named
for a Dr Denzel, who delivered
him. **Denzell, Denzelle,
Denziel, Denzil, Denzill,
Denzille, Denzyl.**

DEODAR. *Sanskrit, 'divine
wood'*. Name of the 'god tree,'
a tall cedar native to India that
also grows in England. Not a
prime baby name candidate,
especially if you want to avoid
odour-related name calling.

DERBY. *English, 'park with
deer'*. It's a hat, it's a race
and it's even been known
to be a name. **Darby, Derbey,
Derbie.**

DEREK. *German, 'the people's
ruler'*. Derek started out as a
sophisticated name, but it
became so common over the
last decades of the twentieth
century that it lost its stylish
edge. **Darriq, Dedrec, Dedreck,
Dedrek, Dedrik, Derec,
Dereck, Deric, Derik, Deriq,
Derreck, Derry, Derryck,
Derryk, Deryk, Deryke,
Dirke, Dyrk, Rick, Ricky.
International: Darrick, Derrick,
Derrig, Derrik** *(Irish)*, **Dirk**
(Dutch), **Darrick, Dedric,
Dedrick, Diederick, Dietrich**
(German), **Derick, Derk,
Derrek, Derrick, Diederik**
(Danish), **Daric** *(Persian)*.

★**DERMOT**. *Irish, Anglicisation
of* **DIARMAID**. This is an
old Irish mythological hero's
name that has long been
popular in Ireland, and has
more recently been imported
elsewhere; we see it in the
next Celtic wave, following
Connor and Liam. **International:
Dermid, Dermit, Dermitt,
Dermod, Dermott, Diarmad**
(Scottish).

DERRY. *Irish place name,
also diminutive of* **DEREK**,
DERMOT, Merry but slight.
Derrie.

DERWIN. *English, 'dear friend'*.
Like Irwin and Merwin, suffers
from terminally anorak sound –
ironically hard to win if your
name ends in *win*. **Darwin,
Darwyn, Derwyn, Derwynn,
Durwin, Durwyn.**

DESCARTES. *(day-CART)
French surname, 'dweller at the
outskirts of town'*. Highly
unlikely philosophical choice.

DESHAN. *Hindi, 'of the
nation'*. Attractive Indian name
unfamiliar to most Western
parents. **Deshad, Deshal.**

DESHAWN. *Modern name,
Shawn with the De- prefix*.
Classically, the *De-* prefix
indicates 'son of,' so any
variation of this name could
work for the child of a dad
named Shawn or Sean. **Dashaun,
Dashawn, Desean, DeShaun,
D'Shawn.**

♀ **DESI**. *Latin, diminutive
of* **DESIDERIO**. **Des, Desito,
Dez, Dezi.**

DESIDERIO. *Spanish, 'desired
one'*. Male form of Desirée, with
less baggage and that familiarly
appealing short form, Desi.
**Deri, Derito, Desi, Desideratus,
Desiderios, Desiderius, Desito,
Diderot, Drio.**

★**DESMOND.** *Latin, 'all creation'.* Well used in England and Ireland but neglected elsewhere, this sophisticated and debonair name, with noble ties to Nobel Peace Prize-winning Bishop Desmond Tutu and with several appealing nicknames, is definitely worth considering. **Des, Desi, Desmund, Desy, Dez, Dezi, Dezmond, Esmond.**

DESTIN. *Latin, 'destiny'.* Synthesised name in the falls into Justin/Dustin mould. **Deston.**

♂ **DESTRY.** *English variation of French, 'war horse'.* Destry rides again.

DEUCE. *Word name.* Trey, yes; Deuce, no.

♂ **DEVERAUX.** *French, 'riverbank'.* Swashbuckling name worthy of a hero in a romance novel. **Deverau, Devereaux, Deverell, Deverill.**

♂ **DEVERE.** *French, 'of the fishing place'.* An original choice for a fisherman's child. **DeVere.**

♂ **DEVIN.** *Irish, 'poet'.* Devilishly handsome, Devin arrived as Kevin was moving out and it's still a popular choice. Not to be confused (though it often is) with the place name Devon (*see below*). **Davin, Davion, Davon, Dev, Devan, Deven, Devinn, Devon, Devyn, Devynn.**

DEVLIN. *Irish, 'fierce courage'.* Fresher and even more devilish than Devin. **Delvin, Devland, Devlen, Devlon, Devlyn.**

♂ **DEVON.** *English place name.* Spelled like the lovely seaside county that inspired the name, this spelling for boys is far behind the more popular Devin, and it is sinking faster in popularity, probably because of its somewhat feminine feel. **Daven, Davin, Davion, Davon, Devan, Devaun, Devawn, Deven, Devin, Devonn, Devyn.**

DEVRAJ. *Hindi, 'ruler of the gods'.* An imposing meaning, an appealing sound.

DEWEY. *Anglicised variation of Welsh* **DEWI.** No more popular than Hughie or Louie. **Dewie.**

DEWI. *Diminutive of* **DAFYDD,** *Welsh variation of* **DAVID.** The name of the patron saint of Wales would not work and play well with others elsewhere.

DEWITT. *Flemish, 'blond'.* If you must, at least call him Witt. **Dewit, DeWitt, Dwight, Witt.**

★**DEX.** *Diminutive of* **DEXTER.** Has lots more energy and sex appeal than the original; it might make an appropriate choice for your son.

♂ **DEXTER.** *Latin, 'right-handed, skillful'.* Former anorak name turned cutie. Do you dare? Diane Keaton single-handedly turned it unisex when she named her daughter Dexter Dean. **Dex.**

♂ **DHANI.** *Hindi, 'rich'.* Transforms Donnie into an exotically appealing name that is also a more masculine alternative for a boy.

DIARMAID. *(DEER-muht) Irish, 'free man'.* This authentic form of the name of an Irish mythological hero with the power to make women fall instantly in love with him would work far better here as the Anglicised Dermot. **Dermid, Dermot, Diarmad, Diarmait, Diarmi, Diarmid, Diarmuid.**

♂ **DIAZ.** *Spanish from Latin, 'days'.* Perfect example of an ethnic surname that would work well as a first.

DICE. *Word name.* Strictly for a casino baby. **Dyce.**

DICK. *Diminutive of* RICHARD. Once-common short form of Richard; replaced by Rick or Richie and finally by the full name itself.

DICKINSON. *English, 'son of Dick'.* Possibility for Richard's boy.

DICKSON. *Scottish, 'son of Dick'.* See *DIXON.*

DIDIER. *(dee-DYAE) French, 'much-desired'.* Desirée for boys; this lively, confident name that's widely used in France has definite possibilities here.

DIEGO. *Spanish variation of* JAMES. Energetic name on the rise along with a lot of other authentically Spanish choices. **Dago, Santiago. International: Diogo** *(Portuguese).*

DIETER. *(DEE-ter) German, diminutive of* **DIETRICH.** Classic German name that gets plenty of satiric exposure in the English-speaking countries. Could conceivably be read as someone on a diet.

DIETRICH. *(DEE-trish) German, 'ruler of the people'.* This form of Theodoric, familiar via Marlene, is a possible German import. **Dedrick, Deke, Derek, Dirk. International: Diderick, Diederick, Tiede** *(Dutch).*

DIGBY. *Norse, 'town by the ditch'.* Place name turned surname turned deservedly obscure first name.

DIJI. *(DEE-jee) Nigerian, 'a farmer'.* Sounds too much like initials (D.G) or deejay.

♂ **DILLON.** *Irish, 'loyal'.* Different origin from the Welsh Dylan, but increasingly used as a variant spelling. **Dillan, Dilon, Dyllon, Dylon.**

DILWYN. *Welsh, 'fair, white, blessed'.* Definite bully victim.

DINGO. *Australian animal name.* These wild dogs eat babies, they do not inspire their names.

DINO. *Italian, diminutive.* Might be reminiscent of dinosaur.

DINSMORE. *Irish, 'dark moor'.* Butler name. **Dinnsmore.**

DIOGENES. *Greek philosopher.* Philosopher who advocated the simple life – though his name is anything but.

DION. *(DEE-on) Greek, 'child of heaven and earth'; also diminutive of* **DIONYSIUS.** In ancient Greece, a student of Plato; elsewhere, a cool guy. **Deion, Deon, Deonn, Deonys, Deyon.**

DIONYSIUS. *Greek mythology name.* Dionysius was the god of wine and revelry, making the

Names for Dark-Haired Babies

Blake	Ebony
Bruno	Hadrian
Carey	Kali
Cole	Keira/
Darcy	Kiera/
	Kieran
Delaney	Kerry
Dolan	Krishna
Donahue	Laila/
Donnan	Layla/
Donnelly	Leila
Douglas	Melanie
Doyle	Merle
Duff/	Nigel
Duffy	Raven
Dunn	Sullivan
Dwayne	Tynan

♂ **DIPLOMACY.** *Word name.* In the Capability Brown vein – not a choice to be made lightly.

DIRK. *Flemish and Dutch, contracted form of* **DEREK.** Both Dirk and cousin Kirk are taking an extended break from maternity wards. **Dierck, Dieric, Dierich, Dierk.**

♂ **DISCOVERY.** *English word name.* Adventurous word choice, but still quite a burden for a child to bear.

♂ **DIVERSITY.** *English word name.* Baby name as political statement.

DIX. *Latin, 'tenth'; also variation of Dick, diminutive of* **DIXON.** Once a birth order name, now might work as a cool *x*-ending nickname.

DIXON. *Scottish, 'son of Dick'.* Inventive way to honour an ancestral Richard or Dick. Use the *x* form. **Dickson, Dix.**

DJANGO. *(JANG-oh) Gypsy, 'I awake'.* The nickname of great Belgian-born jazz guitarist Django (born Jean Baptiste)

Reinhardt makes a dynamic musical choice.

DJIMON. *(gee-MON) African, meaning unknown.* Powerful Benin-born actor Djimon Hounsou made us aware of this African name.

★**DMITRI.** *Russian from Greek* **DEMETRIUS.** Exotic, artistic and attractive Slavic variation of the name of the Greek god of fertility and farming. **Dhimitri, Dimitri. International: Demetrio** *(Italian and Spanish),* **Dymitr** *(Polish),* **Dumitru** *(Romanian),* **Dima, Dimitre, Dmitri, Dmitrik, Mitya** *(Russian),* **Dmitro** *(Ukrainian).*

♂ **DOANE.** *English, 'low, rolling hills'.* Unusual, but clear and strong. **Doan.**

DOBBIN. *Diminutive of* **ROBERT.** Ancient nickname that sounds cuter than its modern alternatives – but be aware that in the days of the horse and buggy, it was most often used for the horse.

DODGE. *English, diminutive of* **ROGER.** Old short form more

name simultaneously heavy and lightweight. One of the short forms much better. **Deion, Deon, Deonn, Deyon, Dion, Dionio, Dionisio, Dioniso, Dionysios, Dionysos, Dionysus.**

than a little dodgy now. **Dod, Dodds, Dodgson.**

DODSON. *English, 'Roger's son'.* Fresh way to pass down Roger. **Doddsen, Dodsen, Dotsen, Dotson, Dottsen, Dottson.**

♂ **DOHERTY.** *Irish, 'not loving'.* Surname that could have pronunciation problems – it's Dorrity – as well as having an off-putting meaning. **Docherty, Dorrity, Dougherty, Douherty.**

DOLAN. *Irish, 'black-haired'.* Fresh choice that could pick up where Dylan and Logan left off. **Doland, Dolans, Dolen, Dolend, Dolens, Dolenz, Dolin.**

DOLPH. *German, diminutive of* **ADOLPH.** All Adolph variations are best avoided, though this takes some of the onus off. **Dolf, Dollfus, Dollfuss, Dollphus, Dolphus.**

DOMINGO. *Spanish, 'born on a Sunday'.* Commonly heard in Hispanic cultures, a rhythmic possibility here. **International: Domenico** *(Italian).*

★♂ **DOMINIC.** *Latin, 'belonging to the lord'.* An upper-crust mainstay that has been popular enough to be in the Top 100. **Dom, Domenic, Domenique, Domini, Dominick, Dominie, Domino, Dominy, Domo, Nick, Nickie, Nicky. International: Dominque** *(French),* **Domenico, Domingo, Menico** *(Italian),* **Chuma, Chumin, Chuminga, Domenico, Domicio, Domingo, Dominguez, Mingo** *(Spanish),* **Txomin** *(Basque),* **Domenge** *(Catalan),* **Domingos** *(Portuguese),* **Dominik, Donek, Niki** *(Polish),* **Deco, Domi, Domokos, Domonokos** *(Hungarian),* **Domek, Dominik, Dumin** *(Czech),* **Domenikos** *(Greek).*

♂ **DOMINO.** *Latin, 'lord, master'.* Don't play games with this one.

DONAHUE. *Irish, 'dark fighter'.* Genial Irish surname, much more current than Donald. **Don, Donaghue, Donahoe, Donohoe, Donohue.**

DONALD. *Scottish, 'proud chief'.* Sorry, Mr Trump, but this is not the greatest name in the world, although it was recently chosen

by Charles and Sarah Kennedy. The Irish Donal has a lot more appeal. **Don, Donaugh, Donel, Donelson, Donnel, Donnell, Donnie, Donny. International: Domhnall** *(Gaelic),* **Donal, Donall** *(Irish),* **Donaldo** *(Italian and Spanish),* **Donalt** *(Norwegian),* **Bogdan, Bohdan, Donya** *(Ukrainian).*

DONAR. *German, 'ancient thunder god'.* Futuristic, in a 1930s kind of way.

DONATO. *Latin, 'given by God'.* Widely used in Italy, Spain and Portugal, has an air of generosity and could easily be adopted here. **International: Donat, Donatien** *(French),* **Donatelli, Donatello, Donati** *(Italian),* **Dodek, Donat** *(Polish).*

DONN. *Irish, 'king' or 'brown'.* Ancient Irish king of the underworld, so much more powerful than Don.

♂ **DONNAN.** *Irish, 'small brown-haired child'.* This Irish saint's name makes an attractive alternative for Dylan or Donald.

♂ **DONNELLY.** *Irish, 'dark, brave one'.* Among the more appealing Irish surname names, less well used than Donovan. **Donnell, Donny, Dony.**

DONOUGH. *(DOH-na) Irish, 'brown chieftain'.* Might be a bit too close to Donna. **Donagh.**

★♂ **DONOVAN.** *Irish, 'dark'.* One of the first of the appealing Irish surnames to take off in this country, has long outgrown its 'Mellow Yellow' association. **Donavon, Donevin, Donevon, Donoven, Donovon.**

DONTE. *Italian, 'lasting'.* Phonetic Dante. **Dantae, Dantay, Dohntae, Dontae, Dontay, Dontey.**

DOOLEY. *Irish, 'dark hero'.* Jokey Irish name, too susceptible to drooling jokes.

♂ **DORAN.** *Irish, 'stranger, exile'.* Strong but gentle Irish last-name-first. Could bring to mind long-running rock group Duran Duran. **Dore, Dorian, Doron, Dorran, Dorren.**

♂ **DORIAN.** *Greek, 'from Doris'.* Still haunted by *The Picture of Dorian Gray*, also sounds somewhat feminine. **Dore, Dorien, Dorrian, Dorrien, Dorryen.**

DORON. *(doh-ROHN) Hebrew, 'gift'.* Benevolent name found in Israel in several forms, including Doran and Doroni. **Doran, Doroni, Dorran.**

♂ **DORSET.** *English place name.* With Devon so overused, consider a move to the undiscovered neighbouring county – though it's nowhere near as euphonious, rhyming with corset.

♂ **DORSEY.** *English from French, 'from Orsay'.* Associated all through the swing years with band-leader brothers Tommy and Jimmy Dorsey. **D'Orsay, Dorsee, Dorsie.**

DOUGAL. *Scottish, 'dark stranger'.* Heard in the Scottish highlands, much more in tune with the times than Douglas. **Doug, Dougal, Dugal, Dugald, Dugall, Duggie. International: Dùghall** *(Scottish Gaelic).*

DOUGLAS. *Scottish, 'black water'.* The surname of a powerful Scottish clan . . . and your mum's date when a teenager. **Doogie, Doug, Dougey, Dougie, Douglass, Dugaid, Duggie, Duglass.**

DOUGRAY. *French surname.* Scottish actor Dougray (born Stephen) Scott took on his French grandmother's surname. Might a family surname of your own work for your son?

DOV. *Hebrew, 'bear'.* Fierce meaning, gentle image. Very common in Israel. **Dovi, Dubi.**

♂ **DOVE.** *Nature name.* A subtle but clear way to signal peace, just as Paloma is for a girl. **Dov, Duv.**

DOVER. *British place name.* Two-syllable place names are stylish and this one is attached to a the city noted for its white chalk cliffs, but there is a minus: it also rhymes with the doggy Rover.

DOVEV. *(doh-VAYV) Hebrew, 'whisper'.* Soft yet strong. **Dov.**

DOW. *Irish, 'dark-haired'.* A bit flat-footed, also too stock-market-related. **Dowan, Dowe, Dowson.**

DOYLE. *Irish, 'black stranger'.* Dark horse Irish surname.

DRACO. *Greek from Latin, 'dragon'.* For as long as we all shall live, Harry Potter's sneering nemesis. **Drago.**

DRAKE. *English, 'dragon'; also word name, 'male duck'.* A simple name that's on the way up, despite references to dragons and ducks.

DRAPER. *English occupational name, 'cloth merchant'.* Other occupational names would be more commonly accepted.

DRAVEN. *Modern invented name.* Inspired by Brandon Lee's character in *The Crow* and Cuba Gooding's in *In the Shadows*. Potential playground rhyming with Craven and Raven make it unsuitable for serious consideration for most boys.

♂ DREAM. *Word name.* Possible middle name inspiration.

DRENNON. *Irish, 'son of Draighnean'.* Brennan alternative.

♂ DRESDEN. *Place name.* Sad tinge to the name of the beautiful German city firebombed during World War II.

★ **♂ DREW.** *Diminutive of* **ANDREW.** Rapidly becoming the Andrew nickname of choice, replacing the past favourite Andy. **Dro, Dru, Drue.**

DRUM. *Word name.* Cool, musical modern choice, especially as a middle name. **Drumm.**

DRUMMOND. *Scottish, 'ridge'.* If you'd like to legitimise Drum.

♂ DRURY. *French, 'dear one, sweetheart'.* A bit thick on the tongue, but rhythmic and energetic. **Drew, Drewry, Dru.**

DRYDEN. *English, 'dry valley'.* Creative inspiration via poet John, but somewhat dry and dusty.

DRYSTAN. *Welsh variation of* **TRISTRAM.** Name of a

counsellor to King Arthur that sounds too much like a nasal decongestant; we'd advise sticking with Tristram or Tristan.

DUALD. *Irish, 'dark, darkness'.* Obscure and quirky, but not without some appeal.

♂ DUANE. *Irish, 'swarthy'.* Duane and his twin Dwayne have become almost a stereotype of an unsophisticated guy.

♂ DUBLIN. *Irish place name.* With Galway and Ireland in play as names (not to mention Shannon and Kerry), there's no reason this one can't work, too.

DUDLEY. *English, 'people's field'.* It's easy to love a name that rhymes with 'cuddly' and is also attached to the surname Do-Right – though there is that 'dud' connection.

♂ DUFF. *Irish, 'swarthy'.* Somewhat rough, rowdy, ragged Celtic name, at home in a noisy pub or out walking on the moors. **Duffey, Duffie, Duffy.**

DUGAN. *Irish, 'swarthy'.* Open, friendly and cheery Irish

If **You Like Dylan**
You Might Love . . .

Bran

Cian

Damon

Darian

Declan

Dillon

Dion

Dixon

Evan

Gareth

Griffin

Killian

Morgan

Owen

Rhys

surname. **Doogan, Dougan, Douggan, Duggan.**

DUKE. *English rank of nobility.* While John Wayne and Duke Ellington are worthy role models, this name sounds like a too-flimsy diminutive. Only someone like Diane Keaton could get away with using it for her son.

DULÉ. *(doo-lay) French, meaning unknown.* Talented Jamaican-American actor Dulé (born Karim Dulé) Hill of TV's The West Wing introduced this name, which may be more invention than genuinely French.

DUMAS. *(DOO-mah) French, 'of the little farm'.* The name of the great French novelist, author of the timeless *The Count of Monte Cristo* and *The Three Musketeers,* would make a surprising middle name choice.

DUNBAR. *Irish, 'castle headland'.* Clear and strong, if a little heavy.

★**DUNCAN.** *Scottish, 'dark warrior'.* Jaunty, confident and open, this Scottish royal name is brimming with friendly charm and makes it into our golden circle of ideal names. **Dun, Dunc, Dunkan, Dunn.**

DUNDEE. *Scottish place name.* A city and river in Scotland; this is upbeat and cheery, but doesn't seem that appropriate as a name.

♂ **DUNE.** *Nature name.* Sibling of Beach and Ocean. **Doon, Doone.**

DUNHAM. *Scottish, 'brown hill homestead'.* Attractive, if somewhat reminiscent of a pipe smoker's tobacco.

DUNN. *Scottish, 'brown'.* Efficient feel. **Dunne.**

DUNSTAN. *English, 'dark stone'.* A two-syllable surname feel puts this name of an important English saint in the running – though it could sound like a confused cross between Duncan and Dustin. **Dunsten, Dunstin, Dunston.**

DURANGO. *Spanish place name.* Tough guy name from Mexican city.

DURANT, DURANTE. *Latin, 'enduring'.* Its meaning signifies staying power. **Dante, Duran, Durand, Durante.**

DURHAM. *English, 'hill peninsula'.* Gentle name that could be used instead of Devon or Dover.

DURWARD. *English occupational name, 'doorkeeper'.* Awkward. **Derward.**

♂ **DURYEA.** *(dur-ee-ay) Irish, 'from the stream'.* Irish name with an intriguing lilt.

DUSHAN. *Czech, 'heartfelt, sincere'.* One of the few Czech names that seems accessible here.

♂ **DUSTIN.** *Norse, 'brave warrior,' 'Thor's stone'.* Its popularity in recent years is probably more due to its similarity to Justin than to idolisation of Dustin Hoffman, who certainly was the one to put it on the name map. **Dustan, Dusten, Duston, Dusty, Dustyn.**

DUVALL. *French, 'of the valley'.* Hard to see it attracting many takers. **Duval, Du Val.**

DWAYNE. *Spelling variation of Duane.* Better off with Wayne. **Duane, Duwain, Duwayne, Dwain, Dwaine.**

DWEEZIL. *Modern invented name.* One of the often-mocked Zappa kid names; it

Stellar Starbabies Beginning with *D*

Damian	Elizabeth Hurley, Natasha Richardson & Liam Neeson
Dashiell	Cate Blanchett, Alice Cooper, Helen *(Bridget Jones)* Fielding, Lisa Rinna & Harry Hamlin
Deacon	Reese Witherspoon & Ryan Phillippe, Don Johnson
Declyn	Cyndi Lauper
Denim	Toni Braxton
Devin	Vanessa Williams
Devon	Nell McAndrew
Dexter	Elvis Costello & Diana Krall
Diezel	Toni Braxton
Donald	Charles & Sarah Kennedy
Draven	Chester *(Linkin Park)* Bennington
Duke	Diane Keaton
Dylan	Pamela Anderson & Tommy Lee, Pierce Brosnan, Nadia Comaneci & Bart Conner, Joan Cusack, Catherine Zeta-Jones & Michael Douglas

supposedly was a nickname his father had for his wife's little toe.

DWIGHT. *German and Dutch, 'white or blond'.* We like Ike better.

♂ **DYLAN.** *Welsh, 'son of the sea'.* Still poetic and romantic after years of popularity, now often used for girls, too. The original Dylan was a legendary Welsh sea god, but its greatest inspirations have been poet Dylan Thomas and singer Bob Dylan. Be aware that it's in the Top 25, so yours may not be the only Dylan in his class. **Dillan, Dillen, Dillon, Dylen, Dyllan, Dylon, Dylonn, Dylun.**

DYSON. *English, contraction of* **DENNISON**. Your son could be mistaken for a vacuum cleaner.

E *boys*

EACHANN. *(AYK-an) Irish, 'keeper of horses'.* Authentic Gaelic name with pronunciation problems – some might assume he was achin'. **Aiken, Aken.**

EAGLE. *Bird name.* Solemn but soaring name.

EAMES. *English, 'son of the uncle'.* Slightly pretentious, but with a nice modern design connection to the creators of the Eames chair.

★**ÉAMON.** *(AY-mon) Irish variation of* **EDMUND**. This friendlier Celtic version of Edmund has an upbeat feel and a good chance of competing with Aidan and Damon sometime soon. **Aimon, Amon, Aymon, Eammon, Éamonn, Eumonn.**

EAN. *Spelling variation of* **IAN**. Phonetic spelling of the British Ian that has earned a share of its own popularity. **Eaen, Eann, Eayon, Eion, Eon, Eyan, Eyon, Iaen, Ian.**

EARL. *English aristocratic title.* It may have a noble ranking, but Earl is likely these days to be either wearing overalls or hunched over his desk crunching numbers with an adding machine. **Airle, Earle, Earlie, Early, Erl, Erle, Errol, Erroll, Erryl, Rollo.**

♂ **EARLY.** *Word name.* Word-turned-name, pleasantly suggesting the start of a bright new day. **Earley, Erly.**

EARVIN. *Spelling variation of* **IRVIN**. Pronunciation could be a problem, if people think of the hearing organ. **Erv, Ervin, Irvin.**

EASTMAN. *English, 'grace protector'.* Solid, old-style surname.

♂ **EASTON.** *English, 'east-facing place'.* Stylish surname name that could be on its way up. **Esten, Wastin.**

♂ **EATON.** *English, 'riverside'.* Similarity to Eton gives it an upscale Old School feel. **Eatton, Eatun, Eton, Eyton.**

★**EBAN, EBEN.** *Hebrew, diminutive of* **EBENEZER**. Affable and creative and perfectly able to stand alone; nothing Scroogish about it. **Ebon, Even.**

EBENEZER. *Hebrew, 'stone of help'.* Dickens's miserly Scrooge character pretty much annihilated this biblical name, but since he *did* reform at the end of *A Christmas Carol*, maybe there's some slight hope for the old name yet. **Eb, Ebbaneza, Eben, Ebeneezer, Ebeneser, Ebenezar, Eveneser, Evenezer.**

EBERHARD. *German, 'brave boar'.* Ever hard and forbiddingly Germanic. **Ebbe, Eberardo, Eberdt, Eberhardt, Ebert, Eburhardt, Everard, Everhard, Evrard, Evreux.** International: **Everet, Everett** *(English),* **Evarado, Everardo** *(Spanish),* **Evert** *(Swedish).*

EBO. *African, Akeradini, 'born on Tuesday'.* A powerful African name that can be used to fit its definition.

♂ **EDAN.** *Irish, 'little fire'.* This alternate spelling of Aidan may get confused with the feminine Eden. **Aedan, Aidan, Aiden, Edain, Edon.**

EDDIE. *Diminutive of* **EDWARD** *et al.* Most parents today call their sons Edward and save Eddie for their pooches.

EDDY. *Diminutive of* **EDWARD** *et al.* Used more often on its own than Eddie, but no better suited to grown-up life.

EDEL. *German, 'noble'.* Rarely used independently, it's more often the start of a multisyllabic German mouthful. **Adel, Adlin, Edelin, Edell, Edlin.**

EDGAR. *German, 'prosperous spearman'.* Though Edgar (and Edgardo) are popular with Latino families and have had such famous forebears as Edgar Allan Poe, most would rate it a distant third to Edward and Edmund. **Eadger, Ed, Eddie, Ned, Neddy, Ted, Teddie.** International: **Eadgar** *(French),* **Edgard** *(French and Hungarian),* **Edgardito, Edgardo** *(Spanish).*

♂ **EDI.** *(Eh-dee) Hebrew, 'my witness'.* A possibility for parents seeking a Hebrew name with an English-language sound.

★ ♂ **EDISON.** *English, 'son of Edward'.* Rhythmic, undiscovered last-name-first-name that projects the creativity and inventiveness of Thomas A. **Eddis, Eddison, Eddy, Edisen, Edson, Edyson.**

EDMUND. *English, 'wealthy protector'.* A neglected classic, both less common and more upscale than Edward. **Eadmund,** **Ed, Eddie, Eddy, Ned, Ted, Teddy, Tedman, Tedmund, Theomund.** International: **Eamonn** *(Gaelic),* **Eames, Eamon,** *(Irish),* **Eumann** *(Scottish Gaelic),* **Edmond** *(French, Dutch),* **Edmondo** *(Italian),* **Edmundo, Mundo** *(Spanish, Portuguese),* **Odön** *(Hungarian),* **Edmunds** *(Latvian),* **Edmon** *(Russian).*

EDMUNDO. *Spanish and Portuguese variation of* **EDMUND.** Livelier Latin form of Edmund. **Admundo, Edmundito.**

EDRIC. *English, 'wealthy ruler'.* Even less likely than Cedric. **Ederic, Ederick, Edrich, Edrick.**

EDSEL. *English, 'wealthy man's estate'.* Besides having an unappealing sound, has long been identified with a much-mocked Ford car model; use of this name is now restricted to the Ford family.

EDUARDO. *Spanish and Italian variation of* **EDWARD.** A stalwart of Latin nomenclature that could work just as well for Anglos. **Duardo, Edrardo, Eduarelo, Eudardo, Guayo.**

If **You** Like **Edward,**

You Might Love . . .

Eamon

Edmund

Eduardo

Elliot

Frederic

Francis

George

Henry

Hugh

Julian

Louis

Patrick

Timothy

Ward

William

★**EDWARD.** *English, 'wealthy guardian'.* Unlike perennials William, John and James, Edward is a classic that moves in and out of fashion. This royal Anglo-Saxon standard is in the Top 50 right now – but whatever its standing we still think it's worth consideration if you're seeking a traditional male name. **Eadward, Ed, Edd, Eddie, Eddy, Edison, Edred, Edson, Ned, Neddy, Ted, Teddy.** International: **Eadbhard** *(Irish),* **Eideard, Eudard** *(Scottish Gaelic),* **Edouard** *(French),* **Edoardo** *(Italian),* **Eduardo** *(Spanish),* **Duarte** *(Portuguese),* **Ede** *(Dutch),* **Eduard** *(German),* **Eatu** *(Finnish),* **Edvard** *(Czech, Russian),* **Ekewak** *(Hawaiian).*

EDWIN. *English, 'wealthy friend'.* Considered outdated by most, but not by the parents who chose it last year. **Eadwinn, Ed, Eddy, Edlin, Ned, Neddy, Ted.** International: **Edwyn** *(Welsh),* **Eduin, Eduino** *(Spanish),* **Edvin, Edvino** *(Eastern European).*

EELIA. *(eel-EE-yah) Russian variation of* **ELIYAHU,** *'the lord is my god'.* Intriguing Russian possibility, even though proper pronunciation would not be obvious. Ilya might be a more manageable option. **Eelusha, Ilya.**

EERO. *Finnish variation of* **ERIC.** Creative gem perfect for an architect's son, in tribute to modern Finnish-American architect Eero Saarinen.

EETU. *Finnish variation of* **EDWARD.** Et tu, Eetu?

EFRAIN. *Spanish variation of* **EPHRAIM.** On the Latino Hit Parade, heard much more often than the English version. **Efra, Efraém, Efraén, Efraine, Efrén, Ephrain, Ifrain.**

EFREM. *Russian variation of* **EPHRAIM.** Phonetic spelling brought to light by actor Efrem Zimbalist Jr. **Efi, Efraim, Efram, Efrayim, Efrim.**

EFRON. *Hebrew, 'bird, lark'.* Biblical name that's not as pleasant sounding as its meaning would suggest. **Efroni, Ephron.**

★**EGAN.** *(EE-ghin or AY-ghin) Irish, 'son of Hugh'.* Likeness to the word *eager* gives this Irish surname a ready-to-please, effervescent energy. **Eagan, Eagen, Eagon, Egann, Egen, Eghan, Egon, Keegan, MacEgan.** International: **Aodhgan** *(Irish Gaelic),* **Iagan** *(Scottish).*

EGBERT. *Anglo-Saxon, 'bright edge of a sword'.* The ultimate anorak name. **Egberto.**

EGON. *(AY-gon) German, 'strong with a sword'.* Muscular, not particularly Germanic German name.

EILAM. *(ehy-lahm) Hebrew, 'eternal'.* One of Noah's biblical grandsons, making it a natural to honour a relative with the name of the ark builder. **Elam.**

EILON. *(ehy-lohn) Hebrew, 'oak tree'.* And since this belonged to a grandson of Jacob's, the same applies here. **Elan, Elon.**

EITAN. *(AY-tahn) Hebrew variation of* **ETHAN.** This Hebrew version of Ethan, also a place name in southern Israel, works well here. **Etan, Eytan.**

♂ **EJA.** *Native American, meaning unknown.* Singer Shania Twain is said to have chosen this name, pronounced as Asia, for her son to honour her father's Native American culture.

ELADIO. *Greek, 'the Greek'.* Musical, with a buoyant beat.

♂ **ELAN.** *(EE-lun) Hebrew, 'tree'; also French word name.* When given the French pronunciation *(ay-LAN)*, has a great deal of esprit and élan.

ELAZER. *Hebrew, 'God has helped'.* In Exodus, a son of Aaron: an interesting, undiscovered Old Testament name. **Elezri.** International: **Eleázar** *(Spanish).*

ELBERT. *English variation of* **ALBERT.** Sitting at the community centre with buddies Hubert, Norbert and Osbert.

ELDEN. *English, 'elf friend' or 'noble friend'.* Elden is definitely an elder. **Eldan, Eldin, Eldwin, Eldwyn.**

ELDON. *English, 'sacred hill'.* Another *El* name lacking any youthful energy.

ELDRED. *English, 'old counsel'.* *Dred* is a syllable that might well invoke dread in children. **Aeldred, Aldred, Eldrid.**

ELDRIDGE. *English, 'old, wise leader'.* Name long associated in the US with Black Panther activist Eldridge Cleaver and

jazz great Roy Eldridge. **Aldrich, Eldredge, Eldrege, Eldrich, Eldrick, Eldrige.**

★**ELEAZER.** *Variation of* **LAZARUS.** Four-syllable names can be tricky, but this rarely used Old Testament name has considerable potential. **Eleasar, Eleazaro, Eli, Elie, Eliezer, Ely.** International: **Aliásar, Elaísar, Elazar, Eleózar, Eliseao, Elizar** *(Spanish).*

♂ **ELEVEN.** *Word name.* Some parents have begun to go beyond word names and move on to numerals, but would you really want your kid to feel like a number?

ELGAR. *Anglo-Saxon, 'elf-spear' or 'spearman'.* Despite its connection to English classical composer Edward Elgar, not a very melodious name. **Algar, Elger, Ellgar, Ellger.**

★**ELI.** *Hebrew, 'ascended, uplifted, height'.* Because it is that rarity – a solid biblical name with lots of spirit and energy – this name is beginning to become more popular in some places. **Eloi, Eloy, Ely.** International **Elie** *(French).*

♂ **ELIA.** *Italian variation of* **ELIJAH.** A multicultural appellation, found in Hebrew, Italian and Zuni, this likable name made famous by director Elia Kazan's only problem is the feminine *a* ending. But then again, that never hurt Joshua. **Eilya, Eliah, Elio, Elya.**

ELIAKIM. *(ee-LI-ah-kim) Hebrew, 'God will raise up'.* Unwieldy name, borne by several biblical characters. **Elika, Elyakim, Elyakum.**

ELIAM. *Hebrew, 'God is my nation'.* Obscure but likeable Hebrew *El-* name. **Elami.**

ELIÁN. *Latin, based on Roman clan name.* A Cuban boy's name that was combined from his parents' names: Elizabeth and Juan. Depending on your own names, this could be worth considering for your baby. **Eliano, Elion.**

★**ELIAS.** *Greek variation of* **ELIJAH.** Following the path of family members Elijah and Eli, the strong and charismatic Elias is also becoming popular. **Elia, Eliasz, Eliaz, Elice, Eliyas, Ellias, Ellice, Ellis, Elyas, Lincha.**

ELIAZ. *Hebrew, 'the Lord is my God'.* The final letter makes the name more unusual and adds some zest.

ELIEZER. *Hebrew, 'God helps'.* Biblical name with a patina of antiquity. **Eleazar, Lazar. International: Elazar** *(Basque),* **Eliazar, Eliécar** *(Spanish),* **Lazer** *(Yiddish).*

ELIHU. *Hebrew, 'the Lord is my God'.* Rarely used in the last two centuries, but might be worth dusting off and holding up to the light. **Elihud, Eliu, Ellihu.**

ELIJAH. *Hebrew, 'the Lord is my God'.* The name of the Old Testament prophet who went to heaven in a chariot of fire has become a fashionable biblical choice, with many parents choosing it in recent years – it could become a top name in future years. **Eli, Elian, Elias, Elijio, Elijuah, Elijuo, Eliot, Eliya, Eliyah, Eljah, Elliot, Ellis, Ely, Elyot, Elyott. International: Élie** *(French),* **Elio** *(Italian),* **Elia** *(Spanish),* **Ilie** *(Romanian),* **Elio, Ilias, Ilya** *(Russian),* **Ilya** *(Greek),* **Elihu, Eliyahu** *(Hebrew).*

★**ELIO.** *Greek, 'sun'.* A sunny and spirited Italian version of Elijah that makes it less biblical, more buoyant.

ELISEO. *Italian and Spanish variation of* **ELISHA.** This Latinate name would have no problem fitting into a classroom elsewhere. **Cheo, Cheyo, Elesio, Elisaeo, Elisio, Eliseo, Licha. International: Elisée** *(French),* **Yelisei** *(Russian).*

♂ **ELISHA.** *Hebrew, 'God is my salvation'.* Creative name whose only limitation is that it sounds a lot like such girls' names as Alicia and Elissa – and in fact rising American actor Elisha Cuthbert is a woman. **Eli, Elisee, Elishah, Elisher, Elishu, Elishua, Eliso, Elysha, Lisha. International: Eliseo** *(Italian and Spanish),* **Elizur** *(Eastern European).*

♂ **ELLERY.** *English, 'island with elder trees'.* Rhythmic old mystery writer/detective name used by Laura Dern and Ben Harper for their son, deserves wider use. **Ellary, Ellerey.**

♂ **ELLINGTON.** *English place name.* Swinging musical name, evoking the jazzy persona of the Duke.

♂ **ELLIOT.** *Anglicisation of* **ELIJAH** *or* **ELIAS.** Has the ideal quality of being neither too common nor weirdly unique, although it is in the Top 100 at the moment. **Eliot, Eliott, Eliut, Elliot, Elyot, Elyott.**

♂ **ELLIS.** *Welsh, 'benevolent'.* A popular surname member of the Elias/Elijah family that is currently in the Top 100. **International: Elis** *(Welsh).*

♂ **ELLISON.** *English, 'son of Ellis'.* Updates Ellis – but also has a lot of feminine potential thanks to Allison/Ellie similarity. **Elison, Elisson, Ellson, Ellyson, Elson.**

ELLSWORTH. *English, 'nobleman's estate'.* Creative only via its connection to artist Ellsworth Kelly, otherwise firmly in the off-puttingly haughty camp. **Ellswerth, Elsworth.**

♂ **ELM.** *Nature name.* Strong, straight and leafy, one of the new tree names used mostly as middles.

ELMER. *English, 'noble and renowned'.* Thanks to Elmer Fudd, this old-fashioned name has become a bit of a joke – making it the quintessential so-far-out-it-will-always-be-out name. **Aylmar, Aylmer, Aymer, Elmar, Elmir.**

ELMO. *Italian from German, 'protector'.* Like fellow *Sesame Street* characters Kermit and Grover, Elmo has a hard time being taken seriously. It isn't easy being red either.

ELMORE. *English, 'moor with elm trees'.* Even writer Elmore 'Dutch' Leonard isn't called Elmore.

ELOI. *(EE-loy) Spanish from the Latin* **ELIGIUS,** *'the chosen'.* Could be misunderstood outside the Hispanic culture. **Eloy. International: Eligio** *(Spanish),* **Alois** *(Czech).*

ELROY. *English variation of* **LEROY.** It may be a variation on the theme of Leroy, but it's not much of an improvement. **Elroi, Elroye.**

ELTON. *English, 'from the old town'.* Even the flamboyant

Elton John can't lift this quiet, drab name. **Alton, Eldon, Ellton.**

ELUL. *Hebrew, sixth month of the Jewish calendar.* Another culture's version of the month-naming tradition.

ELVIN. *English, 'elf friend' or 'noble friend'; variation of* **ALVIN.** Retired along with Alvin and Melvin: try Calvin or Gavin instead. **Elven, Elveryn, Elvyn, Elwin, Elwinn, Elwyn, Elwynne.**

ELVIO. *Latin, 'blond, fair'.* Wearing blue suede gaucho boots.

ELVIS. *Scandinavian, 'all-wise'.* When the King was alive and for years afterwards, few people (except Declan McManus who became Elvis Costello) dared use his singular name, but now there are a number of little Elvi born every year. **Alvis, Alvys, Elvio, Elviss, Elviz, Elvo, Elvys.**

EMANUEL. *See* **EMMANUEL.**

EMERIL. *French, meaning unknown.* A highly unusual name, but it could work elsewhere.

Names That Mean Wise

Alden

Aldo

Alfred

Cato

Conan

Connor

Conrad

Dallas

Elvis

Nestor

Quinn

Raymond

Sage

Shanahan

Solon

♀ **EMERSON.** *German, 'son of the chief'.* Dignified, somewhat serious name sometimes associated with American transcendental thinker Ralph Waldo Emerson – and also the old rock group Emerson, Lake and Palmer. Very occasionally used for girls, as Teri Hatcher did for her daughter. **Emmerson.**

♂ **EMERY.** *German, 'industrious'.* Has potential . . . for girls; consider Amory instead. **International: Amery, Emmerich, Emmo, Emory** *(German)*, **Imre** *(Hungarian)*, **Imrich** *(Czech)*.

EMIL. *Latin, 'industrious'; Teutonic, 'energetic'.* Unlike top girls' name Emily, Emil has a slightly unfriendly feel. **Aimil, Aymil, Emelen, Emilianus, Emilion, Emilyan, Emlen, Emlin, Emlyn, Emlynn. International: Emile** *(French)*, **Emilano, Emilio** *(Spanish)*, **Emelinho, Emilinho** *(Portuguese)*, **Emeli** *(Finnish)*, **Emilian** *(Slavic)*.

EMILIO. *Spanish and Italian variation of* **EMIL.** Dashing and popular Italian and Spanish favourite, as is Emiliano. **Aemilio, Emelio, Emielo, Emileo, Emiliano, Hemilio, Imelio, Llillo, Melo, Milo, Miyo.**

♂ **EMLYN.** *Welsh, from Latin, 'charming, flattering' or 'rival'.* Gentle and poetic and often heard in Wales, but in danger of being perceived as feminine elsewhere. **Emlin.**

EMMANUEL. *Hebrew, 'God is with us'.* Popular with early Jewish immigrants, until overused nickname Manny caused it to fade. Now, this important biblical name is being revived in its full glory. **Eman, Emanual, Emmanual, Emmonual, Emonuel, Imanuel, Immanuele, Mannie, Manny. International: Emanuel, Immanuel** *(French)*, **Emanuele** *(Italian)*, **Mano, Manolete, Manolito, Manolo, Manuel, Manuelo** *(Spanish)*, **Imanol** *(Basque)*, **Manoel** *(Portuguese)*, **Immanuel** *(German)*, **Emanuel** *(Scandinavian)*.

★**EMMET, EMMETT.** *Hebrew, 'truth'; Anglo-Saxon, 'industrious'.* Honest and sincere, laid-back and creative, Emmett is on the rise as a male cognate of the megapopular Emma and Emily. **Emmett, Emmit, Emmitt.**

EMO. *Modern invented name.* If you're not finding Nemo unusual enough, consider the even more eccentric Emo.

EMORY. *See* **EMERY.**

♂ **EMRYS.** *(EM-rees) Welsh, variation of* **AMBROSE**. If you're looking for a Welsh name less common than Dylan, Griffin, Evan or Morgan, you might want to consider this offbeat epithet of the wise wizard Merlin.

ENDICOTT. *English, 'beyond the cottage'.* Upstanding surname name.

ENDYMION. *Greek mythology name.* The name of a mythically handsome youth, but a modern boy could have trouble with this mouthful. **Endimion.**

ENGELBERT. *German, 'bright angel'.* Only for Humperdinks. **Bert, Berty, Ingelbert, Inglebert.**

♂ **ENNIS.** *Irish, 'from the island'.* A variation that doesn't compare with the appealing Scottish original, Angus (though the Heath Ledger character in *Brokeback Mountain* might give it some impetus). **Ennys, Enys.**

ENOCH. *Hebrew, 'dedicated'.* The biblical name of the eldest son of Cain is not one that would have much appeal to the modern ear. **International: Enok** (*Danish*).

ENOS. *Hebrew, 'mankind'.* Don't saddle your son with a name that rhymes with a male body part.

ENRICO. *Italian variation of* **HENRY**. One of several Latin names starting with *E* that would work and play well with others in any family. **Erico, Errico, Rico.**

ENRIQUE. *Spanish variation of* **HENRY**. Scoring high in Hispanic communities, this is an appealing name that could cross ethnic borders and move even higher. **Amrique, Enrigque, Enrigue, Enriques, Enriquillo, Enrrique, Henrico, Henriko, Iniriques, Kiko, Quique.**

★**ENZO.** *Italian variation of* **HENRY**, *also diminutive of* **VINCENZO** *and* **LORENZO**. Like Leonardo and Giacomo, one of the confident and captivating Italian names beginning to be used by parents of all ethnic backgrounds, including Patricia Arquette. **Enzio.**

EÓIN. *(O-en) Irish variation of* **OWEN**. Popular in Ireland, as is the similarly difficult spelling **EOGHAN**, but elsewhere, most would stick with Owen. **Owen.**

EÓNAN *(YOH-nuhn) Irish, 'little Adam'.* Same problem as Eóin – squared.

★**EPHRAIM.** *Hebrew, 'fruitful, fertile, productive'.* We would put this Old Testament name of Joseph's son high on the list of neglected biblical possibilities – solid but not solemn. **Efraim, Efrayim, Efren, Efrim, Efrym, Ephraem, Ephream, Ephrim, Ephrym. International: Efrain** (*Spanish*), **Efram, Efrem, Ephrem, Yefrem** (*Russian*), **Evron** (*Yiddish*).

ERASMUS. *Greek, 'beloved, desired'.* Bearded and bespectacled name of the Dutch philosopher that the audacious may dare to dust off. **Erazmus, Ras, Rastus. International: Érasme** (*French*), **Erasmo, Erasmun, Erazino, Eresmo, Erusmo, Isasmo, Ras, Rasmus** (*Spanish*).

ERIC. *Old Norse, 'eternal ruler'.* The all-time most popular

Scandinavian boys' name in the 1980s period and is now falling out of favour. **Aaric, Aeric, Aerick, Aerric, Aerrick, Aerricko, Aric, Arick, Arik, Arreck, Arric, Arrick, Audrick, Aurick, Erek, Erick, Eriq, Erique, Erric, Errick, Errik, Eryck, Rick, Ricky, Rikky. International: Éric** *(French),* **Erico** *(Italian and Spanish),* **Erich** *(German, Czech),* **Erik** *(Scandinavian),* **Eirik** *(Norwegian),* **Erkki, Eero** *(Finnish),* **Eryk** *(Polish),* **Eriks** *(Latvian, Russian).*

♂ **ERIE.** *American place name.* The kids at school will find this name eerie.

ERNEST. *English from German, 'serious, resolute'.* Too earnest. **Earnest, Ern, Ernie, Erny. International: Earnan** *(Irish),* **Arnesto, Ernestino, Ernesto, Ernio, Necho** *(Spanish, Italian, Portuguese),* **Ernst** *(German, Norwegian, Swedish),* **Estek** *(Polish),* **Erneszt, Ernö,** *(Hungarian).*

ERNESTO. *Spanish and Italian variation of* **ERNEST.** A Latin classic, widely used here and abroad.

ERNST. *German variation of* **ERNEST.** Concise and clipped continental version of the earnest Ernest.

EROS. *Greek, mythology god of love.* Too hot to handle.

♂ **ERROL.** *Scottish, spelling variation of* **EARL.** A swashbuckling name in the Errol Flynn era, still has a trace of jazz cool. **Erroll, Erryl, Erryle, Eryle, Rollo.**

ERSKINE. *Scottish, 'from the high cliffs'.* Rarely used un-Gaelic-sounding Scottish name.

ERVIN. *Scottish variation of* **IRVING.** *See* **IRVING. Erv, Ervyn.**

ERVING. *Variation of* **IRVING.** *See* **IRVING.**

ERWIN. *German, 'respected friend'; also variation of* **IRVING.** You can dress Irwin up, but you can't make him pretty. **Earwin, Earwine, Earwyn, Erwyn. International: Ervin** *(Hungarian).*

ERYX. *Greek mythology name.* This name of the mythic son of

Aphrodite and Poseidon sounds like a sci-fi Eric.

ESAI. *(EE-sye* or *ee-SAY) Spanish from Hebrew, 'wealthy' or 'gift'.* Hebrew-Latin name bristling with electricity that could cross cultural barriers.

ESAU. *Hebrew, 'hairy'.* The name of Jacob's twin brother in the Bible makes an ideal twin choice. **Esav.**

ESMOND. *English, 'graceful protection'.* Haughtier and less accessible than cousin Edmond.

ESSEX. *English place name and surname.* Sex doesn't belong in a baby name.

ESTEBAN. *Spanish variation of* **STEPHEN.** One of several Latino favourites rising in popularity – both solid and strong. **International: Astevan, Estabán, Esteben, Estefan, Estefon, Estiban, Estifan, Estován, Istevan, Teb** *(Spanish),* **Estebe** *(Basque),* **Estevao** *(Portuguese),* **István** *(Hungarian).*

♂ **ESTES.** *Latin surname, 'from a famous ruling house'.* For some, a name more suitable for a girl – although Esther would make a more interesting choice for a daughter. Best to avoid.

ETAN. *Hebrew, 'strong, firm'.* See *ETHAN.*

★ETHAN. *Hebrew, 'strong, firm'.* The name of the Tom Cruise character in the *Mission Impossible* series is a popluar name in this country, where it's in the Top 25 – and it's poised to move up even higher. The biblical Ethan is at once classic and fashionable, serious and cheery, strong and sensitive. What more could a parent want? **Eathan, Eathen, Eathon, Eethan, Ethawn, Ethen, Ethian, Ethon.** International: **Aitan, Eitan, Etan** *(Hebrew).*

ETHELBERT. *English, 'highborn, shining'.* Ethel plus Bert equals ungainly plus obsolete.

ÉTIENNE. *(AY-tee-en) French variation of* **STEPHEN.** Appealingly gentle and romantic.

ETTORE. *Italian variation of*

HECTOR. Has a lot more charm than the ancient Hector.

EUAN. *(YOO-un) Scottish, 'youth'.* See *EWAN.*

EUGENE. *Greek, 'wellborn, noble'.* To quote the American comedian Jim Carrey, whose middle name this is, 'You can never get too cool with a name like Eugene'. **Gene, Gino.** International: **Eugène** *(French),* **Eugenio** *(Spanish, Italian),* **Eugenius** *(Dutch),* **Eugen** *(German),* **Eugen** *(Swedish),* **Eugeniusz** *(Polish),* **Jenö** *(Hungarian),* **Evzen,** *(Czech),* **Evgeni, Yevgeny** *(Russian),* **Yevhen** *(Ukrainian),* **Eugen, Eugenios, Jeno** *(Greek).*

EUGENIO. *Spanish and Italian variation of* **EUGENE.** The name of four popes and several saints: a promising Italian import. **Ahenio, Cheno, Eginio, Euginio, Eujenio, Eujinio, Genio, Geno, Gino, Ugenio.**

EUSTACE. *Greek, 'fruitful, productive'.* A prim and proper choice that sounds more feminine than masculine – not one for the boys. **Eustis, Stacey,**

If You Like Ethan,
You Might Love . . .

Asher
Caleb
Deacon
Eamon
Eben
Elijah
Emmanuel
Esau
Étienne
Ezio
Ezra
Heath
Keenen
Micah
Nathan

Stacy. International: **Eustache** *(French),* **Eustachio** *(Italian),* **Eustaquio** *(Spanish).*

EUSTON. *Irish, 'heart'.* Houston would be an improvement on this in every way.

391

boys' names

Stellar Starbabies Beginning with *E*

Edgar	Melissa Rivers
Edward	Mel Gibson
Eja	Shania Twain
Elijah	Bono, Wynonna Judd, Donnie Wahlberg
Ellery	Laura Dern & Ben Harper
Elliot	Robert De Niro
Enzo	Patricia Arquette
Ethan	Edward Furlong
Euan	Tony Blair & Cherie Blair
Evan	Jenny McCarthy, Bruce Springsteen
Ezekiel	Beau Bridges

♂ **EVAN.** *Welsh variation of* **JOHN.** This Welsh version of John has a mellow nice-guy image that's recently propelled it into the Top 100. **Euan, Euen, Evann, Evans, Even, Evyn, Ewen, Eyvind, Owen. International: Aoibheann** *(Irish Gaelic),* **Eavan, Evin, Ewan** *(Irish).*

EVANDER. *Scottish form of Greek, 'good man'.* Stop at Evan.

♂ **EVELYN.** *English, 'hazelnut'.* Your great-aunt, not your baby boy. **Evelin.**

♂ **EVER.** *Word name.* Its timeless quality would make this word a positive middle name choice.

EVERARD. *English spelling variation of* **EBERHARD.** A character in a 1920s British novel. **Evered, Everhart, Evraud. International: Evrard** *(French),*

Everardo *(Spanish),* **Eberhard, Evert** *(German).*

EVEREST. *Place name, world's tallest mountain.* Lofty.

♂ **EVERETT.** *English variation of* **EBERHARD.** Statesman-like, wintry name that is chosen by hundreds each year. **Evered, Everet, Everhar, Everhard, Everhardo, Everhardt, Everit, Everitt, Evraud, Evret, Evrett, Evrit, Evritt. International: Eberhard** *(German),* **Evert** *(Swedish).*

♂ **EVERLY.** *English, 'wild boar in woodland clearing'.* Evokes 1960s brotherly close harmony. **Everley.**

♂ **EVIAN.** *English variation of* **EVAN.** People might wonder if you were calling your son or ordering a glass of bottled water. **Evyan.**

★**EWAN.** *(YOO-uhn) Scottish variation of* **JOHN.** Appealing Top 100 name, its popularity due to film hunk Ewan McGregor and the trend towards Gaelic names in general. **Euan, Euen, Ewen, Ewyn.**

♂ **EXPLORER.** *Word name.* A bold word name choice for the intrepid baby namer who hopes her son will face the world with a sense of discovery.

EZEKIEL. *Hebrew, 'God strengthens'.* This visionary Old Testament prophet name used to be reduced to its hayseed nickname Zeke, but modern parents now embrace it in full for its power and dignity. **Zeek, Zeke, Ziek.** International: **Ézéchiel** *(French),* **Chaco, Checo, Chequelo, Chequil, Esekial, Esequiel, Esequio, Exechio, Exequiel, Ezechiel, Ezekyel, Ezequiel, Eziechiele, Ezikiel, Ezikyel, Ezykiel, Hesiquio, Hexiquio, Isiwuiel, Isechiel, Quiel** *(Spanish),* **Haskel, Heskel** *(Yiddish).*

EZIO. *(Ā-tzee-o) Greek, 'eagle'.* Operatic Italian option.

★**EZRA.** *Hebrew, 'help'.* Has a lot going for it: the strength of its heroic biblical legacy, its quirky sound and its fresh but familiar feel. **Azariah, Azur, Ezrah, Ezri, Ezurah, Ezyra, Ezyrah.** International: **Esdras** *(French and Spanish),* **Esra** *(German),* **Ezri** *(Israeli),* **Esdra,**
Esdras, Esra, Ezer, Ezzret, Uzair *(Arabic),* **Ezera** *(Hawaiian).*

F *boys*

★**FABIAN.** *Latin clan name, 'bean grower'.* Ancient name of saint and pope best known via a 1960s rocker. Definite cool potential today. **Fabe, Fabeon, Fabion, Faebian, Faebien, Fabyan, Fabyen, Faybian, Faybien, Faybion, Faybionn.** International: **Fabert, Fabien** *(French),* **Fabiano, Fabio** *(Italian),* **Fabián, Fabio** *(Spanish),* **Fabiã** *(Portuguese),* **Faber** *(German),* **Fabek** *(Polish),* **Fabius** *(Latvian, Lithuanian),* **Fabi, Fabiyan** *(Russian).*

♂ **FABLE.** *Word name.* Inventive name for the child of a writer.

♂ **FABRICE.** *French, from Latin, 'skilled craftsman'.* There are plenty of French guys named Fabrice, but elsewhere, it sounds more like a laundry product.

FABRON. *French, 'young blacksmith'.* And this sounds like the synthetic fabric washed with
Fabrice. **Fabre.** International: **Fabbro, Fabroni** *(Italian).*

FACHNAN. *(fahk-nan) Irish, 'malicious'.* This name of four ancient saints is recommended neither for its sound nor its meaning. **Fachtna, Faughnan, Festie, Festus.**

FACTOR. *German and Dutch occupational name, 'agent'.* This name for the steward of an estate sounds too mathematical for most people's taste.

FAGIN. *Irish, 'rustic'.* Forever Dickens's con artist in *Oliver Twist.* **Fagan, Faggan, Feagan, Fegan.**

FAHD. *Arabic, 'panther, leopard'.* Popular name in the Arab world, currently tied to Saudi king Fahd bin Abdulaziz. **Fahad.**

FAIRBAIRN. *Scottish, 'fair-haired child'.* For blonds with ties to Scotland – in theory, anyway.

FAIRBANKS. *English, 'bank along the pathway'.* Place name with a Little Lord Fauntleroy feel.

FAIRCHILD. *English, 'fair-haired child'.* Only if it's a family name and even then, better in the middle. **Fairechild.**

FAIRFAX. *English, 'blond'.* Snotty little rich boy.

FAISAL. *Arabic, 'resolute'.* Another Saudi Arabian royal name. **Faissal, Faysal, Faysl.**

♂ **FALCON.** *English from French, nature name.* There is a whole new species of bird names open to the baby namer, from the light and feminine Lark to the sleek and powerful Falcon. **Falconer, Falconieri.**

FALKNER. *Occupational name, 'falcon trainer'.* Member of a newly chic name genre. Bonus: its relationship to author William Faulkner. **Falconer, Falconner, Falk, Faulconer, Faulconner, Faulkner, Fowler.**

♂ **FALLON.** *Irish, 'leader'.* One of the first of the unisex surname names, but thanks to *Dynasty* in the 1980s it now has a feminine image. **Faolan, Felan, Phelan.**

FANE. *English, 'happy, joyous'.* Used as a nickname in the Middle Ages for someone with a cheerful disposition, this is one of the more offbeat members of the Zane-Kane family. **Fain, Faine, Fayne.**

FARGO. *Place name.* Though we haven't heard of any babies named for this frigid American North Dakota city, it's certainly on the map of possibilities.

FARLEY. *English, 'sheep meadow'.* It could be a gentler alternative to Harley. **Fairlay, Fairlee, Fairleigh, Fairlie, Fanley, Farlay, Farlee, Farleigh, Farlie, Farly, Farrleigh, Lee, Leigh.**

FARMER. *Occupational name, 'farmer'.* Though it fits into a fashionable work-related genre, this one might prove too earthy.

FARO. *Italian word name, 'lighthouse'; also card game.* Better left in the gambling casino.

♂ **FARON.** *French, 'pharaoh'.* Although Faron was a first-century French saint, most people will assume this is a twist on Darren. **Faran, Faren, Farin, Faro, Farren, Farrin, Farryn, Faryn.**

FAROUK. *Arabic, 'seer of truth'.* Name of the last king of Egypt. **Faroq, Farouq, Faruq, Faruqh.**

FARQUHAR. *(far-kar) Scottish, 'friendly man'.* Has never left the Scottish highlands. **Farquar, Farquarson, Farquharson.**

FARRAR. *English occupational name, 'blacksmith, metal-worker'.* Recommended only if it's a family name and then better in the middle position. **Fairer, Farrier, Farrior, Ferrar, Ferrars, Ferrer, Ferrier.**

♂ **FARRELL.** *Irish, 'courageous'.* More modern and more attractive than Darrell. **Farrel, Farrill, Farry, Farryll, Ferrel, Ferrell, Ferrill, Ferryl.**

FAUST. *Latin, 'fortunate one'.* Because the legendary Faust sold his soul to the devil, few parents would choose this for a child, although Fausto is commonly heard in Italy and Spain. **Faustus. International: Fausto** *(Italian, Spanish and Portuguese),* **Faustano, Fausteno,**

Faustín, Faustino, Fausto, Faustulo, Fauztino, Festo *(Spanish)*.

♂ **FAVOURITE.** *Word name.* Maybe if you're planning to have only one child – and iffy even then.

FAVRE. *(farv) French occupational name, 'ironworker'.* Surname of a fifteenth-century saint that doesn't translate for a boy of today. **Fabre, Faivre, Faure, Lefeuvre, Lefèvre.**

FAXON. *English, 'hair'.* Could catch on, thanks to Jaxon.

FEDERICO. *Italian and Spanish variation of* **FREDERICK.** Adds Latin dash to the somewhat formal Frederick. **International: Federigo, Rico *(Italian)*, Fede, Federigo, Federío, Fredericio, Fredico, Fredrico, Friderico, Friderico, Lico, Rico *(Spanish)*.**

FEENY. *Irish, 'little raven'.* Feeble, compared with other Irish surnames. **Feeney, Feichín.**

FEIVEL. *Yiddish, 'brilliant one'.* This comes from Faivish, the Yiddish form of Phoebus, the Greek sun god . . . and it's also the little mouse in *An American Tail*. **Faivish, Fayvel, Feiwel.**

FELIPE. *(feh-LEEP-ay) Spanish variation of Philip.* A royal name in Spain, could make a lively alternative to our Philip. **Filip, Filippo, Fillip, Flip, Lippo, Pip, Pippo.**

★**FELIX.** *Latin, 'happy, fortunate'.* Energetic, upbeat name that deserves to transcend associations with the Cat. The name of four popes and sixty-seven saints, it's fashionable in upscale London and highly recommended for adventurous parents elsewhere. **Fee. International: Felic *(Irish)*, Félicien, Félix *(French)*, Felice *(Italian)*, Feliciano *(Italian and Spanish)*, Felex, Felicio, Felixiano, Feliziano *(Spanish)*, Feliz *(Spanish and Portuguese)*, Feel *(Dutch)*, Bodog *(Hungarian)*, Feliks *(Bulgarian, Polish and Russian)*, Felicjan *(Slavic)*.**

♂ **FENNEL.** *Vegetable and herb name.* Cook's choice. **Fenel, Fenell, Fennell.**

FENNO. *A Finnish tribe and language.* Fenno, a name we'd never heard before or since, was the hero of the acclaimed Julia Glass novel, *Three Junes*.

FERDINAND. *German, 'bold voyager'.* Rather heavy and clumsy feel – most likely because of the bull. **Ferd, Ferdie. International: Fernand, Fernandu, Ferrand, Ferrante *(French)*, Ferdinando, Ferrando *(Italian)*, Ferdi, Ferdinando, Ferdino, Ferdo, Fernán, Fernandeo, Fernando, Ferni, Hernando, Nando *(Spanish)*, Fernão *(Portuguese)*, Nándor *(Hungarian)*, Nandru *(Romanian)*, Ferdynand, Ferdynandy *(Slavic)*.**

FERGALL. *Irish, 'man of valor'.* We'd prefer Fergus. **Fearghall, Fergal, Forgael.**

FERGUS. *Scottish and Irish, 'highest choice'.* In Celtic lore, the ideal of manly courage; Fergus is a charming, slightly quirky Scottish favourite. **Fearghas,**

Fearghus, Feargus, Fergie, Ferguson, Fergusson.

FERMIN, FIRMAN. *French from Latin, 'strong'*. The name of the ancient saint, in whose honour the bulls run at Pamplona, has a sound related to Herman and vermin, so can hardly be recommended. **Ferman, Fernin, Firmilien, Firmin, Firminan, Firmus, Fremin, Furman.**

FERNANDO. *Spanish and Portuguese variation of* FERDINAND. Quintessential Latin lover.

FERRIS. *Irish, 'rock'*. Too closely linked with a certain type of wheel to be seriously considered for a child. **Farris, Farrish, Ferrand, Ferriss.**

FESTUS. *Latin, 'joyous, festive'*. Sounds like something a sore does.

FIDEL. *Latin, 'faithful'*. Almost impossible to detach from Castro. **International: Fidèle** *(French)*, **Fidelis** *(Latin)*, **Fedele, Fidelio** *(Italian)* **Fidel, Fidelio** *(Spanish)*.

★♂ **FIELD.** *Nature name*. Simple, evocative and fresh.

FIELDER, FIELDING. *English, 'dweller in open country'*. Might appeal to a lover of open spaces. **Field, Feilding.**

FIERO. *Italian word name, 'proud'*. Fiery sound and uplifting meaning, but it's also a popular dog name. Spelled Fiyero, it's the hero of the book and musical *Wicked*.

♂ **FIFE.** *Scottish word and place name*. Great middle name choice for music lovers or those with Scottish roots. **Fifer, Fyfe, Fyfer, Fyffe, Pfeiffer, Phyfe.**

50 CENT. *Word name*. So far there's only one . . . and this American rap singer was christened Curtis.

FIGUEROA. *Spanish, 'fig tree'*. Spanish surname that almost could work as a first, if it weren't for that problematic *fig* beginning.

FILBERT. *German, 'very brilliant'*. Like Norbert and Hubert, feels terminally dated – in addition to which it's a nut. **Philbert, Philibert. International: Filberte, Filiberto** *(Italian)*, **Filiberto** *(Spanish)*.

FILIP. *Swedish variation of* PHILIP. Streamlined spelling makes the name seem frivolous and flip. The Spanish Filipo has more zip.

FILMORE. *English, 'very famous'*. A little too geeky sounding for a boy. **Fillmore, Fylmer.**

FINBAR. *Irish, 'fair-haired'.* Ancient saints' name well used in Ireland but unusual elsewhere: there are other appealing *Finn*-ish names. **Bar, Barra, Barry, Finbarr, Finnbar, Finnbarr.**

FINCH. *English word name, 'to swindle'; nature name.* A possible bird name option, though it feels a bit pinched.

FINESSE. *English from French, word name.* This will never have enough sparkle to be considered the finest name for a boy – or girl – but it might make it as one of the worse names.

★FINIAN, FINNIAN. *Irish, 'fair'.* A fair jig of a name, energetic and easy on the ear and familiar through the classic West End musical, *Finian's Rainbow.* **Finan, Fineen, Finien, Finn, Finnan, Finnin, Phinean, Phinian.**

♂ FINLAY, FINLEY. *Irish and Scottish, 'fair-haired hero'.* Scottish royal name (it belonged to Macbeth's father) in Scotland's Top 25, also used by several celebrity parents. It could also be given a gender switch

and used to name a daughter. **Findlay, Findley, Finlea, Finlee, Finn, Finnlea, Finnley, Lee, Leigh.**

★♂ FINN. *Irish, 'bright, fair'.* A name with enormous energy and charm, that of the greatest hero of Irish mythology, Finn McCool. It was chosen by cool supermodel Christy Turlington for her son. **Fin, Fingal, Fingall, Fionn.**

FINNEGAN, FINNIGAN. *Irish, 'fair'.* If you like the *Finn* names and love James Joyce, this one will be an extremely winning candidate. **Finegan.**

FIORELLO. *Italian, 'little flower'.* New York mayor La Guardia made this one famous – in fact he was nicknamed 'the Little Flower' – and the airport was named after him. **Fiore.**

FIORENZO. *Italian, masculine variation of* **FLORENCE.** For lovers of that romantic city. **Fio, Renzo.**

♂ FIRE. *Word name.* Even if you're hoping for a fiery child, this seems like playing with fire.

Fitz Names

Fitzgerald
Fitzgill
Fitzhugh
Fitzjames
Fitzjohn
Fitzpatrick
Fitzroy
Fitzsimmons
Fitzwilliam

FISHER. *Occupational name, 'fisherman'.* As a member of two trendy name categories, animal and occupational, this name has been moving up in popularity. **Fish, Fischer, Fisscher, Visscher.**

FISK. *English, 'fisherman'.* Unusual alternative to Fisher with a brisker surname appeal. **Fiske.**

FITZ. *Diminutive of names beginning with this syllable.* Any number of *Fitz* names – Fitzgerald, Fitzpatrick, Fitzroy, Fitzwilliam – have been used as Christian names, in fact Fitzwilliam was the given name of the dashing Mr Darcy in *Pride and Prejudice*.

♂ **FLAME**. *Word name.* Seen too often in masseuse (not masseur) ads. **Flambeau**.

♂ **FLANN**. *Irish, 'ruddy, red-haired'.* Friendly, cheerful Irish name that originated as a nickname for a redhead. Potential problem: reminiscent of the Spanish custard. **Flainn, Flannan, Flannery**.

FLAVIAN. *Latin, 'yellow hair'.* A Latin clan name that may rise again along with other things Roman. **Flavel, Flavius. International: Flavien** *(French),* **Flavio** *(Italian).*

FLEETWOOD. *English, 'woods with a stream'.* For die-hard Fleetwood Mac fans.

FLEMING. *English, 'man from Flanders'.* Alternative to naming him Ian . . . or 007. **Flemming, Flemyng**.

FLETCHER. *Occupational name, 'arrow-maker'.* Common surname with a touch of quirkiness. **Flecher, Fletch**.

FLINT. *Word name.* You won't find a tougher, steelier-sounding name; on the rise along with macho cousins Stone and Steel. **Flynt**.

FLORENT. *(flor-AHN) French from Latin, 'flowering'.* Way too flowery for most boys. **Flor, Florentine. International: Florentin** *(French),* **Fio, Fiorello, Fiorenzo** *(Italian),* **Flores, Florez** *(Spanish),* **Floris** *(Dutch),* **Florek** *(Polish),* **Flavian** *(Greek).*

FLORIAN. *Latin, 'flowering'.* Popular in Germany – he was the patron saint of those in danger from water – this sounds feminine and floral elsewhere. **Florean, Florien, Florrian, Floryan**.

FLOYD. *Welsh, 'grey-haired'.* A popular name from the 1880s to the 1940s that somehow developed an almost comical persona along with a touch of retro jazz cool; it just might appeal to parents with a strong taste for the quirky.

♂ **FLYNN**. *Irish, 'son of the red-haired one'.* Though Finn is a star of this genre, Flynn is still used only quietly, despite its

easygoing, casual cowboy charm. **Flin, Flinn, Flyn**.

FOGARTY. *Irish, 'exiled one'.* The Old Fogey problem.

FOLEY. *Irish, 'plunderer'.* There are many more appealing Irish surnames and certainly more positive meanings. **International: Foghlaidh** *(Gaelic).*

FOLKE. *Scandinavian, 'people's guardian'.* Too folksy. **Fawke, Folker, Fowke, Fulk, Fulke, Fulker, Volker, Vollker. International: Foulques** *(French).*

FONSO. *German, diminutive of* **ALFONSO**. Better to stick with the original. **Fonzie, Fonzo**.

FORBES. *Scottish, 'field'.* It's a business magazine, long led by Malcolm Forbes, with an image of expensive buttoned-down business suits.

FORD. *English, 'dweller at the ford'.* The car association doesn't stand in the way of this being a strong, independent single-syllable name. **Forde, Forden, Fordon**.

♂ **FOREVER.** *Word name.* Still feels more like a sentiment than a name, and rather feminine at that.

★**FORREST.** *English occupational name, 'woodsman'.* It peaked following the success of the film *Forrest Gump* (although not the greatest role model), but it is still an appealingly sylvan, outdoorsy choice, borne well by American actor Whitaker. **Forest, Forester, Forrest, Forrester, Forster, Foster.**

FORT. *French, 'strong'; also a word name.* There was an ancient Saint Fort and this is a modern, original way to convey a powerful meaning, especially in the middle place. **Forte.**

♂ **FORTITUDE.** *Word name.* The kind of virtue name the Puritans favoured, but would not be easy for a modern boy to carry.

♂ **FORTNEY.** *Latin, 'strong one'.* Not quite as feminine as Courtney – but almost. **Fortenay, Forteney, Forteny, Fortny, Fourtney.**

♂ **FORTUNE.** *Latin, 'luck, fate, wealth'.* Middle name choice designed to generate good luck and prosperity. **Fortunat, Fortunate, Fortuny.** International: **Fortun** *(French),* **Fortunato** *(Italian),* **Fortunado, Fortunato, Fortuno, Tino, Tuno** *(Spanish).*

♂ **FOSTER.** *Occupational name, 'forester'.* This commonly heard last name makes a fine first.

★ ♂ **FOX.** *Animal name.* One animal name that is backed by a longish tradition. Although it is simple and sleek, it can also come across as a little bit wild. **Foxe, Foxen.**

FRANCHOT. *(fron-show) French variation of* **FRANÇOIS.** Old-time film actor Franchot Tone (born Stanislas – Franchot was his mother's maiden name) earned this name its own place in the book. An interesting, provocative choice.

FRANCIS. *Latin, 'Frenchman' or 'free man'.* Famous saints' name pretty much confined to Irish and Italian Catholics (e.g., Francis Albert Sinatra) for decades and still has a starchy feel; likely to stay out of style

due to similarity to the female Frances. **Feri, Fran, France, Frank, Frankie, Franko, Franky, Frann, Frannie.** International: **Proinsias** *(Irish),* **Franchot, François** *(French),* **Francesco, Franco** *(Italian),* **Chicho, Chico, Chilo, Chito, Cisco, Curito, Curro, Farruco, Francilo, Francisco, Frasco, Frascuelo, Paco, Pacorra, Panchito, Pancho, Paquito, Quito** *(Spanish),* **Franciscus** *(Dutch),* **Franken, Frantz, Franz, Franzen, Franzl** *(German),* **Frans, Fransen** *(Scandinavian),* **Frantz** *(Danish),* **Frans** *((Finnish),* **Franio, Franus** *(Polish),* **Ferenc, Ferke, Ferko** *(Hungarian),* **Franc, Franciszk** *(Slavic).*

FRANÇOIS. *(frahn-SWAH) French, 'from France'.* The ultimate sophisticated French name.

FRANK. *Diminutive of* **FRANCIS** *or* **FRANKLIN.** A popular name from the 1880s until the 1920s, Frank has fallen from favour but still has a certain warm, friendly grandpa flavour that could come back into style, like such choices as Jake and Jack. **Franc, Franck, Francke, Frankie.** International:

Franco *(Spanish, Italian)*, **Franz** *(German)*, **Franc** *(Slavic)*.

FRANKLIN. *English, 'free landholder'.* While Frank has a chance at a comeback, Franklin is stuck back in time. **Francklin, Francklyn, Frank, Franklinn, Franklyn, Franklynn.**

♂ **FRASER.** *Scottish from French, 'strawberry'.* TV's *Frasier* made the name famous and Frazier is a well-used variation, but Fraser is the original, used mostly in Scotland. **Frasier, Frazer, Frazier.**

FREDDIE. *Diminutive of* FREDERICK. This shorter, fresher version of the original has been surging up the charts, recently entering the Top 100.

FREDERICK. *German, 'peaceful ruler'.* This is one strong classic chosen by enough parents for the name to recently enter the Top 100. **Fred, Fredd, Freddie, Freddy, Frederic, Frederich, Fredric, Fredrick, Fredricksen, Fredrickson, Fredrik, Fredriksen, Fredrikson, Frido, Fridrick, Ric, Rich, Rickey, Ricky, Rik, Rikki, Rikky. International:** *Frédéric (French),* **Federico, Federigo, Rico** *(Italian and Spanish),* **Frederico** *(Portuguese),* **Frederik, Freek, Frerik, Frits** *(Dutch),* **Fredi, Freidrich, Friedel, Fritz, Fritzchen** *(German),* **Frederik** *(Danish),* **Fredrik** *(Swedish),* **Rieti** *(Finnish),* **Fryderyk** *(Polish),* **Frides, Frigyes, Fritzi** *(Hungarian),* **Bedrich, Fridrich** *(Czech),* **Fredek** *(Eastern European).*

♂ **FREE.** *Word name.* Barbara Hershey and David Carradine gave this name to their son ... who later changed it to Tom.

♂ **FREEDOM.** *Word name.* Like Justice and Peace, this word name makes a very strong statement.

FREEMAN. *Word name.* Another meaningful word name that actually dates back to pre-Emancipation days. **Free, Freedman, Freeland, Freemon, Fried, Friedman.**

FREY. *Scandinavian, 'lord, exalted one'.* Frey is the Norse fertility god, a worthy namesake – though the child might not want to find himself in the thick of the fray.

FRIEDRICH. *German variation of* FREDERICK. One of the most familiar German names, with an uptight Prussian image.

FRIEND. *Word name.* Sociable middle name choice with a Quaker feel.

FRISCO. *Diminutive of* FRANCISCO. Frisky, roguish semi-place name (San Francisco natives never call it that) that might prove to be a bit flimsy.

FRITZ. *German, diminutive of* **FREDERICK.** Still firmly in its liederhosen. **Frits.**

FRODI. *(fro-dee) Norse, 'wise, learned'.* Name of a legendary Danish king who proclaimed universal peace – sounds a bit gnomish here.

FRODO. *Literary name.* Hero of *Lord of the Rings,* better suited to a spaniel than a son.

★♂ **FROST.** *Word name.* A name parents are beginning to warm to; appreciated for its icy simplicity and connection with the venerable poet Robert.

FUENTES. *Spanish, 'springs'.* Common Spanish surname with a lively sound and meaning and literary connection to prominent Latin American writer Carlos Fuentes.

FUJI. *Japanese, 'dweller near the river where wisteria grows'.* To honour the majestic mountain. **Fujikawa, Fujimoto.**

FULBRIGHT. *German, 'bright, famous people'.* No guarantee of a fellowship. **Folbright, Fulbert, Philbert, Philibert, Phillbert.**

FULTON. *English, 'fields of the village'.* One of the surname names used more in the last century, à la Milton and Morton.

♂ **FUTURE.** *Word name.* A forward-looking word name.

FYODOR. *Russian variation of* **THEODORE.** This variation of Theodore is familiar mostly via author Dostoyevsky. **Faydor, Fedor, Feodor, Fyodor, Fyodr.**

G *boys*

♂ **GABI.** *Contemporary variation of* **GABRIEL.** Commonly used in Israel, might tend to sound feminine here.

♂ **GABLE.** *French, 'triangular feature in architecture'.* Gone With the Wind star Clark's surname makes a strong and unusual possibility.

GÁBOR. *Hungarian variation of* **GABRIEL.** Particularly popular in its native land, but elsewhere just getting over Zsa Zsa and her sisters. **Gabi.**

★**GABRIEL.** *Hebrew, 'God is my strength'.* The name of the archangel who heralded the news of Jesus' birth, appearing in Christian, Jewish and Muslim texts, is becoming a biblical favourite; a friendly and appealing alternative to Michael, that other archangel, it's recently entered the Top 100. **Gab, Gabbie, Gabby, Gabbi, Gabe, Gabel, Gabell, Gabi, Gabie, Gabryel, Gaby, Gay. International: Gabriele, Gabrielli, Gabriello** *(Italian),* **Gabian, Gabiel, Gabirel, Gabrial, Riel** *(Spanish),* **Gabirel** *(Basque),* **Gabrielo** *(Portuguese),* **Kappo** *(Finnish),* **Gábor, Gabi** *(Hungarian),* **Gabko, Gabo, Gabris, Gabys** *(Czech),* **Gavrel, Gavril** *(Russian),* **Gaby** *(Israeli),* **Gavirel, Gavriel, Gavril, Jibril** *(Arabic).*

GADIEL. *Hebrew, Arabic, 'God is my fortune'.* Unusual, but possibly confusing, substitute for Gabriel. **Gad, Gaddi, Gadi.**

↑♂ **GAEL.** *(ga-EL) Welsh, 'wild'.* This cross-cultural name, found in Wales, Brittany and Spain, could work in the middle, especially as Gail is no longer active for girls.

GAETANO. *(guy-TAH-no) Italian, 'from the city of Gaeta'.* The progenitor of the English name Guy, Gaetano has a lot more gusto. **Gaetan, Geitano, Guy, Guytano.**

♂ **GAGE.** *French, 'oath, pledge'.* Part of the current craze for one-syllable surnames, Gage is becoming a trendy name in some places, with associations to tasty green gage plums and the mathematical gauge. **Gadge.**

GAHAN. *Hebrew, 'the Lord is gracious'.* Rare Scottish variant of John, with multicultural overtones. **Gehan.**

GAHIJI. *African, 'the hunter'.* A name that originated in Rwanda, rhythmically evocative.

GAIUS. *(GUY-us) Latin, 'to rejoice'.* Ancient Latin names are beginning to form a minitrend – Marcellus, Aurelius, Augustus, Atticus, Magnus, Darius – and this would certainly fit into that category. **Cai, Caio, Guy, Kay, Kaye, Keyes, Keys.**

♂ **GALEN.** *Greek, 'calm, healer'.* The name of the second-century physician who formed the basis of early medicine still projects a scholarly, if somewhat feminine, image. **Gaelan, Gaelen, Gaillen, Galan, Galand,** Gale, Galin, Galon, Galyn, Gaylen, Gaylin, Gaylinn, Gaylon, Jalen, Jalin, Jalon, Jaylen, Jaylon. International: **Galyn** *(Gaelic)*, **Galeno, Galieno, Gallieno** *(Spanish)*, **Galenus** *(Greek)*.

GALIL. *Hebrew, 'rolling hills, cylinder'.* Refers to the hilly region of Galilee, an easily assimilated Israeli name. **Glili.**

GALILEO. *Italian, 'from Galilee'.* The name of the great Renaissance astronomer and mathematician would make a distinctive hero-middle-name for the son of parents involved in those fields.

GALLAGHER. *Irish, 'descendant of foreign helper'.* Gallagher is, like so many of its genre, friendly, open and optimistic.

GALLIO. *Hebrew, 'milky'.* One of the few biblical names ending in the upbeat *o*.

GALLOWAY. *Scottish, 'stranger'.* A contradiction: cheerful and light, yet somewhat heavy, perhaps due to the *gallows* element. **Galway.**

GALO. *Spanish from Latin, 'from Gaul'.* Hispanic name of two saints. **Gallo.**

GALT. *Norse, 'high ground'.* A bit abrupt, as in 'Halt!' **Galtero, Galton.**

GALTON. *English, 'a rented estate'.* A fresher alternative to Dalton. **Galt, Galten, Galton.**

GALVIN. *Irish, 'a sparrow'.* Better than Alvin, worse than Gavin. **Gal, Galvan, Galven.**

♂ **GALWAY.** *place name.* Associated with the poet Galway Kennell, this name of an Irish town, county and bay would make an evocative choice. **Galloway.**

GAMAL. *Arabic, 'camel'; diminutive of Hebrew* **GAMALIEL,** *'God is my reward'.* Near Eastern name with lots of opportunities for variation and improvisation. **Gamali, Gamul, Gemal, Gemali, Gemul, Jamal, Jammal, Jemaal, Jemal.**

GANDOLF. *Teutonic, 'the progress of the wolf'.* Randolph is out of favour and Gandolf – the name of the wizard in *Lord of the Rings* – is out of the question. **Gandolph.**

♂ **GANDY.** *Irish surname.* A dandy, bouncy family name with tap shoes, high hat and cane.

GANESH. *Sanskrit, 'god of the multitude'.* The name of the elephant-headed Hindu god of wisdom is rarely heard outside India.

♂ **GANNET.** *German, 'goose'.* A bird name that could be thought of as an animated spin on Garrett.

♂ **GANNON.** *Irish, 'fair-skinned, fair-haired'.* The name of a historic Irish leader, Gannon has a solid, yet spirited feel. **Gan, Ganen, Ganin, Gannen, Gannie, Gannin, Ganny, Ganon.**

♂ **GARCIA.** *Spanish and Portuguese surname, 'fox'.* A possible hero name inspired by notables from Spanish poet/playwright Federico García Lorca to writer Gabriel García Márquez to the Grateful Dead's Jerry Garcia. **Garcisa.**

★ ♂ **GARDENER, GARDNER.** *English, 'keeper of the garden'.* Surely one of the most pleasant and evocative of the occupational options. **Gardenner, Gardie, Gardiner, Gardnar, Gardnard, Gardner.**

★ **GARETH.** *Welsh, 'gentle'.* This name of a modest and brave knight in King Arthur's court makes a sensitive, gently appealing choice. **Gar, Garith, Garreth, Garrith, Garry, Garth, Gary, Garyth.** International: **Geraint, Gerens** (*Cornish*), **Geronte** (*French*).

GARFIELD. *English, 'triangular field'.* Good enough for an American president.

♂ **GARIAN.** *African place name.* This town in northern Libya could find a spot on the name map.

GARNER. *Latin, 'granary'.* Uncommon word and surname with some prospect of garnering popularity.

GARRET, GARRETT. *Irish variation of* **GERARD.** After being one of the hot upscale surnames of the 1990s, Garrett is dropping in popularity. **Gan, Ganen, Ganin, Gannen, Gannie, Gannin, Ganny, Ganon, Gareth, Garrard, Garreth, Garretson, Garrit, Garrith, Garritt, Garrot, Garrott, Gary, Garyth, Gerity, Gerrit, Gerritt, Jared, Jarod, Jarrot, Jarrott.** International: **Gearoid, Gioroid** *(Irish),* **Gerlad** *(Scottish).*

GARRICK. *Teutonic, 'mighty warrior'.* A rarely used last-name-first-name, never as popular as cousins Garrett or Derek. **Garek, Garick, Garik, Garreck, Garrek, Garrik, Garry, Garryck, Garryk, Gary, Gerek, Gerick, Gerreck, Gerrick, Gerrek, Gerrik, Rick.**

GARRISON. *English, 'son of Garret'.* As Harrison is to Harry, Garrison is to Gary: both of the longer versions sound more modern and appealing. **Gair, Gare, Gari, Garri, Garrie, Garry, Gary.**

GARSON. *French, 'to protect'.* The next Carson? **Garrison.**

GARTH. *Norse, 'groundskeeper, enclosure'.* A name that took on a pronounced country twang via Nashville megastar Garth (born Troyal) Brooks.

GARVAN. *Irish, 'rough little one'.* So much like so many other names, it fails to be itself. **Garbhan, Garv, Garvey, Garvie, Garvy.**

GARY. *English, 'spearman'.* When Gary reached its peak in the 1950s, it was one of the first nonclassic boys' names to do so, largely due to Gary (born Frank) Cooper, who was renamed after Gary, Indiana, his agent's hometown in the US. Now, a half century later, Gary has lost its glitter. **Garey, Gari, Garrie, Garry.**

GASPAR. *Spanish variation of* **CASPER.** The name of one of the Three Wise Men from the East is heard in several continental countries, but rarely elsewhere. **Caspar, Casper, Gasper, Gazpar, Kaspar, Kasper.** International: **Gaspard** *(French),* **Gaspare** *(Italian),* **Gáspár, Gazsi** *(Hungarian).*

GASTON. *French from German, 'the foreigner, the guest'.* Took on an off-putting air via the vain antihero of Disney's *Beauty and the Beast.*

GAUTHIER. *(GO-tee-ay) French variation of* **WALTER.** Fresh, exotic way to honour an ancestral Walter.

GAVI. *Diminutive of* **GABRIEL.** Energetic nickname name.

GAVIN. *Celtic, 'little hawk'.* A Scottish-Welsh name that could stand in for the overused Kevin. **Galvin, Galvyn, Gauvin, Gavan, Gaven, Gavinn, Gavon, Gavvin, Gavyn, Gavynn, Gawain, Gawaine, Gawayn, Gawayne, Gawen, Gawin, Gawyn, Gowen, Gowin.** International: **Gabhan** *(Gaelic),* **Gavino** *(Italian).*

GAVRIEL. *Hebrew, 'God is my strength'.* An Israeli place name as well as being the Hebrew form of Gabriel. **Gabriel, Gavri, Gvaram, Gvarel.**

GAVRIIL, GAVRIL. *(Gav-REEL) Russian variation of* **GABRIEL.** *See* **GABRIEL.** **Ganya, Gavrya.**

GAWAIN. *Welsh, 'May hawk'.* This name of the courteous Knight of the Round Table, the nephew of King Arthur, has long been superseded by its

Scottish form, Gavin. **Gavain, Gavin, Gawain.**

GAY. *French, 'joyful'; diminutive of* **GAETANO.** Don't even think about it.

GAYLORD. *French, 'brisk, high-spirited'. Still* don't think about it – the 'lord' appendage is not a big improvement.

GEDALIAH. *Hebrew, 'made great by Jehovah'.* Long white-bearded image. **Gedalia, Gedaliahu, Gedalya, Gedalyahu.**

♂ **GEMINI.** *Latin, 'twins'.* Might make a boy wonder what happened to his other half.

♂ **GENE.** *Diminutive of* **EUGENE.** Like Ray, a formerly funky nickname name that is newly cool; used for rocker Liam Gallagher's son.

♂ **GENET.** *(zhen-ay) African, 'eden'; French surname.* Appealing French-sounding African name, but also with associations to sometimes scandalous French novelist/dramatist Jean Genet.

GENNARO. *Italian, 'January'.* This name of the patron saint of Naples would make an apt choice for a New Year's baby, or one with Neapolitan roots. **International: Génaro** *(Spanish).*

♂ **GENTRY.** *English, 'aristocracy, the most powerful members of society'.* A distinctive surname that, despite its meaning, has a cowboy swagger, à la Autry.

GEOFFREY. *Anglo-Saxon from French, 'pledge of peace'.* Tonier Anglophile spelling can't make this dad name fit for modern babies. **Geoff, Jeff, Jeffrey, Jeffry, Joffrey. International: Séafra, Siofrai, Siothrán** *(Irish Gaelic),* **Sieffre** *(Welsh),* **Geoffroi** *(French),* **Jaffrez** *(Breton),* **Goffredo** *(Italian),* **Godofredo** *(Spanish, Portuguese).*

★ ♂ **GEORGE.** *Greek, 'farmer'.* Iconoclasts though we may be, we like Fred, we like Frank and we like George, which was a popular name in 1830, it is currently holding steady in the Top 25. Solid, strong, royal, and saintly, yet friendly and unpretentious, we think that –

no matter what your politics – it's in prime position to retain its popularity. **Georgie.**

GEORGI, GEORGII. *Russian variation of* **GEORGE.** The double *i* makes it ultradistinctive and less a generic Georgie. **Egor, Gorya, Gosha, Gunya, Jura, Yura, Yuri, Yurik, Zhora, Zhorz, Zhura.**

GERALD. *English and Irish from German, 'ruler with the spear'.* We've all known dozens of Jerrys and though they're perfectly nice middle-aged guys, we probably won't be naming our babies after them. **Gerard, Gerold, Gerrald, Gerrell, Gerritt, Gerry, Jaryl, Jerold, Jerrald, Jerrold, Jerry. International: Gearald, Gearóidin** *(Irish Gaelic),* **Gearoid** *(Irish),* **Gérald, Géralde, Géaud, Giraud, Girauld** *(French),* **Geraldo** *(Italian and Spanish),* **Girlado** *(Italian),* **Herrado, Jeraldo** *(Spanish),* **Gerrit** *(Dutch),* **Gerhard, Gerhart** *(German),* **Jarel, Jarell** *(Scandinavian),* **Gerek** *(Polish),* **Gellart, Gellert** *(Hungarian),* **Garald, Garold, Garolds** *(Russian).*

George's International Variations

Irish Gaelic	Deorsa, Seoirse, Séoras
Scottish	Geordi, Geordie
French	Georges
Provençal	Joji
Italian	Giorgio
Spanish	Jorge, Jorje, Xorge
Basque	Gorka
Catalan	Jordi
Dutch	Georgius, Joris
German	Jörg, Juergen, Jurgen
Scandinavian	Joran, Joren, Jorg, Jorgen, Jorn, Jory
Swedish	Georg, Goran, Gorin
Finnish	Jorma, Yrjö
Polish	Jerek, Jerzy
Hungarian	György, Gyurgi, Gyuri, Gyurka
Czech	Jiri, Juraz, Jurik, Jurko, Juro
Lithuanian	Jurgis
Russian	Egor, Georgi, Georgii, Gorya, Igoryok, Jurgi, Yura, Yuri, Yurko, Yusha, Zhorka
Estonian	Juri
Greek	Georgios, Giorgis, Giorgos, Iorgas, Iorgos
Hebrew	Yoyi
Arabic	Gevorak
Japanese	Joji
Hawaiian	Keoki, Mahi'ai
Ethiopian	Semer

GERALDO. *(hay-RAHL-doh)*
Spanish variation of **GERALD.**

GERARD. *English and Irish from German, 'spear strength'.* Definitely a grandpa name. **Ged, Gere, Geri, Gerrard, Gerrick, Gerry, Girard, Jerrard, Jerry.** International: **Gérard** *(French)*, **Gerardo** *(Italian)*, **Jerardo** *(Spanish)*, **Gerhard** *(German)*, **Gerik** *(Polish)*, **Gellert** *(Hungarian).*

GERARDO. *(hay-RAHR-doh)* *Spanish variation of* **GERARD.** Widely used in the Latino community.

GERHARD. *(gair-hard)* *German variation of* **GERARD.** There's nothing soft or sensitive about a name ending in *hard*. **Gerd, Gerrit.**

GERIK. *Polish variation of* **EDGAR.** Has possibilities, if only through its kinship with Derek.

GERMAIN. *(zher-MEN) Latin, 'sprout, bud'; French, 'from Germany'.* Saint Germain, the intellectual centre of Paris, lends the name a creative aura. **Germaine, German, Germane,**

Germanicus, Germano, Germanus, Germayn, Germayne, Germin, Jermain, Jermaine, Jermane, Jermayne, Jermaynj.

♂ **GERMAINE, JERMAINE.** *Latin, 'sprout, bud'; French, 'from Germany'.* This French feminine version of Germain was popularised for boys by one of the Jackson Five. **Germain, German, Germane, Germayne, Jermain.**

GERONIMO, JERONIMO. *Native American; Italian variation of* **JEROME.** This name of a renowned Apache leader and mystic would be a difficult choice, since it was used as a rallying cry in so many old western films and by paratroopers jumping out of their planes in World War II.

GERRIT. *Low German variation of* **GERHARD.** The name of several Old Master painters makes an interesting possibility, except for the possible confusion with Garrett.

GERSHOM. *Hebrew, 'stranger, exodus'.* Old Testament name of a son of Moses used by the Puritans and now by Orthodox Jews. **Gersh, Gersham, Gershon, Gerson.**

♀ **GERVAISE.** *French, 'skilled with a spear'.* Unusual saint's name rarely heard outside Roman Catholic rectories; it has an attractive French feel. **Gervase, Gervis, Jarvis, Jervaise, Jervis. International: Gervais** *(French),* **Gervasio** *(Italian, Spanish, Portuguese),* **Gervas** *(German),* **Gervaas** *(Dutch),* **Gerwazy** *(Polish),* **Gervasi** *(Russian).*

GIACOMO. *Italian variation of* **JAMES.** Member of the Giovanni-Gino-Giancarlo-Giacomo gruppo of Italian names beginning to be adopted by parents elsewhere. Singer/creative baby namer Sting chose it for his son.

GIAN. *(Gee-AHN) Italian, diminutive of* **GIOVANNI.** Since it (almost) sounds like John and is the equivalent of John, there's not much advantage to using this spelling. **Gianni.**

GIANCARLO. *Italian combination of* **GIAN** *and* **CARLO.** In Italy, a common melding of two popular names, it could work elsewhere.

GIANNI. *(Gee-AH-nee) Italian, diminutive of* **GIOVANNI.** *See* **GIAN,** as Gianni equals Johnny. **Gian, Giannino.**

♂ **GIBSON.** *English, 'Gilbert's son'.* An undiscovered last-name-first-name, with some appealing nicknames. **Gib, Gibb, Gibbie, Gibby, Gibbson, Gibsen, Gibsyn.**

★**GIDEON.** *Hebrew, 'feller of trees'.* Unjustly neglected Old Testament name, an excellent choice for parents looking to move beyond such overused biblicals as Benjamin and Jacob. **International: Gedeon** *(French),* **Gideone** *(Italian),* **Gedeon, Hedeon** *(Russian),* **Hadeon** *(Ukrainian),* **Gidon** *(Hebrew).*

GIFFORD. *English, 'puffy cheeks'.* Could catch on in tandem with the newfound popularity of Griffin and Griffith. **Giff, Giffard, Gifferd, Gyfford.**

GIL. *Hebrew, 'happiness';* *Spanish and Portuguese variation of* GILES; *diminutive of* GILBERT. Pronounced *zheel*, it's a dashing conquistador; as *gill*, it's the nice and slightly boring guy down the street.

GILBERT. *German, 'shining pledge'.* Considered ultra-debonair in the silent-film era, Gilbert is now eligible for a senior discount ticket at the local cinema – though like Walter and Frank, it could be in for a style revival. **Bert, Gil, Gilburt, Gill, Gilly. International: Gibbon, Gilibeirt (Irish), Gibby, Gilleabart (Scottish), Guilbert (French), Gilberto (Italian, Spanish), Giselbert (German).**

GILBERTO. *(heel-BARE-tō) Spanish variation of* GILBERT. At this point, there are more newborn baby Gilbertos than Gilberts. **Beto, Gelgberto, Geliberto, Gilbero, Gilbirto, Gilio, Gilito, Gilverto, Guilberto, Hilberto, Hillberto, Hilverto, Iberto, Jilberto, Xil.**

GILBY. *Irish, 'blond boy'.* Transformation of the stolid Gilbert into an animated surname name. **Gil, Gilbey, Gillbey, Gillbie, Gillby, Gilley.**

GILEAD. *Hebrew, 'a camel hump'.* Like Bethany and Shiloh, a meaningful biblical place name. **Gilad, Giladi.**

GILES. *(jiles) Greek, 'young goat'.* One of those names that most parents find just too upper class to consider; its meaning has led to occasional use for Capricorn boys. **Gide, Gidie, Gile, Gilean, Gileon, Gilette, Gill, Gillette, Gyle, Gyles, Jiles, Jyles. International: Éigid (Irish Gaelic), Gillie (Scottish Gaelic), Gilles (French), Egidio (Italian), Gil (Spanish), Egidius, (Dutch), Agidius (German), Gillis (Danish), Idzi, Egidiusz (Polish), Egyed (Hungarian).**

♂ **GILI.** *(gee-lee) Hebrew, 'my joy'.* Spirited unisex Hebrew name. **Gil, Gil-Ad, Gilam, Gilon.**

GILLESPIE. *Scottish, 'bishop's servant'.* Sometimes heard as a first name in Scotland, particularly among the Campbell clan. **Gil, Gilley, Gillie, Gilllis.**

♀ **GILMORE.** *Irish and Scottish, 'devoted to the Virgin Mary'.* This has taken on a slightly feminine aspect as it's lately been used as a girl's name. **Gillie, Gillmore, Gillour, Gilmour.**

GINO. *Italian, diminutive of* EUGENIO. Stalwart Italian classic, completely at home in elsewhere.

GIORGIO. *Italian variation of* GEORGE. More enduring than Armani.

GIOVANNI. *(joh-VAHN-nee) Italian variation of* JOHN. Venerable Italian classic that suddenly sounds fresh and cool, is now among a popular boys' name. **Geovanni, Gian, Gianni, Giannino, Gianozzo, Gio, Giovani, Giovannie, Giovanny, Giovanoli, Vannie, Vanny, Vonny.**

★**GIULIANO.** *(jyoo-lee-AH-no) Italian variation of* JULIAN. Less familiar than Giorgio or Giovanni, Giuliano has a lot of captivating Latin charm.

GIULIO. *(JYOO-lee-o) Italian variation of* JULIUS. More manageable than some of the longer Italian appellations, but with less magnetism.

GIUSEPPE. *Italian variation of* **JOSEPH.** Retains some of its old immigrant feel – a remnant of stereotyping. **Beppe, Beppo.**

♂ **GLADE.** *Nature name, 'clearing in a forest'.* Shady, leafy nature-boy name.

♂ **GLASGOW.** *Scottish place name.* An undiscovered place name with an appealing *o*-sound ending.

♂ **GLEN, GLENN.** *Scottish, 'a narrow valley'.* Former cool-boy name now in middle-aged limbo, fresher for girls thanks to Glenn Close. **Glan, Glen, Glin, Glyn, Glynn.**

♂ **GLYN.** *Welsh, 'valley, glen'.* Very popular in Wales; this could make a nice middle name in honour of a Grandpa Glenn. **Glynn, Glynne.**

GODFREY. *Teutonic, 'God's peace'.* Downside: a boy might have difficulty handling a name with *God* as a first syllable. The Italian artist's version Giotto would be more interesting.

Godfry. **International: Gofraidh** *(Irish Gaelic),* **Godefroi** *(French),* **Goffredo, Giotto** *(Italian),* **Godofredo** *(Spanish),* **Godofredo** *(Portuguese and Italian),* **Godfried** *(Dutch),* **Gottfried** *(German),* **Gottfrid** *(Swedish and Hungarian).*

♂ **GOLDEN.** *Word name.* Like Silver, a shimmering metallic colour name, almost too dazzling for an ordinary boy. **Gold, Golding, Goldwin, Goldwyn.**

GOLIATH. *Hebrew, 'exile'.* This Old Testament Philistine giant has always been a pariah to baby namers.

GOMER. *Hebrew, 'to complete'.* Biblical it may be, but not a completely brilliant choice for a baby's name.

GONZALO. *Spanish from German, 'saved from combat'.* Popular among Hispanic parents, it explains the source of the nickname Gonzo. **González, Gonzo, Gonzolito. International: Gonçalvo** *(Portuguese).*

GÖRAN. *Scandinavian variation of* **GEORGE.** *See* **GEORGE. Jüran, Örjan.**

★**GORDON.** *Scottish, 'small wooded dell'.* In this Age of Jordans, both male and female, the neglected Scottish favourite Gordon, with its more distinguished history, could come back; conservative but not stodgy. **Gord, Gordan, Gorden, Gordi, Gordie, Gordin, Gordion,**

Gordius, Gordo, Gordy, Gore, Gorton.

GORE. *English, 'spear', 'wedge-shaped object'.* Surname associated with a recent vice president of the US, but beware of the *gory* connections.

♂ **GOREN.** *Hebrew, 'barn floor, granary'.* Symbolic name given to both boys and girls born on Shavuot, the Feast of the Harvest. **Gorin, Gorren, Gorrin.**

GORKY. *Russian place name and surname.* Perky, quirky literary and artistic name tied to the 'father of Soviet literature' Maxim and influential Armenian-American painter Arshile.

GOWER. *Welsh, 'pure'.* This Old Welsh name associated with blacksmiths has little relevance today.

★♂ **GRADY.** *Irish, 'noble, industrious'.* Following in the footsteps of brother Brady; another lively, ebullient Irish surname name. **Gradey.**

GRAEME. *Scottish variation of* **GRAHAM.** An interesting vowel combination lightens up Graham.

★**GRAHAM.** *English, 'gravelly homestead'.* Well used in England and Scotland since the 1950s, this smooth and sophisticated choice is just beginning to catch on elsewhere. **Ghramm, Graeham, Grahame, Gram, Gramm, Grantham, Granum. International: Graeme** *(Scottish).*

♂ **GRANGER.** *English occupational name, 'worker of the granary'.* If you're seeking a serious, solid last-name-first-name that's not overused, this could be it. **Grainger, Grange.**

♂ **GRANITE.** *Nature name.* There's a whole quarry of rocky names parents are now considering: Slate, Flint, etc., but this one is particularly hard-edged and problematic.

GRANT. *Scottish from French, 'large'.* One-time beach-boy compadre of Glenn, Greg and Gary that originated as a nickname for a tall person, Grant has become a no-nonsense, career-oriented grown-up. **Grantland, Grantley, Grantlen.**

★♂ **GRAY, GREY.** *Colour name, also diminutive of* **GRAYDON.** The limitation of this name is its somberness, but it still could make for a soft and evocative choice, especially in the middle. **Graydon, Graye, Grayson, Greydon, Greyson.**

GRAYDON. *English, 'son of the grey-haired one'.* Preferable to Grayer, but neither would be a good choice. **Grayton Greydon, Greyton.**

GRAYSON. *English, 'the son of the bailiff'.* This Jason-substitute is on the fast track. **Gray, Graydon, Grey, Greydon, Greyson.**

GRAZIANO. *Italian, 'pleasing, beloved, dear'.* Rocky VI, anyone?

GREELEY. *English, 'grey meadow'.* Distinctive option for parents.

♂ **GREEN.** *Colour name.* Middle name possibility for a nature-loving family – Uma Thurman and Ethan

Hawke used it for their son's middle name.

GREGOR. *Greek, diminutive of* **GREGORIOS.** Danger of conjuring up the Kafka character that woke up one day to find himself turned into a cockroach.

GREGORIO. *Italian variation of* **GREGORY.** More dramatic, exotic and energetic spin on Gregory.

GREGORY. *Greek, 'vigilant, a watchman'.* The name of sixteen popes and fifteen saints, gregarious Gregory has slipped sharply over the last decade. **Greg, Gregg, Greggory, Gregori, Gregorie, Gregry.** International: **Greagóir** *(Irish Gaelic),* **Grégoire** *(French),* **Gregorio** *(Italian and Spanish),* **Gregoor** *(Dutch),* **Gredorius, Jörn** *(German),* **Gregos** *(Danish),* **Greger, Gries** *(Swedish),* **Gregor** *(Norwegian),* **Gergo** *(Hungarian),* **Grigor, Grigori, Grigorii, Grisha** *(Russian),* **Gregors** *(Latvian),* **Gregorios** *(Greek).*

GREY. *Colour name. See* **GRAY.** **Greyson.**

★**GRIFFIN.** *Welsh variation of* **GRIFFITH.** One of the newer and most appealing of the two-syllable Celtic surnames (also the name of a mythological creature) and picking up in popularity. **Griff, Griffen, Griffon, Gryffen, Gryffin, Gryffon, Gryphon.**

GRIFFITH. *Welsh, 'strong fighter'.* A classic Welsh name, softer than the Irish Griffin, but its lispy ending makes it a bit more difficult to say – and live with. **Giff, Griffee, Griffeth, Griffey, Griffy, Gryfeth, Gryfith, Gryfudd.**

♂ **GROVE.** *Nature name.* If you find Grover too fusty and furry, this is a much cooler-sounding alternative.

GROVER. *English, 'lives near a grove of trees'.* Forget the furry blue Muppet on *Sesame Street* and consider this name anew. We think it's spunky, a little funky and well worth a second look.

GUIDO. *(GWEE-doe) Italian, 'guide, leader'.* Not likely to top

any 'Most Appealing Italian Names' list.

GUILLAUME. *(gee-YOME) French variation of* **WILLIAM.**

Military Names

Arrow

Bowie

Cannon

Crew

Flint

Garrison

Gunner

Javelin

Jet

Lance

Mace

Major

March

Marine

Marshall

Navy

Rebel

Rocket

Sailor

Scout

Sergeant

An everyday name in France, a charismatic possibility elsewhere.

GUILLERMO. *(ghee-YARE-mo) Spanish variation of* **WILLIAM.** As with Guillaume *(see above),* Liam, Willem and Wilhelm, everyday Williams in their own countries, Guillermo is a captivating possibility here. **Giermo, Gigermo, Gijermo, Gillermo, Gillirmo, Giyermo, Guermillo, Guiermo Guilermón, Guille, Guillelmo, Guillermino, Guillo, Guirmo, Gullermo, Llermo, Memo, Quillermo.**

GULL. *Celtic, 'long-winged swimming birds'.* Suggests the salty, windswept air of the seashore.

GULLIVER. *Irish, 'glutton'.* Obscure Gaelic surname known only through its literary *Travels* until actor Gary Oldman used it for his son, transforming it into a lively option.

GUNNAR, GUNNER. *Scandinavian variation of* **GUNTHER.** A traditional Scandinavian favourite making inroads elsewhere, because or in spite of its macho image, especially with the Gunner spelling. **Guntar, Gunter, Gunther.**

GÜNTER, GUNTHER. *(GOON-ter) German, 'bold warrior'.* Prospective parents tend to respond more to the softer English pronunciation than the harsher German one and even more to the Scandinavian version *(see GUNNAR).* **Gun, Gunn, Gunner, Gunners, Guntar, Gunter, Gunthar, Guntur. International: Guntero** *(Italian),* **Guenther** *(German),* **Gunnar** *(Scandinavian),* **Guenter, Gunder** *(Danish).*

GURI. *Hebrew, 'my lion cub'.* When considering the playground years, might be too close to gory.

GURYON. *Hebrew, 'young lion'.* Hebrew name that is rarely heard outside of Israel, making it a possibly distinctive choice. **Garon, Gorion, Guri, Gurion.**

GUS. *Diminutive of* **AUGUSTUS, ANGUS, GUSTAVE.** Homey grandpa nickname name that's a cutting-edge replacement for Max and Jake. **Gus, Gussie, Gussy.**

GUSTAV. *Teutonic, 'staff of the Goths'.* Grey-bearded name heard primarily in Sweden and Germany. **International: Gustave (French, Polish), Gustavo (Italian), Gustavo, Tabo, Tavo (Spanish), Gustaaf, Gustaff, Staff (Dutch), Gustaof (Danish), Kosti, Kustaa, Kusti, Kyösti (Finnish), Gusztav (Hungarian), Gusti, Gustik, Gusty (Czech), Gustavus (Latvian).**

GUSTAVO. *(goo-STAH-vo) Latinate variation of* **GUSTAV.** Well used in the Latino and Italian communities.

★GUTHRIE. *Scottish, 'windy spot'.* This attractive name has a particularly romantic, windswept aura, with a touch of the cowboy thrown in. **Guthrey, Guthry.**

GUY. *French, 'guide, leader'.* The name of the patron saint of comedians and dancers feels either too upper-class for many parents, or else too everyman for their own little guy. **International: Gui, Vitus (French), Guido (Italian), Guyon, Gye, Veit (Dutch).**

GWILYM. *Welsh variation of* **WILLIAM.** An unusual version of William, helped or hindered by a slight baby-talk feel.

♂ GWYN. *Welsh, 'fair, blessed'.* Although commonly used for boys in Wales, we fear it's far too feminine for use elsewhere. **Guinn, Gwin, Gwynedd, Gwynn, Gwynne.**

GYAN. *(GUY-an) Sanskrit, 'filled with knowledge'.* A traditional name from India combining elements of Guy and Ryan.

H *boys*

HAAKON. *Norse, 'chosen son'.* An ancient name that's been used by the Norwegian royal family; still popular there but not likely to appeal to many British parents. **Haaken, Haakin, Haakon, Hacon, Hagan, Hagen, Hakan, Hako, Hakon.**

HABAKKUK. *Hebrew, 'embrace'.* A minor Old Testament prophet and a (deservedly) even more minor name. **Habacuc, Habbakuk.**

HABIB. *Arabic, 'loved one'.* A North African choice, particularly popular in Tunisia and Syria.

HACKETT. *German occupational name, 'little hewer'.* *Hack* is, unfortunately, both an unappealing word and sound. **Hacket, Hackit, Hackitt.**

HACO. *Celtic and Cornish, 'flame, fire'.* Haco was a mythical Cornish leader who lost his beautiful princess bride by unwittingly promising her to a musician whose songs he admired: a romantic legend to back up a very unusual choice.

♂ HADAR. *Hebrew, 'splendor, ornament, citrus fruit'; also a place name in Israel.* A Hebrew name also used for girls, with many variations to choose from. **Hadaram, Hadarezer, Hadriel, Hadur, Heder.**

HADDEN. *English, 'heathery hill'.* Rarely heard Hayden alternative – though, mark our words, you'll spend your life correcting everyone's pronunciation and spelling. **Haddan, Haddin, Haddon, Haden, Hadon, Hayden.**

♂ HADLEY. *English, 'heather meadow'.* Hemingway readers will recognise this as the name of Papa's first wife (and, eventually, actress Mariel's grandmother). Even without that reference, it's too far in the girls' camp to be viable for boys. **Hadlea, Hadlee, Hadleigh, Hadly, Leigh.**

HADRIAN. *Latin, 'from the Adriatic,' 'dark-haired'.* Most parents would find this old Roman name pretentious compared to the more accessible Adrian, but some history buffs just might want to commemorate the enlightened emperor. **Adrian, Adriano, Adrien, Hadrien.**

HADRIEL. *Hebrew, 'splendour of Jehovah'.* An alternative to the formerly male Ariel, which is now in the grasp of *The Little Mermaid*.

HAGAN. *Irish, 'little fire'.* A little further down the road paved by Aidan and Logan. **Egan.**

HAGRID. *Literary name.* Gentle giant Rubeus Hagrid is the grounds-keeper at Hogwarts in the Harry Potter novels (probably after Hagrid Rubes, the equally kind ancient Greek mythological giant), but that's not the only reason this name could prove a playground liability.

HAIG. *Armenian hero name; also English surname, 'enclosed with hedges'.* This very popular Armenian name represents a grandson of Noah, considered the father of the Armenian nation.

HAIM. *Spelling variation of* **CHAIM.** *See* **CHAIM.** **Hayim, Hayyim.**

HAINES. *German, 'the vined cottage'.* If it's a family name, it could be a decent middle choice, but not worthy as a first name. **Hainey, Hanes, Haney, Haynes.**

HAJI. *Swahili, 'born during the pilgrimage to Mecca'.* A name appropriate for boys born during the hajj, the pilgrimage to Mecca every Muslim is expected to make once in his lifetime.

HAKAN. *Native American, 'fiery'.* Native American choice that could translate easily into mainstream British culture.

HAKEEM. *(ha-KEEM) Arabic, 'judicious'.* Muhammad approved all ninety-nine attributes of Allah as worthy names and this is one of the most popular. **Hakim.**

HAL. *Diminutive of Harold or Henry.* The Jack, Max or Gus of the future?

♂ HALCYON. *Greek, 'kingfisher bird'.* Heaven, Peace, Serenity: parents seem especially attracted to word names that signal paradise, but Halcyon sounds quite feminine and might conjure up the sleeping pill Halcion.

HALDAN. *Scandinavian, 'half Danish'.* If you fit this definition, this might be a clever choice, especially as a middle name. **Haldane, Halden, Halfdan, Halfdane, Halvdan.**

HALDOR. *Norse, 'Thor's stone'.* This, like many Norse and Scandinavian names, remains icebound. **Halldor, Halle.**

★HALE. *English, 'someone who lives in a hollow'.* This name projects a sense of well-being – hale and hearty – and is unusual but accessible, with a clear simple sound and a worthy namesake. It might suit a fisherman's family used to the hearty outdoor sea. **Hal, Hayle.**

♂ HALEY. *English, 'hay meadow'.* This name in all its variations has become too popular for girls to survive as a boys' choice. **Hailey, Haily Halley, Hallie, Hayley.**

HALI. *Greek, 'the sea'.* Like others in this vein, problematic due to the feminine Hailey connection.

HALIAN. *Native American (Zuni), 'youthful'.* A Julian derivative, via Spanish conquistadors, that could be a more unusual yet still reasonable substitute for that current favourite. **Hal.**

HALIFAX. *Place name.* If you want to honour your grandfather Hal but can't work up much enthusiasm for his full name Harold, consider the more stylish (if a bit pretentious) capital of Nova Scotia. **Hal.**

HALL. *English occupational name, 'worker at the hall'.* A simple, self-possessed, somewhat serious surname, which might work better as a middle.

♂ HALLE. *(hah-leh) Norse, diminutive of* **HARALD.** Popular in the Scandinavian countries, but in this country it would surely bring to mind the very feminine Halle Berry.

♂ HALLEY. *Scottish and English, 'hall,' 'woodland clearing'.* While this has a distinguished male namesake – astronomer Edmund Halley and his comet – it still strays far too close to the feminine Hailey family for consideration for a boy.

♂ HALSEY. *English, 'hallowed island'.* Although this was the surname of a rugged World War II admiral, these days it has a feminine feel. **Hallsey, Hallsy, Halse, Halsy.**

HALSTON. *English, 'village near the manor,' 'hallowed stone'.* This choice feels more familiar than other hall-related English surnames, thanks to designer Halston, the single-named disco-era society playmate of Liza and Elton. **Halsten.**

HAM. *Hebrew, 'hot, warm'; diminutive of* **HAMILTON.** Along with Shem and Japheth, a son of Noah with a name that's almost never used – for more obvious reasons than those of his brothers. **Hamm.**

HAMAL. *Arabic, 'lamb'.* Alternative for the popular Jamal. **Amahl, Amal, Hamahl.**

HAMILL. *English, 'scarred'.* Though we usually think a name's image in contemporary culture supersedes its ancient meaning, this is a case where the definition could undermine a child's self-esteem. **Hamel, Hamell, Hammill.**

HAMILTON. *English and Scottish, 'treeless hill'.* Unless it runs in your family, or Alexander Hamilton is your hero, you might consider something less imposing – and without the teasable nickname Ham. **Ham, Hamel, Hamelton, Hamil, Hamill.**

HAMISH. *(HAY-mish) Scottish variation of* **JAMES.** A name that's not unknown here, but still redolent of Scotland. If you're ready to go further than Duncan and Malcolm, way out to Laird and Ewan territory, this may be worth consideration. It also sounds just like the Yiddish word for *homey*.

HAMLET. *Anglicised form of Danish,* **AMLETH.** The 'To Be or Not to Be' jokes, via Shakespeare's tortured prince, will get old by Month Two. **Hammett, Hammond, Hamnet, Hamnett, Hamo, Hanunet.**

HAMLIN. *German, 'little home-lover'.* One you might like for its cozy meaning, but there is that Pied Piper–rat connection. **Hamblin, Hamelin, Hamlen, Hamlyn.**

HAMMETT. *English surname.* A possibility for fans of the mystery writer, but most parents would prefer Dashiell. **Hammet.**

HAMMOND. *English from German, 'mountain home'.* A cross-cultural possibility, but a bit heavy and sombre.

HAMPTON. *English, 'home settlement'.* Names of classy places – Aspen, Paris and yes, Hampton – are in favour with aspiring parents, though they don't always have the intended effect. **Hampden, Hampten.**

HAMZA. *Arabic, 'lion'.* Now even popular in the USA, Hamza was the legendary uncle of the Prophet Muhammad, hero of *The Hamzanama, the Story of Hamza.*

HANAN. *Hebrew, 'graciousness'.* A chief member of the tribe of Benjamin and another obscure Old Testament name that few parents, even those tired of Aaron and Zachary, would consider.

HANCOCK. *English, 'Hans's rooster'; Dutch, 'shellfish-gatherer'.* Surname sure to present playground complications.

HANIF. *Arabic, 'true believer'.* British filmmaker Hanif Kureishi brought this name to the Western world.

HANISH. *Literary name, ' one who forewarns of storms'.* This name from the ancient *Gilgamesh Epic* would be a

challenging choice; Hamish makes a more user-friendly option.

HANK. *Diminutive of* **HENRY.** A mid-century guy nickname of the Al/Frank/Dick school, rarely given on its own, but it does have some earthy cool.

HANNIBAL. *Punic and Assyrian, 'grace of Baal, god of fertility and fortune'.* These days, it's thought of less as the name of the great general and more as the first name of Lecter, the fictional cannibal. Either association is too heavy for a child to bear. **Hanibal.**

HANNO. *German, diminutive of* **JOHANN.** Nicknames ending in *o* are invariably cute, though this one suffers from sounding too much like the popular girls' name Hannah.

HANOCH, HANOKH. *Hebrew, 'vowed, dedicated'.* Variant of Enoch with little appeal.

HANS. *(hons) German, Dutch and Scandinavian, diminutive of* **JOHANNES.** Though familiar to all via such childhood icons as Hans(el) and Gretel and Hans Christian Andersen, few British parents have chosen this name for their sons because of its intractably old-fashioned image. **Hannes, Hanns, Hansel, Hanss, Hanzel.**

HANSON. *Scandinavian, 'son of Hans'.* More familiar and melodic to the British ear than either Hans or Hansen and some might attach it to the three-brother pop-rock band called Hanson. **Hansen, Hanssen, Hansson.**

HARBIN. *German, 'little bright warrior'.* A possible new entry in the Hayden-Corbin two-syllable boys' name club. **Harben.**

♂ **HARBOUR.** *Word name.* If you like names that are not really names – some say, the wave of the future – this one has an attractive sound as well as an appealing meaning and image.

HARDEN. *English, 'valley of the hares'.* While teasing about names is not as bad as it once was, the possibilities presented

by this name would be difficult for any pubescent boy to resist. **Hardin.**

HARDING. *English, 'son of the courageous one'.* A hard name to live with. **Hardinge.**

HARDY. *German, 'bold, brave'.* Spirited and durable un-Germanic German surname and starting to be used elsewhere. **Hardey.**

HARI. *Hindu, 'dark, tawny'.* Familiar via Harry, but much more exotic.

♂ **HARLAN.** *German and English, 'rocky land'.* Pleasant but uninspired surname name somewhat connected to sci-fi writer Harlan Ellison. Might have more edge as a girl's name. **Harland, Harlen, Harlenn, Harlin, Harlon, Harlyn, Harlynn.**

HARLEM. *Place name.* With Brooklyn on the rise, Harlem can't be far behind – it's already been picked by one celebrity and it certainly has a stronger historical and ethnic identity.

London Neighbourhood Names

Barnet

Brixton

Chelsea

Clapton

Docklands

Earlsfield

Fulham

Greenwich

Hampstead

Ilford

Islington

Kensington

Kew

Milwall

Morden

Putney

Richmond

Soho

Streatham

Wembley

boys' names

♂ **HARLEY.** *English, 'the long field'.* You can ride one, you can use it as a baby name – or, as is often the case, both. In spite of its slightly renegade motorcycle image, it recently entered the Top 100. **Arley, Harlea, Harlee, Harleigh, Harly, Hartley.**

HARMON. *Irish variation of* HERMAN. Has a harmonic feel. **Harman, Harmann, Harmonn.**

♂ **HARMONY.** *Word name.* Hippy name with a sweet meaning. But for a boy, Pax or Justice would carry a lot more heft. **Harmonio.**

HAROLD. *Scandinavian, 'army ruler'.* The name of a pipe-smoking, bespectacled grandpa or uncle, rarely a baby, though any latent nerdiness can be counteracted with the relaxed nickname Hal. **Hal, Harrald, Harrold, Harry, Herold, Herrick, Herrold, Herryck. International: Aralt** *(Irish),* **Arailt, Harailt, Harald, Haral** *(Scottish),* **Araldo, Aroldo, Arrigo** *(Italian),* **Haraldo** *(Spanish and Portuguese),* **Heraldo** *(Portuguese),* **Halward** *(German),* **Haral, Harald** *(Scandinavian),* **Heronim, Hieronim** *(Polish),*

Enric *(Romanian),* **Jindra** *(Czech),* **Haraldas** *(Lithuanian),* **Haralds** *(Latvian),* **Garald, Garold, Herahd, Kharald** *(Russian).*

HAROUN. *Arabic variation of* AARON. This name has a sensuous feel that makes it a winner. The Armenian Harout has a similar flavour. **Haroon, Harun.**

♂ **HARP.** *Music name.* Feels as if it's missing a syllable.

★♂ **HARPER.** *English, 'harp player'.* Paul Simon used it years ago for his now-grown son and another American personality recently gave the name to his baby daughter, à la (female) author Harper Lee. A winner, across genders and generations. **Harpur.**

HARPO. *English nickname.* The mute, horn-honking Marx Brother's real name was Adolph – so Harpo represented a huge step up. Also, it's Oprah Winfrey's production company (her first name spelled backwards).

HARRELL. *Hebrew, 'God's mount'.* While everyone may think you said 'Harold,' this name sounds more up-to-date. And if you get tired of explaining, you can always call him Harry.

HARRINGTON. *English, 'family farm'.* On the staff of a manor house.

HARRIS. *English, 'son of Harry'.* When Harrison is too much, but Harry isn't enough. **Harriss, Harrys.**

HARRISON. *English, 'son of Harry'.* This Top 50 name was made viable by Harrison Ford and increasingly popular with parents who want an *H* name that's more formal than Harry or Hank, but doesn't veer into the stiff Huntington-Harrington territory. **Harris, Harriss, Harrisson, Harryson.**

★**HARRY.** *Diminutive of* HENRY. Everyone's elderly uncle until Princess Diana, following British royal tradition, called her son Harry and

Harry Potter became a rage. A Top 100 choice, it's still more popular with parents favouring regular names than those aspiring to royalty.

♂ HART. *English, 'stag'.* Could be the hero of a romantic novel, but on the other hand, it's short, straightforward and strong sounding; its most famous bearer was poet Hart (born Harold) Crane. **Harte.**

HARTIGAN. *Irish, 'descendant of Arthur'.* In *Cool Names,* we cite this as an 'Artist Name,' for twentieth-century abstract painter Grace Hartigan, though for you it may just be an upbeat Irish surname.

♂ HARTLEY. *English, 'stag meadow'.* In these days of Harleys and Hammers, feels a bit limp. **Hartlea, Hartlee, Hartleigh, Hartly.**

HARTMAN. *German, 'hard, strong man'.* A viable choice only if it's growing on your family tree. **Hartmann.**

HARTWIG. *German, 'courageous in battle'.* Baby-naming rule No. 984: forget

any name that contains the syllable *wig*.

HARUKI. *Japanese, 'spring child'.* Japanese writer Haruki Murakami might inspire some namesakes.

HARVARD. *English, 'army guard'.* With Yale and Brown in the mainstream, why not this upscale American college name and surname as well?

HARVEY. *French, 'battle worthy'.* This Norman name is enjoying a style revival in Britain, rising to Number 28. We don't expect it to happen elsewhere. **Harvee, Harvie, Herve, Hervey.**

HAS(S)AN. *Arabic, 'handsome'.* Among the more familiar Arabic choices and also one with an attractive meaning. In one Nigerian tribe, it's used for the first born of a pair of male twins. **International: Hussein** *(Arabic/Middle Eastern),* **Hasani** *(Swahili),* **Husain, Husani, Husayn, Hussain** *(Kiswahili).*

HASKEL, HASKELL. *Yiddish variation* of **EZEKIEL.** Rarely used cerebral-sounding name

that is actually the Yiddish form of Ezekiel.

♂ HAVANA. *Place name.* Vowel ending tilts this sharply towards the feminine and at this point it has some political implications as well.

HAVARD. *Norwegian, 'rock' or 'protector'.* An unusual yet accessible Scandinavian choice, though it might be confused with Harvard. **Halvard.**

HAVELOCK. *Scandinavian, 'sea competition'.* Twentieth-century psychologist/sexologist Havelock (born Henry) Ellis made this name known, but no less forbidding.

♂ HAVEN. *Word name.* Like Harbour, one of the new generation of word names with appealing meanings, though it has been tipped decidedly towards the girls' court. **Hagan, Hagen, Havin, Hogan.**

♂ HAWAII. *Place name.* An actual Hawaiian first name would convey the aura of the islands more originally and effectively.

Carden

Corbin

Emmett

Hadden

Hayward

Holden

Hudson

Kiefer

Lander

Mason

Preston

Slater

Wade

Walker

HAWES. *English, 'hedged area'.* Could be a difficult one to comprehend: Hoss? Or was that horse? **Haws.**

HAWK. *Nature name.* Animal names are on the rise, especially more of the aggressive Hawk-Fox-Wolf variety than cute little Bunnys or Robins.

HAWTHORNE. *English, 'lives where hawthorn hedges grow'.* Nathaniel Hawthorne, the American novelist sets this above many other surnames (and nature names, for that matter), but it's still an imposing choice few would pick. **Hawthorn.**

♂ **HAYDEN.** *English, 'heathen-grown hill'.* Formerly obscure name that's risen to huge popularity – now entering the Top 100. Though this is among the most distinctive of the bunch, it gets lost in the crowd of Jaidens, Bradens, Aidans and endless variations. **Hadan, Haden, Hadin, Hadon, Hadun, Hadyn, Haidan, Haiden, Haidin, Haidon, Haidun, Haidyn, Haydan, Haydin, Haydn, Haydon, Haydun, Haydyn.**

HAYDN. *(HYE-den) German, 'heathen'.* Some music-minded parents might consider this, especially as a middle name, to honour the great Austrian composer.

HAYES. *English, 'hedged area'.* One of those simple, straightforward English surnames that's easy to translate into a first. **Hays, Hazen, Hazin.**

HAYWARD. English occupational name, 'guardian of the hedged enclosure'. Possible Hayden alternative. **Heyward, Heywood, Ward.**

HAZEL. *(HAZ-ay-el) Hebrew, 'one who decides'.* This name of an Old Testament king could easily be mispronounced, bringing it too close to the feminine Hazel for serious consideration.

HAZAIAH. *Hebrew variation of* **CHAZAIAH,** *'God has seen'.* With more parents turning to biblical names like Ezekiel and Isaiah, this could prove a quasi-unique alternative in a similar – if more Orthodox – vein. **Chazaiah, Chazaya, Hazaia.**

♂ **HAZARD.** *French, 'chance, luck'.* Chance has risen on the baby-naming charts, but Hazard has a considerably more dangerous edge. **Hazzard.**

♂ **HAZE.** *Word name.* Trippy variation on Hayes.

HAZELTON. *English,* *'settlement near hazel trees'.* Unless it was your grandmother's maiden name and you're using it in the middle place, we don't think it makes a good choice.

HEATH. *English, 'the heathland dweller'.* Hot Australian actor Heath Ledger has single-handedly made this considerably more than a tract of open land covered with scrubby vegetation. We expect many future parents to be attracted to this name as the actor's star continues to rise.

HEATHCLIFF. *English, 'cliff near a heath'.* Effete name of the original passionate macho hero of Emily Brontë's *Wuthering Heights*, recently chosen by fashionista Lucy Sykes and inspired Heath Ledger's name.

HECTOR. *Greek, 'holds fast'.* This name of the noble hero of the Trojan War is used primarily by Latino families these days. **International: Eachtar** *(Irish),* **Eachann** *(Scottish),* **Ettore** *(Italian),* **Heitor** *(Portuguese).*

HEDDWYN. *Welsh, 'holy peace'.* Takes Edwin one step – make that ten steps – too far. **Edwin, Hedwin, Hedwyn, Hedwynn.**

HEDEON. *Russian variation of* **GIDEON.** A not as appealing variation on an attractive original.

HEINRICH. *(HINE-rish) German, 'home of the king'.* Traditional German names of this ilk have had a difficult time emigrating into the British name pool. One of its nicknames, Harro, might do better. **Harro, Heike, Hein, Heine, Heinecke, Heini, Heinie, Heinz, Henke, Henning, Hinrich.**

HEINZ. *German diminutive of* **HEINRICH.** Heinz has become a cartoonish German name, prone to ketchup teasing. **Hines.**

HELADIO. *Spanish, 'born in Greece'.* Melodic and friendly and similar to a Spanish word for *chilled* and *ice cream*. **Eladio, Eladito Elado, Heladi, Heladito, Helado, Helio.**

HELGI. *Norse, 'productive, successful, happy'.* Unfortunately, to the British ear, a boy named Helgi doesn't *sound* productive, successful or happy. **Helae, Helja, Helje.**

HELIO. *(AY-lee-o) Spanish, 'the sun'.* More familiar to Anglos in the Italian Elio form. **International: Elio** *(Italian),* **Helios** *(Greek).*

HELLER. *German, 'bright, brilliant'.* A li'l hell-raiser name in the Ryder-Rogue-Rebel vein.

HELMUT. *German, 'brave protector'.* Photographer Newton . . . or that hard thing you wear on your head. **Hellmut, Hellmuth.**

HELSINKI. *Finnish place name.* Though lots of obscure place names are now on the map, it's hard to imagine this one inspiring anyone.

HENDERSON. *English, 'son of Henry'.* Bulky surname honouring Grandpa Henry. **Hendrie, Hendries, Hendron, Henryson.**

HENDRIK. *Dutch and Scandinavian variation of* **HENRY.** A bit stiff and formal for British use. **Hendrick.**

★**HENDRIX.** *Dutch and German, from* **HENDRIK.** Like Presley, a better choice than the great musician Jimi's first name.

♂ **HENLEY.** *English, 'high meadow'.* The name of a town on the Thames that hosts a famous regatta, so it could be an appropriate middle name for the son of boat-lovers. **Handley, Hanlea, Hanlee, Hanleigh, Hanley, Hanly, Henlea, Henlee, Henleigh, Henlie.**

HENRY. *German, 'estate ruler'.* Henry's popularity has increased recently, sending it up the Top 50. In upmarket neighourhoods and suburbs, it seems every other boy is named either Jack or Henry. Still, it's a solid name with lots of history and personality. **Hal, Hank, Harry, Heriot, Herriot.** International: **Ánrai, Éinri** *(Irish Gaelic),* **Eanraig** *(Scottish Gaelic),* **Henri** *(French),* **Arrigo, Enrico, Enzio** *(Italian),* **Enrique, Inriques, Quico, Quinto, Quique** *(Spanish),* **Enric** *(Catalan),* **Henrique** *(Portuguese),* **Heiko, Heino, Heinrich, Heinrik, Henrik, Hinrich** *(Dutch),* **Heinz, Henning** *(German),* **Henerik, Henning** *(Danish),* **Heikki** *(Finnish),* **Henryk** *(Polish),* **Henrik** *(Hungarian),* **Henric** *(Romanian),* **Jindrich** *(Czech),* **Hersz** *(Yiddish).*

HERBERT. *German, 'famous army'.* With the possible exception of Robert, all names ending in *bert,* from Egbert to Dilbert, are in permanent exile. **Bert, Bertie, Harbert, Herb, Herbie, Herby.** International: **Hebert** *(French),* **Herberto, Heriberto** *(Italian),* **Eber, Ebert, Eberto** *(Spanish),* **Harbert** *(Dutch),* **Heribert** *(German).*

HERCULES. *Greek, 'glory of Hera'.* Any boy with this name, a synonym for power via the Greek mythology figure, better be strong of body and of psyche. **Ercule, Heracles, Herculies.** International: **Hercule** *(French),* **Ercole** *(Italian),* **Herculano** *(Spanish),* **Heraklees, Herakles** *(Greek).*

HERMAN. *German, 'soldier, warrior'.* It's hard to believe that Herman was once popular and even harder to imagine it making a comeback. But then again, our parents thought the same thing about Max and Jake. Consider the French Armand or Spanish Armando instead. **Herm, Hermie, Hermin.** International: **Heremon, Hermon** *(Irish),* **Armand** *(French),* **Armando, Armino, Ermanno** *(Italian),* **Armando, Armindo, Arminio, Hermá, Hermano, Herminio, Hermino** *(Spanish),* **Ermanos** *(Portuguese and Basque),* **Harman, Harmon, Hermann** *(German),* **Arman, Armen** *(Russian).*

HERMES. *Greek mythology name, 'the messenger god'.* These days, more people will relate to Hermès – pronounced *ayr-MEZ* – as an upscale brand name like Chanel and Porsche than as a Greek god. **Ermes, Herm, Hermite, Hermus.**

HERNANDO. *Spanish, 'adventurer, explorer'.* An exotic and attractive choice for a child of any background. Two early

New World explorers were Hernandos – de Soto and Cortés. **Hernán, Hernandes, Hernandez.**

♂ **HERO.** *Greek mythology name; English word name.* Though the mythological Hero was female, this name might prove too big a responsibility for a little guy to shoulder.

HERON. *Nature name.* The name of the long-legged wading bird might work as a boy's name, having a soft but strong sound. **Herron.**

HERRICK. *German, 'war ruler'.* When you like Eric, but wish it were longer; also the name of a great early English poet. **Herrik, Herryck.**

HERSHEL. *Hebrew, 'deer'.* Gentle meaning and bona fide Hebrew history, but feels old-mannish, like Herman and Menashe. **Hersch, Herschel, Herschell, Hersh, Hertzel, Herzel, Herzl, Hesh, Heschel, Heshel, Hirsch, Hirschel, Hirschl, Hirsh.**

HERVÉ. *(air-VAY) French, 'battle worthy'.* Hervé was a legendary French saint, patron of the blind, who performed many miracles – it's a lot more sophisticated than Harvey. **Hervey.**

HESPEROS. *Greek, personification of the evening star, Venus.* Anyone who's ever heard the phrase 'you look like the wreck of the Hasperus' – from a poem by Longfellow – would want to avoid this one. **Hasperus, Hesperios, Hespero, Hesperus.**

HEWETT. *French, diminutive of* **HUGH.** Hugh plus. **Hewet, Hewie, Hewitt, Hewlett, Hewlitt.**

HEZEKIAH. *Hebrew, 'God gives strength'.* This name of an influential Old Testament king of Judah is one that would challenge even the most adventurous biblical name-seeker, but it does have the modernising short form Zeke.

HIAWATHA. *From Iroquoi, Haio-hw'tha, 'he makes rivers'.* The name of a Native American leader immortalised in a Longfellow poem.

HIDALGO. *Spanish, 'nobleman'.* Hidalgo is the name of a minor planet and, on Earth, the Spanish word for a nobleman, but we don't see much crossover potential.

HIDEKI. *Japanese, 'bright tree'.* A Japanese name popular in its own country but uncommon elsewhere.

HIERONYMUS. *(heer-ON-ee-mos) German variation of* **JEROME.** This cognate of Jerome (of all things), familiar via the Dutch painter of fantastical scenes, H. Bosch, would appeal only to the most audacious, intrepid, attention-seeking baby namer. **Hi, Hiram, Hyram, Jerome. International: Geronimo** *(Native American),* **Heronim, Hieronimos** *(Polish),* **Hieronymos** *(Greek).*

♂ **HILARY.** *Greek, 'cheerful, happy'.* The only version that works for boys anymore is the Latinate Hilario or Ilario. Better to look to Felix for a happy-meaning name. **Hil, Hill, Hillary, Hilliary. International: Hillery, Ilar** *(Welsh),* **Hilaire** *(French),* **Ilario** *(Italian),*

Hilarino, Hilario *(Spanish),* **Ilari** *(Russian),* **Hilarion** *(Greek).*

♂**HILL.** *English, 'someone who lives by a hill'.* Simple and down-to-earth, but would probably work best as a middle name.

HILLEL. *Hebrew, 'greatly praised'.* Hillel the Great was a famous Talmudic scholar, the spiritual and ethical leader of his generation and his name is greatly honoured by parents in Israel and, to some extent, here.

HILTON. *English, 'hill settlement'.* Do you really want to name your baby after a hotel? Or a famous-for-being-famous starlet? **Hillton, Hylton.**

HIPPOLYTE. *(ee-po-LET) French from Greek, 'he who frees horses'.* This name of an unfortunate youth in classical legend, later borne by several saints, is not uncommon in France, but has barely set foot on British soil. **International: Ippolito** *(Italian),* **Hipolito** *(Portuguese),* **Hippolytos** *(Greek).*

HIRAM. *Hebrew, 'most noble'.* One of the few names on which

we disagree. Positive view: biblical name deserving of revival. Negative view: pitching horseshoes with Zeke. **Hi, Hirom, Hy, Hyram, Hyrum.**

HIROSHI. *Japanese, 'generous'.* Several artistic Hiroshis make this one of the more plausible Japanese imports.

♂ **HISTORY.** *Word name.* As a personal name, it may not have much history, but it certainly suggests the subject.

HITCH. *Diminutive of* **HITCHCOCK.** The charming Hitch played by Will Smith in the eponymous film put this into the lexicon. Also known as the nickname of director Alfred Hitchcock.

HOB. *English, diminutive of* **ROBERT.** A Robert nickname out of use for hundreds of years, but now sounds cooler than Bob or Rob for a modern boy.

HOBART. *English and Dutch variation of* **HUBERT.** More user-friendly than the original. **Hobard, Hobert, Hobey, Hobie, Hoebart.**

HOBBES. *English variation of* **ROBERT.** All varieties of Hob are antiquated nicknames for Robert. **Hob, Hobbs.**

HOBSON. *English, 'son of Robert'.* An original way to honour an ancestral Robert. **Hobbson.**

HODGSON. *English, 'son of Roger'.* A possible nod to grandpa Roger, though somewhat stuffy. **Hodge, Hodges.**

HOGAN. *Irish, 'youth'.* Logan is a popular name that came from nowhere in the past few decades, and we think Hogan is a good bet to follow. **Hagan.**

♂ **HOLDEN.** *English, 'hollow valley'.* Parents who loved J. D. Salinger's *The Catcher in the Rye* are flocking to the name of its hero – not coincidentally in tune with the Hayden-Colton field of names.

♂ **HOLLAND.** *Dutch place name.* There are a fair number of Hollands around these days, but most of them are female.

♂ HOLLIS. *English, 'near the holly bushes'.* Another surname-y choice that's gone to the girls. **Hollen, Holley, Hollin, Holling, Hollinger, Holliss, Hollister.**

HOLMES. *English, 'from the island in the river'.* Possible middle name for devotees of detective Sherlock.

HOLT. *English, 'son of the unspoiled forests'.* Has that blunt masculine feel – à la Cole and Kyle – that many modern parents are drawn to.

HOMER. *Greek, 'security, pledge'.* A name that has travelled from the ancient Greek scribe of the great classical epics to Bart Simpson's doltish dad – and lately is the hot celebrity pick of such parents as Richard Gere, Bill Murray and Anne Heche. **International: Homerico, Homero, Omero** *(Spanish),* **Homeros** *(Greek).*

HONOURÉ. *French variation of Latin, 'honoured one'.* A name that is truly honoured in France, as the name of several saints,

artists like Daumier and writers like Balzac. **Honouratus, Honourius.**

HOOKER. *English occupational name, 'shepherd's hook'.* We don't think any parent should get hooked on this name.

HOOPER. *English occupational name, 'hoop-maker'.* Lively, friendly surname that might appeal to netball fans.

HOPPER. *English and Scottish occupational name, 'acrobat'; Dutch, 'hop grower or seller'.* Sean and Robin Wright Penn chose this name for their son to honour their friend Dennis Hopper; others might associate it with the painter Edward.

HORACE. *Latin clan name, 'timekeeper'.* Fustily fuddy-duddy and yet, with the resurrection of Homer and the new interest in old Roman names . . . who knows? **International: Oratio, Orazio** *(Italian),* **Horacio** *(Spanish),* **Horats, Horatz** *(Dutch),* **Horatio, Horatius** *(German).*

Names from Books

Amory

Aram

Atticus

Balthazar

Brick

Chance

Darcy

Dorian

Guitar

Gulliver

Holden

Oliver

Orlando

Levi

Magnus

Malloy

Rhett

Romeo

Tristram

Wolf

Zhivago

★HORATIO. *English variation of* **HORACE.** Like Horace, a variation on the Latin Horatius, but with its Shakespearean and optimistic Horatio Alger pedigree, this is an attractive up-and-comer with its cool final *o*.

♂ **HORIZON.** *Word name.* A name with vision.

HORST. *German, 'a thicket' or 'leap'.* Heavy and horsey. **Hurst.**

HORTON. *English, 'grey settlement'.* This name has a sweet feeling, maybe thanks to the Dr Seuss connection, but still has a harsh sound. **Horten, Orton.**

HORUS. *Egyptian, 'sun god'.* Sounds like Horace, looks like the head of a hawk on the body of a human. **Horis, Horace.**

HOSEA. *Hebrew, 'salvation'.* Since so many of the biblical prophet names – Daniel, Jonah, Nathan, Samuel – are overused, you might want to consider this distinctive alternative. **Hoseia, Hoshea, Hosheia.**

HOUGHTON. *(HOW-tun) English, 'place in an enclosure'.* A family name, a bit haughty. **Hough.**

★♂ **HOUSTON.** *Scottish, 'Hugh's town'; Texas place name.* Here's a fresher, contemporary alternative if you want to honour a Hugh. If you're looking for a place name linked to the American state of Texas, this is a more distinctive choice than other cities such as Austin and Dallas. **Hewson, Huston, Hutcheson, Hutchinson.**

HOWARD. *German, 'high guardian'; English, 'brave heart'.* Howard, once hugely popular from the 1870s to early 1950s, is now a real dad-grandad name, with no sign of a revival in sight. To honour a relative, you might just drop the first syllable and call him Ward. **Howie, Ward.**

HOWE. *German, 'lofty one'; English, 'hill'.* The minimalist Howard. **How.**

HOWEL, HOWELLS, HOWLAND. *English, 'land with hills'.* The Anglophile Howard. **Howlan, Howlen, Hywell.**

HOWELL. *English variation of Hywel, an eminent Welsh king.* A familiar and usable last name turned first, but it might be better as a middle name to avoid it being shortened to How.

HOYT. *English, 'long stick'; originally a nickname for a tall, thin person.* Most prominently borne by country singer Hoyt Axton, problematic because of the *oy* sound. **Hoyce.**

HUBBELL. *English, 'brave heart'.* Memorable as the Robert Redford character who captivated the young Barbra Streisand in the film classic *The Way We Were*: Hubbell Gardiner. **Hubble.**

HUBERT. *German, 'bright, shining intellect'.* A name that sounds so old-fashioned some parents out there might conceivably find it quirky enough for a comeback, along with other fuddie-duddies like Oscar and Homer. **Bert, Eubie, Hubbard, Hube, Hubie. International: Hobard, Hobart, Hoibeard (Irish), Ubert, Uberto (Italian), Huber, Huberto, Uber (Spanish).**

★ **HUDSON.** *English, 'Hugh's son'; place name.* Rising quickly in popularity after in the last decade or so, this surname name has gotten a boost as the surname of the actress Kate Hudson and as the name of a few prominent starbabies. Also would work as a tribute to Rock Hudson, or as a middle name.

HUGH. *English from German, 'mind, intellect'.* Patrician to the core, a name that was particularly popular among the Irish and elsewhere a century ago, but now it is used very quietly. **Hew, Hewe, Howell, Huey, Hughes, Hughie. International: Aodg** *(Irish Gaelic),* **Huw** *(Welsh),* **Hugues** *(French),* **Ugo** *(Italian),* **Hugin, Hugolino, Hugón, Hugues, Huguito, Ugo, Ugolino, Ugone, Uguecria** *(Spanish),* **Hugo** *(Spanish, German, Dutch, Danish).*

★**HUGO.** *German, 'mind, intellect'.* We admit it, we love names that end (or begin, for that matter) with an *o* and this one is especially appealing because it's backed up by lots of solid history and European style. Unlike the original Hugh, its popularity is on the rise. **International: Ugo** *(Italian),* **Ugecria, Ugo, Ugolino, Ugone** *(Spanish).*

HULBERT. *German, 'bright grace'.* No. **Bert, Hulbard, Hulburd, Hulburt.**

HUMBERT. *German, 'renowned warrior'.* A name with two strong literary associations, one negative – *Lolita*'s narrator Humbert Humbert – and one positive, in the preferable European version: Italian author Umberto Eco. **International: Umberto** *(Italian),* **Humbaldo, Humberto, Hunfredo, Hunfrido** *(Spanish).*

HUME. *Scottish variation of* HOLMES. Distinguished actor Hume Cronyn (who shared his father's name) put this unusual choice in the lexicon. **Hulme.**

HUMPHREY. *German, 'peaceful warrior'.* An old name that might have faded completely were it not for Bogie. A royal name in Britain, where it's used most frequently; it might just have some life beyond Bogart elsewhere. **Huffie, Humfrey, Humfroy, Humfry, Humph, Humphery, Humphry. International: Unfrai** *(Irish),* **Wmffre** *(Welsh),* **Onfroi** *(French),* **Onofredo** *(Italian),*

Hunfredo, Onofre *(Spanish),* **Humfried** *(Dutch, German),* **Humfrid** *(Swedish).*

HUNT. *Word name.* Short, strong, manly.

♂ **HUNTER.** *English, 'one who hunts'.* Hunter is one of the leaders of an unusual band of boys' names that combines macho imagery (Hunter, Austin, Harley) with softened masculinity.

HUNTINGTON. *English, 'hunter's settlement'.* If you want to give little Hunt an ultraproper name for his CV. **Hunt, Huntingdon.**

♂ **HUNTLEY.** *English, 'meadow of the hunter'.* A surname name that could work as a first name. **Huntlea, Huntlee, Huntleigh, Huntly.**

HURACAN. *Mayan, 'triple heart of the universe'.* The supreme Mayan god whose name inspired the *hurricane*. If Storm and Sky can make names, why not this?

♂**HURLEY.** *Irish, 'sea tide'.* Middle name possibility, though kids might make malicious fun of the first syllable. **Hurhy, Hurlee, Hurleigh.**

HURST. *English, 'wooded hill'.* Whether spelled like this or as the perhaps-more-familiar Hearst, few would use this surname choice if it wasn't their own family name. **Hearst, Hirst, Horst.**

HUSSEIN. *Arabic, 'small, handsome one'.* Familiar to Westerners as the name of the respected king of Jordan, but also as the surname of Saddam. **Husain, Husayn, Husein.**

♂ **HUXLEY.** *English, 'inhospitable place'.* An X makes almost any name cooler. This one honours author Aldous. **Huxlea, Huxlee, Huxleigh, Huxly.**

HYATT. *English, 'lofty gate'.* Only if you name his brothers Hilton and Marriott. **Hayatt, Hiatt.**

HYDE. *English, 'hide'; a medieval measure of land.* Hyde, of course, is most familiar as a surname – as in Mr Hyde, evil alter ego of Dr Jekyll.

HYMAN. *Anglicised variation of* **CHAIM.** Down at the schvitz with Morty and Myron. This name was commonly used by first-generation Jewish immigrants to Anglicise Chaim, but similarities to terms like *heinie* and *hymen* have taken it out of the realm of modern possibility. **Chaim, Hayim, Hayyim, Hi, Hy, Hymie, Mannie, Manny.**

boys

IAGO. *Welsh variation of* **JAMES** *and* **JACOB.** The villain of Shakespeare's *Othello* was so treacherously evil that his name has hardly ever been heard offstage. **Jago, Yago.**

IAIN. *(EE-ayn) Gaelic variation of* **JOHN.** It's pronounced exactly the same as Ian, making it an unnecessarily confusing spelling. **Ian.**

IAKONA. *Hawaiian variation of* **JASON.** At first hearing, most people would assume this was a girl's name.

★IAN. *Scottish variation of* **JOHN.** Ian Fleming, creator of James Bond, introduced this name to countries outside of Britain, who have been warming more and more to its jaunty charm; it's flying in formation with fellow classic British RAF pilot names, like Derek and Trevor and Colin. **Ean, Eann, Eion, Eon, Iaian, Iain, Iann, Ion.**

IB. *Danish, diminutive of* **JACOB.** Though it sounds insubstantial elsewhere, it's actually a common name in Denmark.

IBO. *(ee-BOW) African, 'my people'.* Short but striking.

IBRAHIM. *Arabic variation of* **ABRAHAM.** Well used by Muslim parents in the Western world as well as in the Middle

East. **Ibrahaim, Ibraham, Ibraheem, Ibrahem.**

♂ IBSEN. *Danish, 'son of Ib'.* A literary hero name possibility, after the great Norwegian dramatist, Henrik I. **Ib, Ibsan, Ibsin, Ibson.**

ICARUS. *Greek mythology name.* The mythological figure famous for flying too close to the sun has a couple of negatives: his rash reputation and those 'icky' nicknames. **Ikaros, Ikarus.**

ICHABOD. *Hebrew, 'the glory is gone'.* This eccentric Old Testament name is forever tied to the character of Ichabod Crane – and worse, the teasing possibilities of 'icky bod'. **Ikabod, Ikavod.**

ICHIRŌ. *(ee-chee-ro) Japanese, 'firstborn son'.* A good classic choice for the first boy in a Japanese family.

♂ IDAN. *(ee-dohn) Hebrew, 'era, time'.* A Hebrew unisex place name rarely heard in this country.

IDI. *African, 'born during the Idd festival'.* Adverse associations

with the ruthless Ugandan dictator Idi Amin.

IDO. *Hebrew, 'to evaporate'; Arabic, 'to be mighty'.* Multicultural name unheard of in the West, has a bit of a weirdo aura. **Iddo.**

IEUAN. *Welsh variation of* **JOHN.** Scrabble-rack full of impossible vowels. **Iefan, Ifan.**

IFOR. *Welsh, 'archer'.* Seems to make more sense in its Anglicised version, Ivor.

IGASHU. *Native American, 'wanderer, seeker'.* Has a primitive feel that doesn't quite fit into the mainstream. **Igasho.**

IGGY. *Latin, diminutive of* **IGNATIUS.** Would only work for a pop star.

IGNACIO. *(eeg-NAH-see-o) Spanish, 'fiery'.* Frequently heard in the Latino community, though in English that *Ig-* beginning – as in ignoble and ignorant – doesn't make it. **International: Egnacio, Hignacio, Ignacius, Ignasi, Ignasio, Ignatio, Ignazio, Ignocio, Ingnacio,**

Trouble Ahead

Names Projected for Tropical Storms in 2008 & 2009

Arthur	Ana
Bertha	Bill
Cristobal	Claudette
Dolly	Danny
Edouard	Erika
Fay	Fred
Gustav	Grace
Hanna	Henri
Ike	Ida
Josephine	Joaquin
Kyle	Kate
Laura	Larry
Marco	Mindy
Nana	Nicholas
Omar	Odette
Paloma	Peter
Rene	Rose
Sally	Sam
Teddy	Teresa
Vicky	Victor
Wilfred	Wanda

Nacho, Nas, Ygnasio, Ygnocio *(all Spanish)*.

IGNATIUS. *Latin, 'fiery'.* This name of several saints, including the founder of the Catholic Jesuit order, is more apt to be borne by churches and schools than babies. **Iggie, Iggy. International: Ignatz** *(German),* **Ignati** *(Irish),* **Ignace** *(French),* **Ignazio** *(Italian),* **Ignacio, Ignado, Ignazio, Nacho, Nacio** *(Spanish),* **Iáaki, Inigo** *(Basque),* **Ignaas** *(Dutch),* **Ignacius, Ignate, Ignatz** *(German),* **Ignacek, Ignacy, Nacek** *(Polish),* **Ignác** *(Czech),* **Ignat, Ignati, Ignatiy** *(Russian),* **Ignatios** *(Greek).*

IGNATZ. *German variation of* **IGNATIUS.** Natz recommended.

IGOR. *(EE-gor) Russian variation of* **IVOR.** Musical association with Igor Stravinsky, but also Dr Frankenstein's right-hand man. **Gorik, Gosha, Iga, Igoryok, Inge, Ingemar, Ingmar, Yegor, Ygor.**

IKE. *Diminutive of* **ISAAC.** The rise of Isaac and the stylishness of short down-to-earth nicknames like Max and Gus means that many parents like Ike once again.

IKU. *(EE-koo) Japanese, 'nourishing'.* Easily assimilated Japanese name.

ILAN. *Hebrew, 'tree'.* Because of its meaning, a symbolic name given to boys born on TuB'Shevat, the New Year of the Trees, or Arbor Day. **Eilon, Elam, Elan, Ilan, Ilani, Ilanya, Ilon.**

ILARI. *Basque, 'cheerful'.* See *ILARIO.*

ILARIO. *(ee-LAH-ree-o) Latin, 'cheerful, glad'.* Its merry, jovial sound reflects a shared root with the word *hilarious.* **International: Iara, Ilario** *(Basque),* **Illarion** *(Russian).*

ILIE. *Romanian variation of* **ELIAS.** *See* **ELIAS.**

♂ **ILYA.** *Russian variation of* **ELIJAH.** A rare example of an *a*-ending boy's name that sounds masculine, Ilya has a large measure of creative Slavic charm. **Ilia, Illya.**

♂ IMARI. *Modern invented name.* Name with an Asian feel, thanks to a Japanese city and Imari porcelain.

IMMANUEL. *German variation of* **EMMANUEL.** *See* *EMMANUEL.* Imannuel, Imanoel, Imanuel.

IMRE. *(EEM-reh) Hungarian, from German, 'strength'.* Commonly heard in its native country, would take a bit of explaining elsewhere. Imric, Imrie, Omri.

♂ INDIANA. *Place name.* This American state name emerged in the 1980s along with Dakota and Montana and it's still used occasionally by parents such as superstar-sib couple Summer Phoenix and Casey Affleck.

★INDIO. *Place name.* This name of a California desert town in the US, used by Deborah Falconer and Robert Downey Jr for their son, makes a much livelier and more individual – not to mention more masculine – improvisation on the themes of India and Indiana.

INGMAR, INGEMAR. *Norse, 'son of Ing'.* Ing was the powerful Norse god of fertility and peace, Ingmar is known here almost solely through Swedish director Ingmar Bergman. **Ingamar, Inge.**

INGRAM. *German, 'angel-raven'.* An undiscovered surname possibility with upscale overtones, could be enlivened with nickname Ingo. **Ingamar, Inglis, Ingmar, Ingo, Ingra, Ingraham, Ingrim.**

★INIGO. *(IN-i-go) Basque, medieval Spanish variation of* **IGNATIUS.** Almost unknown outside Spain, an attractive choice, with its strong beat, creative and evocative sound and association with the great early British architect, Inigo Jones.

INIKO. *Nigerian, 'time of trouble'.* African name with Niko-nickname option.

INNES. *Scottish, 'from the river island'.* This Scottish place name turned surname is used occasionally in first place. **Ennis, Iniss, Inness, Innis, Inniss.**

INNOCENT. *Latin, 'harmless, innocent'.* This name of thirteen popes is rarely heard in a secular setting, where loaded meaning opens the door to ridicule. **International: Inocenzio, Inocenzo** *(Italian),* **Chencho, Chente, Enesenico, Enicencio, Enocencio, Incencio, Innocensio, Innocentio, Inocencio, Sencio, Ynocencio, Ynocente** *(Spanish),* **Innokenti, Kenya, Kesha** *(Russian).*

IOAN. *(yo-ahn) Romanian variation of* **JOHN.** Less confusing with phonetic Johann spelling. **Iancu, Ion, Ionel.**

IOLO. *(YOH-loh) Welsh diminutive of* **EDWARD.** Rhythmic Welsh nickname-name, perilously close to yo-yo. **Iolyn.**

ION. *Romanian and Basque variation of* **JOHN.** A cross between Ian and a group of atomic particles.

IRA. *Hebrew, 'watchful one'.* Now considered more retirement-account acronym than proper name.

IRVIN. *Scottish, 'handsome, fair of face'.* Losing the final *g* in Irving makes the name *slightly* less dated. **Earvin, Ervin, Irv, Irvine.**

IRVING. *Scottish, 'green river, sea friend'.* A popular choice for first-generation Jewish-American boys whose parents looked to surnames from the British Isles to confer a measure of assimilation and class. **Earvin, Erv, Ervin, Ervine, Irv, Irven, Irvin, Irvine, Irvyn, Irwin, Irwyn, Ving. International: Inek** *(Welsh).*

IRWIN. *English, 'boar friend'.* Son of Irving. **Erwin, Erwinn, Erwyn, Irwinn, Irwyn.**

★ISAAC. *Hebrew, 'laughter'.* Isaac has shaved off its biblical beard and leaped into the Top 100, showing signs of heading even higher. A Puritan favourite, the Old Testament Isaac was the long-awaited son of the elderly Sarah and Abraham, so old that their news provoked laughter. **Ike, Ikey, Ikie, Isa, Isac, Isack, Isi, Issa, Itzak, Izik, Izsak, Zack, Zak. International: Iosóg** *(Irish),* **Isaak** *(Spanish, German, Russian, Greek),* **Isaco, Issac, Izaac, Ysaac, Ysaach, Yssac** *(Spanish),* **Itzaak, Itzik** *(Dutch),* **Izaak** *(Dutch, Czech),* **Izak** *(Scandinavian),* **Izák** *(Hungarian),* **Isak, Izaac** *(Czech),* **Aizik, Eisaak, Isak** *(Russian),* **Isaakios** *(Greek),* **Sahak** *(Armenian),* **Ishaq, Shaqil** *(Arabic).*

ISAAK. *Variation of* **ISAAC.** Cool spelling of the venerable Isaac used in several different cultures.

ISAI. *(EE-say* or *EE-sigh) Diminutive of* **ISAIAH** *and* **ISAIAS,** *spelling variation of* **ESAI.** This form, coming from various elements, has started to take off on its own. **International: Isaï** *(French).*

★ISAIAH. *Hebrew, 'God is salvation'.* Like Elijah, a once-neglected name of an Old Testament prophet, the appealing Isaiah is coming back into favour, already surpassing such long-popular brethren as Aaron and Adam. **Essaiah, Isai, Isia, Issiah, Izaiah, Iseyah, Iziah. International: Esaias** *(Latin),* **Isaïe** *(French),* **Isaia** *(Italian),* **Isaias, Ysai, Ysais** *(Spanish),* **Esa** *(Finnish),* **Yeshaya** *(Hebrew),* **Isiah, Issa** *(Arabic),* **Isa** *(Persian),* **Ikaia** *(Hawaiian).*

ISAIAS. *Latin variation of* **ISAIAH.** Widely used in the Hispanic community, as is the shorter Isai.

ISANDRO. *Spanish, from the Greek, 'liberator'.* A more distinctive alternative to Alejandro.

ISHAAN. *Hindi, 'the sun'.* Double vowel adds interest. **Ishan.**

ISHAM. *English, 'from the Iron One's estate'.* Wishy-washy.

ISHAQ. *Arabic from Hebrew* **YITZCHAK.** Unique, but made user-friendly by incorporating the familiar *shaq* sound.

ISHMAEL. *Hebrew, 'listen to God'; Arabic, 'outcast'.* 'Call me Ishmael' is the opening line of *Moby-Dick,* but few parents have followed that advice. **International: Ichmaël, Ismaël, Ismâîl** *(French),* **Esmael, Isamel, Ishmael, Ismael, Ismeal, Melito, Ysmael** *(Spanish),* **Ismail, Ismeal, Ismeil** *(Arabic).*

ISIAH. *Variation of* **ISAIAH.** Here is an increasingly popular streamlined spelling of the biblical name.

ISIDORE. *Greek, 'gift of Isis'.* A common ancient Greek name belonging to several saints, Isidore was adopted by Spanish Jews. Could be time for a more widespread revival. **Dore, Dory, Isador, Isadore, Izzy. International: Cedro, Chidro, Cidro, Ecedro, Ecidro, Esidor, Esidore, Esidoro, Esidro, Hisidro, Isidoro** *(Italian),* **Icidro, Isadoro, Ishico, Isidoro, Isidro, Izidro, Sidro, Ysidor, Ysidoro, Ysidro** *(Spanish),* **Ixidor** *(Basque),* **Isdro** *(Portuguese),* **Isidor** *(German),* **Izydor** *(Polish),* **Isidorios, Isiforos** *(Greek).*

ISMAEL. *Spanish variation of* **ISHMAEL.** High on the Latino hit parade.

ISRAEL. *Hebrew, 'he who struggles with God'; place name.* The founding of the modern Jewish state in 1948 transformed Israel from a traditional Jewish favourite into an icon of Judaism, which has limited its appeal. Still, in recent years it

has been given to hundreds of baby boys born in the US. **Issy, Izrael, Izzy, Yisrael. International: Isareal, Isra, Israh, Israil, Isreal, Ysrael** *(Spanish),* **Israil** *(Russian,)* **Iser, Issur, Sroel** *(Yiddish).*

ISSAC. *Hebrew, 'laughter'.* A contemporary play on the spelling of Isaac, currently catching on.

ITALO. *Italian, 'from Italy'.* You can't get more Italian than this name of the daddy of legendary twins Romulus and Remus.

IVAN. *Russian variation of* **JOHN.** One of the few Russian boys' names to become fully accepted into the naming pool, though some might find it a bit harsh and heavy-booted. Inevitable: Ivan the Terrible

teasing. **Van. International: Eyvan, Eyvind** *(Irish Gaelic),* **Iwan** *(Welsh),* **Yvan** *(Breton),* **Ivánek, Váňa, Váňuška** *(Czech),* **Ioann, Vanya, Vanusha** *(Russian).*

IVANHOE. *English, possible variation of* **IVAN.** So identified with the hero of the Sir Walter Scott novel, it would be almost impossible for any boy to carry.

IVAR. *(EE-vahr) Norse, 'yew wood, archer'.* Part of a small group of similar names – Ivor, Iver, Ivo – all worthy of consideration. **Ive, Ivor, Yvar. International: Ibhar, Ivo** *(Irish),* **Iver** *(Danish),* **Ivarr** *(Norse),* **Yvor** *(Russian).*

IVES. *Teutonic variation of* **YVES.** Smooth and sleek one-syllable surname, sometimes suggested for Sagittarius boys. **International: Yves** *(French)*, **Ivo** *(German)*.

★**IVO.** *German, 'yew wood, archer'*. Unusual, catchy name with the energetic impact of all names ending in *o*. **Ivair, Ivar, Iven, Iver, Ives, Yves, Yvo. International: Ibon** *(Basque)*, **Ivor** *(Scandinavian)*.

IVOR. *Scottish variation of* **IVAR**. A favourite for upscale characters in novels by Wodehouse and Waugh. **Ifor, Ivair, Ivar, Ive, Iver, Yvor. International: Yves, Yvet, Yvon** *(French)*, **Ibon** *(Basque)*, **Ivo** *(German)*.

♂ **IVORY.** *Word name.* Extremely attractive colour name chosen by some African-heritage parents for its reference to the West African Ivory Coast; more commonly used for girls.

IZAIAH. *Hebrew, 'God is salvation'. See* **ISAIAH.**

IZAK. *Polish variation of* **ISAAC.** *See* **ISAAC.**

♂ **IZAR.** *Basque, 'star'.* Used more for girls in Europe, but definitely sounds masculine enough for a boy here.

IZIDOR. *Hungarian variation of* **ISIDORE.** *See* **ISIDORE.**

♂ **IZZY.** *Nickname.* Multipurpose pet name serving Isidore, Isaac, Israel and – increasingly – Isabel.

J *boys*

JABARI. *Swahili, 'comforter, bringer of consolation'.* Coolly attractive African name, with distinguished representatives in sports and literature. **Jabaar, Jabahri, Jabar, Jabarae, Jabare, Jabaree, Jabarei, Jabarie, Jabarri, Jabarrie, Jabary, Jabbar, Jabbaree, Jabbari, Jaber, Jabiari, Jabier, Jabori, Jaborie.**

★**JABEZ.** *Hebrew, 'borne in pain'.* Biblical name popular with the Puritans, the rarely used Jabez now has a distinct accent and a far from puritanical image; it is an interesting alternative to Jacob or Jason. **Jabe, Jabes, Jabesh.**

JACE. *Hebrew, diminutive of* **JASON.** May sound like only half a name – or a spelling-out of the initials J.C. – but it's a popular choice in some places. **JC, J.C., Jacee, Jacek, Jacey, Jacian, Jacie, Jaice, Jaicee, Jayce.**

JACINTO. *(Hah-SEEN-to) Spanish, 'hyacinth'.* Less familiar and appealing than the feminine Jacinta. **Jacint.**

JACK. *English, diminutive of* **JOHN.** Long the Number 1 name in England, this durable, cheery everyman form of John has been chosen by dozens of celebs, including Meg Ryan and Dennis Quaid, and is a favourite for TV and films characters. Dads especially seem to like it. **Jackie, Jacko, Jackub, Jacqin, Jak, Jaq, Jax, Jock, Jocko.**

JACKSON. *English, 'son of Jack'.* When Dad agitates for Jack, Mom suggests this compromise. It's a popular choice and is another favoured Starbaby name (Bill Murray, Spike Lee, etc.). **Jack, Jackie, Jacksen, Jacksin, Jacky, Jacson, Jakeson, Jakson, Jaxen, Jaxon, Jaxson.**

JACO. *Portuguese variation of* **JACOB.** Intriguing twist on Jacob, but may be too strongly associated with Michael Jackson. **Jacko.**

JACOB. *Hebrew, 'he who supplants'.* A popular name recently entering the Top 25, Jacob was the Old Testament patriarch of the tribes of Israel. Strong, honest and venerable, but at this point way overused. **Cob, Cobb, Cobby, Cobey, Coby, Jachob, Jack, Jackie, Jacko, Jackob, Jackub, Jacky, Jaco, Jacobb, Jacobe, Jacobi, Jacoby, Jacolbi, Jacolby, Jacub, Jaecob, Jaicob, Jake, Jakie, Jakob, Jock, Jocob, Jocobb, Jocoby, Jocolby.**

JACOBO. *Spanish variation of* **JACOB.** Charming way to freshen up Jacob.

JACQUES. *French variation of* **JAMES** *and* **JACOB.** Classic French name that becomes pretentious when used for a British baby. **Jacot, Jacque, Jaq, Jaques.**

JADEN, JADON. *Hebrew, 'God has heard'.* While Jadon is the authentic biblical name,

Jacob's International Variations	
Scottish	Hamish
French	Jackquet, Jacquan, Jacquel, Jacquelin, Jacques, Jacquez
Italian	Giaco, Giacobbe, Giacobo, Giacomo, Giacopo
Spanish	Diego, Jacobo, Tiago
Basque	Yakobe
Portuguese	Jaco, Jacopo, Jago, Jaime
Dutch	Jaap
German	Jakob, Jockel
Finnish	Jaako, Jouko
Polish	Jakub, Jakubek, Jalu
Hungarian	Jakab, Kobi
Czech	Jakub, Jolubas, Kuba, Kubes, Kubik, Kubo
Lithuanian	Jecis, Jekebs, Jokubas
Bulgarian	Ikov
Latvian	Akkub, Akkubian, Akoub, Akoubian
Russian	Jakiv, Jakov, Jasha, Yakov, Yanka, Yashko
Greek	Iakovos
Hebrew	Jacobe
Yiddish	Koppel
Arabic	Akib, Akiv, Yocoub
Hindu	Akoobjee
Hawaiian	Iakopa

Jaden is by far the more popular spelling, first noticed when Will and Jada Pinkett Smith used it for their son. It has since become popular for both sexes, in a wide variety of spellings and rhyming cousins. **Jaden, Jadrien, Jadyn, Jaedon, Jaiden, Jayden, Jaydon.**

♂ **JAEL.** *(yah-el) Hebrew, 'mountain goat'.* A unisex Hebrew name sometimes given in Israel to kids born under the goat sign of Capricorn; it's also spelled Yael.

JAGGER. *English occupational name, 'carter'.* A swaggering Rolling Stone of a name that had a flicker of popularity in the late 1990s.

JAGO. *(jay-go or yay-go) Spanish and Cornish variation of* **JACOB.** Dashing alternative to overused favourite. **Jacut, Jagu, Jegu.**

JAGUAR. *Animal name.* Grrrrrr. **Jagguar.**

JAHAN. *Sanksrit, 'the world'.* Indian emperor Shah Jahan built the Taj Mahal. **Jehan.**

JAIDEN. *Hebrew variation of* **JADON.** This spelling is now more popular than the original. **Jaidan, Jaidon, Jaidyn.**

JAIME. *(HI-may) Spanish variation of* **JAMES.** Hispanic classic, could be misunderstood by others as Jamie. **Chago, Haime, Jaimee, Jaimey, Jaimie, Jaimito, Jaimy, Jayme, Jaymie, Mito, Xaime.**

JAKE. *Hebrew, diminutive of Jacob.* This unpretentious, accessible and optimistic (in the 1920s, 'everything's jake' meant everything's OK) short form of the popular Jacob is itself moving up the Top 25. **Jakie, Jayk, Jayke.**

JALEN. *Modern invented name.* The new Jason, spelled many different ways. **Jaelan, Jaelaun, Jaelen, Jaelin, Jaelon, Jailen, Jailin, Jaillen, Jaillin, Jailon, Jailyn, Jalan, Jaleen, Jalend, Jalene, Jalin, Jallen, Jalon, Jalyn, Jayelan, Jayelen, Jaylan, Jaylen, Jaylin, Jaylon, Jaylonn.**

JAMAL. *Arabic, 'handsome'.* Popular in the Mideast and among Muslim parents, though slightly less than it was a decade ago, after appearing as a character in Disney's *Aladdin* – albeit an evil one. **Jahmal, Jahmeal, Jahmeel, Jahmeil, Jahmel, Jahmelle, Jahmil, Jahmile, Jaimal, Jam, Jamaal, Jamael, Jamahl, Jamail, Jamaile, Jamala, Jamale, Jamall, Jamar, Jamaul, Jameel, Jamel, Jamell, Jamiel, Jamil, Jamile, Jammal, Jamor, Jamual, Jarmal, Jaumal, Jemaal, Jemahl, Jemal, Jemall, Jermal, Jimahl, Jimal, Jomahl, Jomal, Jomall. International: Cemal** *(Turkish),* **Gamal** *(Arabic).*

JAMAR. *Invented variation of* **JAMAL.** Attractive twist on Middle Eastern favourite – with further twists listed below. **Jam, Jamaar, Jamaari, Jamahrae, Jamair, Jamar, Jamaras, Jamaraus, Jamarl, Jamarr, Jamarre, Jamarrea, Jamarree, Jamarri, Jamarvis, Jamaur, Jamir, Jamire, Jamiree, Jammar, Jarmar, Jarmarr, Jatnarr, Jaumar, Jemaar, Jemar, Jemarr, Jimar, Jimarr, Jomar.**

JAMARI. *Invented elaboration of* **JAMAR.** Sleek and modern.

♂ **JAMES.** *Hebrew, 'supplanter'; English variation of* **JACOB.**

Classic New Testament name common among British royals, shared by great writers and entertainers. It is a longtime favourite, still in the Top 10. There are fewer Jimmys or Jamies these days: the most fashionable form of the name is James itself. **Jaimes, Jaimey, Jaimie, Jameson, Jamesie, Jamesy, Jamey, Jamez, Jameze, Jamies, Jamison, Jamse, Jamyes, Jamze, Jas, Jasha, Jay, Jayines, Jaymes, Jaymie, Jaymz, Jem, Jemes, Jim, Jiminy, Jimmy, Jocko.** International: **Séamas, Seumas, Seumus, Shamas, Shamus, Shay** (*Irish*), **Hamish, Jamie, Jock, Seumas** (*Scottish*), **Jago** (*Cornish*), **Jacque, Jacques** (*French*), **Giacomo** (*Italian*), **Diego, Iago, Jaime, Santiago, Yago** (*Spanish*), **Jaap** (*Dutch*), **Hagop** (*Armenian*).

♂ **JAMESON.** *English, 'son of James'.* Strong new James varietal, though sometimes shared by girls. A good choice to honour Grandpa Jim. **Jaimison, Jamerson, Jamesian, Jamieson, Jamison, Jaymeson.**

♂ **JAMIE.** *Scottish, diminutive of* **JAMES.** The cool form of James in the 1970s and 80s for both sexes, still holding steady in the Top 50. **Jaime, Jaimey, Jaimie, Jame, Jamee, Jamey, Jameyel, Jami, Jamia, Jamiah, Jamian, Jamiee, Jamme, Jammie, Jammy, Jamy, Jamye, Jayme, Jaymee, Jaymie.**

JAMIL. *Arabic, 'beautiful, handsome'.* Peaked in the 1990s. **Jameel, Jamen, Jamian, Jamien, Jamion, Jamionn, Jamon, Jamun, Jamyn, Jarmin, Jarmon, Jaymin.**

♂ **JAN.** *Dutch variation of* **JOHN.** Properly pronounced *yahn*, but Americans will equate it with the girls' name Jan. **Hans, Jaan, Janek, Jann, Janne, Jano, Janos, Janson, Jenda, Yan.**

JANEK. *(YAHN-ek) Polish variation of* **JOHN.** A bit too continental for a British boy. **Janak, Janik, Janika, Janka, Jankiel, Janko.**

JÁNOS. *(YAHN-os) Hungarian variation of* **JOHN.** Even more continental, especially with that accent. **Jancsi, Jani, Jankia, Jano.**

JANSON. *Scandinavian, 'Jan's son'.* Intriguing way to honour an ancestral John. **Jansen, Janssen, Jansson, Jantzen, Janzen, Jenson, Jensen.**

♂ **JANUARY.** *Word name.* Cooler than the older month names like April and May, but would be very unusual to use for a boy. International: **Janvier** (*French*), **Gennaro** (*Italian*), **Jenaro** (*Spanish*), **Januario** (*Portuguese*), **Janiusz, Janiuszek, Januarius, Jarek** (*Polish*).

JANUS. *Greek, 'gateway'.* Rather than the two-faced Roman mythological god of beginnings and ends, modern Westerners might relate this to the dated girls' name Janice. **Janan, Janiusz, Jannese, Jannus, Janusz.**

JAPHETH. *(JAY-feth) Hebrew, 'he expands'.* This name of the youngest son of Noah is one of the few biblical names that's still and forever *too* Old Testament. **Japeth, Japhet, Japhy.**

JAREB. *Hebrew, 'he will struggle'.* Unfortunately, everyone will just hear Jared. **Jarib.**

JARED. *Hebrew, 'he descends'.* Second-wave Old Testament name supplanted now by such choices as Jonah and Noah, though still an appealing option. **Jahred, Jaired, Jarad, Jaredd, Jareid, Jaren, Jarid, Jarod, Jarrad, Jarrard, Jarred, Jarrett, Jarrid, Jarrod, Jarryd, Jerad, Jered, Jerod, Jerrad, Jerred, Jerrod, Jerryd, Jordan.**

JAREK. *(YAHR-ek) Slavic, 'spring'.* Diminutive for all the Slavic names that start with *Jar-*. If for family or ethnic reasons you're seeking such a name, then this is a reasonable short form. **Janiuszck, Januarius, Januisz, Jarec, Jarrek, Jarric, Jarrick.**

JARETH. *Hybrid name.* For that rare parent who's torn between Jared and Gareth. **Jarreth, Jereth, Jarreth.**

JARMAN. *English from French* GERMAIN. A more modern-sounding alternative to Harman. **Jarmann, Jerman.**

♂ **JARON.** *Hebrew, 'to sing out'.* Not a biblical name, but one with authentic Hebrew roots that's used in Israel; would fit in with the current trend for two-syllable *J* names. **Jaaron, Jairon,** Jaran, Jaren, Jarin, Jarone, Jarran, Jarren, Jarrin, Jarron, Jaryn, Jayron, Jayronn, Je Ronn, J'ron.

JARRELL. *German variation of* GERALD. Briefly faddish a few decades ago when Darrell was cool. **Jarel, Jarell, Jarrall, Jarrel, Jerall, Jerel, Jerell.**

JARRETT. *English variation of* GARRETT. Got some notice as a Jared alternative, has musical association with pianist Keith Jarrett. **Jairett, Jairot, Jareth, Jarett, Jaretté, Jarhett, Jarratt, Jarret, Jarrett, Jarrette, Jarrot, Jarrott, Jerrett, Jerrot, Jerrott.**

JARVIS. *German, 'servant of the spear'.* One of the original two-syllable nouveau boys' names, this saint's name has a certain retro charm. **Jaravis, Jarv, Jarvaris, Jarvas, Jarvaska, Jarvey, Jarvez, Jarvie, Jarvios, Jarvious, Jarvius, Jarvorice, Jarvoris, Jarvous, Jarvus, Jary, Javaris, Jervey, Jervis.**

JAS. *(yash) Polish variation of* JOHN. Jas? No. **Jasio.**

JASON. *Hebrew, 'the Lord is salvation'.* A once popular name for the entire decade of the 1970s – thus the title of our original baby-naming book, *Beyond Jennifer & Jason* – this is more likely to be dad's name than baby's. It still hangs in, but has recently slipped out of the Top 100. **Jace, Jacen, Jaeson, Jahson, Jaisen, Jaison, Jasan, Jasaun, Jase, Jasen, Jasin, Jasson, Jasten, Jasun, Jasyn, Jathan, Jathon, Jay, Jayce, Jaysen, Jayson.**

★**JASPER.** *English variation of* CASPAR. As an unusual yet distinctly masculine name that represents a variety of quartz and is the first name of the great modern artist Jasper Johns, this has a lot going for it. Our only caveat: it's a favourite of a lot of hip parents. **Caspar, Gasper, Jas, Jaspar, Jaz, Jazper, Jespar, Jesper.**

JAVIER. *(hah-bee-AIR) Spanish variation of* XAVIER. A popular Latino choice that's embodied for some people in the magnetic persona of Spanish-born Oscar-nominated actor Javier Bardem. **Haviero, Jabier, Javer, Javere, Javi, Javiar, Javiero, Xabier, Xaverio, Zavier.**

JAVON. *Hebrew variation of* JAVAN, *'Greece'.* While the biblical Javan, the son of Japheth, is spelled with two *a*'s, the *on* version is by far the favourite among contemporary parents. Variant spellings and pronunciations abound. **Jaavon, Jaevin, Jaevon, Jaewan, Jaewon, Jahvaughan, Jahvaughn, Jahvon, Jaivon, Javante, Javaon, JaVaughan, JaVaughn, Javen, Javeon, Javian, Javien, Javin, Javine, Javion, Javionne, Javohn, Javon, Javona, Javone, Javoney, Javoni, Javonn, Javonne, Javonni, Javonnie, Javonnte, Javonte, Javoun, Jayvin, Jayvon, Jevan, Jevon.**

JAX. *Modern invented name.* The Dex-Jex-Bix type of cool – maybe too cool – variation of Jack or nickname for Jaxon or Jackson.

JAXON, JAXSON. *Spelling variations of* **JACKSON.** Many parents have decided to rev up the cool factor of Jackson and give it one of these streamlined spellings. We prefer the original. **Jaxen, Jaxsen, Jaxsin, Jaxsun, Jaxun.**

♂ **JAY.** *Latin, 'jaybird'.* Though it feels like a modern invention, Jay dates from the Middle Ages.

Now less popular than modern cousins like Jayden, Jalen and Jayce and slippind down the Top 100 though variant Jai is a hit Down Under. **Jae, Jai, Jave, Jaye, Jeays, Jeh, Jeyes.**

♂ **JAYCE.** *(jay-see) Modern invented name.* When you're choosing the single name your child will bear forever and ever, do you really want it to be one that's just a fancy form of the initials J.C.? We didn't think so. **J.C., Jace, Jacee, Jacey, Jaece, Jaecee, Jaecey, Jaecy, Jaycee.**

♂ **JAYDEN.** *Variation of* **JADON.** This popular spelling is rocketing up the Top 100 and was chosen by Britney Spears. **Jaydan, Jaydin, Jaydn, Jaydon.**

♂ **JAYLEN.** *Modern invented name.* Almost as popular as the Jalen version. Like other names with many variant spellings, when you count up all the alternatives, the name will be *much* more popular than it first appears. **Jaylaan, Jaylan, Jayland, Jayleen, Jaylend, Jaylin, Jayln, Jaylon, Jaylun, Jaylund, Jaylyn.**

♂ **JAZZ.** *Word name.* Sometimes used as a nickname for Jasper,

much more often for Jasmine or Jazlyn. Could work as a middle name. **Jaz, Jazze, Jazzlee, Jazzman, Jazzmen, Jazzmin, Jazzmon, Jazztin, Jazzton, Jazzy.**

JEAN. *(zhahn) French variation of* **JOHN.** In Paris, it's charming, but in Britain, it's still Jean, as in blue jean. **Jéan, Jeane, Jeannot, Jeano, Jeanot, Jeanty, Jene.**

★**JEB.** *Diminutive of* **JEBEDIAH.** This is a very attractive Old Testament short form, which we think will have a long and bright future. **Jebb, Jebi, Jeby.**

JEBEDIAH. *Hebrew, 'beloved friend'.* Still sporting a long white beard, but the modern-sounding Jeb solves that problem. **Jeb, Jebadia, Jebadiah, Jebadieh, Jebidia.**

★**JED.** *Diminutive of* **JEDIDIAH.** Here's a short form that's both macho and cool. It got television exposure on *The West Wing.* **Jedd, Jeddy, Jedi, Jedidiah.**

JEDAIAH. *(jeh-DI-ah) Hebrew, 'invoker of the Lord'.* More manageable than the Jebediahs and Jedidiahs, this name of several biblical characters would make an interesting, undiscovered Old Testament choice. **Jedaia, Jedaiah, Jedeiah, Jedi, Yedaya.**

JEDIDIAH. *Hebrew, 'beloved of the Lord'.* Old Testament name, with a touch of *Gunsmoke*-era western panache, that could be revived à la Jeremiah. **Jebediah,** Jed, Jedadiah, Jedd, Jeddediah, Jedediah, Jedediha, Jedidia, Jedidiah, Jedidiyah, Yedidya.

JEFF. *Diminutive of* **JEFFREY, JEFFERSON.** The ultimate dad name. **Jef, Jefe, Jeffe, Jeffey, Jeffie, Jeffy, Jhef.**

JEFFERSON. *English, 'son of Jeffrey'.* Like Harrison and Jackson, sounds more modern than its root name. **Jeferson, Jeff, Jeffers, Jeffersson, Jeffey, Jeffie, Jeffy.**

JEFFREY. *Spelling variation of* **GEOFFREY.** Yes, there actually were Jeffreys/Geoffreys in the Middle Ages . . . but now they're just middle-aged. **Geoff, Geoffry, Geofrey, Geofry, Godfrey, Jeff, Jefferey, Jefferies, Jeffre, Jeffree, Jeffrie, Jeffries, Jeffry, Jeffy, Jefre, Jefri, Jefry. International: Séafra, Siofrai** *(Irish Gaelic),* **Sheary, Sheron** *(Irish),* **Searthra** *(Scottish Gaelic),* **Joffrey** *(Scottish),* **Sieffre** *(Welsh),* **Geoffrey, Geoffroi, Geoffroy, Jeffroi, Jeoffroi** *(French),* **Jaffrez** *(Breton),* **Geofredo, Giotto** *(Italian),* **Fredo, Godofredo, Gofredo** *(Spanish),* **Friedl, Gottfried** *(German),* **Gotfryd** *(Polish),* **Frici, Gottfrid** *(Hungarian),* **Godoried** *(Romanian),* **Gotfrids** *(Latvian),* **Gitfrid** *(Russian).*

♂ **JEM.** *Diminutive of* **JAMES** *or* **JEREMIAH.** This name of the ten-year-old boy in the much loved and acclaimed modern classic *To Kill a Mockingbird* could find favour along with that of the character's sister, Scout. **Jemmie, Jemmy.**

JENKIN. *Flemish, 'little John'.* Possible (and offbeat) middle name twist when honouring a familial John. **Jenkins, Jenkyn, Jenkyns, Jennings.**

JENS. *Scandinavian variation of* **JOHANNES** *or* **JOHN.** Short but substantial Nordic name that travels well – although it runs the risk of being confused with all the feminine *Jen* names. **Jense, Jensen, Jenson, Jenssen, Jensson, Jensy, Jentz.**

JEREMIAH. *Hebrew, 'the Lord exalts'.* Old Testament prophet name that is still popular today, gradually taking the place of the overused Jeremy. **Geremiah, Jaramia, Jem, Jemeriah, Jemiah, Jemmie, Jemmy, Jer, Jeramiah, Jeramiha, Jere, Jereias, Jeremaya,**

Jeremi, Jeremial, Jeremiya, Jeremy, Jerimiah, Jerimiha, Jerimya, Jermiah, Jermyn, Jerry, Yeremia, Yeremiya, Yerenuyah. International: Hiram, Irimias *(Irish),* Jérémie *(French),* Geremia *(Italian),* Jeremias *(Spanish, Greek, Dutch, German),* Jeremia *(Swedish),* Jorma *(Finnish),* Ember, Jeremiah, Katone, Nemet *(Hungarian),* Jeramie, Jeramy, Jeremie, Jermija, Yeremy, Yerik *(Russian),* Heremias, Hieremias *(Greek).*

JEREMY. *English vernacular form of* **JEREMIAH.** The sun is setting on this recently trendy form of Jeremiah, which was popular throughout the 1970s and 80s. **Jaremay, Jaremi, Jaremy, Jem, Jemmie, Jemmy, Jer, Jerahmy, Jeramee, Jeramey, Jeramie, Jeramy, Jere, Jereamy, Jeremee, Jeremey, Jeremry, Jeremye, Jereomy, Jeriemy, Jerime, Jerimy, Jermey, Jeromy, Jerr, Jerremy, Jerrie, Jerry.**

♂ **JERICHO.** *Biblical place name.* Intriguing alternative if you want a biblical name but have rejected all the usual suspects. **Jeric, Jerick, Jericko, Jerico, Jerik, Jerric, Jerrick,** Jerrico, Jerricoh, Jerryco, Jherico.

♂ **JERMAINE.** *Variation of* **GERMAINE.** A Jackson brother name. **Germain, Germaine, Jarman, Jeremaine, Jeremane, Jerimane, Jermain, Jerman, Jermane, Jermanie, Jermanne, Jermany, Jermayn, Jermayne, Jermiane, Jermin, Jermine, Jer-Mon, Jermone, Jermoney, Jermyn, Jhirmaine.**

JEROME. *Greek, 'sacred name'.* Has a bespectacled, serious, studious image, just like its namesake saint, who was a brilliant scholar. **Gerrie, Gerry, Hierome, Hieronun, Jairo, Jairome, Jere, Jerom, Jeromo, Jeromy, Jeron, Jerrome, Jerromy, Jerron, Jerrone, Jerry.** International: **Iarom** *(Irish),* **Jereme, Jeremie, Jérôme** *(French),* **Gerome, Geronimo, Girolamo** *(Italian),* **Jerónimo** *(Spanish),* **Jeroen** *(Dutch),* **Hieronymous** *(German).*

JERRELL. *Modern variation of* **GERALD.** Yesterday's Jaylen. **Gerall, Gerrall, Jerall, Jerel, Jeril, Jeroll, Jerrill, Jerroll, Jerryll.**

JERRICK. *Variation of* **DERRICK, DEREK.** A product of the contemporary Scrabble approach to baby naming.

♂ **JERRY.** *Diminutive of* **GERALD** *or* **JEROME.** Most Jerrys are geriatric. **Gerrey, Gerry, Jehri, Jere, Jefree, Jeris, Jerison, Jerre, Jerrey, Jerri, Jerrie, Jery.**

♂ **JERSEY.** *Place name.* Neither the Channel island nor the American state should be considered, particularly for boys.

JERZY. *Polish variation of* **GEORGE.** Writer Jerzy Kosinski put this foreign variation on the map. **Jersey, Jerzey, Jurek.**

JESSE. *Hebrew, 'the Lord exists'.* King David's father turned 1980s cowboy, now way down in popularity, though still rising in Australia. **Jese, Jesee, Jesi, Jess, Jessé, Jessee, Jessie, Jessy, Yishai.**

JESTIN. *Welsh variation of* **JUSTIN.** Unusual twist – but everyone will hear it as Justin –

or jester. **Jessten, Jesten, Jeston, Jesstin, Jesston.**

JESÚS. *(hay-SOOS) Spanish variation of* **JESUS,** *from* **JOSHUA.** Used exclusively and extensively in the Latino community. **Hesús, Jechú, Jessús, Jesú, Jesulito, Jesúso, Jezús, Josú, Josue.**

JETHRO. *Hebrew, 'preeminence'.* The father-in-law of Moses but some really adventurous parents might consider updating and urbanizing its image. **Jeth, Jethroe, Jetro, Jett.**

JETT. *Mineral name.* Aviation enthusiast John Travolta put this fast-paced name in the lexicon when he chose it for his son and film producer George Lucas, of *Star Wars* fame, soon followed suit. **Jet, Jetson, Jetter, Jetty.**

♂ **JEVIN, JEVAN.** *Modern invented name.* This recent riff on the theme of Kevin has a pleasant sound but no real history or meaning.

★**JEX.** *English surname derived from* **JACQUES.** Decidedly offbeat name that combines jauntiness with sex appeal and would certainly set your son up for life outside the mainstream.

JIM. *English, diminutive of* **JAMES.** Peaked in the 1940s, but still an amiable classic, à la Joe and Tom – though rarely used on its own. **Jimbo, Jimi, Jimm, Jimmee, Jimmey, Jimmie, Jimmy, Jimson.**

JIRO. *Japanese, 'second son'.* Commonly used Japanese name – and not only for a second son.

JOAB. *Hebrew, 'praise Jehovah'.* Biblical name – of an advisor of David, who led many military victories – that's more usable than the burdened Job. **Joabe, Joaby.**

JOACHIM. *(jo-AE-kim or jo-AH-kum) Hebrew, 'God will judge'.* Another undiscovered biblical name with potential, although most modern parents would probably prefer the more lively Spanish version, Joaquin. **Jachim, Jakim, Joacheim, Jokin, Josquin, Jov.** International: **Gioachino** *(Italian),* **Joaquin**

(Spanish), **Joaquim** *(Portuguese),* **Jochim** *(German),* **Joakim, Jockum, Jokum** *(Scandinavian),* **Jáchym** *(Czech),* **Akim, Kima, Yackim** *(Russian).*

★**JOAQUIN.** *(wah-KEEN) Spanish variation of* **JOACHIM.** Actor Joaquin Phoenix (brother of River, Rain, Liberty and Summer) highlighted this one, and it's now one of the hottest multicultural choices – a mixture of Spanish and Hebrew – albeit a judgemental name. **Jehoichin, Joachín, Joachino, Joakín, Jocquinn, Jocqun, Joquin, Juaquín, Quaquín, Yoaquín.**

JOB. *Hebrew, 'the afflicted'.* We don't think any parents would want to lay the trials of Job on their son. **Joab, Jobe, Jobert, Jobey, Jobie, Joby.**

JOCK. *Scottish variation of* **JACK.** Not even if you're dying for an athlete. **Jocko, Joco, Jocoby, Jocolby.**

♂ **JODY.** *Variation or diminutive of* **JOSEPH.** Quintessentially sweet and innocent unisex name of the 1960s and 70s, now gone the way of hot pants and disco balls. **Jodey, Jodi, Jodie, Jodiha, Joedy.**

JOE. *Diminutive of* **JOSEPH.** Still the ultimate good-guy name, but slowly descending the Top 100. **Jo, Joley, Joey.**

JOEL. *Hebrew, 'Jehovah is the Lord'.* Parents a half-century ago jazzed up and formalised old standby Joe by reviving this Old Testament prophet name, and it remains steady in the Top 100. However, at this point, we're back to basics and Joe sounds much more honest and straightforward. **Joell, Joelle, Joely, Jole. International: Jöel** *(French),* **Yoel** *(Hebrew).*

JOHAN, JOHANN, JOHANNES. *(yo-hahn* or *yo-hannis) German variations of* **JOHN.** Very continental, conjuring up the image of a classical composer. **Joahan, Joan, Joannes, Johahn, Johanan, Johane, Johannan, Johanthan, Johatan, Johathan, Johathon, Johaun, Johon.**

JOHN. *Hebrew, 'the Lord is gracious'.* For centuries the most popular of all boys' names, borne by saints, kings and

John's International Variations

Irish	Eoin, Sean, Seann, Seghan
Scottish	Ian, Iain, Eòin, Seathan
Welsh	Bevan, Evan, Ieuan, Ifan, Jone, Siôn
French	Jean, Jeannot, Jehan
Breton	Yann, Yannick
Italian	Gian, Gianni, Giannini, Giovanni, Nino, Vanni
Spanish	Juan
Basque	Ion, Yon
Catalan	Joan
Portuguese	João
Dutch	Jan, Joop
German	Hans, Hansel, Johann, Johannes
Danish/Norwegian	Jens, Johan, Jan
Swedish	Johan, Jon, Jöns,
Norwegian	Jan, Jens, Johan
Finnish	Hannes, Hannu, Juhani, Jussi
Polish	Iwan, Jan, Janek, Janusz
Hungarian	Janos
Czech	Jan, Janek, Jano, Johan
Bulgarian	Ioan, Ivan

Russian	Ivan, Vanka, Vanya, Yanka
Greek	Giannis, Giannos, Ioannes, Ioannikios, Yannis
Turkish	Ohannes
Armenian	Hovhannes, Ohari
Arabic	Yahya, Yohannan
Persian	Jehan
Hawaiian	Keaka, Keoni

countless other illustrious notables. Steady in the Top 100, but many of today's baby Johns get their names for family rather than stylistic reasons. Celebrities who have gone with this timeless choice include Michelle Pfeiffer, Bono and Rob Lowe. **Jack, Jackie, Jahn, Jaxon, Jhan, Jhon, Jian, Jianni, Jock, Joen, Johan, Johne, Johnee, Johnie, Johnnie, Johnny, Johnson, Johon, Jon, Jones, Jonni, Jonnie, Jonny, Jonté, Jovanney, Jovanni, Jovonni, Juwan.**

JOHNNY. *Diminutive of* **JOHN.** The ultimate mid-century nickname, retaining a good measure of retro charm. **Jonny.**

JOHNSON. *English, 'son of John'.* No competition for Jackson. **Johnsen, Johnston, Jonson.**

★**JONAH.** *Hebrew, 'dove'.* The name of the Old Testament prophet who was swallowed by the whale is increasingly appreciated by parents looking for a biblical name less common than Jacob or Joshua – and it comes with a ready-made nursery-decorating motif. **Giona, Jona, Yonah, Yunus.**

JONAS. *Greek variation of* **JONAH.** Has a slightly more grandfatherly image than the English version, but that only adds to its retro appeal. **Jonah, Jonahs, Jonaso, Jonass, Jonaus, Jonelis, Jonukas, Jonus, Jonutis, Joonas.**

JONATHAN. *Hebrew, 'gift of Jehovah'.* Old Testament name – he was the loyal friend of King David – almost as widely used as John. Although it's just left the Top 100, it's a perenially appealing choice. **Janathan, Johnathan, Johnathon, Jon, Jonatan, Jonatha, Jonathen, Jonathin, Jonathon, Jonathun, Jonathyn, Jonethen, Jonnatha, Jonnathan, Jonnathun, Jonothan, Jonthan.**

JONES. *English surname derived from* **JOHN.** Quintessentially common last name makes distinctive first. **Joenns, Joness, Jonesy.**

JOOP. *(yoop) Dutch, diminutive of* **JOHANNES.** Has an almost comical enthusiastic feel that may not translate to this culture. **Jopie.**

JOOST. *(yoost) Dutch variation of* **JUSTUS.** Ditto.

♂ JOPLIN. *English surname related to* JOB. Musical middle name possibility for fans of Janis . . . or Scott.

♂ JORDAN. *Hebrew, 'flowing down'.* First used by Crusaders recently returned from the river Jordan; in modern times, nearly equally used for boys and girls. It's recently dropped out of the boys Top 100. Jardan, Jordae, Jordain, Jordaine, Jordane, Jordani, Jordanio, Jordann, Jordanny, Jordano, Jordany, Jordayne, Jordian, Jordin, Jordun, Jordy, Jordyn, Jori, Jorrdan, Jory, Jourdan, Jud, Judd. International: Jorden, Jordon, Jourdain *(French)*, Giordano *(Italian)*, Jordão *(Portuguese)*, Jordaan, Joord *(Dutch)*, Jarden *(Hebrew)*.

JOR-EL. *Modern invented name.* Just because Nicolas Cage gave his son Superman's birth name, Kal-el, that doesn't give you permission to use the name of Superman's father. Jorel, Jorell, Jorelle, Jorl, Jorrel, Jorrell.

JORGE. *(hor-hay) Spanish variation of* GEORGE. One of the more popular names in the Latino community. Better to stick with the English version here – it's easier for an Anglo tongue to pronounce. Jorrín.

JORGEN. *(yor-gen) Danish variation of* GEORGE. Anglicising it to a phonetic pronunciation might make it easier. Joergen, Jorgan, Jörgen.

♂ JORY. *Diminutive of Jordan.* Cute. For a girl. Joar, Joary, Jorey, Jori, Jorie, Jorrie.

JOSÉ. *Spanish variation of* JOSEPH. Another name hugely popular in the Latino population – but still rarely used by Anglos. It could be mistaken for the girl's name Josie. Cepito, Che, Cheche, Chepe, Josean, Josecito, Josee, Josefe, Joseito, Joselito, Josey, Pepe, Pepito, Pepo.

★JOSEPH. *Hebrew, 'Jehovah increases'.* One of the top boys' names for. . . . well, forever, Joseph, with its substantial Old and New Testament provenance, has more style currency these days among yuppie parents. It's currently in the Top 20. Jodi, Jodie, Jody, Joe, Joeseph, Joey, Jojo, Jopie, Jos, Josephus, Josheph, Josif, Josiff, Joss, Jozef, Jozeff.

JOSH. *A diminutive of* JOSHUA. Not as popular as the original, recently leaving the Top 100 though still in Scotland's Top 40.

JOSHUA. *Hebrew, 'the Lord is salvation'.* A Top 10 name, the biblical Joshua manages to retain a relaxed image. But with so many Joshuas born in recent years, yours would have a tough time standing out from the crowd. Jeshua, Johsua, Johusa, Josh, Joshau, Joshaua, Joshauh, Joshawa, Joshawah, Joshia, Joshu, Joshuaa, Joshuea, Joshuia, Joshula, Joshus, Joshusa, Joshuwa, Joshwa, Jousha, Joushua, Jozshua, Jushua. International: Josue *(French)*, Giosia, Giosue *(Italian)*, Joaquin *(Spanish)*, Joaquim *(Portuguese)*, Josua, Joshuah, Jozua *(Dutch)*, Josua *(German and Swedish)*, Jozsua *(Hungarian)*, Iosua *(Romanian)*, Yehoshua *(Israeli)*, Yeshua *(Yiddish)*, Yushua *(Arabic)*.

★JOSIAH. *Hebrew, 'fire of the Lord'.* A biblical name with a quaint, old-fashioned charm, would make a fresher alternative to either Joseph or Joshua,

Joseph's International Variations

Irish	Seosamh
Scottish Gaelic	Iòseph
Italian	Beppe, Giuseppe, Pino
Spanish	José, Josecito, Pepe, Pepito, Pipo
Basque	Joseba, Josoba
Catalan	Josep
German, Swedish, Dutch, Scandinavian, Polish, Czech	Josef
Finnish	Joosef, Jooseppi
Polish	Józef
Russian	Iosif, Osip
Greek	Iosif
Hebrew	Yosef
Yiddish	Yousef
Arabic	Yazid, Yusef
Japanese	Jo
Hawaiian	Iokepa, Kep
Swahili	Yusuf

combining the best of both. **Josiah, Josia, Josiahs, Josian, Josias, Josie.**

♂ **JOSS.** *English diminutive of* **JOCELIN,** *'the merry one'.* Hadn't been heard much in this country before the emergence of Joss (born Joseph) Whedon, creator of *Buffy the Vampire Slayer, Angel,* et al.; it would make a catchy middle name choice.

JOTHAM. *Hebrew, 'the Lord is upright'.* Old Testament name that would certainly be the only one in its class.

JOVAN. *Latin, 'Jove-like, majestic'; Slavic, variation of* **JOHN.** This name of the supreme Roman deity seems more extraterrestrial now – and it's also firmly attached to a perfume label. **Johvan, Johvon, Jovaan, Jovane, Jovani, Jovanic, Jovann, Jovanni, Jovannis, Jovanny, Jovany, Jovaugn, Jovaun, Joven, Jovenal, Jovenel, Jovi, Jovian, Jovin, Jovito, Jovoan, Jovon, Jovone, Jovonn, Jovonne, Jowan, Jowaun, Yovan, Yovani.**

JUAN. *Spanish variation of* **JOHN.** Second only to José in popularity among Hispanic names and familiar to all ethnicities via such references as Don and San Juan. **Juanch, Juanchito, Juane, Juanito, Juann, Juaun, Juwan.**

JUBAL. *Latin, 'joyous celebration'; Hebrew, 'ram's horn'.* A possibility for musical families: Jubal was credited in Genesis with the invention of the lyre, harp and organ. It also has a jubilant feel through its sound and meaning.

JUDAH. *Hebrew, 'praise'.* Strong, resonant Old Testament name of the eponymous ancestor of one of the tribes of Israel that owes its newfound popularity to Jude Law. **Jud, Juda, Judas, Judd, Jude.**

JUDAS. *Greek variation of* **JUDAH.** Though there were two apostles named Judas, everyone remembers the one who betrayed Jesus and the name has been permanently shunned.

JUDD. *Variation of* **JORDAN** *or* **JUDAH.** Strong but sensitive short form that can easily stand on its own. **Jud, Judson.**

★♂ JUDE. *Latin diminutive of* **JUDAH.** Hey, Jude Law, take your bow: You've erased old connections to Judas and Thomas Hardy's tragic *Jude the Obscure.* Jude recently left the Top 100. **Jud, Judah, Judas, Judd, Judsen, Judson.**

JUDGE. *Word name.* A legal-oriented word name, this could cause a lot of confusion, especially if your son ends up on the wrong side of the law.

JUDSON. *English, 'son of Jordan'.* With Hudson gaining in popularity, Judson – a possible alternative to Justin – could follow its path. **Judsen**

♂ JULES. *Latin, 'youthful'; Greek, 'soft, downy'.* Jules is way more romantic than, say, Jim. These days, though, it's more apt to be heard as a nickname for the feminine Julia or Julie. **Jewels, Joles, Jule.**

★JULIAN. *English from Latin, variation of* **JULIUS.** A rising star – picked for their sons by Jerry Seinfeld, Robert De Niro and Lisa Kudrow – Julian has overcome the somewhat pale, aesthetic image it projected in the past and become a solid, handsome, recommended choice. **Julean, Juliaan, Juliano, Julianus, Julie, Julion, Jullian, Julyan.** International: **Jolyon, Julien** *(French),* **Giuliano, Giulio** *(Italian),* **Julián, Julio** *(Spanish),* **Juià** *(Catalan),* **Jule** *(Dutch),* **Juli** *(Hungarian),* **Halian** *(Zuni).*

JULIO. *(HOO-lee-oh) Spanish variation of* **JULIUS.** What with Paul Simon's classic lyric about Julio down by the schoolyard and several distinguished bearers, this livelier Spanish version of Julius is completely familiar to the non-Hispanic community and would make a great choice for a bicultural family.

JULIUS. *Latin clan name, 'youthful'.* Immortal through its association with the ancient Caesar (it was his clan name), Julius is lagging behind Julian, but making a bit of a comeback. **Jolyon, Juie, Julas, Jule, Julen, Julian, Julias, Julie, Jullius, Juluis,**

Stellar Starbabies Beginning with *J*

Jack	Johnny Depp & Vanessa Paradis
Jackson	Susannah *(The Bangles)* Hoff, Spike Lee, Bill Murray, Patti Smith
Jacob	Robbie Fowler
Jaden	Steffi Graf & Andre Agassi, Christian Slater, Jada Pinkett Smith & Will Smith
James	Gorden Brown, Colin Farrell, Mick Jagger & Jerry Hall, Sarah Jessica Parker & Matthew Broderick
Jasper	Bryan Ferry, Don Johnson, Wynton Marsalis
Jayden	Britney Spears & Kevin Federline
Jermajesty	Jermaine Jackson
Jett	George Lucas, Kelly Preston & John Travolta
Joe	Kate Winslet & Sam Mendes
Johan	Heidi Klum & Seal
Judah	Lucy Lawless
Jude	Kelsey Grammer
Julian	Robert De Niro, Lisa Kudrow, John Lennon, Jerry Seinfeld
Junior	Jordan & Peter Andre

Yul. International: Jules, Julien *(French),* **Giulio** *(Italian),* **Julio** *(Spanish),* **Juliusz** *(Polish),* **Gyula, Juli** *(Hungarian).*

JUN. *Chinese, 'truthful'; Japanese, 'obedient, pure'.*

A spring-like Asian choice that seems possible here. **Junnie.**

Junior. *Latin, 'young'.* Don't be cruel to your son. **Jr., Junious, Junius, Junor.**

♂ **JUNIPER.** *Plant name.* We really like this name. For a girl. **International: Junipère** *(French),* **Junípero** *(Spanish).*

JUNIUS. *Latin, 'born in June'.* A combination of the least attractive elements of Junior and Julius. **June, Juneau, Junot, Junto.**

♂ **JUNOT.** *(zhoo-no) Spanish variation of* **JUNIUS.** The literati will recognise the unusual name of writer Junot Diaz.

JUPITER. *Roman mythology name.* The name of the supreme Roman deity and the largest planet probably has too hippy a feel for most mortals. **Juppiter.**

♂ **JUSTICE.** *Word name.* Parents' search for names implying virtue has led to a minirevival of this long-neglected name in both its German form, Justus and in the word itself. **Justic, Justiz, Justyc, Justyce. International: Juste, Justis** *(French),* **Justo, Justino** *(Spanish),* **Justus** *(Dutch).*

JUSTIN. *Latin, 'fair, righteous'.* This crisp British-inflected name has been widely popular in recent years, sounding fresher than choices like Jason and Jeremy, but has suffered from overexposure (just think Justin Timberlake). **Giustin, Jastin, Jaston, Jestin, Jobst, Joos, Jost, Justain, Justan, Justen, Justian, Justice, Justinian, Justinius, Justinn, Justis, Juston, Justton.** International: **Juste** *(French)*, **Giustino** *(Italian)*, **Justino, Justo, Tuto** *(Spanish)*, **Joost** *(Dutch)*, **Just, Justus** *(German)*, **Justinus** *(Swedish)*, **Inek, Justek, Justyn** *(Polish, Czech)*, **Jusa, Ustin, Yust, Yustyn** *(Czech)*, **Iustin** *(Bulgarian, Russian)*, **Justins, Justs** *(Latvian)*, **Justas, Justinas, Justukas** *(Lithuanian)*.

K *boys*

KADE. *Spelling variation of* **CADE.** A prime example of the new trend for substituting *K*'s at the beginning of traditionally *C*-starting names.

KADEEM. *Arabic, 'servant'.* A fresher alternative to the better known Kareem.

♂ KADEN. *Spelling variation of* **CADEN.** Popular member of popular family. Kadin, Kaeden, Kaiden and Kayden – along with Caden, Caiden and Cayden, as well as Cade and Kade are all variations that have been favoured by parents. **Caden, Caidan, Caiden, Caidin, Caidon, Caydan, Cayden, Caydin, Caydon, Kadan, Kadeen, Kadein, Kadin, Kadon, Kaeden, Kaedon, Kaedyn, Kaidan, Kaiden, Kaidin, Kaidon, Kaydan, Kayden, Kaydin, Kaydon, Kaydn.**

KADIR. *Arabic, 'capable'.* Deriving from Qadir (many Arabic *K* names are phonetic versions of *Q*-starting names), a classic Muslim name reflecting one of the ninety-nine attributes of Allah. **Kadar, Kedar, Qadir.**

♂ KAEDEN. *Spelling variation of* **KADEN** *or* **CADEN.** *See* **KADEN.**

♂ KAELAN. *Spelling variation of* **KELLEN.** The *ae* spelling gives the name a distinctly feminine feel.

KAHLIL. *Arabic, 'friend'; Hebrew, 'crown, garland'.* Spelled in various ways, this name was first brought into the Western consciousness by the poet Kahlil Gibran, author of *The Prophet.* **Cahil, Kaheel, Kahil, Kahleel, Kaleel, Kalil, Khaleel, Khalil.**

★**♂ KAI.** *(Kye) Hawaiian 'sea'; also Japanese, 'forgiveness'; Navajo, 'willow tree'; Scandinavian, 'earth'.* An exotic multicultural name that packs a lot of power in its single syllable, famous as the boy enchanted by the fairy-tale Snow Queen and now currently a favourite that's in the Top 100 and zooming upwards in Australia. **Kaj, Kye.** International: **Kája, Kájin** *(Czech).*

KAIDEN. *See* **KADEN.**

KAIIS. *Derivation and meaning unknown.* Geena Davis picked this ancient Roman-sounding name (which would have been spelled then with a *C*) for one of her twin boys.

KAJ. *(kye) Danish, 'earth'.* A name that looks great on paper, but is sure to be pronounced by most people to rhyme with 'raj' or, much worse, 'Madge'.

♂ **KALE.** *Modern invented name.* Whether you think of it as Cale with a *K*, or a pet form of Kalen or Kaleb, this is just the kind of short, synthetic name finding a lot of favour now, but remember – it's also the name of a vegetable.

KALEB. *Spelling variation of* **CALEB.** A modernised spelling of Caleb that is beginning to gain in popularity among parents. **Kaeleb, Kalab, Kale, Kalib, Kalob.**

♂ **KALEN.** *Modern invented name.* One of the new *K* boys' names that emerged in the 1990s, it's now slipping off the radar. **Kalan, Kalin.**

KÁLMÁN. *Hungarian variation of* **COLMAN.** One of the few stylish names, along with Roman and Truman, that end in *man*.

KAMAL. *Hindi, 'lotus'; Arabic, 'perfect, perfection'.* Two positive associations with this name: one of the ninety-nine qualities of Allah listed in the Koran and the evocative lotus flower. **Cemal, Kamaal, Kamahl, Kamali, Kameel, Kamil, Kemal.**

♂ **KAMARI.** *Meaning unknown.* A melodic name that's taking off among parents who like new-fangled choices.

♂ **KAMDEN.** *See CAMDEN.*

♂ **KAMERON.** *Spelling variation of* **CAMERON.** Now that there are more and more girl Camerons, this has become a very popular spelling for boys – as are the condensed **KAMRON** and **KAMREN.** *See CAMERON.*

KAMIL. *Arabic, 'perfect'.* Although popular in the Muslim community, this could be confused with the female Camille.

♂ **KANE.** *Celtic, 'warrior'; Welsh, 'beautiful'; Japanese, 'golden'; Hawaiian, 'man of the eastern sky'.* A name of multiple identities: a somewhat soap-operatic single-syllable surname, a homonym for the biblical bad boy Cain and, when found in Japan and Hawaii, it transforms into the two syllable *KA-neh.* **Caen, Cahan, Cahane, Cain, Kahan, Kahane, Kain, Kaine, Kayne, Keane, Keyne.**

KANIEL. *Hebrew, 'the Lord supports me'.* Unusual Daniel relative.

KANO. *Japanese, 'the god of the waters'; African place name.* Pleasing crossover possibility.

KANYE. *African place name, Tswana, 'hill of the chief'.* Rapper Kanye West's name has become popular in the USA.

KAREEM. *Arabic, 'noble, distinguished'.* A favourite Muslim name that's becoming familiar in Westernised countries. **Karam, Karem, Kareme, Karim, Karriem.**

♂ **KAREL.** *Czech variation of* **CHARLES.** A name that seems to switch genders when it switches nationalities. **Kája, Kájik, Karlík.**

♂ **KARI.** *Norse, 'puff of wind' or 'curly hair'.* In Norse mythology, the son of the giant who ruled the wind and air; in modern times, recalls a 1970s girl's nickname name, à la Carrie and Keri.

KARL. *German and Scandinavian variation of* **CHARLES.** Manly almost to the point of macho. **Carl, Kale, Karlan, Karlens, Karli, Karrel.** International: **Carlo** *(Italian)*, **Carlos** *(Spanish)*, **Karel** *(Dutch)*, **Kalle** *(Swedish)*, **Kaarle, Kaarlo** *(Finnish)*, **Karol** *(Polish)*, **Karcsi, Károly** *(Hungarian)*, **Karole** *(Russian)*.

♂ **KARSON.** *Spelling variation of* **CARSON.** An increasingly popular spelling of Carson, bringing it into the new century. **Karrson, Karsen.**

KARSTEN. *Spelling variation of* **CARSTEN.** *See CARSTEN.* **Carsten, Karstan, Karstin, Karston.**

KASE. *Spelling variation of* **CASE.** *See CASE.*

♀ **KASEY** *Spelling variation of* **CASEY.** *See CASEY.*

KASON. *Modern invented name.* Jason with a *K* or Kase with an *N* or Karson without the *R.* **Case, Kase, Kasen.**

KASPER. *Persian, 'treasurer'; Polish variation of* **CASPAR.** Initial change eliminates the ghostly aspect of the name. International: **Gaspard** *(French)*, **Gasparo** *(Italian)*, **Kaspar** *(German and Scandinavian)*.

KATO. *African, Uganda, 'second of twins'.* Infamous name of O. J. Simpson trial witness Kaelin.

KAVAN. *Breton, 'battle'.* Rarely heard and all too likely to be confused with Kevin. **Cavan, Kayvan, Kayven.**

KAVANAGH. *Irish, 'son of the monk'.* If you're looking for an Irish last name that moves beyond Casey and Cassidy, this one is pleasant sounding and worth considering. **Cavanagh, Cavanaugh, Kavanaugh.**

KAYDEN. *See KADEN.*

KAYSON. *Modern invented name.* Popped up when Jason dropped down. **Kasen, Kason, Kaysen.**

♂ **KEA.** *(KAY) Cornish, from Roman* **CAIUS.** This name of an ancient saint and one of the

first knights of King Arthur's Round Table has a modern, if feminine, feel.

♂ **KEAGAN.** *Spelling variation of* **KEEGAN.** An increasingly popular spelling of the energetic and bouncy Irish family name. **Keagen, Keaghan, Keagyn, Keegan.**

KEAN. *Spelling variation of* **KEEN** *and* **KEANE.**

KEANE. *Anglicised form of Irish Gaelic* **CIAN.** Has a sharp investigative quality that's not a bad thing to impart to a child. **Cian, Kean, Keen, Keene, Kian.**

KEANU. *Hawaiian, 'cool breeze over the mountains'.* An evocatively exotic name brought from Hawaii to the mainland by film star Keanu Reeves, who was born in Beirut to a part-Hawaiian, part-Chinese father.

★♂ **KEATON.** *English, 'where hawks fly,' 'shed town'.* An engaging surname with warmth, energy and a sense of humour. **Keatan, Keaten, Keatin, Keatton, Keatyn, Keeton, Keetun.**

Celebrity-Inspired Names

Aidan

Ashton

Cillian

Colin

Denzel

Donovan

Ewan

Harrison

Hayden

Heath

Joaquin

Jude

Keanu

Kiefer

Leonardo

Liam

Orlando

Owen

Taye

Tupac

Tyson

Vin

KEATS. *English literary name, 'kite'.* Poetic and easier to pronounce (it's *keets*) than Yeats (which is *yates*).

KEEFE. *Irish, 'handsome and noble'.* Energetic Irish surname occasionally used as a first. But will people think your little Keefe is a Keith with enunciation problems? **Keeffe.**

♂ **KEEGAN.** *Irish, 'son of Egan'.* Animated, spirited Irish surname. **Keagan, Keagen, Keegen, Keeghan, Keegon, Keegun, Kegan, Keigan.**

♂ **KEELEY.** *Irish, 'slender'.* One of the more feminine Irish surnames. **Kealey, Kealy, Keelie, Keely.**

♂ **KEEN.** *Word name.* Sharp. An appropriate name for a son whose father is a woodworker that hones the blades on his tools.

♂ **KEENAN.** *Irish, 'ancient'.* The name of three ancient saints makes an energetic choice. **Keanan, Keen, Keenen, Kenan, Kienan, Kienen. International: Cianán** *(Irish Gaelic).*

KEES. *(keys) Dutch diminutive of* **CORNELIUS.** Has a lot of charm, giving the sense of opening the door to life. **Cees, Kies.**

KEIR. *(KEE-er) Irish, 'dark, black'.* Single-syllable name that packs a lot of punch, might suggest a caring person. **Kear, Keer.**

KEIRAN. *See KIERAN.*

KEITH. *Scottish, 'wood'.* Strong, gentle Keith was cool in the 1970s but no longer.

♂ **KELBY.** *English, 'dweller at the farm by the stream'.* This British last-name-first-name could make a more masculine alternative to Shelby. **Kelbey, Kelbie, Kellby.**

KELLAM. *Modern invented name.* Definite twenty-first-century possibilities, with its stylish *K* opening, strong first syllable and softer second.

♂ **KELLEN.** *German, 'swamp'; Irish, 'slender'.* German in origin, Irish in spirit, this name is now popular among some parents. **Kelan, Kelen, Kelin, Kellan,**

Kellin, Kellon, Kellyn, Kelon, Kelyn. International: **Caolán** *(Irish Gaelic)*.

♂ **KELLY.** *Irish, 'war'.* Kelly was a perfectly acceptable, virile male name in the 1960s; by the time of *Charlie's Angels* a decade later it had become almost exclusively feminine. **Keighley, Keiley, Keilly, Keily, Kelley, Kelli, Kellie.**

♀ **KELSEY.** *English, 'island'.* Kelsey (ex-*Frasier*) Grammer aside, this is an almost completely feminine name. **Kelcy, Kelsie, Kelso, Kelsy.**

KELSO. *Scottish place name.* This name of a town in Scotland has more vitality – and is more boyish – than the feminised Kelsey.

KELTON. *English, 'town of the keels'.* This unusual two-syllable *K* name relates to ship-building. **Keldon, Kelltin, Kellton, Kelten, Keltin, Keltonn.**

KELVIN. *Scottish river name.* Kevin-Melvin hybrid cloned in the 1920s and still alive. **Kellven, Kelvan, Kelven, Kelvon,** Kelvyn, Kelwin, Kelwinn, Kelwyn.

KEMUEL. *Hebrew, 'helper of God'.* If you're seeking a biblical name somewhat similar to the popular Samuel but way more distinctive, this could be the one.

KEN. *Diminutive of* **KENNETH.** Permanently wed to Barbie.

♂ **KENDAL, KENDALL.** *English, 'valley of the river Kent'.* This English Lake District beauty spot makes a better choice for a girl. **Ken, Kendal, Kendel, Kendell.**

KENDRICK. *English and Scottish, 'royal ruler, champion'.* Harsh name that found some favour in the last couple of decades, less so now. **Kendric, Kendricks, Kendrik, Kendrix, Kendryck, Kenrick, Kenricks, Kenrik.**

KENELM. *English, 'brave helmet, protection'.* One of the least known of the *Ken* names – for good reason. **Kenhelm, Kennelm.**

KENJI. *Japanese, 'second son'.* One of several Japanese names that refer to a child's place in the family birth order.

KENN. *Welsh, 'bright water'.* Occult name for babies born under water signs – Pisces, Cancer and Scorpio.

♂ **KENNEDY.** *Irish, 'misshapen head'.* This has become such a trendy name for girls in recent years that its manpower has diminished, despite its obvious tie to the popular American president and the once-shining image of Camelot. **Canaday, Canady, Kennedey.**

KENNETH. *English, 'born of fire, handsome'.* It may sound lacklustre now, but Kenneth had its moments of glory as the first king of Scotland, a Sir Walter Scott hero and a Top 20 name from the 1920s through the 1950s. **Ken, Keneth, Kennith, Kenny, Kennyth. International: Kennet, Kennett, Kent** *(Scandinavian).*

KENNY. *Diminutive of* **KENNETH.** Believe it or not, there were more baby boys christened Kenny last year than there were Kadins or Kolbys.

KENT. *English surname and place name, 'edge'.* No-nonsense, brief, brisk one-syllable name, almost as curt as Kurt. **Kennt, Kentt.**

KENTON. *English, 'the royal settlement'.* Although it has the trendy *K* beginning and *on* ending and a jazz reference to Stan Kenton, it still manages to sound stiff and old-fashioned. **Kentan, Kentin, Kenton.**

♂ **KENYA.** *African place name, Russian diminutive.* A bold, evocative and meaningful east-central African place name. **Kenyatta.**

♂ **KENYATTA.** *African hero name.* Used to honour Jomo Kenyatta, the first president of the independent Kenyan republic.

★**KENYON,** *English, 'white-haired or blond'.* A very engaging British surname name and the middle *y* gives it a kind of canyonesque undertone. **Kenyan.**

KENZO. *Japanese, 'strong and healthy'.* This common Japanese name has several creative bearers – the single-named fashion designer, prize-winning architect Kenzo Takada and painter Kenzo Okada.

KEON. *Modern invented name, variation of* **KIAN.** This neo-name has been chosen by parents for a decade and a half, following in the wake of cousin Kiana. **Keion, Keonn, Keyawn, Keyon, Kion, Kionn, Kyan, Kyon.**

KERMIT. *Irish, 'son of Dermot'.* If it wasn't for the powerful Muppet connection, this would make an ideal choice.

KEROUAC. *Breton literary name.* Modern literary inspiration, from *On the Road* author Jack.

♂ **KERR.** *Scottish, 'someone who lived near wet ground'.* When this surname name entered the scene, there was a debate over it's pronunciation. *Car* or *Ker?* Your choice.

♂ **KERRY.** *Irish, 'dark, dark-haired'.* An Irish county name almost exclusively used for girls now. Kerrigan would be a more modern and masculine choice. **Keary, Kerrey, Kerrie, Kerrigan.**

KESEY. *Irish literary name, variation of* **CASEY.** A possible literary hero name honouring Merry Prankster Ken Kesey, whose characters flew over the cuckoo's nest.

KEVIN. *Irish, 'handsome'.* Even though Kevin is almost as popular as it was fifteen years ago, Kevin seems more a young man's than a baby's name these days. **Keaven, Kev, Kevan, Keve, Keveen, Keven, Keveon, Kevian, Kevien, Kevinn, Kevn, Kevon, Kevonne, Kevvy, Kevyn, Keyvan, Keyvon, Kivon, Kyven.**

KEYON. *English, 'guide, leading'.* This rising name, possibly a variation of the Irish Kian, has been associated with several accomplished athletes.

KEYSHAWN *Modern invented name.* One of the most popular of the creative spellings of this name. **Kayshaune, Keeshaan, Keeshaun, Keeshaune, Keeshawn, Keeshon, Kesean, Keshaan, Keshaun, Keshaune, Keshawn, Keshon, Keyshaan, Keyshaun.**

KHALÍL. *Arabic, 'friend'.* One of several similar names well used in the Muslim community. **Kahlil, Kaleel, Kalil, Khahlil, Khailil, Khailyl, Khaleel, Khaleil.**

KIAN *(KEE-ahn) Irish, variation of* **CIAN.** Friendly Irish name chosen for one of her twin boys by Geena Davis and in the Top 100. **Kayan, Kayen, Kyan, Kyen.**

KIEFER. *German, 'barrel maker'.* An occupational name made famous by actor Kiefer Sutherland. **Keefer, Kiefert, Kieffer, Kieffner, Kiefner, Kuefer, Kueffner.**

KIER. *Diminutive of* **KIERAN,** *alternate spelling of* **KEIR.** *See* **KEIR.**

★♂ **KIERAN.** *Irish, 'little dark one'; Anglicised variation of* **CIARÁN.** Long popular in Ireland and England, this name of Ireland's firstborn saint has just slipped out of the Top 50. Strong and attractive, with a fashionable Irish brogue, its only drawback is confusion with such female choices as Karen and Kyra. **Keiran, Keiren, Keirnon, Keiron, Kiaron, Kiarron, Kier, Kieren, Kierian, Kierien, Kiernan, Kieron, Kierr, Kierre, Kierron, Kyran. International: Ciarán** *(Irish Gaelic).*

KILLIAN. *Irish, 'war strife' or 'church'.* A spirited yet resonant Gaelic surname that was borne by several Irish saints and could make a distinctive replacement for the feminised Kelly. Possible downsides an unsavoury first syllable. **Cillian, Kilean, Kilian, Kilien, Killie, Killiean, Killien, Killion, Killy.**

♂ **KIM.** *English, diminutive of* **KIMBALL.** Forever feminised, despite memories of the Rudyard Kipling character.

♂ **KIMBALL.** *Welsh, 'warrior chief'.* Unlikely choice, since its short form's been co-opted by the girls. **Kim, Kimbal, Kimbel, Kimbell, Kimble.**

Irish Names That Aren't Overused

Baird

Beacán *(BEH-kan)*

Cian *(keen)*

Carbry

Colm

Conall

Cormac

Declan

Duff

Eamon *(AY-mun)*

Egan

Jarlath

Keegan

Keir *(care)*

Killian

Laughlin *(lauf-lin)*

Lucan

Malachy

Ronan

Tiernan

Tierney

Tully

KING. *English, 'monarch'.* While some might think of it as more fitting for a canine, others see it as a strong name with offbeat style and a full court of rich associations, from Dr Martin Luther King Jr to Elvis.

KINGSLEY. *English, 'king's meadow'.* Haughty.

KINGSTON. *English place name.* Chosen by Gwen Stefani and Gavin Rossdale, this Jamaican place and elegant British surname also boasts the more regal yet user-friendly short form, King.

KIPP. *English, 'pointed hill'.* Full name that sounds more like a short form; more likely to be spelled Kip. **Kip, Kipper, Kyp.**

♂ **KIRAN.** *Sanskrit, 'ray of light'* Though it sounds like a modern invention, or even an Irish name, Kiran is a traditional Hindu name from India.

♂ **KIRBY.** *Norse, 'church settlement'.* Attractive British place name with a sense of humour. Fun fact: John Wayne played five characters with the first or second name of Kirby. **Kerbey, Kerbie, Kerby, Kirbey, Kirbie, Kirkby.**

KIRK. *Norse, 'church'.* Far more friendly and open than similar one-syllable names like Kent, Kurt and Karl, it's been associated for more than half a century with actor Kirk Douglas. **Kerk, Kirke.**

♂ **KIT.** *English, diminutive of* **CHRISTOPHER.** Nickname occasionally used on its own, has a bit of a western twang thanks to Kit Carson. Actress Jodie Foster used it for her son. **Kitt.**

♂ **KITO.** *(KEE-to) Swahili, 'precious jewel'.* An energetic African name that verges on the canine.

KITTO. *Cornish, diminutive of* **CHRISTOPHER.** Sounds a bit like a board game.

KLAUS. *German variation of* **CLAUS,** *diminutive of* **NICOLAS.** Two drawbacks: some unpleasant World War II associations and the Santa clause. **Claus, Klaas, Klaes.**

♂ **KLEE.** *(clay) Swiss artist name.* The whimsical quality of the work of Swiss artist Paul Klee is somehow reflected in his name, although many would mispronounce it to rhyme with *key.*

KLEMENS. *German and Swedish variation of* **CLEMENT.** Soft, gentle and non-Germanic, but the final *s* almost makes it sound plural. **Clemens. International: Kliment** *(Russian).*

KNUT. *(noot) Old Norse, 'knot'.* The *K* is silent in this royal but common Scandinavian name that is in most other countries unknown. It could easily be confused with Newt. **Canute, Cnut, Knute. International: Knud** *(Danish).*

KOBE. *Swahili, 'tortoise'.* An African name that sounds like it could also be Japanese, makes a possible multicultural choice. It also sounds similar to Koby.

KOBY. *Polish, diminutive of* **JACOB.** More distinctive nickname for Jacob than the ubiquitous Jake. **Cobe, Cobi, Cobie, Coby, Kobe, Kobey, Kobi, Kobie, Koby.**

KODA. *Japanese surname.* This Japanese last-name-first-name has become popular among some parents elsewhere.

KODY. *Spelling variation of* CODY. More and more parents are choosing to use this trendier spelling of Cody.

KOFI. *African, Twi, 'born on Friday'.* This African day name is very much associated with the Ghanaian Kofi Annan, the seventh secretary general of the United Nations.

KOJO. *Ghanaian, 'born on Monday'.* The Ashantis of Ghana traditionally use this animated name for boys born on Monday.

KOLBY. *See COLBY.*

KOLE. *See COLE.*

KOLTON. *See COLTON.*

KOLYA. *Russian, diminutive of* NIKOLAI. Could be seen as an affectionate continental take on Kole.

KONNER, KONNOR. *See CONNOR.*

KONRAD. *See CONRAD.*

KORBEN, KORBIN. *See CORBIN.*

♂ **KOREN.** *Hebrew, 'gleaming'.* An unusual, sensitive and gently attractive Hebrew name.

♂ **KOREY.** *Spelling variation of* COREY. *See COREY.* **Korrey, Korry, Kory.**

KORT. *Dutch, variation of* KURT. *See KURT.* **Cort.**

KOSTYA. *Russian, diminutive of* KONSTANTIN. An accessible Russian nickname . . . but could 'cost ya'.

♂ **KRISHNA.** *Sanskrit, 'dark, black'.* The name of the supreme Hindu god is still considered secular enough for mortal children and is often found in Hindu families.

KRISTIAN. *Danish and Greek variation of* CHRISTIAN. *See*

CHRISTIAN. **Khristos, Kit, Kris, Krist, Kristan, Kristien.**

KRISTOF. *Slavic variation of* CHRISTOPHER. Attractive attenuated form of the popular Christopher, well used on the Continent, appearing as **Christophe** in France and

---

Names That Mean Handsome

Adonis

Alan

Ara

Beal

Beau

Bellamy

Bello

Cavan

Hassan

Hassim

Jamal

Jamil

Keefe

Keeley

Kenneth

Kevin

Kyle

Christoph in Germany. **Kristoff, Krystof, Krystoff.**

KRISTOFFER. *Scandinavian variation of* **CHRISTOPHER.** This Scandinavian spin on Christopher gives that enduring classic a lighter, more individual twist. **Kristof, Kristofer, Kristoff, Kristofor, Kristopher, Krystof, Krystopher.**

KRISTOPHER. *Greek variation of* **CHRISTOPHER.** *See* **CHRISTOPHER.** **Khristopher, Kit, Kris, Krisstopher, Kristapher, Kristepher, Kristfer, Kristfor, Kristof, Kristofer, Kristoffer, Tophe, Topher.**

KUMAR. *Sanskrit, 'a boy, a son'.* Exotic name often heard in India.

KURT. *German, diminutive of* **KURTIS** *or* **KONRAD.** A name that defines itself. **Curt.** International: **Kort** *(Dutch).*

KWAME. *African, Ghanaian, 'born on Saturday'.* A popular name among the Akan of Ghana, especially for boys born on Saturday.

KWAN. *Korean, 'strong'.* An Asian name that would be easily understood in this country.

KYAN. *Modern invented name.* A quintessential twenty-first-century name, a twist on the twentieth-century standard Ryan, used by an increasing numbers of parents.

KYD. *English surname.* Téa Leoni and David Duchovny named their kid Kyd Miller, but the little boy is usually called by his middle name – a wise choice.

KYLAN. *Modern invented name.* A new-style name based on Kyle and a cousin of Dylan, in spelling if not sound or image.

♂ **KYLE.** *Scottish, 'narrow spit of land'.* Still appreciated by many parents each year for its combination of simplicity, strength and style, Kyle remains popular and is in the Top 50. **Kilan, Kile, Kilen, Kiley, Ky, Kye, Kylan, Kylar, Kylen, Kyler, Kyll, Kyrell.**

KYLER. *Dutch, 'bowman, archer'.* A favourite among younger parents, this is one of the names that rose to the surface when Tyler and Kyle started to sink. **Cuyler, Kylor.**

KYNASTON. *English, 'royal peace settlement'.* A dignified yet gentle surname name occasionally heard in England and the West Indies.

L *boys*

LABAN. *Hebrew, 'white'.* An Old Testament name used by the Puritans, less well known than female relatives Rebecca, Rachel and Leah and as deserving of revival. **Labe, Labon, Laeb, Lavan, Lebaan, Leban. International: Liban** *(Hawaiian).*

LACHLAN. *(LAHK-lan) Scottish, 'belligerent' or 'from the fjord-land'.* Scottish favourite used through the British world: it's made Number 1 in Australia. **Lache, Lachlann, Lachunn, Lakelan, Lakeland.**

LACROSSE. *French, 'the cross'.* Could be used by fans of the game, but it is far from the easiest of names to carry.

LADD. *English, 'manservant, young man'.* Seems like a redundant name for a lad. **Lad, Laddey, Laddie, Laddy.**

LAEL, LA'EL. *Hebrew, 'belonging to God'.* Although this is an ancient Old Testament name, it has a contemporary feel that might appeal to parents.

LAFAYETTE. *French, 'faith'.* Foppish name with a distinguished forebear, French general Marquis de Lafayette, who fought for the Americans during their Revolution. It accounts for the *L* in L. Ron Hubbard. Not bound to be a popular boy's name here. **Lafaiete, Lafayett, Lafette, Laffyette.**

LAIRD. *Scottish, 'lord of the land'.* Scottish title for wealthy landowners, with a pleasantly distinctive Scottish burr that must have appealled to Sharon Stone, who chose it for her son.

♂ **LAKE.** *Nature name.* Evocative modern choice that feels a bit feminine for a boy. **Laike, Laiken, Laikin, Laken, Lakon. International: Lac** *(French),* **Lago** *(Spanish).*

♂ **LAKOTA.** *Native American tribal name.* Would work better for a girl. **Lakoda.**

LAMAR. *English from French, 'dweller by a pool'.* Surname borne by several famous athletes. **Lamair, Lamario, Lamaris, Lamarr, Lamarre, Larmar, Lemarr. International: Lemar** *(French).*

LAMBERT. *German, 'land brilliant'.* Ancient saint's name. **Bert, Lambard, Lambart, Lamberto, Lambirt, Lampard, Landbert.**

LAMONT. *Scandinavian, 'man of law'.* Not heard much elsewhere. **Lamaunt, Lamond, Lamonta, Lamonte, Lamontie, Lamonto, Lamount, Lemond, Lemont.**

LANCASTER. *English place name.* British place name unlikely to evoke much passion in any baby namer. **Lancashire, Lancester, Lanchester, Lankester.**

LANCE. *Diminutive of* **LANCELOT***; also word name.* Despite the heroic achievements

Writers' Names

Anaïs
Austen
Ayn
Beckett
Brontë
Carson
Cheever
Colette
Cormac
Dashiell
Djuna
Ellison
Fitzgerald
Flannery
Harper
Kerouac
Langston
Márquez
Paz
Poe
Salinger
Truman
Willa
Zadie
Zane
Zora
Zola

of astronaut Lance Armstrong, has a rather limp-wristed image. **Lancy, Lantz, Launce. International: Lanz** *(Italian).*

LANCELOT. *French, 'servant'.* Dashing Knight of the Round Table who seduced Queen Guinevere: romantic story but overly romantic, too-loaded name. **Lance, Lancelott, Launcelet, Launcelot.**

LANDER. *English from German, 'territory'.* Possibility in the Landon vein. **Land, Landers, Landis, Landiss, Landor, Landry.**

LANDO. *Portuguese and Spanish diminutive of* **ORLANDO, ROLANDO.** Lively nickname, but we'd prefer the more substantial Orlando.

LANDON. *English, 'grassy plain'.* A surname name that's recently become popular among parents in some places. **Land, Landan, Landen, Landin, Landyn.**

♂ **LANDRY.** *French and English, 'ruler'.* Too redolent of laundry. **Landre, Landré, Landrue.**

♂ **LANE.** *English, 'a small roadway or path'.* A name that could be used for either gender, but is much more popular for boys. Metallica's Lars Ulrich used the Layne spelling for his son. **Laine, Laney, Lanie, Layn, Layne, Laynee.**

LANFORD. *English, 'narrow way'.* Surname choice that could be used to honour the playwright Lanford Wilson.

LANGDON. *English, 'long hill'.* Classy-sounding surname name usually bypassed in favour of the simpler Landon. **Landon, Langden, Langsdon, Langston.**

♂ **LANGLEY.** *English, 'long meadow'.* Might lead to teasing if your son grows up to be tall and thin. **Langlea, Langlee, Langleigh, Langly.**

LANGSTON. *English, 'tall man's town'.* African-American writer Langston Hughes puts this one on the map; actor Laurence Fishburne adopted it for his son. **Langsden, Langsdon, Langton.**

♂ **LANIER.** *French occupational name, 'wool worker'.* The fashionable occupational last name category gets some French flair with this, Tennessee Williams's middle name.

♂ **LARAMIE.** *French, 'canopy of leafy boughs'; Wyoming place name.* Swaggering American place name with a lot of bravado and panache. **Larami, Laramy, Laremy.**

LARDNER. *Occupational name, 'servant in charge of a larder'.* The surname name is a new entry in the trendy occupational class – but watch the *lard.*

LAREDO. *Place name.* Like Laramie, an unexplored place name with a twang.

LARKIN. *Irish, 'rough, fierce'.* The additional syllable makes Lark a masculine surname name. **Larklin.**

LARRY. *Diminutive of* **LAWRENCE.** Your friendly next-door neighbour . . . not your baby.

★**LARS.** *Scandinavian variation of* **LAURENCE.** A perfect candidate for a cross-cultural passport: Lars has been heard often enough here to sound familiar and friendly, yet it retains the charisma of a charming foreigner. **Laris, Larris, Larse, Larsen, Larson, Larsson, Larz, Lasse, Laurans, Laurits, Lavrans, Lorens.**

♂ **LASHAWN.** *American, a combination of the prefix La- and* **SHAWN.** The prefix *La-* was historically used by the Free Blacks of New Orleans in the nineteenth century to indicate paternity. Thus, someone named Lashawn was the son of Shawn. **Lasaun, Lasean, Lashajaun, Lashan, Lashane, Lashaun, Lashon, Lashun.**

LASZLO. *Hungarian, 'famous ruler'.* Intriguing name with *Casablanca* overtones. **Laci, Lacko, Laslo, László, Lazlo.**

LATHAM. *Scandinavian, 'the barn'.* Familiar surname with a surprising meaning. **Laith, Lathe, Lathom, Lay.**

LATIF. *Arabic, 'gentle, kind'.* Classic Muslim name representing one of the ninety-nine attributes of Allah; Queen Latifah has drawn attention to the feminine form of the name. **Lateef.**

LAUGHLIN. *(lauf-lin) Irish, 'dweller at the fjord-land'.* First used for Norse invaders, this name, along with the similar Lachlan, is an attractive, exotic and unusual choice. **Lanty, Lauchlin, Leachlainn, Loughlin.**

♂ **LAURENCE.** *Spelling variation of* **LAWRENCE.** Spelling refines but doesn't update original. Great option, though, for girls. **Lanny, Lauran, Laurance, Laureano, Lauren, Laurencho, Laurentiu, Laurentius, Laurentz, Laurentzi, Laurie, Laurin, Laurits, Laurnet, Laurus, Lurance. International: Laurent** *(French),* **Laurencio** *(Spanish),* **Laurens** *(Dutch),* **Lauris** *(Swedish),* **Lauro** *(Filipino).*

LAURENT. *(law-RAHNT) French variation of* **LAWRENCE.** A French accent makes almost everything sound better. **Laurentin.**

LAWRENCE. *Latin, 'from Laurentium'.* Has survived from Roman times, when Laurentium was a city noted for its laurel trees. One of the favourite names from the 1890s through the 1950s and still popular for decades longer, but now used less for babies than Landon or Lorenzo. Nickname Lauro perks it up. **Lanny, Lanty, Larance, Laranz, Laren, Larenz, Larian, Larien, Laris, Larka, Larrance, Larrence, Larrens, Larrey, Larry, Lary, Larya, Laurance, Lauren, Laurence, Laurentios, Laurentius, Laurenz, Laurie, Laurits, Lavrans, Lavrens, Lavrenti, Law, Lawerence, Lawrance, Lawren, Lawrey, Lawrie, Lawron, Lawry, Lena, Lencho, Lon, Lonnie, Lonny, Loran, Loreca, Loren, Lorence, Lorene, Lorentz, Lorenzen, Lorin, Loritz, Lorn, Lorne, Lorrence, Lorrenz, Lorrie, Lorry, Lourenco, Lowrance.** International: **Labhras, Lochlann, Lorcan** *(Irish),* **Laurent** *(French),* **Lorenzo, Renzo** *(Italian),* **Laurencio, Lorenzo** *(Spanish),* **Laudalino, Laurencho, Lorenco, Lourenco** *(Portuguese),* **Laurens** *(Dutch),* **Lorenz** *(German, Danish and Polish),* **Lauritz, Lorens** *(Danish),* **Lars,** Larse, Laurans, Lorens *(Swedish and Danish),* **Lauri** *(Finnish),* **Inek** *(Polish),* **Lenci, Lorant, Lornic** *(Hungarian),* **Brencis, Labrencis, Labrentsis, Larka, Larya, Lavr, Lavrik, Lavro** *(Latvian).*

LAWSON. *English, 'son of Lawrence'.* Appealing way, à la Dawson, to honour an ancestral Lawrence. **Lawsen, Layson.**

♂ **LAWYER.** *Occupational name.* One professional surname that won't do in a legal family.

LAYNE. *See LANE.*

♂ **LAZARUS.** *Greek variation of Hebrew ELIAZAR.* Name that could possibly be raised from the dead, like its Biblical bearer. **Eleazer, Lazar, Lázár, Lazarillo, Lazarius, Lazaros, Lazear, Lazer, Lazorus, Lazzaro.** International: **Lazare** *(French),* **Lazaro** *(Italian),* **Lázaro** *(Spanish).*

♂ **LEAF.** *Nature name.* If you must, spell it Leif and claim you're Norwegian.

LEANDER. *Greek, 'lion-man'.* Heroic name from Greek myth that adventurous parents might want to consider, gingerly, as an alternative to the overused Alexander. **Ander, Leandres, Leanther, Lee, Leiandros, Leo, Liander, Liandro.** International: **Léon, Léandre** *(French),* **Leandro** *(Italian and Spanish),* **Leandros** *(Greek).*

♂ **LEARY.** *Irish, Anglicisation of LAOGHAIRE, 'herder'.* We'd be leery of this one.

L**E**BRON, LEBRUN. *French, 'brown-haired one'.* Not that many boys have borne this name outside of France. **Labron, Labrun.**

LECH. *(lek) Polish, 'a Pole'.* Lech (brother of Czech and Rus) was the mythical father of the Poles and also the name of the Polish worker-president Lech Walesa, but it still isn't a name that travels well. **Leszek.**

♂ **LEE.** *English, 'pasture, meadow'.* A name with a feeble shouldn't-I-be-a-middle-name? image. **Lea, Leigh.**

♂ **LEGEND.** *Word name.* A word name possibility with a nice story-telling quality.

LEIB. *(leeb) Yiddish, 'roaring lion'.* Appealing name because, in German and Yiddish, it also means 'dear'. **Leibel.**

LEIF. *(leef or layf) Scandinavian, 'heir, descendant'.* One of the most widely known Scandinavian names, thanks to Norwegian explorer Leif Ericsson and still one of the best, with a pleasant association with the word *leaf*. **Laif, Leife, Lief.**

♂ **LEIGHTON.** *(LAY-ton) English, 'meadow settlement'.* Not as hardy as Haden-Caden cousins. **Lay, Layton, Leigh, Leyton.**

♂ **LEITH.** *Scottish, 'broad'.* Unusual Scottish surname that might serve as a possible alternative to the ageing Keith, but it's a little tough on the tongue.

♂ **LELAND.** *English, 'meadow land'.* Although last had its day in the 1920s, it seems to be coming back to life. **Lealand, Lee, Leeland, Leigh, Leighland, Lelan, Lelann, Lelend, Lelund, Leyland.**

★**LEMUEL.** *Hebrew, 'devoted to God'.* Unjustly neglected Old Testament option for those who've known too many Samuels. **Lem, Lemmie, Lemmy.**

★♂ **LENNON.** *Irish, 'small cloak or cape'.* A growing number of high-profile (and other) parents are choosing to honour their musical idols: Presley, Jagger, Dylan – and Lennon. **Lenan, Lenen, Lenin, Lennan, Lennen, Lennin, Lennyn, Lenon, Lenyn.**

★**LENNOX.** *Scottish, 'with many elm trees'.* An aristocratic and powerful surname name made truly special by that final *x*. **Lennix, Lenox.**

★**LEO.** *Latin, 'lion'.* A strong-yet-friendly name common among the Romans, used for thirteen popes, that is rising up the Top 50, partly via the Leonardo fallout factor. **Lee, Leib, Leibel, Léo, Leon, Leond, Lion, Lyon. International: Leone, Leonello, Leonzio** *(Italian),* **Leão** *(Portuguese),* **Lev** *(Russian),* **Leos** *(Slavic),* **Lio** *(Hawaiian).*

LEON. *Greek variation of* **LEO.** Steady in the Top 100 and hot

in Germany. **Leonas, Leoncio, Leondris, Leone, Leonek, Leonetti, Leoni, Leonidas, Leonirez, Leonizio, Leonon, Leons, Leontes, Leontios, Leontrae, Lioni, Lionisio, Lionni, Liutas. International: Léon, Léonce** *(French),* **Leone, Leonzio** *(Italian),* **Leoncio** *(Spanish),* **Leo** *(German),* **Leonid** *(Russian),* **Leonti, Leos** *(Slavic).*

LEONARD. *German, 'brave lion'.* Medieval saint's name – he's the patron of prisoners – now popular only in Leo and Leonardo forms. **Leanard, Lee, Lena, Lenn, Lennerd, Lennie, Lenny, Leno, Leo, Léonard, Leonardis, Leonart, Leonerd, Leondaus, Leone, Leoperd, Leonides, Leonis, Leonnard, Leontes, Lernard, Lienard, Linek, Lon, Lonard, Londard, Lonnard, Lonny, Lonya, Lynnard. International: Leonardo, Lionzio** *(Italian),* **Leonardo** *(Spanish),* **Len, Lenard, Lennard, Leonhard** *(German),* **Lennart** *(Swedish),* **Leonid** *(Russian),* **Leonti, Leos** *(Slavic),* **Leon, Leonida, Leonidas, Leonides** *(Greek).*

LEONARDO. *Italian and Spanish variation of*

Cool Middle Names

Cruz

Flynn

Fox

Green

Heath

Lars

Levi

Lincoln

March

Miles

Oak

Smith

Thor

West

Zane

LEONARD. There's one reason this version is on the rise: Leonardo DiCaprio. He was supposedly given the name because his pregnant mother felt a kick while looking at a da Vinci painting.

LEONID. *Russian, 'son of a lion'.* This form got noticed as the first name of Russian president Brezhnev; it's unlikely to join the pride of lion-related names here. **Lyenya, Lyeka.**

LEOPOLD. *German, 'brave people'.* This European royal name might appeal if you want to move way beyond Oscar and Gus. **Leo, Leorad, Leupold, Lopolda, Luepold, Poldi. International: Léopold** *(French),* **Leopoldo** *(Italian and Spanish),* **Luitpold** *(German).*

LEROY. *French, 'the king'.* A name that's a joke in England but a fashion hit in Germany. **Elroi, Elroy, Lee, Leeroy, LeeRoy, Leigh, Lerai, Leroi, LeRoi, LeRoy, Roy.**

♂ **LESLIE.** *Scottish, 'garden by the pool'.* Plunging as a boy's name even as its popularity for girls begins to rise once again. **Lee, Leigh, Les, Leslea, Leslee, Lesley, Lesli, Lesly, Lezlie, Lezly.**

LESTER. *English place name; phonetic form of* **LEICESTER.** Has gone the way of Hester, Esther and Sylvester: an anorak name. **Leicester, Les.**

LEV. *(leev) Hebrew, 'heart'; Russian and Czech, 'lion'.* This concise one-syllable form of Leo has definite potential. **Leb, Leva, Levka, Levko, Levushka, Lyeka, Lyenya, Lyeva.**

★**LEVI.** *Hebrew, 'joined, attached'.* Lighter and more energetic than most biblical names, with its up vowel ending; combines Old Testament gravitas with the casual flair associated with Levi Strauss jeans. Now being rediscovered in a major way. **Leavi, Leevi, Leevie, Lev, Levey, Levie, Levin, Levitis, Levon, Levy, Lewi, Leyvi.**

LEVITICUS. *Greek, 'belonging to the Levites'.* Old Testament book way too heavy to carry.

LEWIS. *English variation of* **LOUIS.** This more formal and phonetic spelling of the French Louis is the Number two name in Scotland and in the Top 25 in England and Wales. **Lew, Lewes, Lewie, Lewy, Lou, Louis.**

LEX. *English, diminutive of* **ALEXANDER.** Trendy short form of Alexander; like all the names that rhyme with sex, it has a seductive edge. **Lexi, Lexie, Lexin.**

♂ **LEXUS.** *Greek variation of a diminutive of* **ALEXIS.** Do you really want to name your baby after a car when there are so many other *lex* possibilities? **Lexis.**

LIAM. *Irish variation of* **WILLIAM.** Actor Liam Neeson was instrumental in driving his name up the Top 50. It's both jaunty and richly textured, but now feels a tad trendy. **Liem, Lliam, Lyam.**

LIBERATO. *Spanish and Portuguese, 'freedom'.* An offbeat way to celebrate this virtue. **Liberato, Liberaratore, Liberatus, Liberto. International: Liborio** *(Spanish).*

♂ **LIGHT.** *Word name.* A shimmering day name in the old African tradition, with a bit of hippy residue.

★**LINCOLN.** *English, 'town by the pool'.* This place name with a two-syllable sound (and the name of the honest US president) has a stylish image

and the cool nickname Linc. Bill Murray is father to a son named Lincoln. **Linc, Lincon, Link, Lyncoln.**

♂ **LINDSAY.** *English, 'island of linden trees'.* The girls have definitely filched this one out of the male box. **Lind, Lindesay, Lindsee, Lindsey, Lindsie, Lindsy, Lindy, Lindzy, Linsay, Linsey, Linzie, Linzy, Lyndsay, Lyndsey, Lyndsie, Lynzie.**

LINK. *Word name or diminutive of* **LINCOLN.** Here is a groovy name that still sounds retro cool.

LINTON. *English, 'flax settlement'.* In *Wuthering Heights,* Cathy's milquetoast husband; Heath is so much more appealing. **Lintonn, Lynton, Lyntonn.**

★**LINUS.** *Greek, 'flax'.* The mythological Linus taught music to Hercules and Orpheus – an inspired background for a melodic name, and a suitable choice for a son born into a musical family. **Linas, Lino, Linux.**

★**LIONEL.** *Latin, 'young lion'.* Jazzy name and daring choice. **Lional, Lionell, Lionnell, Lionnello, Lynel, Lynnell, Lyinell, Lyonel, Lyonelo, Lyonnel, Lyonnell, Lyonnello. International: Leonel, Leonello, Leonila, Linnel, Lio, Lionello, Lionellu, Lionnel, Lyonell** *(French),* **Leonel** *(Spanish).*

LITTON. *English, 'settlement on the hill'.* Slightly less stiff and small if spelled Lytton. **Liton, Litten, Littonn, Lytten, Lytton.**

LIVINGSTON. *English, 'dear friend's place'.* Will grow up using phrases like 'I presume'. **Livingsten, Livingstin, Livingstone.**

LLEWELLYN. *Welsh, 'resembling a lion'.* A common first name in Wales, with its distinctive Welsh double *LL*'s; would make a daring choice, though some might find the *ellen* sound slightly feminine. **Lew, Lewellen, Lewellyn, Lewis, Llewelin, Llewellen, Llewelleyn, Llewellin, Llewlyn, Llywellyn, Llywellynn, Llywelyn.**

LLOYD. *Welsh, 'grey'.* Originally a nickname for a grey-haired man, the name itself now seems pretty grey. **Floyd, Loy, Loyd, Loydie.**

LOCHLAINN. *(LOK-lin) Irish, 'land of the Vikings'.* Conjures up pleasant images of lakes, but the pronunciation challenge makes the Anglicised Loughlin preferable. **Laughlin, Lochlain, Lochlan, Lochlann, Lochlin, Locklynn.** International: **Lochner** *(German)*.

LOCKE. *English, 'enclosure' or 'fortified place'.* Stylishly strong, supermasculine one-syllable name. **Loch, Lock, Locker, Lockwood.**

LODGE. *English, 'shelter'.* Sounds upper-class yet macho: a winning combination.

LOEB. *German, 'lion'.* Historic association with Leopold damns it. **Loeber, Loew, Loewe, Loewy.**

LOEWY. *Swiss and German nickname for brave person.* Enigmatic choice of enigmatic John Malkovich.

♂ **LOGAN.** *Scottish, 'small hollow'.* This bright and cheerful Scottish surname is megapopular, now quickly rising up the Top 100. **Llogen, Loagan, Loagen, Loagon, Logann, Logen, Loggan, Loghan, Logon, Logn, Logun, Logunn, Logyn.**

LOMAN. *Irish, 'small bare one'; Serbo-Croatian, 'delicate'.* May be too reminiscent of Willy in *Death of a Salesman*.

LON. *Diminutive of* **ALONZO.** For older generations this still summons silent horror star Chaney; for others it's a pleasant if slight nickname name. **Llon, Loni, Lonie, Lonn, Lonnell, Lonney, Lonni, Lonnie, Lonniel, Lonny.**

LONAN. *Irish, 'blackbird'.* This name of several early Irish saints makes a nice Logan/Conan alternative. **Lonen, Lonhan, Lonin, Lonyn.**

♂ **LONDON.** *Place name.* On the rise for both sexes, replacing Paris. **Londen, Londyn, Lunden, Lundon.**

LONGFELLOW. *English, 'tall one'.* It's hard to imagine anyone using this except as a middle name to honour the poet.

LONZO. *Diminutive of* **ALONZO.** Adds some dash and substance to Lon. **Lonso.**

★**LORCAN.** *Irish, 'little, fierce'.* Name of several legendary Irish kings that seems destined – like compatriots Aidan and Logan and Finn – for much wider use.

LORD. *English, 'loaf-keeper'.* If it's royalty you're after, stick with Earl or Prince – this is too deified.

♂ **LOREN.** *Variation of* **LORENZO.** To similar to the girl's name Lauren. **Lorin, Lorren, Lorrin, Loron.**

★**LORENZO.** *Italian variation of* **LAWRENCE.** Latinising Lawrence gives it a whole new lease on life; would work well with a simple one-syllable Anglo name. **Chencho, Latent, Laurencio, Lauro, Lencho, Lerenzo, Lewrenzo, Loren, Lorence, Lorenco, Loreno, Lorens, Lorenso, Lorento, Lorenza, Lorenzino, Loretto, Lorinzo, Loritz, Lorrenzo, Lorrie, Lorry, Lourenza, Lourenzo, Lowrenzo, Nenzo, Renzo, Zo.** International: **Larenzo** *(Italian, Spanish)*, **Lorenz** *(Scandinavian)*.

LORNE. *Variation of* LAWRENCE. A name that's oddly more popular in Canada than in Britain or the US.

LOTHAR. *German, 'famous army'.* Cloddish, till you add a dashing *io* to the end . . . **Lotaire, Lotarrio, Lothahr, Lothair, Lothaire, Lothario, Lotharrio, Lother, Lothur.**

LOUDON. *German, 'from the low valley'.* This unusual name is not normally heard outside of Germany. **Loudan, Louden, Loudin, Lowden.**

LOUIE. *A variation of* LOUIS. Although not as popular as Louis, it's briefly appeared in the Top 100 in recent years.

LOUIS. *German and French, 'renowned warrior'.* While this classic royal name is just slipping out of the Top 50, we think it is still a strong choice. **Aloysius, Lashi, Lasho, Lew, Lewes, Lewis, Lou, Louie, Louies, Lucho, Ludis, Ludovicus, Ludvik, Luki. International: Lughaidh** *(Irish),* **Ludovic** *(Scottish),* **Clovis** *(French),* **Lodovico, Luigi** *(Italian),* **Luis, Luiz** *(Spanish),* **Ludwig** *(German),* **Lothar, Ludvig** *(Scandinavian),* **Ludwik, Lutek** *(Polish),* **Lude, Ludek, Ludko, Ludvik** *(Czech),* **Ludis** *(Russian),* **Lui** *(Hawaiian),* **Lash** *(Gypsy).*

LOWELL. *French, 'young wolf'.* Rich and poetic surname name. **Lovel, Lovell, Lowe, Lowel.**

LOYAL. *English, 'faithful, loyal'.* One of the few virtue names for boys, this one has a long, distinguished history. **Loy, Loyall, Loye, Lyall, Lyell.**

LUC. *French variation of* LUKE. If you want to know the difference in the pronunciations of Luc and Luke, watch Kevin Kline's hilarious description in the film *French Kiss*.

★♂ **LUCA.** *Italian variation of* LUKE. A venerable Italian name with considerable charm, very popular throughout the Continent, though some might fear it could sound too feminine. Colin Firth and his Italian wife chose it for their son.

LUCAN. *Irish from Latin, 'light'.* Irish name, a *luke* form with the trendy *an* ending. **Loucan, Louccan, Luca, Lukan.**

LUCAS. *Latin variation of* LUKE. Long a favourite of screenwriters, Lucas is gaining in popularity with parents who want something similar to but more substantial than Luke, just making it into the Top 50 and up 27 places to make the Australian Top 25. **International: Labhcás** *(Gaelic),* **Chano, Lucho, Luciano, Luciliano, Lucino, Lucio** *(Spanish),* **Loucas, Loukas, Lucais, Lukas** *(Greek).*

★**LUCIAN.** *Latin, 'light'.* A sleeker, more sophisticated version of Lucius, picked by Indie actor Steve Buscemi. **International: Lucan** *(Irish),* **Lucien** *(French),* **Luciano** *(Italian, Spanish and Portuguese),* **Lucio** *(Spanish).*

LUCIANO. *Italian, 'light'.* A vibrant, operatic Latin choice. **Lui, Luiggi, Luigina.**

LUCIUS. *Latin, 'light'.* Exotic old Roman clan name that has lots of religious and literary resonance and is still vital today. **Loukas, Luc, Lucais, Lucanus, Luccheus, Luce, Lucian, Lucias, Lucious, Lucis, Lukas, Luke, Lukeus, Lusio. International:**

Ancient Roman Names

Atticus
Augustus
Aurelius
Caesar
Cassius
Cato
Cicero
Claudius
Cornelius
Decimus
Felix
Julius
Justus
Lucius
Magnus
Marcus
Marius
Maximus
Nero
Octavius
Philo
Quintus
Rufus
Seneca
Septimus

Lúcás *(Irish, German, Dutch and Danish),* Lucien *(French),* Luca, Lucio *(Italian, Spanish).*

♂ LUCKY. *Word name.* Better suited to a pet fish. Luckee, Luckie, Luckson, Lucson.

LUCRETIUS. *Latin clan name, 'wealth'.* The name of the Roman philosopher who invented Epicureanism doesn't sound very appetizing.

LUDLOW. *English, 'ruler's hill'.* Lands with a thud. Ludlo, Ludlowe.

LUDOVIC. *Italian variation of* LUDWIG. Euro-cool. Ludo.

LUDWIG. *German, 'famous warrior'.* As heavy as a marble bust of Beethoven. Ludo, Ludovic, Ludovico.

LUIGI. *Italian vernacular form of* LOUIS. Long seen as stereo-typically Italian, still could sound spiffy with an Anglo surname.

LUIS. *French and German variation of* LOUIS. One of the most popular Hispanic names; familiar yet would add

an exotic touch to an unexotic surname.

LUKAS. *German variation of* LUCAS. A Top 10 name in Germany and a spelling that translates well.

★LUKE. *Greek, 'from Lucanus'.* Cool-yet-strong biblical name that's in the Top 25, Luke has been on the rise since the advent of Skywalker. The New Testament Luke, a physician, is the patron saint of artists and doctors. Lookaa, Lucan, Lucas, Luchok, Lucian, Locior, Lucius, Luck, Lucky, Luhacs, Luk, Luka, Lukaa, Luken, Lukes, Lukyan, Lusio. International: Luc *(French),* Lukas, Lukus *(Swedish, Czech and Greek).*

♂ LUNDY. *Scottish, 'grove near the island'; French, 'Monday's child'.* Lively and engaging Scottish surname, particularly appropriate for a boy born on Monday.

LUTHER. *German, 'army people'.* Once restricted to evangelical Protestants honouring Martin Luther, more recently favoured by parents wishing to pay a tribute to Martin Luther King Jr. **Lotario, Lothahr. Lothar, Lothario, Louther, Lutero, Luthor.**

♂ **LYLE.** *Scottish and English from French, 'someone who lives on an island'.* Straight-forward single-syllable name, but be warned that by the time he's in school, he'll be sick of hearing 'Lyle, Lyle, Crocodile'. **Lisle, Ly, Lyall, Lyell, Lysle.**

LYMAN. *English, 'meadow-dweller'.* Almost as passé as Hyman. **Leaman, Leeman, Lymon.**

LYNCH. *Irish, 'mariner'.* One Irish surname that will never make it as a first. **Linch.**

LYNDON. *English, 'linden tree hill'.* The shortened version would be too close to the girls' Lynn. **Lin, Linden, Lindon, Lindy, Lyden, Lyn, Lyndan, Lynden, Lynn.**

♂ **LYNN.** *English, 'waterfall, brook'.* Long gone to the girls. **Lyn, Lynell, Lynette, Lynnard, Lynne, Lynoll.**

♂ **LYNX.** *Animal name.* Slinky.

LYON. *French, 'lion'.* The *y* makes it seem more like a name and less like an animal, but it's still not as appealing as several Leo choices. **Lion, Lyons.**

LYSANDER. *Greek, 'liberator'.* This name of a character in Greek history and a Shakespeare play is sometimes heard in Mayfair and Belgravia. **Leandro, Lesandro, Lezandro, Lyzander, Sander, Sandros. International: Lysandros** *(Greek).*

M *boys*

MAC. *Scottish, 'son of'.* In Ireland and Scotland, Mac and Mc mean 'son of'; elsewhere, Mac is a generic fella, or a short form cooler than either Matt or Max. **Mack, Mackey, Mackie.**

MACAULAY. *Scottish, 'son of righteousness'.* Made famous by former child star Macaulay Culkin, one of the more popular Mac names. **Macalay, Macaulee,**

Mac Names

Macaulay

MacCarter

MacDonald

Mackenzie

McAdam

McAlaster

McArthur

McCabe

McCallum

McConnal

McCormack

McDermot

McDonnell

McDougal

McDuff

McGeorge

McGregor

McKee

McLeod

McNeill

McPhee

McQueen

McRory

McTavish

Macauley, Macaully, Macauly, Macawlay, MacCauley, McCauley.

MACDONALD. *Scottish, 'son of Donald'.* Between 'Old MacDonald' and Big Mac allusions, this would be a risky choice. **MacDonald, McDonald, Mcdonald, McDonnell, Mcdonnell.**

MACE. *English, 'heavy club'.* Has a slight aura of danger, from its being two types of weapons and a looming character in the *Star Wars* films. Best left as a nickname for Mason. **Macean, Macer, Macey.**

MACGREGOR. *Scottish, 'son of Gregor'.* Interesting possibility for the son or grandson of a Gregory. **Macgreggor.**

★**MACK.** *Scottish, diminutive of names beginning with 'Mac' or 'Mc'.* When 'formalised' with the final *k,* it makes an engagingly amiable choice.

♂ **MACKENZIE.** *Scottish, 'son of Comeley'.* One Mac name that's been pretty much taken over by the girls, though short form Kenzie is popular for boys in Scotland. **Mackensy, Mackenze, Mackenzey, MacKenzie, Mackinsey, Mackinzie, Makenzie.**

♂ **MACLEAN.** *Scottish, 'servant of Saint John'.* Whether you pronounce it *Mac-cleen* or *Mac-clayn,* this is one of the crispest and most appealing of the Mac names. **MacClain, MacClayn, MacLain, MacLayne, McLain, McLayne, McLean.**

♂ **MACON.** *Place name.* Attractive American place name, with a thick Georgia accent, it has played major roles in two novels, Anne Tyler's *The Accidental Tourist* and Toni Morrison's *Song of Solomon.*

MADDOX. *Welsh, 'fortunate, benefactor's son'.* This previously obscure Welsh family name, with its powerfully masculine image, suddenly came into the spotlight when Angelina Jolie chose it for her son; now many other baby namers are following her lead. **Maddock, Maddocks, Maddux, Madock, Madocks, Madog, Madox.**

♂ **MADIGAN.** *Irish, 'little dog'.* A jovial and jaunty Irish name that would make an appealing choice. Slight downside: sharing the nickname Maddy with many little Madelines.

♂ **MADISON.** *English, 'son of the mighty warrior'.* When a name has been popular as a girl's name for a decade, would you really want to inflict it on a son?

MADOC. *Welsh, 'fortunate, benefactor's son'.* Maddox is stronger and more familiar. **Maddoc, Maddock, Maddox, Madog, Madok, Maidoc.**

♂ **MAGEE.** *Irish, 'son of Hugh'.* Magee has a broad and bouncy appeal for the sons of anyone from Adam to Zachary. **MacGee, McGee.**

MAGGIO. *Italian, 'May'.* Interesting ethnic last-name-first possibility, evoking the springtime month.

MAGNUS. *Latin, 'greatest'.* Powerful name with a commanding quality, Magnus is one of the newly unearthed ancient artefacts – it dates back to Charlemagne being called Carolus Magnus, or Charles the Great. A royal name in Scandinavia, it was picked for his son by Will Ferrell. **Magnes, Manius, Manyus.** International: **Maghnus** *(Irish Gaelic),* **Manus** *(Irish),* **Mánas, Magnuss** *(Scottish Gaelic),* **Mogens** *(Danish),* **Mäns** *(Swedish),* **Mauno** *(Finnish).*

★♂ **MAGUIRE.** *Irish, 'son of the beige one'.* Popular Irish surname with a lot of verve as a first. But don't spell it McGwire. **McGuire, McGwire.**

MAHMOUD. *Arabic, 'praiseworthy'.* Historic name commonly found in the Arab world. **Mahmood, Mahmūd, Mehmood, Mehmud.**

MAHOMET. *Variation of* **MUHAMMAD.** *See* **MUHAMMAD.**

♂ **MAISON.** *French word name, 'house'.* Mason with a French accent.

MAJID. *Arabic, 'illustrious'.* This evocative Arabic name is often heard in India. **Magid, Maj, Majdi, Majeed.**

♂ **MAKARI.** *Russian from Greek, 'blessed'.* This name associated with several saints would make a truly distinctive choice for a child with a Russian heritage. International: **Macaire** *(French),* **Macario** *(Italian, Spanish, Portuguese),* **Makary** *(Polish),* **Makar** *(Russian).*

MALACHI. *Hebrew, 'my messenger, angel'.* An Old Testament name with a Gaelic lilt that's on the rise in some places. Two other popular spellings are Malakai and Malaki. **Makequi Malachie, Malachy, Malaki, Malakie, Malaquias, Malechy, Maleki.**

★**MALACHY.** *(MAL-ah-kee) Irish variation of* **MALACHI.** This spelling, associated here with writer Malachy McCourt, lends the biblical name a more expansive, almost boisterous image.

★**MALCOLM.** *Scottish, 'devotee of Saint Colomba'.* This warm and welcoming Scottish appellation fits into that golden circle of names that are distinctive but not odd; a royal name in Scotland and a hero name for many via radical civil rights activist Malcolm X. **Mal, Malcalm, Malcohm, Malcolum Malcom, Malkolm.**

MÁLIK. *(MAH-lick) Arabic, 'lord, master'.* For several years this name ranked high as a Michael alternative, but it's definitely started to slide. **Maalik, Mailik, Malak, Malic, Malick, Malicke, Maliek, Maliik, Malik, Malike, Malikh, Maliq, Malique, Mallik, Malyk, Malyq.**

MALIN. *English, 'strong, little warrior'.* Rarely used name without much personality. **Mallen, Mallin, Mallon.**

MALO. *(MAH-lo) Breton, 'hostage shining'.* This name of an important Breton saint – St Malo is a charming port town in Brittany – is worth considering as a highly unusual alternative to Milo.

MALONE. *Irish, 'a devotee of Saint John'.* Classic Irish surname with a lot of character and some interesting associations, including the title character of a Samuel Beckett novel.

MALONEY. *Irish, 'devotee of the church'.* Too close to baloney.

★♂ **MANDELA.** *African surname.* An African family name ripe for adoption in honour of Nelson Mandela, the South African activist imprisoned for almost thirty years for his antiapartheid activities.

MANDO. *Spanish, diminutive of* **ARMANDO.** Nickname that just might be man enough to stand on its own.

MANFRED. *German, 'man of peace'.* Hipsters might consider reviving this old German name, though we're not sure their sons will thank them. **Fred, Freddie, Freddy, Mannfred, Mannfryd, Manny. International: Manfredo** *(Italian),* **Manfried, Manfrid** *(German).*

MANLEY. *English, 'shared wood'.* Not manly enough.

MANNIX. *Irish, 'a little monk'.* Grandparents might still remember the name; today's parents would probably prefer the more modern Maddox.

MANNY. *English, diminutive of* **EMMANUEL.** Manuel might be a better choice.

MANO. *Italian, 'hand'; diminutive of* **EMMANUEL.** A nickname that sounds like a nickname.

MANOLO. *Variation of* **MANUEL.** Because of shoe designer Manolo Blahnik, this has become a generic term for pricey stilettos, as in 'I must have those Manolos!' **Mano, Manollo.**

MANSUR. *Arabic, 'divine aid'.* Prevalent Arabic name that suggests a man who is sure of himself.

MANU. *Polynesian, 'bird of the night'; Sanskrit, 'man'.* Has the exotic texture of batik.

MANUEL. *Spanish variation of* **EMMANUEL.** A staple of Hispanic naming, much more common than the English Emmanuel. **Mango, Mani, Mannie, Mannuel, Manny, Manolete, Manolito, Manolo, Manue, Manuelito, Manuelo, Nelo. International: Manoel** *(Portuguese),* **Maco, Mano**

(Hungarian), **Manuil, Manuyil**
(Russian).

MANUS. *Irish variation of*
MAGNUS. Not as pleasing or
impressive as Magnus.

MANZO. *Japanese, 'third son'.*
Strong and vital Asian birth
order name.

MANZU. *Italian artist name.*
Could make a singularly creative
choice inspired by modern
Italian sculptor Giacomo
Manzù.

MAOZ. *(mah-ohz) Hebrew,*
'fortress, strength'. Symbolic
name given to boys born at
Hanukkah because of the song
'Maoz Tzur' – 'Rock of Ages' –
which is sung at that time.
Maazya, Maazyahu, Maosya,
Ma'oz.

MARC. *French variation of*
MARK. Designer (as in Marc
Jacobs) form of Mark. *See*
MARK.

MARCEL. *French variation of*
MARCELLUS, *'little warrior'.*
Despite distinguished
namesakes, including Proust
and Duchamp, suffers from a

terminal headwaiter image in
trendy restaurants. **Marcellus,**
Marcely. International: Marceau,
Marcellin *(French),* **Marcelino,**
Marcello *(Italian),* **Marcelino,**
Marcelo *(Spanish and Portuguese).*

MARCELO *Spanish variation*
of **MARCELLUS.** Both the
Spanish Marcelo and Italian
Marcello would work well
outside their ethnic
neighbourhoods. **Marcello.**

♂ **MARCH.** *Word name.* Along
with August, one of the few
month names available to boys;
this brisk single-syllable name
might be worth considering as
either a first or middle option.
International: Marc, Mars
(French), **Marzo** *(Italian and*
Spanish), **Marz** *(German),* **Maret**
(Indonesian), **Machi** *(Swahili).*

★**MARCO.** *Italian and Spanish*
variation of **MARK.** Simple and
universal, Marco is a Latin
classic that is worthwhile
considering for your son.

MARCOS. *Portuguese and*
Spanish variation of **MARK.**
Another culture's slant on
Mark, sometimes associated
with former president of the

Philippines Ferdinand Marcos
and his shoe-collecting wife,
Imelda. **International: Marcano,**
Marco, Marcolino, Marko
(Spanish).

MARCUS. *Latin, 'warlike'.* A
popular choice with many
parents, this ancient Roman
name briefly entered the Top
100 in recent years, some
perhaps honouring Marcus
Garvey, leader of the Back
to Africa movement. **Marc,**
Marco, Marius, Marko,
Markus. International:
Marcos *(Spanish),* **Markus**
(German), **Markos** *(Greek).*

MARINO. *Latin, 'of the sea'.*
Italian surname with distinct
crossover possibilities, having
pleasant seaside undertones.

MARIO. *Italian variation of*
MARIUS. Familiar via such
notable Marios as Lanza, this
Italian name could be a
possiblity when combined
with a more bland surname.
Marios, Marius, Marrio.

♂ **MARION.** *French variation*
of **MARY.** Would John Wayne
have become a mythic screen
hero if he had kept his unisex

birth name of Marion? Very doubtful.

MARIUS. *Latin, from a Roman family name of uncertain derivation.* Frequently heard in Germany and France, this fusty yet accessible name has been a favourite of novelists from Victor Hugo to Anne Rice and could suit a boy in this country.

International: Mariano, Mario *(Italian, Spanish),* **Marian** *(Polish).*

MARK. *Latin, 'warl-ike'.* After centuries of lagging behind other apostle names Peter and Paul, Mark suddenly caught on in the early 1950s. But though it was a big baby-boomer name, their offspring are beginning to think it doesn't have as much spark – it recently left the Top 100. **Marc, Markey, Markie, Marko, Markus, Marky, Marq, Marque, Marquus.** International: **Marcas** *(Irish and Scottish Gaelic),* **Mawrth** *(Welsh),* **Marc, Marcel, Marcellin, Marcellus** *(French),* **Marcellino, Marcello, Marco** *(Italian, Spanish),* **Marcano, Marcas, Marcelino, Marcelo, Marciano, Marcio, Marcos, Marko** *(Spanish and Portuguese),* **Markell, Markus, Marx** *(German),* **Markku** *(Finnish),* **Marek** *(Polish),* **Marku** *(Romanian),* **Mareček, Marek, Mareš, Mařík, Maroušek** *(Czech),* **Marko** *(Ukrainian),* **Markos** *(Greek),* **Maaka** *(Maori).*

MARKUS. *German variation of* **MARCUS.** *See* **MARCUS.**

♂**MARLEY.** *English, 'pleasant woods'.* Opposite in image from the similar-sounding Harley, this name has a soft and gentle, almost feminine aura; also, many might associate it with reggae great Bob Marley.

MARLON. *English, 'little hawk'.* Associated for half a century with Marlon Brando, who inherited the French-inflected name from his father, Marlon has been used occasionally by ordinary folk, but much less so now than it was in the 1970s. **Marlen, Marlin, Marlinn, Marlonn.**

♂ **MARLOW.** *English, 'hill near the lake'.* Caveat: sounds just like the feminine Marlo. **Marloe, Marlowe.**

MARMADUKE. *Irish, 'devotee of Maedóc'.* Suitable only for oversized dogs.

MARQUEZ. *Spanish, 'nobleman'.* This Spanish spelling of Marquis is popular in its own right.

MARQUIS. *English rank of nobleman between duke and count.* There are ordinary folk named Prince, Earl and Duke, so why not this rank of nobility as well? Many spellings compete, the most common being Marquis, Marquise and Marquez. Rapper 50 Cent chose the Marquise version for his son; David Caruso, Marquez. **Markese, Markess, Markis, Markise, Markiss, Markise, Markquise, Markwees, Marques, Marquess, Marquez, Marquise, Marquiz, Marquise.**

MARS. *Roman mythology god of war.* Intimidating.

MARSDEN. *English, 'boundary valley'.* Stuffy surname. **Marsdin, Marsdon.**

♂ **MARSH.** *English nature name.* Soft and mellifluous nature-surname name, situated miles away from the dated Marshall.

MARSHALL. *French, 'one who looks after horses'.* Being the real name of rapper Eminem doesn't make Marshall any cooler. **Marchall, Marischal, Marischall, Marsh, Marshal, Marshell.**

MARSTON. *English, 'residence near a marshy place'.* Fussy. Streamline it to Marsh, Mason, or Carson.

MARTEZ. *Spanish, variation of* **MARTIN.** Adds some spunk and Latin rhythm to mundane Martin.

MARTIN. *Latin, 'war-like'.* One of those balding middle-aged names that, like Raymond and Vincent and George, are just starting to sound possible again. Stylish in London. **Mart, Marten, Martie, Marton, Marty,** International: **Mártan, Máirtín** *(Irish Gaelic),* **Mártainn** *(Scottish Gaelic),* **Marcin, Märtel, Marten** *(French),* **Martino** *(Italian),* **Martinez, Martiniano, Martino, Marto, Tin, Tino** *(Spanish),* **Martí** *(Catalan),* **Martinho** *(Portuguese),* **Maarten, Martijn** *(Dutch),* **Martel, Merten** *(German),* **Morten** *(Danish, Norwegian),* **Martti** *(Finnish),* **Marcin, Marcinek** *(Polish,* **Márton** *(Hungarian),* **Martins** *(Latvian),* **Martyn** *(Russian),* **Martinos** *(Greek).*

MARVIN. *Welsh, 'sea fortress'.* Hard to believe that this now Jewish-sounding name has windswept Welsh roots. **Marv, Marve, Marven, Marwin, Marwynn, Mervin, Mervyn, Merwin, Merwyn, Murvin, Murvynn.**

MASO. *Italian, diminutive of* **TOMASSO.** Appealing, lively and distinctive. **Mazo.**

★♂ **MASON.** *English occupational name, 'worker in stone'.* Occupational surname which has been rising quickly in the Top 100, was chosen by a number of celebs for their sons (and Kelsey Grammer for his daughter): a fresher sounding replacement for the Jason we've moved beyond, in step with the new style Cason/Kason.

MASSAI. *African tribe; also Italian, 'owner of land and farms'.* Unusual name not often heard elsewhere.

MASSEY. *English, Scottish and French place name.* Some definite downsides: Massive? Messy?

MASSIMO. *Italian variation of* **MAXIMUS.** Latin charmer, much more appealing than the old-fashioned Mario, if a tad boastful.

★**MATEO, MATTEO.** *Latin variations of* **MATTHEW.** These attractively energetic Spanish and Italian versions of the classic Matthew are primed to move further into mainstream nomenclature. Actor Colin Firth has a son called Matteo. **Matejo, Matheo, Mattheo, Teo.**

MATTHEW. *Hebrew, 'gift of God'.* A popular boys' name throughout the 1980s and 90s and still standing strong on the Top 20, the New Testament Matthew is the epitome of the fashionable classic – safe and sturdy, yet with a more engaging personality than John or James. It's so common by now, though, that parents are starting to look elsewhere for fresher choices, such as its variations Matthias and Mateo. **Matai, Matek, Matfei, Mathe, Matheson, Mathew, Mathian, Mathias, Mathieson, Matro, Matt, Matteus, Matthaeus, Matthaios, Matthaus, Mattheus, Matthews, Mattie, Matty,** Matvey, Matyas, Mayhew. International: **Maitias, Maitiú** *(Irish Gaelic),* **Mata, Matha** *(Scottish Gaelic),* **Mathieu** *(French),* **Matteo, Mattia** *(Italian),* **Mateo, Matejo, Matheo, Matias, Teo** *(Spanish),* **Mateu** *(Catalan),* **Mateus** *(Portuguese),* **Matthijs** *(Dutch),* **Mattäus** *(German),* **Mads, Mathies** *(Danish),* **Mats, Matteus** *(Swedish, Norwegian),* **Matti** *(Finnish),* **Maciej, Mateusz** *(Polish),* **Mátyás, Matyi, Matyo** *(Hungarian),* **Matheiu** *(Romanian),* **Matej, Matyás** *(Czech),* **Matei** *(Bulgarian),* **Matvei, Motka, Motya** *(Russian),* **Matvi** *(Ukrainian),* **Matthaiso** *(Greek).*

★**MATTHIAS.** *Ecclesiastic Greek variation of* **MATTHEW.** With Matthew sounding somewhat exhausted and ancient endings sounding new again, this New Testament apostolic name makes an appealing and recommended choice. Both Mathias and Matias are well used in the Hispanic community and throughout Europe. **Mathias, Mathis, Matthieus, Mattias.** International: **Maitias** *(Gaelic),* **Mathías, Mathios, Matías, Matíos, Mattáes, Mattías** *(Spanish),* **Matteus** *(Portuguese),* **Mathais, Mathi, Matthaeus, Matthaus, Matthis, Matz** *(German),* **Mattathias, Matthaios** *(Greek).*

MAURICE. *Latin, 'dark-skinned'.* Last popular in the 1870s, Maurice (pronounced *morris* in the UK, *more-EESE* elsewhere) isn't planning a return any time soon. **Maureese, Mauriece, Maurin, Mauritz, Mauro, Maury, Mo, Moreese, Moris, Morrice, Morris, Morry, Moss.** International: **Muiris** *(Irish Gaelic),* **Meurig, Morys** *(Welsh),* **Maurizio** *(Italian),* **Mauricio** *(Spanish and Portuguese),* **Maricio, Maurecio, Maurisio, Mauritio, Maurizio, Richo** *(Spanish),* **Maurids, Mauridsje** *(Dutch),* **Mortiz** *(German),* **Maurits** *(Scandinavian),* **Maury, Maurycy** *(Polish),* **Moricz** *(Hungarian),* **Mavriki** *(Russian),* **Moris** *(Greek).*

MAURICIO. *Spanish variation of* **MAURICE.** *See* **MAURICE.**

MAVERICK. *American, 'independent, nonconformist'.* At the rate it's growing, Maverick soon won't seem like such a maverick anymore. Heard first in a 1950s and then as the Tom Cruise character in *Top Gun,* Maverick symbolises an unfettered, free spirit. **Maverik, Mavric, Mavrick.**

MAX. *English and German diminutive of* **MAXIMILIAN** *or* **MAXWELL.** Holding steady in the Top 50, Max was transformed from cigar-chomping grandpa to rosy-cheeked baby in the 1980s, becoming one of the starbaby names of recent years. **Maxey, Maxie, Maxx, Maxy.**

MAXEN. *Welsh, from* **MAXIMUS.** Max plus the trendy *-en* ending equals not a good idea.

MAXIM. *Russian variation of* **MAXIMUS.** Best known now as a men's magazine title. *See* *MAXIMUS.* **Maksim.**

MAXIME. *French variation of* **MAXIMUS.** Common in France, but could be confused with the feminine Maxine here. **Maximien, Maximin.**

MAXIMILIAN, MAXIMILLIAN. *Latin, 'greatest'.* Might seem a bit grand for a British baby boy, but some parents do prefer it as a substantial platform for the nickname Max. **Mack, Maks, Maksim, Maksym, Max, Maxemilian, Maxemilion, Maxey, Maxi, Maxie, Maximilianus, Maximus, Maxy, Maxymilian.** International: **Maxim, Maxime, Maximilien** *(French),* **Massimo, Maximiliano, Maximino, Maximo** *(Italian),* **Chilano, Macimilian, Mancho, Mascimiliano, Maximiano, Maximiliano, Maximillano, Maximilliano, Maximino** *(Spanish),* **Maksym, Maksymilian** *(Polish),* **Maksim, Maxim** *(Russian),* **Maximos** *(Greek).*

MAXIMO. *Spanish variation of* **MAXIMUS.** The Max born to Latino families.

MAXIMUS. *Latin 'greatest'.* The powerful name of the powerful character played by Russell Crowe in the 2000 film *Gladiator* first appeared on the popularity charts that same year. Max to the max. International: **Màmus** *(Gaelic),* **Maxime** *(French),* **Massimo** *(Italian),* **Masimiano, Másimio, Máxcimo, Maximiano, Máximo, Maxsimiano, Méssimo, Miximino** *(Spanish),* **Maximino** *(Portuguese),*

Film Character Names

Amsterdam

Castor

Chili

Cotton

Devlin

Draven

Ferris

Forrest

Hitch

Korben

Mace

Maximus

Napoleon

Nemo

Neo

Roux

Makimus *(Polish),* **Maximos** *(Greek).*

MAXWELL. *Scottish, 'great stream'.* A happy medium between the weighty Maximilian and the laid-back Max.

MAYER. *Hebrew variation of* **MEIR.** More common – when it was common – with the Meyer spelling. **Maier, Meir, Meyer.**

MAYNARD. *German, 'hardy, brave, strong'.* Sometimes pronounced *MAY-nerd*, which is death to a name. **International: Meinhard** *(German).*

MAYO. *Irish place name, 'yew-tree plain'.* When ordering a baby name, hold the mayo.

McCOY. *Irish variation of* **McKAY**, *'fire'.* Too vulnerable to 'real McCoy' jokes.

McEWAN. *Scottish, 'son of Ewan'.* Shows promise via connection to growing interest in Ewan. **MacEuan, MacEwen, McEuan, McEwen.**

♂ **MEAD.** *English, 'from the meadow'.* Undiscovered single-syllable surname option, a friendly alternative to Reed. **Meade, Meed, Meede, Meid.**

MEIR. *Hebrew, 'bringer of light'. See MEYER.* **Maier, Mayer, Mayr, Meier, Meiri, Meyer, Myer.**

MEKHI. *(me-KYE) Derivation and meaning unknown.* An unusual first name that could well prove to be an interesting alternative to Michale or Micky.

♂ **MEL.** *English, diminutive of* **MELVIN** *or* **MELVILLE.** There was a Saint Mel, though most Mels are playing pinochle with Murray and Morris.

MELCHIOR. *Polish, 'city of the king'.* This name of one of the Three Wise Men is rarely used, for good reason. **Malchior, Malkior, Melker, Melkior.**

MELOR. *Russian, modern invented name.* Historical oddity: name composed of the initial letters of the words Marx, Engels, Lenin, October and Revolution.

MELVILLE. *Scottish, 'settlement on infertile land'.* All names ending in *ville* are in nowheresville.

MELVIN. *English and Scottish, 'council protector'.* This once perfectly respectable surname has suffered decades of abuse, not least by Jerry Lewis's demented, spastic character in the 1950s. **Malvin, Malvyn,** Malvynn, Mel, Melvyn, Melwin, Melwyn, Melwynn, Vinnie.

MENACHEM. *Hebrew, 'the comforter'.* A middle-aged, if not elderly, name associated with Israeli statesman and onetime prime minister Begin, this is a symbolic appellation for boys born on the holiday of Tishah-b'Ab. **Menahem, Menchem, Nachum, Nahum. International: Mende, Mendele** *(Yiddish).*

MENASHE. *Hebrew, 'causing to forget'.* An Old Testament name – he was the eldest son of Joseph – that's still used in the Jewish community.

MENDEL. *Yiddish variation of* **MENACHEM.** Another Old World Jewish name, also the surname of the founder of genetics.

★**MERCE.** *Diminutive of* **MERCER.** Loaded with creative charm, associated with dancer-choreographer Merce Cunningham.

MERCER. *French occupational name, 'a merchant'.* Attractive possibility with musical links to songwriter Johnny Mercer and bandleader-musician Mercer Ellington. **Merce.**

♂ **MERCURY.** *Roman mythology name, the messenger of the gods.* Adventurous parents are starting to look back to names of ancient gods like Mercury, Zeus and Apollo. This one is also a planet and a metallic element and has a friendly nickname, Merc. **Merc.**

♂ **MEREDITH.** *Welsh, 'great chief'.* Has been considered a girl's name since the 1950s. **Meridith.**

♂ **MERLE.** *French, 'blackbird'.* Originally a nickname for someone who loved to sing or whistle, Merle is even less masculine than Meredith.

MERLIN. *Welsh, 'sea fortress'.* This name of the famous fifth-century sorcerer and mentor of King Arthur is a bit wizardy for a real-life modern child. **Marlin, Marlon, Merle, Merlen, Merlinn, Merlyn, Merlynn.**

MERTON. *English, 'town by the lake'.* Sounds like a displaced Dr Seuss character. **Merwyn, Murton.**

MERVYN. *Welsh, 'sea hill'.* Terminally outmoded. **Marv, Marvin, Marvyn, Merfyn, Merv, Merven, Mervin, Mervynn, Merwin, Merwinn, Merwyn, Murvin, Murvyn.**

MESHACH. *Hebrew, 'agile'.* Old Testament name with a rousing, gospel feel.

METEOR. *Word name.* A beyond-bold shooting-star name choice, sure to raise some relatives' eyebrows.

MEYER. *Hebrew, 'bringer of light'.* A name favoured by Jewish families a hundred years ago, now more likely morphed back into the original Moses or Malachi.

♂ **MICAH.** *Hebrew, 'who is like God?'* Growing numbers of parents are looking at the biblical Micah as a more unusual alternative to Michael, projecting a shinier, more lively image. **Mycah.**

MICHAEL. *Hebrew, 'who is like God?'* Holding steady in the Top 50 in recent years, this popular boys' name for almost half a century. It's phenomenal record is probably due to its use by parents of diverse ethnic and religious groups and its all-around likability, strength and sincerity. **Micael, Mickie, Micko, Micky, Mike, Mikey, Mikkeli, Mitch, Mitchel, Mitchell.**

MICHEÁL *(MEE-haul) Irish variation of* **MICHAEL.** This Gaelic version of the enduring Michael was chosen by Natasha Richardson and Liam Neeson for their first son.

MICHELANGELO. *Combination of* **MICHAEL** *and* **ANGELO.** The ultimate artist's name would make an unforgettable impression.

MICK. *English, diminutive of* **MICHAEL.** Most often associated with Rolling Stone Jagger, Mick is a common nickname found here, although it is sometimes used in a derogatory way. **Mickey, Micky.**

MICKEY. *Diminutive of* **MICHAEL.** Pugnacious and spunky like the young Mickey Rooney and the original Mickey

Michael's International Variations

Irish/Scottish Gaelic	**Mícheál**
Scottish	**Micheil**
Welsh	**Meical, Mihangel**
French	**Michel, Michon**
Italian	**Michele**
Spanish/Portuguese	**Micho, Miguel**
Basque	**Mikel**
Catalan	**Miquel**
Danish/Norwegian	**Mikael, Mikkel**
Swedish	**Mikael**
Finnish	**Mikko**
Polish	**Michal, Mietek**
Hungarian	**Mihály, Misi, Miska**
Romanian	**Mihai**
Russian	**Mikhail, Mischa, Misha**
Estonian	**Mihkel, Mikk**
Greek	**Makis, Mikhos**
Hebrew	**Mica, Micah, Micha, Misha**

Mouse, but more often used as a nickname today.

MIES. *Dutch, diminutive of* **BARTHOLOMEUS.** Apt choice for an architect's child, honouring German-born Ludwig Mies van der Rohe, a central figure in modern design and universally referred to as Mies.

MIGUEL. *Spanish and Portuguese variation of* **MICHAEL.** A Spanish classic popular in the Latino communities.

MIKE. *English, diminutive of* **MICHAEL.** Unlike Jake or Sam, few parents put Mike on the birth certificate. **Mikey.**

MIKEL. *Basque and Scandinavian variation of* **MICHAEL.** Although this is a legitimate continental form of Michael, parents who choose it see it as a streamlined, simplified spelling. **Mikle, Mykel, Mykle.**

MIKHAIL. *Russian variation of* **MICHAEL.** *See* **MICHAEL.**

MIKLÓS. *Czech and Hungarian variation of* **NICHOLAS.** Surprisingly, attached to the Greek Nikolaos rather than Michael.

♂ **MILAN.** *Slavic, diminutive of names beginning with* mila, *or Italian place name.* With the first syllable pronounced *mee*, this could also suggest the Italian city, although the native version Milano is a lot livelier.

MILES. *Latin, 'a soldier'; German, 'merciful, generous'.* Jazz great Miles Davis applied a permanent veneer of cool to this confident and polished name; it has been appreciated in particular by celebrity baby namers. **Myles.**

MILLARD. *Latin, 'caretaker of the mill'.* Might be too reminiscent of a duck – keep looking.

★**MILLER.** *English occupational name, 'grinder of grain'.* An up-and-coming choice in the stylish occupational genre; chosen by Stella McCartney and by Téa Leoni and David Duchovny. **Millar, Myllar, Myller.**

★**MILO.** *German, 'mild, peaceful, calm'; also Irish diminutive of* **MILES.** A highly recommended author favourite; with its German, Greek and jaunty British input, Milo combines the strength of the ancient Greek Olympic wrestler with the debonair charm of a World War II RAF pilot.

Among the celebrity mums who share our enthusiasm is Liv Tyler who has bestowed this name on her son.

MILTON. *English, 'settlement with a mill'.* Once an upper-class British surname conjuring up the epic poetry of John Milton, now summons up the image of a gran-dad in a dusty cardie. **Millton, Milt, Milten, Miltie, Miltin, Miltun, Milty, Mylten, Mylton.**

MINGUS. *Scottish, variation of* **MENZIES.** Supermodel Helena Christensen named her son in honour of jazz great Charles Mingus, opening up a whole category of jazzy possibilities: Kenton, Calloway, Ellington, Gillespie, Mulligan, Tatum and Thelonius.

♂ **MIRÓ.** *(meer-O) Spanish artist name.* Unique option honouring Spanish surrealist painter Joan Miró. Could have some pronunciation problems, but preferable to calling your little boy Joan.

MISAEL. *Hebrew, 'who is what God is?'* Old Testament name all but unknown outside the Latino community.

♂ **MISHA.** *Russian, diminutive of* **MIKHAIL.** Brought into the British consciousness as the nickname of ballet great Mikhail Baryshnikov, it more recently took on a unisex air via the screen actress Mischa Barton. Could become the next Sasha. **Mischa.**

MITCHELL. *English variation of* **MICHAEL.** Had some panache in the 1940s and 50s, when it was seen as a sharper alternative to Michael with its cool Mitch nickname. It then went to sleep, though it's showing signs of a comeback – no thanks to the Mitchell brothers on *Eastenders'.* **Michell, Mitch, Mitchel, Mitchill, Mytch.**

MOE. *English, diminutive of* **MOSES.** Vying with Gus to become the next Max. **Mo.**

MOHAMMED. *Arabic, 'greatly praised'.* The most popular spelling over here. *See* **MUHAMMAD.**

MOISÉS. *(moy-SASE) Spanish variation of* **MOSES.** Well used in the Hispanic culture. *See* **MOSES.**

MOISHE. *Yiddish variation of* **MOSES.** *See* **MOSES.** Moshe.

MOJAVE. *(moe-HAV-ay) Native American tribal and place name.* Resonant place name of the beautiful Southern California desert. **Mohave.**

♂ **MOLLOY.** *Irish, 'a venerable chieftain'.* There are many dynamic three-syllable Irish surnames; this is one of the rarer two-syllable ones.

MONGO. *Yoruba, 'famous'.* Associated with famed percussionist Mongo Santamaria, but it's too close to the word *mongrel* to ever have widespread success in this country.

MONROE. *Scottish, 'mouth of Roe'.* A surname name with links to the actress Marilyn we don't see zooming to popularity. **Monro, Munro, Munroe.**

MONTAGUE. *French, 'pointy hill'.* The family name of Shakespeare's Romeo has an effete, monocled image. **Montagew, Montagu, Monty.**

♂**MONTANA.** *Spanish place name; 'mountainous'.* Relaxed American place name that still has some masculine punch, but be warned: this whole posse of similarly trendy names, like Sierra and Dakota, will soon ride towards the sunset.

MONTEL. *Modern invented name.* Parents who like this kind of fabricated name usually want to invent their own. **Montell, Montelle.**

MONTEZ. *Spanish, 'dweller in the mountains'.* Sensuous and rhythmic.

MONTGOMERY. *Norman, 'man power'.* Fusty and formal.

MONTY. *Diminutive of* **MONTAGUE,** **MONTGOMERY.** Rarely used on its own; has a World War II feel.

♂ **MOORE.** *English place name, 'the moors'.* Recommended as a rich and satisfying middle name choice. **Moor.**

MORANDI. *Italian artist name.* The last name of the twentieth-century Italian painter of quietly expressive still lifes presents an artistic possibility.

MORDECAI. *Hebrew, from the Persian, 'warrior'.* A symbolic name for boys born on the holiday of Purim, Mordecai has a rather mournful tone. **Mordacai, Mordachai, Mordechai, Mordy, Mort. International: Motke, Motl (Yiddish).**

♂ **MORGAN.** *Welsh, 'circle' or 'sea'.* Once split evenly between the sexes, this attractive Welsh favourite is quickly slipping down the Top 100 in the boys chart – perhaps because it has been a popular girls' name for more than a decade. **Morgen, Morghan, Morgin, Morgon, Morgun, Morgunn, Morgyn, Morrgan.**

♂ **MORLEY.** *English, 'moor, meadow clearing'.* Gently pleasant English family name. **Moorley, Moorly, Morlee, Morleigh, Morly, Morrley.**

MORPHEUS. *Greek mythology name, god of sleep and dreams.*

Though you may pray to the god of sleep for your baby to slumber through the night, a drowsy image is not the greatest one to inflict on your little boy.

♂ **MORRIE.** *Latin, diminutive of* **MAURICE.** Soft and sensitive and elderly, associated with mega-best-seller *Tuesdays with Morrie.* **Maury, Morey, Morry.**

MORRIS. *English variation of* **MAURICE.** As quiet and comfortable as a Morris chair, also as old-fashioned. **Maurey, Maurie, Maury, Morey, Morice, Morie, Moris, Moritz, Morrie, Morrison, Morriss, Morrisson, Morry, Moss.**

♂ **MORRISEY.** *Irish, 'sea taboo'.* When British rocker Steven Patrick Morrissey decided to use his last name alone, it became a viable option for baby namers, a lot cooler than Morris or Maurice. **Morrissey, Morrissy.**

MORRISON. *English, 'son of Morris'.* Possible alternative to Harrison.

MORTIMER. *English, 'dead sea'.* Other kids might see a teasible connection to mortician or mortuary. **Mort, Mortmer, Morty.**

MORTON. *English, 'town near the moor'.* Another death name that could be turned into mortuary in the playground. **Mort, Morten, Mortin, Mortun, Morty.**

MOSES. *Egyptian, 'saviour,' 'delivered from the water'.* Gwyneth Paltrow and Chris Martin's choice of this white-bearded Old Testament name brings it into the modern age, along with brethren Elijah, Isaiah and Isaac. User-friendly nicknames include Moe and Mose. **Mo, Moe, Moise, Moises, Moishe, Moishye, Moke, Mose, Moshe, Mosheh, Mosie, Moss, Moyses, Moze, Mozes. International:** Maois *(Irish Gaelic),* Moïse *(French),* Moises *(Spanish, Portuguese),* **Mosze, Moszek** *(Polish),* **Mojzesz, Mózes, Mozses** *(Hungarian),* **Moze** *(Lithuanian),* **Moisei** *(Bulgarian),* **Moisey, Moisse, Mosya** *(Russian),* **Móises** *(Slavic),*

Moisis, Moyses *(Greek),* **Moishe, Moshe, Mosheh, Moyshe** *(Hebrew, Yiddish),* **Mousa, Mozes, Musa** *(Arabic).*

MOSHE. *Hebrew variation of* **MOSES.** Old-fashioned name. **Moyse.**

MOSS. *English, 'descendant of Moses'; word name.* Evocative, green combination nature surname, associated with playwright Moss Hart.

MOZART. *German musical name.* A daring middle name possibility for classical concert-goers.

MUHAMMAD. *Arabic, 'praiseworthy'.* There are over five hundred names for the Arab prophet who founded the Muslim religion (some of which are listed below), making it the most common boys' name in the world and explaining the Muslim adage, 'If you have a hundred sons, name them all Muhammad'. This version has just entered the Top 50. **Ahmad, Hamid, Hammad, Mahmood, Mahmoud, Mahmud, Mahomet,**

Stellar Starbabies Beginning with M

Maddox	Angelina Jolie
Magnus	Will Ferrell
Malachy	Cillian Murphy
Mandla	Stevie Wonder
Marcel	Stella Tennant
Marlon	Dennis Miller
Marlon	Lou Doillon
Marquez	David Caruso
Marquise	50 Cent
Mason	Cuba Gooding Jr
Mateo	Colin Firth
Matteo	Talisa Soto & Benjamin Bratt
Mattias	Will Ferrell
Miles	Joan Cusack, Susan Sarandon & Tim Robbins
Miller	Stella McCartney
Milo	Ricki Lake, Liv Tyler
Mingus	Helena Christensen
Moses	Gwyneth Paltrow & Chris Martin
Myles	Eddie Murphy

♂MUIR. *(myoor) Scottish, 'dweller near the moor'.* A family name in Scotland, occasionally used as a first.

♂MULLIGAN. *Irish, 'descendent of the bald-headed'.* This is less appealing than some other Irish surnames, such as Malone and Sullivan.

MUNGO. *Scottish, 'kind, gentle'.* Here's a lesson in not choosing a name just for its meaning. **International: Munga** *(Gaelic).*

♀♂MUNRO. *Scottish, 'mouth of the river Ro'.* Although it's been around, it has a fresh, new sound to it. **Munroe.**

♂MURPHY. *Irish, 'hound of the sea'.* This jaunty Irish surname is the most common family name in Ireland.

♂MURRAY. *Scottish, 'from the land by the sea'.* More often given to dogs than babies these days, but it sounds cute – à la Sydney – when used for girls. **Moray, Murrey, Murry.**

MYLES. *English spelling variation of* **MILES.** This

Mehmet, Mehmood, Mehmoud, Mehmud, Mihammad, Mohamad, Mohamed, Mohamet, Mohammad, Mohammed, Muhamet, Muhammed.

alternate spelling of Miles has its fans, among them Myles-parents Eddie Murphy and Lars Ulrich. *See **MILES.***

MYRON. *Greek, 'fragrant, an aromatic shrub, myrrh'.* One of many *M* names – including Murray, Melvin, Morton, Milton and Marvin – given to first-generation Jewish boys to replace the old-fashioned Moses. Now we'd pick Moses over any of them. **Miron.**

N boys

NAAMAN. *Hebrew, 'pleasant'; Nigerian, Hausa, 'sweet herbs'.* The double *a* makes it special. **Nahman, Nahmon, Namon.**

NABIL. *Arabic, 'highborn'.* Pleasant and exotic and not as common as some other African names. **Nabeel, Nabiel.**

NACHUM. *(nay-KAHM) Hebrew, 'comforter'.* This name of a minor Hebrew prophet in the Old Testament is not recommended as a first name, but maybe in the middle. **Menachem, Menahem, Nacham,**

Nachman, Nachmann, Nachum, Nahum.

NACIO. *(NAH-see-o) Spanish diminutive of **IGNACIO.*** Attractive and energetic – one of the most appealing Spanish nickname names.

NADIM. *Arabic, 'friend'.* Friendly option: has also been defined as 'drinking companion'. **Nadeem.**

NADIR. *Arabic, 'precious, scarce'.* Try Zenith instead. **Nadeer, Nadeir, Nader.**

NAEEM. *(nah-eem) Arabic, 'benevolent'.* Could present pronunciation problems. **Naem, Naim, Naiym, Nieem.**

NAGEL. *German occupational name, 'maker of nails'.* Only if it's a family name and then, best in the middle. **Naegel, Nageier, Nagelle, Nagle, Nagler.**

NAHIR. *Hebrew, 'clear, bright'.* Positive meaning – and a choice of spelling variations. **Naheer, Nahur, Namir, Nehor, Nohar.**

NAHMA. *Native American, 'sturgeon'.* Fish – or caviar –

lover's choice, though it would tend to sound like a girl's name.

NAIM. *Scottish, 'river with alder trees'.* May give rise to some teasing problems: 'What's your name?' 'Naim'. 'Yes'. 'Naim'. 'That's what I'm asking you'. **Naime.**

♂ **NAIRN.** *Scottish, 'river with alder trees'.* Scottish nature name that could prove a tongue-twister for the younger set. **Naern, Nairne.**

♂ **NAIROBI.** *African place name.* The capital of Kenya makes a melodic and exotic name.

NAJI. *Arabic, 'safe'.* Spelled Najee, this was chosen by rapper LL Cool J for his son several years ago. **Najae, Najee, Najei, Najiee, Najih.**

NAJIB. *Arabic, 'wellborn'.* Regal feel. **Nageeb, Nagib, Najeeb, Najíb, Nejeeb.**

NAKIA. *Arabic, 'pure'.* Attractive name, but it does sound feminine. Some have changed it to Nakari. **Nakai, Nakee, Nakeia, Naki, Nakiah, Nakii.**

NAKOS. *Native American, Arapaho, 'sage, wise'.* Interesting Native American choice that could be taken for Greek.

♂ NAKOTAH. *Sioux, 'friend to all'.* This name of a subtribe in the Great Sioux Nation could make an inventive twist on the overused Dakota. **Nakota.**

NALDO. *Spanish, diminutive of* **REINALDO.** Manages to make Reginald sexy.

NALIN. *Hindi, 'lotus'; also Apache, 'maiden'.* Extremely meaningful in the Buddhist culture, where a lotus symbolises the victory of the spirit over the senses. **Naleen.**

♂ NAMAKA. *Hawaiian, 'eyes'.* For a baby with beautiful eyes.

NAMID. *Ojibwa, 'star dancer'.* Fanciful image distinguishes this Native American name.

NAMIR. *Hebrew, 'leopard'.* Exotic choice that translates well. **Nameer, Namer.**

NANDO. *Spanish, diminutive of* **FERNANDO.** O-ending short forms are almost invariably appealing, though this might seem slight as the child grows up. **Nandor.**

NANSEN. *Swedish, 'son of Nancy'.* Feminist twist on Hansen and Jansen.

NAOKO. *Japanese, 'straight, honest'.* Admirable meaning.

NAOR. *(nah-ohr) Hebrew, 'cultured and enlightened'.* Certainly qualities desired for our sons. **Nehorai.**

NAPHTALI. *Hebrew, 'wrestling, struggling'.* Rarely used biblical choice – he's a son of Jacob – with a bit of a white-bearded image. **Naftali, Naftalie, Naphtalie, Naphthak, Naphthali, Neftali, Nefthafi, Nephtali, Nephthali.**

NAPIER. *Scottish occupational name, 'producer or seller of table linens'.* The surname of the influential early Scottish inventor of logarithms could make an inspiring middle name choice for a mathematically inclined family. **Neper.**

NAPOLEON. *Greek, 'lion of the new city'.* Overly ambitious choice. **Leon, Leone, Nap, Napolean, Napoléon, Napoleone, Nappie, Nappy.**

NAQUAN. *Modern invented name.* Further along the Dewayne, Dejuan, Daquan continuum. **Naqawn, Naquain, Naquen, Naquon, Naqwan.**

NARAIN. *Hindi, 'protector'.* Another name for the Hindu god-Vishnu. **Narayan.**

NARCISSUS. *Greek, 'daffodil'.* Mythological young man who fell in love with his own image: the first narcissist. Don't make your son another one **Narcis, Narciso, Narcissus, Narkis, Narkissos, Narses. International:** Narcisse *(French),* Narciso *(Italian, Spanish and Portuguese),* Narcis *(Catalan),* Narcyz *(Polish).*

NARDO. *Spanish, diminutive of* **BERNARDO.** Possible 'nerd' temptation for nicknamers makes Nando a preferable choice.

NAREN. *Sanskrit, 'superior man'.* Might translate, thanks to Darren connection.

NARVE. *Dutch, 'healthy, strong'.* Harv and Marv are out and this difficult Dutch choice doesn't fare any better.

NASH. *English, 'by the ash tree'. Beautiful Mind* mathematician John Nash make this name seem possible, even dashing.

NASHUA. *Place name.* The name of a city in the American state of New Hampshire that might attract some Joshua refugees – though we can conceive of nausea-connection bullying.

NASIM. *Arabic, 'breeze, fresh air'.* Traditional Arabic choice. **Naseem, Nassim.**

NASSER. *Arabic, 'the winner'.* Commonly used Muslim name, also sometimes chosen to honour Egyptian president Gamal Abdel-Nasser. **Naseer, Naser, Nasier, Nasir, Nasr, Nassir, Nassor.**

NAT. *English, diminutive of* **NATHAN** *or* **NATHANIEL.** Just the kind of old-fashioned nickname coming back into style. **Natt, Natty.**

NATAL. *(Nah-TAHL) Spanish variation of* **NOEL.** Because of its relationship to the English word, better lengthened to Natalio. **Nataho, Natale, Natalie, Natalino, Natalio, Nataly.**

NATE. *English, diminutive of* **NATHAN** *or* **NATHANIEL.** Very much in style.

NATHAN. *Hebrew, 'given'.* Old Testament name that's been on the upswing for forty years and is in the Top 50. Strong, solid and attractive, it was chosen for his son by Jon Stewart. **Naethan, Nat, Nate, Nathann, Nathean, Nathen, Nathian, Nathin, Nathon, Nathyn, Natthan, Naythan, Nethan. International: Natan** *(Spanish, Hungarian, Polish, Russian),* **Natanael** *(Swedish).*

★**NATHANIEL.** *Hebrew, 'given by God'.* Although Nathan's more popular, this has a firm following. Despite the profusion of *Nat* names around, this remains singularly appealing and distinctive. Parents finding it overused might opt for the apostle Nathaniel's other name – Bartholomew. **Nat, Nataniel, Nate, Nathan, Nathanial, Nathanie, Nathanielle, Nathanil, Nathanile, Nathanuel, Nathanyal, Nathanyel, Nathanyl, Natheal, Nathel, Nathinel, Nethanel, Nethaniel, Nethanyel, Thaniel. International: Nathanael** *(French),* **Nataniele** *(Italian),* **Natanael** *(Spanish and Swedish).*

NAVARONE. *Spanish, meaning unknown.* Known for the film *The Guns of Navarone,* chosen by Priscilla Presley.

NAVARRO. *Spanish, 'from Navarre'.* Dashing surname for the Basque kingdom. **Navarre.**

NAVEED. *Persian, 'auspicious news'.* Attractive Middle Eastern choice. **Navid.**

NAVIGATOR. *Occupational name.* Adventurous and unusual choice from this trendy group in the wild new world of baby names.

NAVIN. *Hindi, 'new, novel'.* Would fit right in with the currently popular *in/an/en/on-*

ending boys' names. **Naveen, Naven.**

NAYLAND. *English, 'island-dweller'.* Intriguing meaning, but stuffy sound.

NAYLOR. *English occupational name, carpenter or 'nailer'.* Unique name for the son of a wood-worker. **Nailer, Nailor.**

NAZAIRE. *(nah-ZAHR), French from Latin, referring to Nazareth.* Saint-Nazaire is a harbour town in France; the name relates to Nazareth, where Jesus lived as a child. Two possible variations: Nazarius, an Italian martyr and Nazario. **Nasareo, Nasarrio, Nazario, Nazarius, Nazaro, Nazor.**

NAZARETH. *Hebrew place name.* For purists. **Nazaire, Nazaret, Nazarie, Nazario, Nazerene, Nazerine.**

NAZIH. *Arabic, 'pure, chaste'.* A *z* almost always adds zest to a name. **Nazeeh, Nazeem, Nazeer, Nazieh, Nazim, Nazir, Nazz.**

NEAL. *Irish, 'champion' or 'cloud'.* Always the second-best spelling of the name (*see NEIL*), Neal has been slipping in popularity in recent years. **Neale, Neall, Nealle, Nealon, Nealy, Neel, Niall. International: Niall** *(Irish),* **Njal** *(Scandinavian).*

NEANDER. *Greek, 'new man'.* Following a custom among scholars in Renaissance Germany, Neander is the classical form of the surname Newman. But the bullies at school are sure to call him Neanderthal.

NEBO. *Babylonian mythology name.* Sounds like a name from an old science fiction film – but this god of letters invented writing and so might interest parents who are writers or professors.

NECTARIOS. *Greek, 'of nectar'.* A twentieth-century Greek saint's name redolent of the beverage of the gods that imparted immortality. **Nectaire, Nectarius, Nektario, Nektarios, Nektarius.**

★**NED.** *English, diminutive of* **EDWARD.** Gently old-fashioned short form that's been enjoying a small style Renaissance in recent years. **Neddie, Neddy, Neddym, Nedrick.**

NEEL. *Hindi, 'sapphire blue'.* If you want people to appreciate this choice, you're going to have to explain how it's not Neil.

NEGASI. *Amharic, 'he will wear a crown'.* Ethiopian name that would be difficult here.

NEHEMIAH. *Hebrew, 'the Lord's comfort'.* Old Testament name, last used by the Puritans, of the prophet assigned the rebuilding of Jerusalem – a venerable possibility for an architect or building contractor. **Nahemiah, Nechemia, Nechemiah, Nechemya, Nehemias, Nehemie, Nehemyah, Nehimiah, Nehmia, Nehmiah, Nemo, Neyamia.**

NEHRU. *Hindi, 'canal'.* A name associated with the Indian prime minister.

NEIL. *Irish, 'champion' or 'cloud'.* Always the top spelling of the name; Neil peaked in the 1950s, but then enjoyed a second coming following the fame of such Neils as astronaut Armstrong and singers Sedaka, Diamond and Young. Now semi-retired. **Neal, Neale, Neall, Nealle, Nealon, Neel, Neihl, Neile, Neill, Neils, Nellie, Nels, Niall, Niel, Niele, Niels, Nigel, Nil, Niles, Nilo, Nils.** International: **Niall** *(Irish),* **Nyle** *(Scandinavian).*

NELIUS. *Latin, diminutive of* **CORNELIUS.** A lot more substantial than Corny or Nellie.

♂ **NELLY.** *English, diminutive of* **CORNELIUS, CORNELL, NELSON.** Naming a child Cornelius or Nelson might prove character building – but naming him Nelly (even the rap star was christened Cornell) is just cruel. **Nell, Nellie.**

NELO. *Spanish, diminutive of* **DANIEL.** Lively nickname form of overused biblical favourite. **Nello, Nilo.**

NELS. *Norwegian and Swedish variation of* **NICHOLAS.** One of those simple Norse names, like Lars, that is definitely worth thinking about. **Nelse, Nelson, Nils.**

NELSON. *English, 'son of Neil'.* It's not modern or particularly masculine, but there are several noteworthy Nelsons you might want to honour, from the British admiral to South African president Mandela. **Nealson, Neillson, Neils, Neilson, Nellie, Nels, Nelsen, Niles, Nils, Nilson, Nilsson.**

NEMESIO. *Spanish, 'justice'.* The meaning makes this name interesting, but the sound is too related to nemesis. **Nemi.**

NEMO. *Greek, 'from the glen'.* The original Nemo was the captain in *Twenty Thousand Leagues under the Sea,* while the more familiar modern one is the animated little fish in the Disney movie. Unusual name well worth considering.

NEN. *Egyptian, 'ancient waters'.* Couldn't be simpler . . . or more exotic – though it could lead to some head-scratching.

NEO. *Latin, 'new'.* This nouveau name of Keanu Reeves's character in *The Matrix* has not enjoyed the same burst of popularity as its female counterpart, Trinity.

NEPTUNE. *Roman god of the sea.* This Roman mythology name would be very hard to handle.

NEREUS. *Greek mythology name.* The name of the father of the sea nymphs – or one of its shorter forms – would be somewhat easier for a child to carry than Neptune. **Nereo, Nerio.**

NERO. *Latin, 'stern'.* The association with the infamous Nero, the fiddling Roman emperor, would be unavoidable. **Neron, Nerone, Nerron.**

NERUDA. *Literary name.* Evocative of the great Nobel Prize-winning poet Pablo Neruda, real last name Basoalito, who took on the surname Neruda to honour a Czech poet of that name.

NESBIT. *English, 'land or river bend shaped like a nose'.* A family name that wouldn't appeal to many parents. **Naisbit, Naisbitt, Nesbitt, Nisbet, Nisbett.**

NESTOR. *Greek, 'traveller, voyager'.* A wise ruler of legend whose name is a possibility for the adventurous, though related in sound to the dated Lester-Hester family. **Nester, Nesterio, Nestore, Nestorio.**

♂ **NEVADA.** *Spanish place name, 'covered in snow'.* American place name whose final *a* makes it feminine,

though it still retains some cowboy punch. **Navada, Nevade.**

NEVILLE. *French, 'new town'.* More often used in Britain than elsewhere, though fans of the musical Neville Brothers might make it their own. **Nev, Nevil, Nevile, Nevyle.**

NEVIN. *Irish, 'holy'.* Possible Gaelic alternative to Kevin and Devon. **Nefen, Nev, Nevan, Nevean, Neven, Nevins, Nevon, Nevyn, Niven.**

NEWBOLD. *English, 'new building'.* Surname choice that's neither new nor bold.

NEWBURY. *English, 'new borough, new settlement'.* A name only a bully could love. **Newberry, Newbery.**

NEWELL. *English variation of* **NEVILLE.** One of several surnames beginning with *New* that nevertheless sound anything but. **Newall, Newel, Newhall, Newyle.**

♂ **NEWLAND.** *English, 'new land'.* Some will see this as spirited, others stuffy. **Newlan.**

♂ **NEWLIN.** *Welsh, 'new pond'.* An obscure possibility . . . for a girl. **Neulin, Neulyn, Newlinn, Newlinne, Newlyn, Newlynn, Newlynne.**

NEWMAN. *English, 'newcomer'.* Family name best used in the middle, even with the popularity of the American actor Paul. **Neiman, Neimann, Neimon, Neuman, Neumann, Newmann, Numan, Numen.**

NEWPORT. *English place name, 'new port'.* For sailors or jazz lovers.

NEWT. *English, 'a small salamander'; Scottish, diminutive of* **NEWTON.** Rarely used on its own and with good reason – who would want to be named after a lizard?

NEWTON. *English, 'new town'.* Named after Isaac? Or Wayne? **Newt.**

NGUYEN. *(new-win) Vietnamese, 'sleep'.* One of the most familiar Vietnamese names, yet still hard on the Western tongue.

NIALL. *(neel) Irish, 'champion'.* This Irish spelling brings Neil into the twenty-first century. **Nial, Nialle.**

NICABAR. *Gypsy, 'stealthy'.* Rhythmic and intriguingly unusual.

NICANDRO. *Spanish variation from Greek, 'man of victory'.* Might be of interest as a blend of two Anglo favourites – Nicholas and Andrew. **Nicandreo, Nicandrios, Nicandros, Nikander, Nikandreo, Nikandrios.**

NICASIO. *Spanish from Greek, 'victory'.* Closer to Nike than to Nicholas, this is an attractive, viable import that could be used elsewhere. **International: Nicaise** *(French),* **Nicasi** *(Catalan),* **Nikasios** *(Greek),* **Nicasius** *(Latin).*

★**NICHOLAS.** *Greek, 'people of victory'.* It recently slipped out of the Top 100, but Nicholas is still one of the top boys' names, with great historical depth – what child wouldn't appreciate being named after Old Saint Nicholas? – and masculine panache. If you're not put off by its mass popularity, Nicholas makes an attractive, solid choice. **Cole, Collin, Nic, Niccolas, Nichalas, Nichelas, Nichlas, Nichlos, Nichola, Nicholaas, Nicholaes, Nicholase, Nicholaus, Nichole, Nicholias, Nicholl, Nichollas, Nicholos, Nicholus, Nick, Nickalus, Nickey, Nickie, Nickolas, Nicky, Niclas, Niclasse, Nico, Nicolaas, Nicoles, Nicolet, Nicolis, Nicoll, Nicollet, Nik, Nikki, Nikkolas, Nikky, Nycholas. International: Neacal** *(Gaelic),* **Nioclas, Niocol** *(Irish),* **Nicol** *(Scottish),* **Colas, Colin, Nicol, Nicolas** *(French),* **Niccolò, Nicola** *(Italian),* **Nicolao, Nicolás** *(Spanish and Portuguese),* **Mikolas** *(Basque),* **Nicolau** *(Portuguese),* **Claus, Nicolaes, Nikolaas** *(Dutch),* **Klaas, Nicolaus, Niklaus** *(German),* **Klaus** *(German, Danish, Swedish),* **Niklas, Nils** *(Scandinavian),* **Niels** *(Danish),* **Lasse, Launo, Niilo** *(Finnish),* **Mikolaj, Milosz** *(Polish),* **Miklós, Nicolae** *(Hungarian),* **Mikolás** *(Czech),* **Kolya, Nicolai, Nikita, Nikolos** *(Russian),* **Niko, Nikolaos, Nikolos, Nikos,** *(Greek),* **Nikolao** *(Hawaiian).*

If You Like Nicholas, *You Might Love . . .*

Alexios
Andreas
Christos
Cole
Homer
Lucas
Marcus
Milo
Nico
Nicol
Nikos
Noam
Plato
Spencer
Theo

NICHOLSON. *English, 'son of Nicol'.* Unusual but not outlandish Nicholas alternative that still gets you to Nick; associated with writer Nicholson Baker. **Nicholsen, Nickelsen, Nickelson, Nicklesen, Nickleson,**

Nikkelsen, Nikkelson, Nikklesen, Nikkleson.

NICK. *English, diminutive of* **NICHOLAS** *and* **DOMINICK;** *also used independently.* The classic strong-yet-sexy nickname name, much used for charming film characters. **Nic, Nik.**

NICKLEBY. *English, 'Nicholas's village'.* Charming Dickensian route to Nick. **Nickelbee, Nicklebee, Nickelby, Nikkelby, Nikkleby.**

NICKOLAS. *Spelling variation of* **NICHOLAS.** Nouveau spelling that's rising in popularity, though a child bearing it could be accused of misspelling his own name.

★**NICO.** *Greek, diminutive of any of the* Nico- *names.* One of the great nickname names, full of charm, energy and sex appeal. A neo-Nick. **Neco, Neko, Nicco, Nicos, Niko, Nikos.**

NICODEMUS. *Greek, 'victory of the people'.* Rarely used New Testament name; we say just skip to Nico. **Nicodem, Nicodemius, Nicodemo,** Nikodem, Nikodema, Nikodemious, Nikodemus, Nikodim.

NICOL. *Scottish and English, medieval variation of* **NICHOLAS.** Often used here, but it could be confused with the feminine Nicole. **Nichol, Nicholl, Nicoll.**

NICOLAS. *Spelling variation of* **NICHOLAS.** French and Spanish form, or streamlined spelling of Nicholas, popularised by actor Nicolas Cage, that's still on the rise. **Nic.**

NICOLÒ. *Italian variation of* **NICOLA.** Rhythmic form of popular name, for those who want an exotic spin on Nicholas. **Niccolò.**

NICOMEDES. *Greek, 'pondering victory'.* Even more daunting than Nicodemus. **Nicomedo, Nikomedes.**

NIELS. *Danish variation of* **NICHOLAS;** *Dutch diminutive of* **CORNELIUS.** Gives middle-aged Neil a new lease on life. **Niel, Nielsen, Nielson, Niles, Nils.**

NIGEL. *Irish, 'dark, black-haired'.* A name that combined with the right surname, may have a little Sherlock Holmes about it. But there might be some playground teasing about 'waiting for plans from …' **Niegel, Nigal, Nigale, Nigele, Nigell, Nigiel, Nigil, Nigle, Nijel, Nye, Nygel, Nygell, Nyigel, Nyjil. International: Niguel** *(Spanish).*

♂ **NIGHT.** *Word name.* An ubercool and mysterious name that's recently entered the lexicon via an American director.

♂ **NIKE.** *Greek, 'victory'.* Cool goddess name, but be braced for lots of trainer jokes. **Nikka.**

♂ **NIKITA.** *Russian cognate of Greek* **ANIKETOS,** *'unconquered'.* Redolent of Khrushchev and la femme.

NIKKO. *Diminutive of* **NICHOLAS.** Unique spelling chosen by an American singer for his son.

NIKOS. *Greek, diminutive of various names beginning with the element* Niko-. Attractive, approachable and more striking Nick alternative.

★**NIKOLAI.** *Russian variation of* **NICHOLAS.** Russian forms, like Russian supermodels, are hot these days. This is a strong, exotic way to make Nicholas new. **Kolya.**

NIKOSTRATOS. *Greek, 'army of victory'.* A lengthy continental route to Nick. **Nicostrato, Nicostratos, Nicostratus.**

♂ **NILA.** *Hindi, 'blue'.* To the Western ear, a girl's name.

♂ **NILE.** *Greek, 'river valley'.* Water names are a cool category these days and this one of the famous Egyptian river streamlining the fussier Niles is no exception.

NILES. *Scandinavian, 'son of Neil'.* Perfect name for TV Frasier's effete brother. **Nilesh, Nyles.**

NILS. *Norwegian variation of* **NICHOLAS** *and* **NILSSON.** Like Lars, Sven, Niels and

Nels, an unjustly neglected straightforward Scandinavian name. **Nills.**

NILSSON. *Scandinavian, 'son of Nils'.* The *son* at the end of many Scandinavian names makes them more consistent with modern British name tastes. **Nilsen, Nilson, Nilssen.**

NIMROD. *Hebrew, 'we shall rise up, we shall rebel'.* Our kids laughed when they saw this name. Enough said.

NIN. *Literary name, meaning unknown.* Better hold off and hope for a daughter you can name Anaïs.

NINIAN. *Scottish and Irish, meaning unknown.* Ancient Irish saint's name that's unlikely, because of its similarity to 'ninny,' to join cousin Finian in popularity. **Ninnian.**

NIÑO. *Spanish, 'young child'.* Too child-like, in addition to the objectionable association with the el niño phenomenon.

NINO. *Italian, diminutive of* **GIANNINO** *and of* **GIANNI.**

Old-time Italian pet name, now mostly seen on pizzeria signs.

NIR. *(neer) Hebrew, 'ploughed field'.* Short, simple foreign-flavoured names like this make distinctive middle name possibilities. **Niral, Nirel, Niria.**

NIRAN. *Thai, 'eternal'.* Simple, attractive and exotic, would fit in with the Kierans and Kylans in the preschool class.

NISHAN. *Armenian, 'cross, sign, mark'.* A gentle name well used in Armenian families, unfamiliar elsewhere. **Nishon.**

NISSAN. *Hebrew, 'miracle'.* Though the accent falls on the second syllable, people will mistake this name of the first month of the Jewish calendar for the Japanese car. **Nisan, Nissim, Nissin, Nisson.**

NIVEN. *Scottish, 'little saint'.* Excellent candidate for use as an undiscovered surname name.

NIXON. *English, 'son of Nicholas'.* Too closely linked to the former American president to foist this on a child. **Nixan, Nixson.**

NJORD. *(nyord) Scandinavian, 'north'*. Pronounced to rhyme with *fjord,* the Norse god of the sea's name, this would make an unorthodox choice for sea-lovers and fishermen. **Njorth.**

★**NOAH.** *Hebrew, 'rest' or 'wandering'*. This name of the Old Testament patriarch of the ark is one of those unexpected fashion hits, shaking off its ancient image and rising rapidly up and into the Top 50. **Noach, Noak, Noe, Noé, Noi. International: Noë** *(French),* **Noé** *(Spanish),* **Nuh** *(Arabic).*

♂ **NOAM.** *Hebrew, 'pleasantness, charm, tenderness'*. If you like Noah but want something less popular, this would make a highly distinctive choice; also a place name in south Israel. **Naam, Naaman, Naim, Naum.**

NOAZ. *Hebrew, 'bold'*. And this would take it from distinctive to unique.

NOBLE. *Latin, 'aristocratic'*. A virtue name used by the Puritans and with Honor and Justice back in fashion, this

might be revived too. **Nobe, Nobie, Noby.**

♂ **NOEL.** *French, 'Christmas'*. Fey and sophisticated, connoting wit and creativity, but not the most masculine of choices. Indeed, the female versions of the name are more popular. **Nata, Natal, Natale, Noël, Noél, Noell, Nole, Noli, Nowel, Nowell. International: Nollaig** *(Irish Gaelic),* **Novelo** *(Italian and Spanish).*

NOHEA. *Hawaiian, 'handsome'*. Any name that means handsome has something going for it, though this would cause some head-scratching. **Noha, Nohe.**

NOLAN. *Irish, 'renowned'*. One of the rising Irish surname names, in the spirit of Logan and Dillon. **Noland, Nolande, Nolane, Nolen, Nolin, Nollan, Nolyn.**

♂ **NOLLIE.** *Latin and Scandinavian variation of* **OLIVER.** Unconventional nickname option that's best kept as a nickname. **Noll, Nolli, Nolly.**

♂ **NOON.** *Word name*. Cool middle name possibility. **Noone.**

NORBERT. *German, 'renowned northerner'*. This one comes with a sign on it reading 'Kick me'. **Bert, Bertie, Berty, Norberto, Norbie, Norby.**

NORFOLK. *English, 'place of the northern people'*. Would make a difficult choice even for those with ties to the British county.

♂ **NORI.** *Japanese, 'doctrine' or 'seaweed'*. Attractive, simple Japanese choice that, while not strictly unisex, could work even better for a girl.

NORMAN. *English, 'northerner'*. One of those names that has become an almost stock choice, indicating a normal, earthbound, guy – not an image many parents seek for their sons. **Norm, Normand, Normen, Normie, Normy. International: Norrie** *(Scottish).*

♂ **NORRIS.** *French, 'northerner'*. Somehow more modern and likable than Morris or Doris. **Norice, Norie, Noris, Norreys, Norrie, Norry, Norrys.**

★ ♂ **NORTH.** *Word name.* Word name that's long been used, albeit very quietly and so has a certain purity and strength. Good choice if you're from, say, Cumbria or Yorkshire, love winter or are an avid skier, or if you just want a name that's both familiar and unusual. **Northcliffe, Northcote, Northrop, Norton, Norval, Norwood.**

NORTHCLIFF. *English, 'northern cliff'.* Stick with North. **Northcliffe, Northclyff, Northclyffe.**

NORTHROP. *English, 'northern farm'.* North is so much crisper. **North, Northrup, Northup.**

NORTON. *English, 'northern town'.* Linked today with the Irish TV presenter Graham – need we say more? **Nortan, Norten, Nortin.**

NORVILLE. *Scottish, 'northern town'.* A nice enough last name that turns supercilious as a first. **Norval, Norvel, Norvell, Norvil, Norvill, Norvylle.**

NORVIN. *English, 'northern friend'.* Alvin, Melvin, Norvin – most *vin* names, except maybe Kevin and Gavin – are not vinners. **Norvyn, Norwin, Norwinn, Norwyn, Norwynn.**

NORWOOD. *English, 'woods in the north'.* Another stiff northerly choice. **Norward, Norwerd, Norwett.**

♂ **NOVEMBER.** *Latin, 'ninth month'.* The only month name that's really boy-worthy is August.

NOYCE. *English, 'walnut tree'.* As always, that *oy* sound is problematic.

NUMAIR. *Arabic, 'panther'.* Projects an air of power and speed.

NUNCIO, NUNZIO. *Italian, diminutive of* **ANNUNZIO**, *'messenger'.* Attractive Latinate choice, a lively possibility for the child of a journalist. **Nunzi.**

♂ **NURI.** *Arabic, 'light'; Hebrew, 'my fire'.* To the British ear, a cute nickname name that could work for either sex. **Nery, Noori, Nur, Nuriel, Nuris, Nuris, Nury.**

NURIEL. *Hebrew, 'fire of God'; related to the Arab* **NUR.** Too much like Muriel. **Nooriel,**

O' Names

O'Brian/O'Brien
O'Callahan
O'Casey
O'Connor
O'Donnell
O'Donovan
O'Fallon
O'Grady
O'Hara
O'Keefe
O'Neal/O'Neill
O'Reilly/O'Riley
O'Ryan
O'Shea
O'Sullivan

Nuria, Nuriah, Nuriya, Nuriyah, Nurya.

NURU. *Swahili, 'born in daylight'.* Evocative African choice.

NYE. *Welsh diminutive of* **ANEURIN.** This can make an unusual yet simple middle name choice, especially for anyone with family ties to Wales. **Nyle.**

O boys

OAK. *Nature name.* A symbol of solidity, strength and longevity, Oak is joining Cedar and Pine as a viable name and it would work especially well in the middle.

OAKES. *English, 'near the oaks'.* A single Oak is sufficient. **Oaks, Okes.**

♂ **OAKLEY.** *English, 'from the oak tree meadow'.* As sturdy as Oak, with deeper roots. **Oakie, Oaklea, Oaklee, Oakleigh, Oaklie, Oakly.**

OAN. *Breton, 'lamb'.* A too-literal spin on Owen.

★**OBADIAH.** *Hebrew, 'servant of God'.* For the seriously audacious biblical baby namer who wants to move beyond Elijah and Jeremiah, this name has considerable old-fangled charm. **Obadia, Obadias, Obadius, Obedia, Obediah, Obie, Ovadiah, Ovadya, Oved.**

OBERON. *English spelling variation of* **AUBERON.** Fey, like Shakespeare's king of the fairies. **Auberon, Oberen, Oberron, Oeberon, Oeberron.** International: **Obéron** *(French).*

OBI. *African, Nigerian-Ibo, 'heart'.* Return of the Jedi: strongly linked to the complex *Star Wars* character, Obi Wan Kenobi. **Obbi, Obbie, Obe, Obie, Oby.**

★♂ **O'BRIEN.** *Irish, 'descendant of Brian'.* The use of *O* prefixes could create the next wave of Irish-inflected names, offering an innovative way of honouring a relative with an old-fashioned moniker. **O'Brian, O'Bryan.** *For more O' names, see sidebar.*

♂ **OCEAN.** *Nature name.* Last heard in the hippy-dippy 1960s and 70s, names like Ocean and River are flowing back into favour, especially with nature lovers and green-oriented parents. **Oceanus, Oshun.**

★**OCTAVIO.** *Spanish variation of* **OCTAVIUS.** The most popular of the number names used by Hispanic parents, open to all. **Actaviano, Actavio, Octave, Octavian, Octavianno, Octavino,**

Octavión, Octavo, Octavius, Octovio, Ottavio.

OCTAVIUS. *Latin, 'eighth'.* Has the worn leather patina of all the ancient Roman names now up for reconsideration. **Octaveus, Octavian, Octavious, Octavous, Octavus, Tavey. International: Octave** *(French),* **Ottavio** *(Italian),* **Octavio, Tavio** *(Spanish).*

ODELL. *English, 'of the valley'.* Bland compared to the Irish-sounding *O*-starting names. **Del, Dell, Odale, Odall, Odayle, Odel, Odelle, Odey, Odie.**

ODILIO. *German, 'possessor of enormous wealth'.* German name with a Latin rhythm. **Odilón.**

ODIN. *Old Norse mythology name.* The name of the supreme Norse god of art, culture and magic projects a good measure of strength and power and has excellent assimilation potential. **Odan, Oddin, Oddon, Oden, Odo, Odon, Odran.**

ODION. *(o-dee-OHN) African, 'first born of twins'.* Strong Nigerian name that could work for a twin of any ethnicity.

ODISSAN. *(oh-DEES-sahn) African, 'thirteenth born son'.* If you choose this name, it's not likely to be for the meaning.

ÖDÖN. *(OO-dun) Hungarian variation of* **EDMOND.** Properly pronounced, an agreeable, almost witty name. **Odi, Odin, Ody.**

ODYSSEUS. *Greek mythology name, 'wrathful'.* The name of the brave, resourceful hero of Homer's epic saga has almost always been considered too weighty for a child to bear, but some brave, resourceful parents out there might be willing to take it on. **Ulysses. International: Odyssée** *(French).*

OEDIPUS. *Greek, 'swollen foot'.* Sure to give a complex.

OGDEN. *English, 'from the oak valley'.* Rarely used surname, associated with humorous poet Ogden Nash. **Ogdan, Ogdon.**

OGUN. *(OH-gun) African, Yoruba, 'god of war'.* Militaristic.

Armenian Names

Ara

Aram

Arathoon

Armen

Arno

Arshile

Berj

Deron

Garo

Haig

Haroutoun

Jirair

Keran

Ohan

Rafik

Sero

Vano

Vartan

Zeroun

Zori

OHAN. *Armenian variation of* **JOHN.** Strong and appealing Armenian choice, but could be confused with Owen. **Ohann.**

♀ OHARA. *(oh-hah-rah) Japanese, 'small field'.* Perfect for a child of Japanese-Irish heritage.

OISÍN. *(ush-een) Irish Gaelic, 'little deer'.* The name of the son of the legendary Finn McCool is often Anglicised to Ossian, but the original has recently been revived in Ireland. **Osheen, Ossian, Ossin.**

OJAI. *(Ō-hī) California place name.* This name of an attractive and arty California town could make an exotic but friendly choice.

OKELLO. *Ugandan, 'born after twins'.* Mellow and musical.

OLAF. *Norse, 'ancestor's relic'.* Sainted and regal in Norway, slightly oafish here. **Ola, Olaff, Olan, Olav, Olave, Ole, Olef, Olev, Olin, Olof, Oluf. International: Auley, Auliffe** *(Irish),* **Olav, Ole** *(Danish, Norwegian),* **Ola** *(Norwegian, Swedish),* **Olof, Olov, Oluf** *(Swedish),* **Olay** *(Norwegian),* **Olavi, Olli** *(Finnish),* **Olafur** *(Icelandic).*

OLEG. *Russian, 'holy'.* This common Russian name has a somewhat effete pencil-thin-moustached image here. **Olezka.**

OLIMPIO. *Greek, 'pertaining to the Mount Olympus of Greek mythology'.* Bold and muscular. **Olimios, Olimpo, Olympios, Olympos, Olympus.**

OLIN. *Swedish, 'ancestor'; English, 'to inherit'.* Would fit right in with the trendy Colins and Owens. **Olen, Olinn, Olyn, Olynn.**

★OLIVER. *Latin, 'olive tree'.* Everybody likes the energetic, good-natured Oliver; this Top 10 name is stylish, just like its trendy twin-sister Olivia, with a meaning symbolising peace and fruitfulness. Works particularly well with single-syllable surnames, as in Olivers Stone, North and Short (son of Martin). **Noll, Ollie, Olliver, Ollyver, Olyver. International: Oilibhear** *(Irish),* **Olivier** *(French),* **Oliviero** *(Italian),* **Oliverio** *(Spanish),* **Olivieros** *(Portuguese),* **Oliwjer** *(Polish).*

OLIVIER. *(o-LIV-ee-ay) French, 'olive tree'.* More and more frequently heard Gallic version of Oliver, could be seen as a tribute to great British actor, Sir Laurence O. **Lell, Noll, Ol, Olier, Ollie, Ollier, Ollivier.**

OLLIE. *Diminutive of* **OLIVER.** A comfortable nickname name, once associated as part of a comedy duo, with his partner Stan. **Olly.**

OLSEN. *Scandinavian, 'Olaf's son'.* A name not likely to become popular here. **Olson.**

OLYMPOS, *Greek, 'from Mount Olympus'.* Mythical, yet limp. **Olympio.**

OMAR. *Arabic, 'flourishing, thriving'; Hebrew, 'eloquent'.* To British people, Omar has an interesting blend of exoticism and familiarity, plus a strong, open initial *O*. Long associated with Persian poet Omar Khayyan, it sounds anything but ancient now. **Odemar, Odomar, Omaire, Omari, Omarr, Omavi, Omer, Ommar, Ommo, Omri, Oomer, Othmar, Otmar, Ottmar, Umar, Ummo.**

♂ OMARI *Swahili variation of* **OMAR.** This name, like Omar and Amari, has been gaining in popularity.

♂ **OMARION.** *Elaboration of* **OMARI.** Another increasingly popular member of the Omar family.

OMER. *Hebrew, 'sheaf of corn'.* A symbolic name for boys born during a period between Passover and Shavuot, but to most it would sound like Homer with a Cockney accent.

OMRI. *Hebrew, 'servant of Jehovah' or 'my sheaf'.* Old Testament name of a king of Israel, looks a bit like a bad Scrabble hand. **Omrey, Omry.**

♂ **O'NEAL, O'NEIL.** *Irish, 'from the chief's line'.* Perfect as an updated namesake for Great-Uncle Neal (or Neil). **Oneal, Oneall, O'Neall, O'Neel, Oneil, Oneill, O'Neill.**

ONSLOW. *English, 'from the zealous one's hill'.* Baby-naming rule Number 101: steer clear of names containing the word *slow*. **Onslowe.**

♂ **ONTARIO.** *Place name.* This geographical name with Iroquois

roots has a lot going for it: a strong sound, a vigorous *o* ending and – a quality prised today – rarity.

♂ **ONYX.** *Gem name.* Unlike Pearl and Ruby, this is one gem name suited for boys, the final *x* making it sound strong and virile.

ORAN. *Aramaic, 'light'; also Irish, 'pale little green one'.* Gentle and calm multicutural Jewish-Irish choice.

OREL. *Russian, 'eagle'; also Russian place name.* With a name like this, but give your son a really strong nickname – like Bulldog. **Oral, Orrel.**

OREN. *Hebrew, 'pine tree'.* Soft and sensitive name often heard in Israel. **Oran, Orin, Orni, Orran, Orren, Orrin.**

ORESTES. *Greek, 'from the mountain'.* Another baby-naming rule: don't name your son after a character in Greek drama who murdered his mother. **Oreste.**

OREV. *Hebrew, 'raven'.* Idiosyncratic Hebrew choice.

ORFEO. *Italian variation of* **ORPHEUS.** *See* **ORPHEUS.**

♂ **ORI.** *Hebrew, 'my light'.* Friendly but substantial. **Or, Orad, Oran, Or-Chayim, Orie, Oron, Ory, Oryan, Oryon.**

♂ **ORION.** *Greek mythology name.* The mythical Greek hunter turned into a heavenly constellation has an ever-so-slight sci-fi feel, plus a Gaelic connection to O'Ryan, all of which make it a rising star. **International: Zorian, Zorion** *(Basque).*

★**ORLANDO.** *Italian variation of* **ROLAND.** This ornate Italianate twist on the dated Roland, with a literary heritage stretching back to Shakespeare and Virginia Woolf, has appealing book-ended *o*'s and is open to combination with almost any last name, à la young British actor Orlando Bloom. **Arlando, Landi, Lando, Olo, Orlan, Orland, Orlandito, Orlondo, Roland, Rolando.**

ORNETTE. *Musical name.* Long associated with jazz great Ornette Coleman, this name's main problem is that almost all other *ette*-ending names – from Annette to Paulette – are unequivocally feminine.

ORO. *Spanish, 'gold'.* Rare name choice , with a gleaming, golden image.

ORPHEUS. *Greek mythology name.* Name of the legendary ancient Greek poet and musician – whose music was so beautiful it made trees dance and rivers stop to listen – would provide a child with a challenging but indelible identity. **International: Orfeo** *(Italian).*

ORSON. *Latin and English, 'bearlike'.* Has a rotund teddy-bear image, à la Orson (birth name George) Welles, who seemed to own it during his lifetime. No longer a single-person signature, it's now an interesting possibility for any parent seeking an unusal yet solid name. **Orsen, Orsin, Orsis, Orso, Urson. International: Ourson** *(French),* **Orsino** *(Italian).*

ORTEGA. *Spanish name, 'dweller at the sign of the grouse'.*

Dashing Latin surname name. **Ortege, Ortego.**

ORVILLE. *French, 'gold town'.* Only if you're an aviation buff. **Orvelle, Orvil.**

OSBERT. *English, 'divinely brilliant'.* Poor Osbert suffers from the double whammy of a soft beginning and the wimpy *bert* ending.

OSBORN. *English, 'divine bear'.* Future CEO – or add an *e* for a hard rocker? **Osbern, Osborne, Osbourn, Osbourne, Osburn, Osburne, Oz, Ozborn, Ozborne, Ozzie, Usborn.**

★**OSCAR.** *English, 'God's spear'; Irish, 'deer-lover'.* Round and jovial, Oscar is a grandpa name that's fast taking over for such trendies as Max and Sam, rising up the Top 50. Actor Hugh Jackman chose it for his son. **Oscarito, Oskar, Osker, Osqui, Osquitar, Ozcar. International: Osgar** *(Scottish Gaelic),* **Osckar, Oskar** *(German),* **Okko, Oskari** *(Finnish),* **Oszkar** *(Hungarian).*

OSGOOD. *Teutonic, 'divine creator'.* Future CFO.

♂ O'SHEA. *Irish, 'son of Séaghdha,' 'hawk-like, stately'.* One of the jauntiest o' the *O* names, the birth name of actor/rapper Ice Cube. **Oshae, Oshai, O'Shane, Oshaun, O'Shay.** *See list on page 496 for other* **O'** *names.*

OSHEEN. *Anglicised variation of Gaelic* **OISÍN.** *Shiny.*

OSIAS. *Greek, 'salvation'.* Has biblical feel without making an appearance in the Bible. **Osías, Ozias.**

OSIRIS. *Egyptian, 'with strong eyesight'.* Name of Egyptian mythology god-king who died and was reborn every year.

OSKAR. *German variation of* **OSCAR.** Oskar is to Oscar as Jakob is to Jacob: harsher and more Old World, but no better. **Osker.**

OSMAN. *Arabic, 'son of snake'.* Its most famous bearer was Prince Osman the First, founder of the Ottoman Empire.

OSMOND. *English, 'divine protection'.* Too tightly tied to the ageing musical clan featuring Donny and Marie. **Osman,** Osmand, Osment, Osmin, Osmonde, Osmont, Osmund, Osmunde, Oz, Ozzie, Ozzy. **International: Osmundo** *(Spanish),* **Asmund** *(Scandinavian),* **Osmanek, Osmen** *(Polish).*

OSRIC. *English, 'divine ruler'.* Clad in armour. **Osrick.**

OSSIAN. *(OH-see-un) Anglicised variation of* **OISÍN.** Too easily confused with Ocean. **Ossin.**

OSVALDO. *Spanish variation of* **OSWALD.** Popular in the Hispanic community, unlike its English cousin. **Oswaldo.**

OSWALD. *English, 'divine power'.* It has been a weak choice for more than a century and it doesn't look like there's any chance of it becoming popular any time soon. **Ossie, Oswaldo, Oswall, Oswell, Oswold, Ox, Ozzie, Waldo. International: Osvaldo** *(Italian, Spanish and Portuguese),* **Osvald** *(Scandinavian).*

OTHELLO. *Hebrew, 'he has the sound of God'; also a variation of* **OTTO.** Shakespeare's moor has exclusive ownership of this name. **Otello. International: Othão** *(Portuguese).*

★**OTIS.** *German, 'wealthy'; variation of* **OTTO.** Cool and bluesy à la Otis Redding, but also an upscale high-society name of the past, Otis has real appeal for parents attracted to its catchy *O* initial and combination of strength and spunk.

OTTAVIO. *Italian, from* **OCTAVIUS.** Spirited and seductive Italiano. **Octavio.**

OTTO. *German, 'wealthy'.* Some truly cutting-edge parent might consider this German classic a so-far-out-it-could-come-back name à la Oscar: a nice round palindrome. **International: Odon, Othon** *(French),* **Otello, Ottone** *(Italian),* **Otilio, Otman, Oto, Oton, Tilo** *(Spanish),* **Otfried, Otho, Ottocar, Ottomar** *(German),* **Audr, Odo** *(Norwegian),* **Onek, Otek, Oton, Otton, Tonek** *(Polish),* **Otik,** *(Czech).*

★**OWEN.** *Welsh, 'young warrior' or 'wellborn'.* This resonant Celtic name is firmly planted in the Top 50, with every indication it will stay

Ocean	Forest Whitaker
Oliver	Bridget Fonda
Oscar	Hugh Jackman
Owen	Phoebe Cates & Kevin Kline, Ricki Lake

there for a while. The name of a legendary saint, it's hot in Hollywood and televisionland, picked by such celebrities as Kevin Kline and Ricki Lake. **Owain, Owin, Owyn. International: Eóghan, Eoin** *(Gaelic),* **Ouen, Owain** *(French).*

OXFORD. *English place name; 'from the oxen crossing'.* High-collared and straitlaced, with the deadly 'Ox' nickname.

OZ. *Hebrew, 'strength, powerful, courageous'.* This may be a legitimate Hebrew name denoting power, but to any Western kid, it will evoke ruby slippers and a yellow brick road. **Ozi, Ozzi, Ozzie, Ozzy.**

OZNI. *Hebrew, 'my hearing'.* This Old Testament name borne by a grandson of Jacob would not rate high in the classroom.

OZURU. *Japanese, 'big stork'.* Has good vibes via the stork's intimations of longevity.

P *boys*

PAAVO. *Finnish variation of* **PAUL.** This exotic variation deserves its own listing for a winning combination of distinctiveness and simplicity. **Paaveli.**

PABLO. *Spanish variation of* **PAUL.** Names that end in *o* are cool and Pablo has the added bonus of some fantastic artistic bearers: painter Picasso, cellist Casals and poet Neruda. **Pable, Pablos, Paublo.**

♂ **PACE.** *Word name.* Calm, straightforward, patrician sounding: one new-style name that's well grounded. **Paice, Payce, Payse.**

PACIANO. *Spanish from Latin, 'peaceful'.* An appealing twist on all the newly fashionable names that suggest peace.

PACIFIC. *Ocean name; from Latin, 'tranquil'.* An adventurous kind of place name, with the added bonus of the association with peace. **International: Pacifico** *(Spanish),* **Pacificus** *(Latin).*

PACKARD. *English, 'pack, bundle,'* could refer to a peddler. As hefty and weighty as the old car. **Packer, Packert.**

PACO. *Spanish, diminutive of* **FRANCISCO;** *Native American, 'eagle'.* Another winning and relaxed but energetic *o*-ending Latin name, sometimes associated with designer Paco Rabanne. **Pacorro, Panchito, Pancho, Paquito.**

PADDY. *Irish, diminutive of* **PATRICK.** Because it's a generic (and often derogatory) term for an Irishman, Paddy fell out of use as a diminutive or given name, though actress Mare Winningham used it not long ago. **Paddey, Paddi, Paddie, Padraic, Padraig.**

PADEN. *English, 'path hill'.* This could be a new variation on the megapopular Braden-Caden-Haden bunch, or a nonmilitaristic form of Patton.

♂ **PADGET, PADGETT.** *English, diminutive of* **PAGE.** A masculine way to honour a feminine Page – although that *ett* ending is typically found in girls' names. **Paget, Pagett.**

PÁDRAIC. *(PAW-rik) Irish variation of* **PATRICK.** This form, common in Ireland, could create confusion. **Paddrick, Paddy, Padhraig, Padrai, Pádraig, Padraigh, Padreic, Padriac, Padric, Padron, Padruig.**

PÁDRAIG. *(PAW-dreeg) Gaelic variation of* **PATRICK.** Once considered too sacred to give to children in Ireland, it is now among their most common names and this attention-getting form could be imported. Could be used to honour an ancestral

Patrick. **Pára, Pádair, Páidean, Páidín, Páraic.**

♂ **PAGAN.** *English, 'heathen,' from Latin, 'from the country, countryman'.* Writer Anne Tyler gave this name to the hippy child in her novel *Amateur Marriage,* but she wasn't the first – it was also used by the Puritans. Today it would be quite a loaded choice.

♂ **PAGE.** *French, 'page, attendant'.* Strictly for the girls. **Padget, Padgett, Paget, Pagett, Paggio, Paige, Payge.**

PAGIEL. *Hebrew, 'God allots'.* Undiscovered, but somewhat awkward Old Testament choice: he was the head of the tribe of Asher.

PAINE. *Latin, 'villager, country-dweller'.* The mere association with 'pain' knocks this name out-of-bounds. **Pain, Payne.**

★ ♂ **PAINTER.** *Occupational name.* A creative choice in this very fashionable category of names, with a pleasant sound. **Paynter.**

♂ **PAISLEY.** *Scottish, 'church, cemetery'.* This name of an intricately patterned fabric is too swirly for a boy.

♂ **PALACE.** *Word name.* Too similar to the female Pallas and Alice.

PALADIN. *French, 'of the palace'.* This title of honour given to Charlemagne's twelve best knights would be prized as a name by most sword-loving little boys. **Paladine, Palatin, Palatine, Palladin, Pallatin, Pallatine, Pallaton, Palldin, Palldine, Palleten, Palleton.**

PALADIO. *Spanish from Greek, 'follower of Pallas'.* Although Pallas was a goddess, a noted male bearer of this name was Saint Palladius, the first Christian bishop of Ireland and the name has an appealing swagger. **Palladius.**

PALANI. *Hawaiian variation of* **FRANK.** One of the Hawaiian names being discovered by stylish parents, especially Californians.

PALASH. *Hindi, 'flowery tree'.* Could be used in an Indian family for a garden-lover's son.

PALBEN. *Basque, 'blond'.* There are many names that mean redhead or dark, fewer that mean blond, but this one would have little appeal.

PALERMO. *Place name.* Son of Sicily.

PALEY. *English, possibly originated as a nickname for pale eyes.* Strong, friendly surname choice, à la Bailey.

PALMER. *English, 'pilgrim' or 'one who holds a palm'.* Pilgrims often carried palms, thus the double meaning. A fresher sounding twist on such upper-class surname names as Porter and Parker. **Pallmer, Palmar, Palmerston.**

PALOMO. *Spanish, 'dove'.* The feminine form, Paloma, is more popular, but this has potential.

PALTI. *Hebrew, 'God liberates'.* Outlook in this country: paltry. **Palti-el, Paltiel, Platya, Platyahu.**

PAN. *Greek, 'all'; Hindi, 'leaf' or 'feather'.* Pan is the Greek god with the legs of a goat and the body of a pipes-playing man

known for his mischievousness. Use of his name is not recommended.

PANAS. *Russian, 'immortal'.* Enviable meaning, but off-putting sound.

PANCHO. *Spanish, diminutive of* **FRANCISCO.** A bit more problematic than such similar names as Pablo and Paco because of the Pancho Villa association. **Panchito, Pancholo, Panzo.**

PANOS. *Greek variation of* **PETER.** Straightforward choice for parents looking to honour their Greek ancestry. **Panagiotis, Panajiotis, Panayioti, Panayiotis, Panayoti, Panayotis, Petros.**

★PAOLO. *Italian variation of* **PAUL.** An irresistibly lush name worlds more romantic than its spare English equivalent.

PAQUITO. *Spanish, diminutive of* **FRANCIS.** The minimising *ito* ending could make your child feel insignificant. **Paco.**

PARAMESH. *Hindi, 'greatest'; another name for the Hindu god Shiva.* Though meaningful in its

own culture, would make a challenging crossover.

PARC. *French, 'park'.* Of course, you can just name him Park. But that's so pedestrian. **Park.**

♂ **PARIS.** *French place name.* The first famous Paris was a mythological prince of incredible beauty. The most recent was media darling Paris Hilton, inspirer of a generation of baby-girl namesakes. But since Pierce Brosnan and other celebs have continued to use it for their sons, the name retains some masculine identity. **Paras, Paree, Pares, Parese, Parie, Parris, Parys.**

♂ **PARISH, PARRISH.** *French, 'ecclesiastical locality'.* More masculine than Paris for a boy, but in danger of being misunderstood as that name; has a slightly churchy feel. **Parrie, Parrisch, Parriss, Parry, Parrysh.**

♂ **PARK.** *Word name.* A grassy place with trees is a nice image to attach to a name. **Parke, Parkes, Parkey, Parks.**

♂ **PARKER.** *English occupational name, 'park-keeper'.*

One of the first generation of surname names, along with Porter and Morgan and still one of the most appealing. The association with Charlie Parker gives it a jazzy edge. **Park, Parke, Parkes, Parkman, Parks.**

PARKIN. *English, 'little Peter'.* To honour an ancestral Peter. **Parken.**

PARNELL. *French, 'little Peter'.* Likable choice for history-minded parents who might want to honour Irish patriot Charles Parnell. **Nell, Parle, Parnel, Parrnell, Pernell.**

PARR. *English, 'enclosure'.* Above par middle name possibility.

PARREN. *Modern invented name.* Darren with a *P*.

♂ **PARRY.** *Welsh, 'son of Harry'.* Quite common in Wales, but would inevitably be misunderstood as Perry or even Harry. **Panie, Parrey, Parrie, Pary.**

PARSON. *English occupational name, 'clergyman'.* This name might have seemed ridiculous even a few years ago, but when

Reese Witherspoon and Ryan Phillippe named their son Deacon, they opened up a whole new field of ecclesiastical cool. **Parsons, Person, Persons.**

PARTHALÁN. *Irish, 'ploughman'.* Familiar in Ireland, strange here. **Parlan, Parth.**

PARTHENIOS. *Greek mythology name.* This name of a Greek river god is draped in a toga. **Par, Parthenius.**

PARTON. *English, 'pear orchard'.* For now at least, conjures up the larger-than-life image of Dolly.

PARVAIZ. *Persian, 'lucky, happy'.* Would certainly stand out in a British classroom. **Parvez, Parviz, Parwiz.**

PASCAL. *French, 'of the Passover'; English, 'Easter'.* Historically used for sons born at Easter, this can make an interesting choice for a boy with Gallic roots arriving around that holiday. **Pace, Pascalle, Paschal, Paschalis, Pascoe, Pascow, Pasquall.** International: **Pascale** *(French)*, **Pasquale** *(Italian)*,

If You Like
Parker,
You Might Love . . .

Asher
Baker
Carter
Colton
Gardener
Judson
Marlon
Palmer
Patrick
Paxton
Peter
Pierce
Powell
Preston
Sawyer
Sayer
Slater

Pascual, Pascul *(Spanish)*, **Pascoal** *(Portuguese)*.

PASCOE. *English variation of* **PASCAL.** Popular in medieval times and definitely deserving of revival. **Pasco.**

PASHA. *Russian, diminutive of* **PAVEL.** Your little Pasha will rule the roost. In Russia, traditionally given to a boy born on Good Friday. **Pascha Pashenka, Pashka.**

PASQUAL. *Spanish, 'Easter,' from Hebrew* **PESACH.** The ultimate Eastertime name. **Paco, Pascalo, Pasco, Pascualo, Pasquel, Pazcual, PazQual.** International: **Pasquale** *(Italian).*

PASTOR. *Latin, 'spiritual leader'.* Brother for Parson and Deacon.

♂ **PAT.** *English, diminutive of* **PATRICK.** The ultimate androgynous name. Stick with the long form. **Pattie, Patty.**

♂ **PATRICE.** *French variation of* **PATRICK.** Still common for boys in France, this has long been feminine elsewhere.

PATRICIO. *(pah-TREE-see-o) Spanish variation of* **PATRICK.** The final *o* adds a bit of masculine punch and pizzazz.

Pachi, Patricius, Patrico, Patrizio, Richi, Ticho.

PATRICK. *Latin, 'noble, patrician'.* Long tied to a hyper-Irish image, Patrick's star has waned as a favourite, recently slipping out of the Top 100, while at the same time enjoying a renaissance as a stylish classic, along with such choices as Henry, Charles and George, that have escaped overuse in the past several decades. **Paddey, Paddie, Paddy, Pat, Patek, Patrece, Patric, Patrice, Patrickk, Patricus, Patrik, Patrique, Patrizius, Pats, Patsy, Patten, Patton, Pattrick, Patty.** International: **Patricius** *(Latin, Dutch),* **Pádraig, Páraic** *(Irish Gaelic),* **Patrizio** *(Italian),* **Patricio** *(Spanish, Portuguese),* **Patek, Patryk** *(Polish),* **Padrik** *(Slavic).*

PATRIN. *Gypsy, 'leaf trail'.* A truly unusual yet easily comprehended choice. **Pattin.**

♂ **PATSY.** *English and Irish, diminutive of* **PATRICK.** Rarely heard for half a century, for either gender.

PATTERSON. *English, 'son of Peter'.* An upscale name worth

considering if you're looking to continue a line of Peters. **Paterson, Patteson, Pattison.**

PATTON. *English, 'fighter's town'.* Attractive name in the fashionable Haden-Peyton mould, though there is that association with the severe war-time general. **Paden, Paten, Patin, Paton, Patten, Pattin, Patty, Payton, Peyton.**

PATXI. *Basque variation of* **FRANCIS.** Basque names are like no others, though this one would be pronounced too much like Patsy.

PAUL. *Latin, 'small'.* An ancient name – popular in Roman and medieval times – that's not very fashionable now, which can work in its favour – scarcity balancing simplicity. It also boasts a wide range of name-sharing heroes, from Revere to Newman, Cézanne to McCartney. **Pall, Pauley, Pauli, Paulie, Paulo, Pauly, Pawl.**

PAULIN. *German and Polish variation of* **PAUL.** The *-in* suffix and the two-syllable rhythm make this a fashionable alternative to the original, but

it looks like an abbreviation of
Pauline. **Paulen.**

PAULO. *Portuguese, Swedish and
Hawaiian variation of* **PAUL.**
Suffers in comparison to the
richer and more authentic-
sounding Paolo.

PAVEL. *Russian variation of*
PAUL. Widespread in the
former Soviet Union, but has a
somewhat impoverished image
here. **Paavel, Panya, Pasha, Pava,
Pavils, Pavlik, Pavlo, Pavlusha,
Pavlushenka, Pawl, Pusha.**

♂ **PAWNEE.** *Native American
tribal name.* The name of this
Plains tribe seems cartoonish as
a first name.

♂ **PAX.** *Latin, 'peaceful'.* One of
the variations of peace newly
popular in these less-than-
peaceful times, chosen by
Angelina Jolie and Brad Pitt for
their adopted son. **Paxx, Paz.**

♂ **PAXTON.** *Latin and English,
'peace town'.* Combines a
fashionable peace association
with equally fashionable two-
syllable surname feel. **Packston,
Pax, Paxon, Paxten, Paxtun.**

Paul's International Variations

Irish Gaelic	**Pól**
Scottish Gaelic	**Pál, Poll**
French	**Paulin**
Italian	**Paolo**
Spanish	**Pablo**
Spanish/Portuguese	**Paulo, Paulino**
Catalan	**Pau**
Dutch	**Pauel**
Danish	**Poul**
Swedish	**Pål, Påvel, Pol**
Norwegian	**Pal**
Finnish	**Paavali, Paavo**
Polish	**Pawel, Pawelek**
Hungarian	**Pál, Pali**
Czech	**Pavilček, Pavlík, Pavloušek**
Russian	**Pasha, Pashenka, Pava, Pavel, Pavlusha, Pusha**
Ukrainian	**Pavlo**
Greek	**Pavlos**

PAYNE. *English, 'villager, country-dweller'.* The *y* helps a bit, but still a painful image. **Paine, Paynn.**

♂ **PAYTON.** *English variation of* **PATTON** *or* **PEYTON.** Though Peyton is the more popular spelling for both sexes, this version of the name is wildly popular too. **Paiton, Pate, Payden, Peaton, Peighton, Peyton.**

♂ **PAZ.** *Hebrew, 'golden'; Spanish, 'peace'.* A less familiar but equally appealing form of peace.

♂ **PAZEL.** *Hebrew, 'golden'; Spanish, 'peace'.* The abbreviated version, Paz, is far more modern and attractive. **Paz.**

PEABODY. *English, 'having the body of a gnat'.* Here is a quintessential surname that your child won't thank you for – either the *pea* part or the *body* part, or its meaning.

♂ **PEACE.** *Word name.* The translated and thus more subtle versions, like Pax or Placido, work better.

PEADAIR. *(PAY-tuhr) Irish variation of* **PETER.** One way to reinvent a classic, though insisting on the authentic pronunciation could cause problems.

♂ **PEAK.** *English word name.* Here is an ambitious geographical name.

PEALE. *English occupational name, 'bell ringer'.* Child may have to endure more than a few banana jokes, but the Peales were a distinguished family of artists. **Peal, Peall, Pealle, Peel, Peele.**

PEARCE. *English and Irish, 'son of Piers'.* This spelling softens the name's sharper edges, though we prefer the original Piers. **Pierce, Piers.**

PEDER. *Scandinavian variation of* **PETER.** You'll have to do a lot of spelling and explaining of this one. **Peadar, Pedey.**

PEDRO. *Spanish variation of* **PETER.** One of the most familiar Spanish names. **Pedrin, Pedrín, Pedrio, Pepe, Petrolino, Petronio, Piero.**

PEEL. *English, 'tower, stockade'.* A peel was a tower that sheltered humans and animals against attack, though these days it's better known as the skin of a banana. **Peele.**

PEERLESS. *Word name.* This name would certainly exert undue pressure.

♂ **PEI.** *(pay) Chinese surname.* For admirers of modernist architect I.M.

PELAGIOS. *Greek, 'from the sea'.* One of the more outré of the sea-related names. **Pelagius, Pelayo.**

PELÉ. *Athlete name.* The name of the Brazilian-born football great (whose name at birth was Edson) is popular in France and could make it here too.

PELHAM. *English, 'tannery town'.* This place name surname could work well as a first, despite its slightly arrogant air.

PELÍ. *Latin and Basque, ' happy'.* Cute as a nickname, slight as a first.

PELL. *English occupational name, 'dealer in furs'.* Unusual middle name choice. **Pall.**

PELLE. *Scandinavian variation of* **PETER.** One of several possible Peter-related Scandinavian choices.

PELLEGRINO. *Italian variation of* **PEREGRINE.** The water – that's it.

PELLO. *Greek and Basque, 'stone'.* Creative variation on Peter. **Peru, Piarres.**

PEMBROKE. *English, 'bluff, headland'.* Better suited to a stuffy school than a little boy. **Pembrook.**

PENDLETON. *English, 'overhanging settlement'.* Pembroke's brother.

PENLEY. *English, 'enclosed meadow'.* And if it's triplets: Pembroke, Pendleton and Penley. **Penlea, Penleigh, Penly, Pennlea, Pennleigh, Pennley.**

★**PENN.** *English, 'enclosure, hill'; occupational name indicating a writer.* This simple, elegant name offers something for many kinds of parents, from writers and history buffs to Pennsylvania-dwellers and fans of Sean. **Pen, Penn, Penney, Pennie, Penny.**

PENROD. *German, 'famous commander'.* This name of a famous Booth Tarkington novel is alien in today's world. **Penn, Pennrod, Rod.**

PEPA. *Czech variation of* **JOSEPH.** Much too feminine in this country. **Pepek, Pepik.**

PEPE. *Spanish variation of* **JOSÉ.** It's a megacommon nickname name in Latino countries but not likely to become come elsewhere. **Pepillo, Pepito, Pequin, Pipo.**

PEPIN. *German, 'determined petitioner'.* Most famous as the name of King Pepin the Short, this choice might feel somewhat belittling. **Pepi, Peppie, Peppy.**

♂ **PEPPER.** *Sanskrit, 'berry'.* There's an American football player called Pepper (given the childhood nickname for sprinkling pepper on his cereal) Johnson – but this sounds more like the name of a teenage girl. **International: Pepe** (*Italian*), **Peppar** (*Swedish*), **Pfeffer** (*German*), **Biber** (*Turkish*), **Koshoo** (*Japanese*), **Meritja** (*Indonesian*).

PER. *Scandinavian variation of* **PETER.** So simple, yet so exotic: a prime candidate for export. **Pelle.**

PERCIVAL. *French, 'pierce the vale'.* In today's world, Percival is seen as an almost laughably effete name, but the original Percival was the one perfectly pure Knight of the Round Table, a worthy hero. **Parsafal, Parsefal, Parsifal, Parzival, Perc, Perce, Perceval, Percevall, Percey, Percivall, Percy, Peredur, Purcell.**

PERCY. *French, 'from Percy'.* A bit more down-to-earth than Percival. Believe it or not, we think it could make a comeback down the road. **Pearcey, Pearcy, Percey, Percie, Piercey, Piercy.**

PERDIDO. *Spanish, 'lost'.* The feminine version, Perdita, is more familiar here.

PEREGRINE. *Latin, 'traveller, pilgrim'.* Elegantly aristocratic here, extravagantly eccentric, even foppish, elsewhere. **Peregrin, Peregrino, Peregryn, Peregryne, Perine, Perry. International: Pellegrino** *(Italian),* **Perine** *(Latin).*

PEREZ. *Spanish from Hebrew, 'to blossom'.* The newest trendy surname names are ethnic, and this is an excellent example. **International: Peretz** *(Hebrew).*

PERFECTO. *Spanish, 'perfect'.* Spanish speakers use this name for Jesus Christ only. Probably a good policy.

PERICLES. *Greek, 'far-famed'.* Ancient Athenian statesman whose name was once used in the USA mostly for slaves. Deserves to be liberated for use by the population at large – though it might take a few generations.

PERICO. *Spanish variation of* **PETER.** Cooler and sexier than Pedro, but also has a slightly industrial sound. **Pequin, Perequin.**

PERKIN. *English, 'little Peter'.* Sounds like a Hobbit. **Perka, Perkins, Perkyii, Perkyn, Perrin.**

♂ **PERRY.** *English, 'pear tree'.* A casual but suave name in velvet-throated singer Perry Como's day . . . about fifty years ago. These days, most cool Perrys (or Peris) are girls. **Parry, Peri, Perrie, Perrye.**

PERSEUS. *Greek mythology name.* A godly Greek hero (he was a son of Zeus) whose name has more muscle than Percy.

♀ **PERSIA.** *Place name.* Exotic and sexy . . . and feminine.

PERTH. *Scottish, 'thornbush thicket'; place name.* There's a Perth in Scotland and a bigger one in Australia; this name could make a statement similar to Heath.

★ ♀ **PERU.** *place name.* An unexplored choice, evocative of the snowcapped Andes, with a pleasant, catchy sound.

PERVIS. *Latin, 'passage'.* The *perv* connection crosses this name off the list. **Pervez.**

PESAH. *Hebrew, 'spared'.* The Hebrew name for Passover, making this the Jewish version of naming your child Christmas or Easter. **Pesach, Pessach.**

PETER. *Greek, 'rock'.* New Testament name that has recently slipped out of the Top 100, which makes it a good choice if you're seeking a less-used classic with many nice childhood associations, like Peter Rabbit and Peter Pan. More fashionable versions of this name are the Italian Piero and Pietro. **Pearce, Peers, Peeter, Peirce, Perico, Perion, Perkin, Pero, Perrin, Perry, Pete, Péter, Petey, Peto, Pierce, Pierson.**

PETERSON. *English, 'son of Peter'.* To honour an ancestral Peter. **Peteris, Petersen.**

PETEUL. *Aramaic, 'vision of the Lord'.* Old Testament name that deserves its obscurity.

PETIRI. *Shona, 'where we are'.* Unknown in this country, it has some exotic appeal. **Petri.**

PEVERELL. *French, 'piper'.* Effete. **Peverall, Peverel, Peveril.**

♂ **PEYTON.** *English, 'fighting-man's estate'.* The most-used spelling of this ever-more-popular name, but now thought of as a female name. **Payton, Peyt, Peyten, Peython, Peytonn.**

PHARAOH. *Latin, 'ruler'.* Overstretching, in the Prince and Pope mould. Famous jazz saxophonist Pharoah [*sic*] Saunders was really named Ferrell. **Faroh, Pharo, Pharoah, Pharoh.**

♂ **PHELAN.** *(FAY-lin) Irish, 'wolf'.* Appealing Irish surname name. **Felan, Felin, Palan, Palin, Phaelan, Phelin.**

PHELIX. *Latin variation of* **FELIX.** Phar-phetched.

PHELPS. *English, 'son of Philip'.* Solid Philip middle name alternative.

♂ **PHILADELPHIA.** *Greek place name, 'brotherly love'.* Not nearly as popular as other American city names, but occasionally used for girls. Shirley Temple played a

Peter's International Variations

Irish Gaelic	**Peadar**
Scottish Gaelic	**Peadair, Peidearan**
Welsh	**Pedr**
French	**Pierre**
Italian	**Piero, Pietro**
Spanish/Portuguese	**Pedro**
Basque	**Peio, Pello, Peru**
Catalan	**Pere**
Dutch	**Piet, Pieter, Pietr**
Danish	**Peder, Perben**
Swedish	**Pär, Pehr, Per, Petter**
Norwegian	**Peder, Per, Petter**
Finnish	**Pekka, Petteri**
Polish	**Piotr**
Romanian	**Petar, Petru**
Czech	**Péťa, Peťka, Petr, Petríček, Petrik, Petroušek**
Lithuanian	**Petras**
Russian	**Petenka, Petya, Pyotr**
Ukrainian	**Petro**
Latvian	**Peteris**
Greek	**Panos, Petrini, Petrino, Petros**
Armenian	**Bedros**
Hawaiian	**Pekelo**

Philadelphian in the old western movie *Fort Apache*.

PHILANDER. *Greek, 'loving mankind'.* Old name too close to 'philanderer'.

PHILBERT. *French from Greek, 'dear, beloved'.* Varying Filbert does not improve the name: it still makes one think of a nut. **Filbert, Philibert, Phillbert.**

PHILEMON. *Greek, 'affectionate' or 'kiss'.* Rarely heard New Testament name – he was a friend of Saint Paul – that might conceivably stand up to modern usage.

PHILIP. *Greek, 'lover of horses'.* The name of one of the twelve apostles, Philip is still favoured by parents in search of a solid boys' classic that is less neutral than Robert or John and more distinctive than Daniel or Matthew and has many historic, royal ties. **Fillip, Flip, Fyllip, Phelps, Phil, Phillip, Phillipp, Phillips, Philly, Philp, Phylip, Phyllip, Pip, Pippo. International: Pilip** *(Irish Gaelic),* **Filib** *(Scottish Gaelic),* **Philbin, Pilbin** *(Scottish),* **Philippe**

(French), **Filippo** *(Italian),* **Felipe** *(Spanish),* **Felip** *(Catalan),* **Philipp** *(German),* **Filip** *(Norwegian and Czech),* **Vilppu** *(Finnish),* **Fülöp** *(Hungarian).*

PHILIPPE. *French variation of* **PHILIP.** Philip with Gallic flair. **Philipe, Phillepe, Phillipe, Phillippe, Phillippee, Phyllipe.**

★**PHILO.** *Greek, 'loving'.* We love the *o* ending and sweet meaning of this dynamic and distinctive Greek name, often used in literature, but never particularly popular. Possible substitute for the increasingly popular Milo. **Phylo.**

PHILOSOPHY. *Word name.* Far-fetched, but friends can always call him Phil.

PHINEAN. *Irish variation of* **FINIAN.** Julia Roberts's choice of Phinnaeus gives a boost to all *Ph* forms. Or should we say, phorms. **Phinian.**

PHINEAS. *Hebrew, 'oracle'.* Julia Roberts drew this biblical name into the limelight when she chose it – with the even-more-antique spelling Phinnaeus – for her twin son, now called

Finn. It had last been heard from via circus impresario Phineas T. Barnum and would appeal to parents with a sense of humour as well as adventure. **Fineas, Phinehas, Phinnaeus, Phinneas, Phinny, Pincas, Pinchas, Pinchos, Pincus, Pinhas, Pinkus.**

PHIPPS. *English, 'son of Philip'.* Possible middle name to honour an ancestral Philip. **Philips, Philipson, Phips.**

PHOEBUS. *(FEE-bus) Greek, 'shining, brilliant'.* One of the names of the sun god Apollo, this is better known in its feminine form, Phoebe. **Phoibos.**

♂ **PHOENIX.** *Greek, 'dark red'; also Arizona place name.* Phoenix rolls a lot of cool trends into one: it's a place name and a bird name, it ends in the oh-so-hip letter *x* and as the mythic bird that rose from the ashes, it's a symbol of immortality. It's also got celebrity chops, via the acting family that includes Joaquin and the late River and as the child of an ex-Spice Girl. **Fenix, Phenix, Pheonix, Phynix.**

♂ **PIANO.** *Music name.* If Banjo can be a name, why not Piano?

♂ **PICABIA.** *Artist name.* A middle name idea to honour surrealist painter Francis.

PICARD. *French from Basque, 'from Picardy'.* Associated with the *Star Trek* commander of the USS *Enterprise*. **Pecard, Pecardo, Picardo.**

PICASSO. *Spanish artist name.* A worthy honouree that would place a too-heavy expectation on a child, probably subjecting him to ridicule. Try Pablo instead.

PICKFORD. *English, 'from the ford at the peak'.* One surname name unlikely to cross over to first.

★**PIERCE.** *English 'son of Piers'.* Actor Pierce Brosnan brings a strong helping of charm to this name. **Pearce, Pears, Pearson, Pearsson, Peerce, Peirce, Piers, Pierson, Piersson.**

PIERLUIGI. *Italian, combination of* **PIERO** *and* **LUIGI.** If one exotic name won't do.

★**PIERO.** *Italian variation of* **PETER.** Elegant, melodic, appealing. Think Piero della Francesca. **Pero, Pierro, Pietro.**

PIERRE. *French variation of* **PETER.** One of the most familiar – if stereotypical – Gallic names. **Peiree, Piere, Pierrot.**

PIERRE-LUC. *French, combination of* **PIERRE** *and* **LUC.** French for Pierluigi. **Piere Luc.**

PIERS. *Greek, 'rock'.* The first version of Peter to reach the English-speaking world, via the Normans, but it never been as popular as the English version, despite its large measure of understated panache. **Pearce, Pears, Pearson, Pierce, Pierson, Piersson.**

PIET. *(Peet) Dutch, diminutive of* **PIETER.** Most often associated in this country with Dutch modernist painter Mondrian.

PIETRO. *Italian variation of* **PETER.** Yet another winning international form of Peter.

★**PIKE.** *English nature name.* Cool choice for sons of fishermen. **Pyke.**

PILI. *African, Swahili, 'second born'.* Will be frequently misunderstood as Pelé or, worse, 'pilly'.

PILOT. *Occupational name.* One celebrity baby Pilot put this occupational choice into the pool – together with the middle name Inspektor, something we wouldn't advise following.

PINCHAS. *(pink-us) Hebrew, 'oracle'; Egyptian, 'dark-skinned'.* Famous violinist-conductor Pinchas Zuckerman is the most famous modern bearer; the biblical Pinchas was the son of Eleazar and the grandson of Aaron – both preferable name choices. **Phineas, Pincas, Pinchos, Pincus, Pinkas, Pinkus, Pinky.**

♂ **PINE.** *Nature name.* Fresh.

PINO. *Italian, diminutive of names such as* **GIUSEPPINO.** There are many more substantial Italian choices.

PIO. *Latin, 'pious'.* Though the variation Pius is too, well, popeish, Pio might work for an ordinary boy. **Pius.**

PIP. *English, diminutive of* **PHILIP.** The original Pip was the main character in *Great Expectations* (full name Philip Pirrip). Cute for a tike, problematic for a man.

♂ **PIPER.** *English occupational name, 'one who plays the pipes'.* Girly.

PIPPIN. *German, 'father'.* Childish name that was the title of a West End musical – but best known as a type of apple. Keep this one as a term of affection.

PIRAN. *Irish, 'prayer'.* Could be a future Kieran, which looks like the next Conor. Piran is the patron saint of miners. **Peran, Pieran.**

PITNEY. *English, 'island, dry ground in moss'.* Unless this is a family name, give it a pass. **Pittney.**

PITT. *English, 'pit, ditch'.* You have to be Brad to pull off this name.

PLACIDO. *Spanish, 'serene'.* Opera star Domingo was responsible for giving this popular Spanish name international attention. **Placedo, Placide, Plácido, Placidus, Placijo, Placydo, Plasedo. International: Palacido** (*Spanish*), **Placyd** (*Slavic*).

PLATO. *Greek, 'broad-shouldered'.* The name of one of the greatest Western philosophers is often used in Greece and would make a really interesting, thought-provoking choice elsewhere.

PLATT. *French, 'flat land'.* Flat. **Platte.**

♂ **PLENTY.** *Word name.* Wishful thinking.

PLUTO. *Greek, 'rich'.* The Roman god of the underworld, the former ninth planet, a cartoon dog . . . but *not* a baby.

♂ **PO.** *Italian river name.* A river (in Italy), a writer (Bronson), a Teletubby: the Bo of the new millennium.

♂ **POE.** *English, 'peacock'.* With its literary reference, it feels

much more distinguished and complete, if less cowboyish, than cousin Po.

POLDI. *German diminutive of* **LEOPOLD.** If you must name your child Leopold, at least call him Leo. **Poldo.**

POLLARD. *English, 'shorn head'.* Clumsy when used as a first name. **Poll, Pollerd, Pollyrd.**

POLLOCK. *Scottish, 'pool' or 'pit'.* If used at all these days, it would be to honour artist Jackson, whose first name would be far preferable. **Pollack, Polloch.**

POLLUX. *Greek, 'crown'.* Castor's twin in the constellation Gemini. That final *x* makes this name modern and cool. **Pollock.**

POLO. *Tibetan, 'brave wanderer'; Greek, diminutive of Apollo; also word name.* If Portia can become Porsche, then Apollo can morph into Polo – the imprint of designer Ralph Lauren.

POM. *French diminutive, 'apple'.* Not much used in

France, but cute and familiar here as one of Babar (the Elephant's) triplets.

POMEROY. *French, 'apple orchard'.* Baroque and sissified. **Pommeray, Pommeroy, Ponuneray, Potnmeroy.**

POMPEY. *Latin, 'five'.* Roman statesman and Caesar rival whose name, like other classical choices, was occasionally used for slaves. The Pompeo version could rise again. **Pompei, Pompeo, Pompeyo, Pompi, Pompilio, Pomponio.**

PONCE. *Spanish, 'fifth'.* Spanish explorer Ponce de León may be a worthy namesake, but 'poncey' is British slang for effeminate. Better go with Quintus, this name's Latin equivalent, or one of its variations.

PORAT. *Hebrew, 'fruitful, productive'.* A name that is used to describe a handsome or clever boy and is also an Israeli place name.

PORFIRIO. *Greek, 'purple stone'.* This ancient saint's name was borne by the infamous mid-

century playboy, Porfirio Rubirosa. **Porphirios, Prophyrios.**

PORIEL. *Hebrew, 'fruit of God'.* An obscure Hebrew name that would not be many parents' first choice.

PORTER. *Latin, 'gate-keeper'; occupational name.* A quintessential yuppie name, one of the many *P* surnames to catch on in the early 1990s. **Port, Portie, Porty.**

PORTHOS. *Literary name.* One of Alexandre Dumas' *Three Musketeers,* probably better than the perfume-scented Aramis.

♂ **PORTLAND.** *English, 'land near the port'; place name.* There are two lovely Portlands in the US, in Maine and Oregon, but not many babies with their name.

POSEIDON. *Greek mythology name.* This version of the sea god's name may be more ready for prime time than the Roman version, Neptune – slightly.

POTTER. *English, 'maker of drinking and storage vessels'.*

Could join such up-and-comers as Miller and Gardener.

POWELL. *English, 'alert'; Welsh, 'son of Howell'.* Powerful surname choice with many distinguished bearers, fresher sounding than Parker. **Powel.**

POWER. *Word name.* One of the new crop – Justice, Liberty, Peace – of strong, clear-cut, declarative choices, though this lacks their virtuous attributes.

POWERS. *Word name.* The singular version sounds more contemporary.

POWHATAN. *Native American, Algonquin, 'powwow hill'.* Powhatan is identified with the powerful chief and father of Pocahontas; not likely to be adopted by others.

PRADEEP. *Hindi, 'light, lantern'.* One of the more familiar Hindu choices, with built-in depth and a suggestion of enlightenment.

♂ **PRAIRIE.** *Nature name.* An evocative, windswept choice that is part of the third generation of American-influenced names, picking up where first Jesse and then Dakota left off, though with a slight feminine edge.

PRANAV. *Hindi, 'primordial'.* This Indian name represents Aum, or Om, the most sacred syllable in Hinduism, symbolising the entire universe.

PRATT. *English, 'trick, craft'.* In British slang, a 'prat' is an idiot – enough said. **Prat.**

♂ **PRENTICE.** *English, 'apprentice'.* Long-used surname name that's up for promotion to greater popularity. **Prent, Prentis, Prentiss, Printes, Printiss.**

PRESCOTT. *English, 'priest's cottage'.* The *scott* part makes it more approachable than other upper-class surname names. **Prescot, Prestcot, Prestcott.**

♂ **PRESLEY.** *English, 'priest's meadow'.* More universal than Elvis. . . . and more attractive, too. Cindy Crawford used it for her son, though it's on the rise mainly for girls. **Presleigh, Presly, Presslee, Pressley, Prestley, Priestley, Priestly.**

PRESTON. *English, 'priest's estate'.* Britney Spears put this old-fashioned surname name back on the map when she chose it as son Sean's middle name. For now, a fine choice – but it could become overexposed. It's already shot up nearly 800 places! **Prestan, Presten, Prestin, Prestyn.**

PREWITT. *French, 'brave little one'.* Common surname rarely used as a first. **Preuet, Prew, Prewet, Prewett, Prewit, Pruit, Pruitt.**

PRIAM. *Greek mythology name.* In ancient Greek mythology, a Trojan king with fifty children; in the modern world it sounds more like a computer language or environmentally correct car.

PRICE. *Welsh, 'son of Rhys'; word name.* Some names referring to expensive things – Tiffany, Armani, Porsche – are in fact déclassé, but Price transcends that label with its simplicity and strength. **Brice, Bryce, Pryce, Prys.**

PRIEST. *Occupational name.* An extreme example of the newly possible ecclesiastical brotherhood

that includes Deacon and Bishop. This one might work better in the middle spot.

PRIMO. *Italian, 'first'.* Would make your son number one. **Preemo, Premo, Prymo. International: Prym** *(Polish).*

PRIMUS. *Latin, 'first'.* The revival of long-dormant Roman names could put this back in the lexicon.

PRINCE. *Latin, 'chief, prince'.* The singer once again known as Prince once had sole dominion over this name, but then Michael Jackson chose it for not one but *two* of his sons – more evidence of his dubious parenting ideas. **Prence, Prinz, Prinze.**

PRINCETON. *English, 'princely town'.* American college name. **Prenston, Princeston, Princton.**

PROCTOR. *Latin, 'official, administrator'.* With the new fashion for occupational names, we may hear more of this one. **Prockter, Procter.**

PROSPER. *Latin, 'favourable, prosperous'.* In France,

pronounced *PRO-spare,* it's a fairly common name; elsewhere it presents a worthy message for a child. **Prospero, Próspero.**

PROSPERO. *Italian, Spanish and Portuguese variation of* **PROSPER.** Shakespeare's *Tempest* has kept this name alive.

PROUST. *French literary name.* For remembrance of books past, a meaningful middle name.

PROVO. *Place name.* Conservative city in the US state of Utah, it's unlikely to be a fashionable place name.

PRYOR. *Latin, 'head of the monastery, prior'.* For those in search of an unusual occupational name . . . or in memory of comedian Richard. **Prior, Pry.**

PRYS. *Welsh, 'son of Rhys'.* The Welsh way to spell Price, which is more complicated but elevates it beyond the monetary realm.

PUCK. *Literary name.* Shakespeare's mischievous pixie would be better left in the world of literature.

PURVIS. *French and English, 'providing food'.* This spelling does not dispel the 'perv' connection. **Pervis, Purves, Purviss.**

PUTNAM. *English, 'dweller by the hollow'.* Perhaps if there's a Putnam in your background. **Putnem.**

PYOTR. *(pee-O-ter) Russian variation of* **PETER.** For British people, may prove too much of a twist on Peter. **Petenka, Petinka, Petrusha, Petya, Piotr, Pyatr.**

PYRAMID. *Word name.* Spiritually resonant, but will definitely raise grandparents' eyebrows.

Q boys

QADAR. *(kah-DAHR) Arabic, 'decree, destination'.* One of several Arabic names that can be spelled with a *Q* or a *K*, rarely heard outside the Muslim community.

QADIM. *(kah-DEEM) Arabic, 'ancient'.* More frequently seen with the Kadeem spelling. **Kadeem, Kadim, Qadeem, Quadeem, Quadim, Quadym.**

Q Names
New to the Mix

Qaeshaun

Qajon

Qashon

Qequon

Quadarius

Quadrees

Quamaine

Quandarrius

Quandre

Quantavius

Quantay

Quantrell

Quashaun

Quashon

Quesean

Quindarius

Quintavis

Quintavius

Quintay

Qweshon

QĀDIR. *(kah-DEER) Arabic, 'capable, powerful'.* A name that represents one of the ninety-nine attributes of Allah. **Kadir,**

Qaadirm, Qadar, Qadeer, Qadry, Qadyr, Quaadir, Quadeer, Quadir, Quadyr, Quaida.

QAMAR. *(kah-MAR) Arabic, 'moon'.* Appealing in part because of its similarity to the likable Omar. **Quamar, Quamir.**

QASIM. *(kah-SIM) Arabic, 'charitable, generous'.* Name of a son of the Prophet Muhammad, with a particularly positive meaning. **International: Kasim, Qassim, Qassen** *(French).*

♂QUADE. *Latin, 'fourth' or 'born fourth'.* A confident, contemporary-sounding name that would fit right in with classmates Cade, Zade and Jade. **Quaden, Quadin, Quadon, Quaid, Quaide, Qwade.**

QUAID. *See QUADE.*

♂ QUAIN. *French, 'clever, quick'.* Truly offbeat, but just on the brink of outré.

♂ QUANAH. *(KWAN-NAH) Native American, 'sweet smelling, fragrant'.* Name of a major figure in American Indian

history, Quanah Parker, a Comanche chief who became a judge on the Court of Indian Affairs. **Quan.**

QUANTAVIUS. *English, modern combination of* **QUAN** *(a variation of Juan) and* **OCTAVIUS.** One of the more imposing and intriguing of the combo names. **Quantavious, Quantavis, Quantavous, Quatavius.**

♂ QUARRY. *Nature name.* Has the offbeat quality and macho feel – like Stone and Flint – that appeals to increasing numbers of modern parents.

♂ QUAY. *(kay) French word name, 'wharf'.* A name that looks intriguing and masculine on paper, but is, unfortunately, a homonym for a girl's name. **Quaye. International: Qué** *(French).*

♂ QUEBEC. *place name.* An interesting Canadian province and city name that has some literary history as the name of a character in Dickens's *Bleak House;* could make a distinctive choice for parents with literary roots.

♂ **QUENNEL.** *(ken-ell) French, 'dweller at the little oak tree'.* We can think of two drawbacks to this name: the slightly feminine *el* ending and the resemblance to the delicate dumpling called a quenelle. **Quenal, Quenall, Quenel, Quenell, Quennell.**

★**QUENTIN.** *Latin, 'fifth'.* An offbeat name with lots of character, Quentin is the most usable of the Latin birth-order names, masculine as well as stylish and distinctive. Trivia tidbit: Saint Quentin is the protector against coughs. **Quantin, Quent, Quentan, Quenten, Quenton, Quint, Quintin, Quinton, Quintus, Quentyn, Qwentin.** International: **Caointean, Caoidhean** *(Scottish Gaelic),* **Quentilien, Quintien** *(French),* **Quito** *(Spanish).*

♂ **QUEST.** *Word name.* Suggests a sense of curiosity and purpose.

QUICO. *(KEE-ko) Spanish, diminutive of* **ENRIQUE.** Kinetic nickname name, might just be more suited to a Chihuahua.

QUIGLEY. *Irish, 'from the mother's side'.* The spoiled only son of the richest family in town in a 1950s movie. **Quiglea, Quiglee, Quigleigh.**

♂ **QUILL.** *Irish, diminutive of* **QUILLAN** *or* **QUILLER;** *also English word name.* Unique possibility for the child of writers – even if they do use computers rather than pens; could also serve as a rhyming tribute to an ancestor named Gil, Phil or Bill (or Jill).

♂ **QUILLAN.** *(KILL-an) Irish, 'cub'; Zodiac sign of Leo, the lion.* If you like Dylan but find it too popular, this could be a distinctive alternative. **Killan, Quilan, Quilen, Quilin, Quillen.**

♂ **QUILLER.** *English occupational name, 'scribe, writer with a quill pen'.* Heard in a 1960s spy movie, *The Quiller Memorandum,* this name has an offbeat charm.

QUILLIAM. *Irish, 'son of William'.* A really unusual choice that could be used to honour Grandpa Will.

QUILLON. *(KILL-on) Latin, 'crossing swords'; Greek, 'strong'. See* **QUILLAN.** **Killon, Quilen, Quill, Quillen, Quillo, Quilon.**

♂ **QUIMBY.** *Norse, 'from the woman's estate'.* Virtually never heard in this country – and probably not very often in Scandinavia – with a quirky quality. **Quemby, Quenbey, Quemby, Quinby.**

♂ **QUINCE.** *Latin, 'apple-like fruit'.* The girls have Apple, Plum, Peaches, Cherry and Berry: here's one variety of fruit suitable for a boy.

♂ **QUINCY.** *French, 'estate of the fifth son'.* Quirky in the way that all *Q* names are quirky, Quincy was once a buttoned-up, patrician New England name, an image countered in recent years by the talented and ultracool musician Quincy Jones (middle name: Delight; nickname: Q). **Quency, Quin, Quince, Quincey, Quinn, Quinncy, Quinnsy, Quinsey, Quinsy, Quinzy.**

♂ **QUINLAN.** *Irish, 'graceful, fit, shapely, strong'.* An Irish last-name-first-name that could make a child feel distinctive, while still having the regular guy nickname of Quinn. Christine Taylor and Ben Stiller spelled their son's name Quinlin. **Quindlan, Quindlen, Quindlyn, Quinlen, Quinlin, Quinlyn, Quinn.**

♂**QUINN.** *Irish, 'descendant of Conn'.* Engaging Celtic surname that has some history as a unisex first name and some power from 'The Mighty Quinn', the name of a film, a band and a Bob Dylan song. **Quin.**

♂ **QUINNEY.** *Manx, 'son of Crafty'.* Sounds like an endearment of Quinn.

QUINT. *English from* **QUINTUS;** *diminutive of* **QUINTON.** Clint with a glint; used for flinty characters in old TV westerns.

QUINTAS. *Spanish, 'small estate'.* Sounds a bit like an Australian airline.

QUINTEN. *See* **QUENTIN** *and* **QUINTIN.**

QUINTERO. *Spanish, 'five'.* Adds some salsa to the Latin root. **Quinterro.**

QUINTIN. *Latin, 'fifth'.* Both this form and Quentin are authentic modern forms of the Roman family name Quintus. Your choice. **Quentin, Quiliano, Quinn, Quinnton, Quinten, Quintiliano, Quintilio, Quintino, Quintion, Quintten, Quiton, Qwinton. International: Quintilin, Quintille, Qutien** *(French).*

QUINTO. *(KEEN-tō) Spanish variation of* **QUINTIN.** Quint doing the samba. **Queeto, Quinino, Quintin, Quintó, Quyto, Qyto.**

QUINTON. *English, 'queen's manor'.* As Clinton is to Clint, Quinton is to Quint: a bit less commanding. **Quinntan, Quinnten, Quinntin, Quinnton, Quintain, Quintan, Quintyn, Quintynn.**

QUINTUS. *Latin, 'fifth'.* A literary name – figuring in the story of *Ben Hur* and the novels of Anthony Trollope – with the feel of Roman antiquity that's beginning to appeal to many

parents. One of only about twenty male first names in ancient Rome.

♂ **QUIRIN.** *(KEER-in) Origin unknown.* A child might like to have a name connected to the legendary Quirin stone, which, when placed on a sleeping person's head, prompts him to expose his secret thoughts.

QUIRINAL. *Roman mythology name, son of Mars.* Major problem: drop just two letters and you have a direct path to bathroom humour. **Quirinus.**

QUIRINO. *Latin, 'a spearman, a warrior'; also Italian variation of* **CORIN.** An adolescent boy might have problems with the first syllable.

QUIRT. *Spanish, 'riding whip,' from Spanish word 'cuarta'.* Add an *s* and you've got squirt.

QUITO. *(KEE-toe) Spanish variation of* **QUENTIN;** *capital of Ecuador.* A place name with lots of lively energy. **Qeeto, Qito, Queeto, Quyto, Qyto.**

♂ **QUIXLEY.** *English, 'clearing'.* Only if you don't mind hearing yourself saying, 'Come quickly, Quixley!' **Quix.**

QUIXOTE. *(kee-HOE-tay) Spanish literary name.* Tied to the hero of the classic Spanish novel *Don Quixote*, likely to produce a quixotic daydreamer.

QUON. *(KWAN) Chinese, 'bright'.* A well-used name in China has some potential for assimilation.

R boys

RA. *Egyptian, 'sun'.* The name of the sun god of Egyptian mythology could only be used in combination with a longer name.

RAANAN. *(rah-ah-nahn) Hebrew, 'fresh, luxuriant'.* This strong name and its variations are well used in Israel. **Ranan, Renan, Renon.**

RABI. *Arabic, 'gentle wind'.* Could cause pronunciation problems. Robbie? Or Rabbi? **Rabbi, Rabee, Rabeeh, Rabiah, Rabie, Rabih.**

RACER. *Word name.* New, fast, cool and chosen by a film director whose other sons are Rebel, Rocket and Rogue – all somewhat risky options. **Race, Racel, Rayce, Raycer.**

RACHAM. *Hebrew, 'mercy, compassion'.* This name – the basic form is Rachamim – is especially popular among Sephardic Jews. **Rachaman, Rachim, Rachman, Rachmiel, Rachum, Raham, Rahamim, Rahim.**

RAD. *English, 'advisor'.* Radical, man. **Raad, Radd, Raddie, Raddy, Rade, Radee, Radell, Radey, Radi.**

RADBURN. *English, 'reedy stream'.* Upper-class surname name. **Radborn, Radborne, Radbourn, Radbourne, Radburne.**

RADCLIFF. *English, 'red cliff'.* Harvard's sibling – another elite American college. **Radcliffe, Radclyffe, Ratcliff, Ratcliffe.**

RADLEY. *English, 'red meadow'.* Radical Bradley. **Radlea, Radlee, Radleigh, Radly.**

★**RAFAEL.** *Spanish variation of* **RAPHAEL.** Perhaps the ultimate sexy Latino name, not a bad gift to give your son. **Fallo, Falo, Felio, Rafaelle, Rafaello, Rafaelo, Rafal, Rafe, Rafeal, Rafeé, Rafel, Rafello, Rafer, Raffael, Raffaelo, Raffeal, Raffel, Rafffaello, Raffiel, Rafi, Rafiel, Rafo, Raphael, Raphel. International: Raffaele** *(Italian).*

RAFE. *Variation of* **RALPH.** Used almost exclusively in England; would make an equally amiable short form elsewhere for Raphael or Rafferty – and could also stand on its own.

★**RAFFERTY.** *Irish, 'flood-tide, abundance, prosperity'.* Jaunty and raffish, one of the most engaging of the Irish surnames; used by Jude Law for his son. **Rafe, Rafer, Raferty, Raff, Raffarty, Raffer, Raffertey.**

RAFI. *Arabic, diminutive of* **RAFIQ;** *Spanish, diminutive of* **RAFAEL.** Some people will associate it with a well-known children's singer. **Rafee, Raffe, Raffee, Raffi, Raffy, Rafi.**

RAFIQ. *Arabic, 'friend, companion, gentle, kind'.*

Confident Middle Eastern choice. Children will relate to the Rafiki form via the wise guru in Disney's *The Lion King*. **Raafiq, Rafeeq, Rafi, Rafic, Rafik, Rafiki, Rafique.**

RAGNAR. *Norse, 'powerful army' or 'warrior or judgment'.* Historical name in Scandinavia (Ragnar Shaggybritches is a Danish warrior). Easier versions here would be Raynor or Rainier, as in the late prince of Monaco. **Ragnor, Rainer, Rainier, Rainor, Raneir, Ranier, Rannier, Raynar, Rayner, Regner, Reiner, Reinold. International: Ranieri** *(Italian),* **Raynor** *(Scandinavian),* **Reinhold** *(Swedish).*

RAHIM. *Arabic, 'empathetic, merciful'.* To Muslims, an auspicious name. **Raaheim, Rahaeim, Raheam, Raheem, Raheim, Rahiem, Rahiim, Rahime, Rahium, Rakiim, Rakim.**

RAIDEN. *Japanese, 'thunder and lightning'.* The name of the Japanese god of thunder makes an assertive choice, very much at home in the Western world. **Raidan, Raidin, Rayden, Raydun, Rayedon.**

RAINER. *German, 'wise army'.* Starting to sound like a good possibility here, as opposed to the more Teutonic Reiner. **Rainart, Raine, Rainhard, Rainhardt, Reinart, Reiner, Reinhard, Reinhardt, Reinhart, Renke.**

RAINES. *English, 'from Rayne or Rennes'.* The final *s* turns a nature name into an upper-class surname. **Rain, Raine, Rains, Rayne, Raynee, Raynes, Rayno.**

RAINIER. *German, 'wise army'.* European royal name and to Americans a place name evoking the majestic mountain in Washington state. **Rainar, Raine, Rainee, Rainer, Rainey, Rainie, Rainney, Rainor, Rainy, Rayner, Raynier, Reinier, Reiny.**

RAJAH. *Hindi, 'prince, chief'.* Indian princely title, more exotic than Prince or Duke. **Raj, Raja, Rajaah, Rajaahn, Rajae, Rajahe, Rajain, Rajan, Raje, Rajeh, Rajen, Raji, Rajin.**

RAJIV. *Sanskrit, 'striped'.* Known elsewhere via the son of Indira Gandhi, who himself became prime minister of India.

★ ♂ **RALEIGH.** *English, 'meadow of roe deer'.* Attractive place name in the US state of North Carolina and surname of explorer Sir Walter Raleigh. Distinctive choice for either sex. **Ralegh, Raleigh, Rawle, Rawleigh, Rawley, Rawling, Rawly, Rawylyn.**

RALPH. *English, 'wolf-counsel'.* Ralph has a double image: the suave Ralph Fiennes–type often pronounced Rafe, and the blue-collar version with the more common pronunciation. It's all in the eye (or ear) of the beholder. **Radolphus, Rafe, Raff, Ralf, Ralpheal, Ralphel, Ralphie, Ralphy, Ralston, Raoul, Raul, Rolf, Rolfe, Rolle, Rolph, Rolphe.**

RALSTON. *English, 'Ralph's settlement'.* Down-to-earth surname name, but it is also associated with cereal and dog food in the US.

RAM. *Sanskrit, 'pleasing'.* One of the most familiar and assertive Indian names, but it can also be linked to a certain wooly animal. **Rahm, Rame, Ramee, Ramey, Rami, Ramie, Ramih, Ramy.**

RAMIRO. *Portuguese, 'great judge'.* Familiar as a Latin surname but has potential as a first. **Ramario, Rame, Ramee, Rameer, Rameir, Ramere, Rameriz, Ramero, Ramey, Rami, Ramih, Ramires, Ramirez, Ramos.**

RAMÓN. *Spanish variation of* RAYMOND. Dashing Latin classic, familiar and functional elsewhere. **Moncho, Ramón, Remon, Remone, Romone.**

RAMSAY, RAMSEY. *English, 'low-lying land'.* A surname occasionally used as a firs. **Ram, Ramsee, Ramsey, Ramsie, Ramsy, Ramzee, Ramzey, Ramzi, Ramzy.**

RANCHER. *Occupational name.* Any name that combines two big trends in the US – in this case, occupational and western names – has potential.

RAND. *English, 'living on riverbank'.* The new Randy – though a bit commercial, as in Rand Corporation, Rand McNally, et al.

RANDALL. *English, 'shield-wolf'.* Medieval name without much of a future. **Rand, Randahl, Randal, Randale, Randel, Randell, Randey, Randi, Randie, Randl, Randle, Randy, Randyll.**

RANDOLPH. *English, 'shield-wolf'.* Had its last hurrah in the 1940s. **Randal, Randall, Randell, Randol, Randolf, Randolfo, Randolpho, Randy, Ranolph.**

RANDY. *Diminutive of* RANDALL, RANDOLPH. Ever since Austin Powers reminded film-goers that 'randy' meant 'horny', it's been hard to take this name seriously. **Randdy, Randee, Randey, Randi, Randie, Ranndy.**

RANGER. *French, 'forest guardian'.* Where trends collide. **Rainger, Range.**

RANI. *Hebrew, 'my song, my joy'.* Too bad some people will tend to hear Ronnie. **Ran, Ranen, Ranie, Ranon, Roni.**

RANJIT. *Sanskrit, 'charmed, beguiled'.* Intriguing import. **Ranjeet.**

RANSOM. *English, 'shield's son'.* Rakish and handsome, but unavoidable association with holding someone for ransom. **Rance, Rand, Ransome, Ranson.**

RAOUL. *French variation of* **RALPH.** A lot more appealing and exotic than the original. **Raol, Reuel, Roul, Rowl. International: Raul** *(Spanish).*

RAPHAEL. *Hebrew, 'God has healed'.* Romantic archangel name that sounds both artistic and powerful. **Falito, Rafael, Rafaelle, Rafaello, Rafaelo, Rafal, Rafe, Rafel, Raffaello, Raffello, Raphaél, Raphaello, Raphale, Rapheal, Raphel, Raphello, Raphiel, Ravel, Ray, Rephael. International: Rafaele** *(Italian),* **Rafal** *(Polish).*

RASHAD. *Arabic, 'having good judgment'.* One of the most popular and best-known Arabic names that's readily understood on our shores. **Raashad, Rachad, Rachard, Rachaud, Raeshad, Raishard, Rashaad, Rashadd, Rashade, Rashaud, Rashaude, Rashead, Rashed, Rasheed, Rashid, Rashod, Rashoda, Rashodd, Rashoud, Raychard, Rayshad, Rayshard, Rayshaud, Rayshod, Reshad, Reshade, Reshard, Resharrd, Reshaud,** Reshawd, Reshead, Reshod, Rhashad, Rhashod, Rishaad, Rishad, Roshad, Roshard.

RASHID. *Arabic, 'righteous, rightly advised'.* Widely used Arabic choice – but Rashad is more popular. **Rasheed, Rasheid, Rasheyd, Rashida, Rashidah, Rashidi, Rashied, Rashieda, Raushaid.**

RAÚL. *Spanish variation of* **RALPH.** Heard much more frequently now than the English Ralph and could work well with an Anglo surname. **Raol, Raoul, Raulio, Rulo.**

♂ **RAVEN.** *Word name.* A bird name that works for both genders, but that is far more popular for girls. **Ravan, Ravean, Raveen, Raveon, Ravin, Ravine, Ravinn, Ravion, Ravon, Ravone, Ravonn, Ravonne, Rayvan, Rayvaun, Rayven, Rayvin, Rayvn, Rayvon, Rayvone, Reven, Revon, Reyven, Reyvon, Rhaven.**

RAVI. *Hindi, 'sun' or 'conferring'.* A title of the Hindu sun god, made cross-culturally famous by sitar player Ravi Shankar. **Ravee, Ravijot.**

RAWLINS. *British surname.* Drawlin'. **Rawlinson, Rawson.**

★**RAY.** *Diminutive of* **RAYMOND.** Still and forever, one of the hippest names and the Ray Charles biopic only polished its cool image. **Rae, Rai, Raye, Reigh.**

RAYBURN. *English, 'roe-deer brook'.* If you feel a burning need to gussy up Ray – think again. **Burney, Raeborn, Raeborne, Raebourn, Raeburn, Ray, Rayborn, Raybourn, Raybourne, Rayburne.**

RAYMOND. *German, 'wise-protector'.* Long dormant, but some parents – including Jack Nicholson – are finding its cool component, largely through the nickname Ray. **Mundo, Radmond, Rae, Raemon, Raemond, Raemondo, Raemonn, Raimon, Raimond, Raimonds, Raimund, Ramon, Ramond, Ramonde, Ramone, Ramonte, Ray, Rayman, Raymand, Raymann, Raymen, Rayment, Raymon, Raymone, Raymont, Raymun, Raymund, Raymunde, Raymundo, Reamonn, Redmond, Reimond, Reimonde,**

Reimundo, Remone, Reymon, Reymond, Reymound, Reymund. International: Réamann *(Irish Gaelic)*, Raimondo *(Italian)*, Raimundo, Ramón, Raymundo *(Spanish, Portuguese)*, Erramun *(Basque)*, Raimund, Reimund *(German)*, Raimo, Reima *(Finnish)*, Rajmund *(Polish)*.

RAYNOR. *Norse, 'mighty army'.* Original and straightforward, but with little appeal. **Ragnar, Rainer, Rainor, Ranieri, Raynar, Rayner.** International: **Ranier** *(French)*.

READ. *See* **REED.**

READING. *(red-ing) English, 'son of the red-haired'.* Inventive way to honour a ginger ancestor, though, like the English city, some people will mispronounce it *reed*ing, making it sound to some kids like a school assignment: Redding is a preferable spelling. **Redding, Reeding, Reiding.**

♂ **REAGAN.** *(REE-gun or RAY-gan) Irish, 'little king'.* Used much more often for girls. **Regan, Reegan.**

REBEL. *Word name.* Asking for trouble. **Reb.**

REBOP. *Word name.* Chosen by one musician, Todd Rundgren, for his son, but unlikely to be emulated by others.

RED. *Colour name.* Fiery but slight middle name choice; much more apt to be a redhead's nickname. **Redd.**

REDFORD. *English, 'red ford'.* Everyone will assume you're honouring actor Robert, which isn't too probable. **Ford, Radford, Radfurd, Readford, Red, Redd, Redffurd.**

REDMOND. *Irish variation of* **RAYMOND.** We love this for purely personal reasons *(see cover)*. **Radmond, Radmund, Reddin, Redman, Redmen, Redmon, Redmund.** International: **Réamann, Reamon** *(Irish)*.

♂ **REECE.** *Spelling variation of* **RHYS.** The most common boys' version of this attractive name, which is in the Top 100, but there is that Reese Witherspoon feminising alert. **Reace, Rease, Rece, Rees, Reese, Reice, Reis,** Reise, Reiss, Reyce, Reyes, Reyse, Rhett, Rhyce, Rhys, Rhyse, Rice, Riese, Riess, Ryese, Ryez, Ryse.

★**REED.** *English, 'red-haired'.* Slim, elegant, silvery surname: Reed could be a banker or a sculptor and therein lies the appeal of this simple yet distinctive name. **Raed, Raede, Raeed, Read, Reade, Reid, Reide, Reyd, Reyde, Rheed.**

REEF. *Word name.* Modern surfer boy. Just don't call him Reefer.

♀ **REESE.** *Spelling variation of* **RHYS.** On the rise for girls, thanks to the high-profile Ms Witherspoon.

♀ **REEVE.** *English occupational name, 'bailiff'.* Cool and dignified, an excellent combination and a name being seen as a more masculine alternative to Reese. **Reave, Reaves, Reeves.**

♀ **REGAN.** *Irish, 'little king'.* Going, going, gone to the girls now. **Raegan, Reagan, Reagen, Reaghan, Reegan, Reegen, Regen, Reigan, Reighan, Reign, Rheagan.**

If You Like Reed,

You Might Love . . .

Blake

Drew

Eames

Heath

Keen

Leif

Quinn

Reeve

Rhys

Roan

Roman

Ross

Ryder

Slade

Tate

REGINALD. *English, 'counsel power'.* The chap in the smoking jacket in a 1930s drawing-room comedy. **Reg, Reggie, Regginald, Reggis, Reggy, Regi, Regie, Regin, Reginal, Reginaldo, Reginale, Reginalt, Reginel, Reginold, Reginuld, Reynold,**

Reynolds, Ronald. International: Raghnall *(Irish)*, Raynold, Regnauld, Regnault, Renaud, Renault, René *(French)*, Renato, Rinaldo *(Italian)*, Naldo, Reinaldo, Reinaldos, Renato, Reynaldo *(Spanish)*, Reinald, Reinhold, Reinwald *(German)*, Reinhold *(Swedish)*.

REGIS. *French, 'kingly'.* Venerable old saint's name, but it sounds more like a dog's name. **Reeg, Reege.**

REID. *English, 'red-haired'.* This spelling is the most popular by a hair. *See REED.* **Read, Reade, Reed, Reide, Reyd, Ried.**

REILLY. *See RILEY.*

REINALDO. *Spanish variation of REGINALD.* Used in the Hispanic community. **Raynaldo, Renaldo, Renardo, Reynaldo, Rinaldo.**

REMBRANDT. *Dutch artist name.* The name of the most renowned of the Old Masters is a potential, if problematic, option for families who put an emphasis on the creative.

♂ **REMINGTON.** *English, 'place on a riverbank'.* Remington is the perfect name for an upper-class action hero, as played by Pierce Brosnan. **Rem, Reminton, Remy, Tony.**

★**REMUS.** *Latin, 'swift'.* One of the legendary twins who, with brother Romulus, founded Rome. An unusual yet classic name for the extremely adventurous who can put aside the stereotyped image of Uncle Remus. **Remo.**

★♂ **RÉMY.** *French, 'oarsman'.* Dashing unisex saint's name sometimes associated with the Cajun cadences of New Orleans. **Ramey, Remee, Remi, Rémi, Remie, Remmie, Remmy, Renuney, Renuny.**

REN. *Diminutive of RENÉ or any other Ren- name.* Your child will wonder why you forgot the rest of the name. **Renne, Renny.**

RENATO. *Italian, 'reborn'.* Elegant and exotic.

RENAUD. *(ren-OH) French variation of REGINALD.* Attractive if phonetically confusing; also pronounced exactly the same as the Renault car.

♂ **RENÉ.** *French, 'reborn'.* Hard to get past the image of the main character on 'Ello 'Ello, though Celine Dion's boy René-Charles reminded us of its masculine origins. **Ren, Renat, Renato, Renatus, Renault, Renay, René, Renee, Renn, Renne, Rennie, Renny.**

♂ **RENNY.** *Anglicised variation of Irish* **RAITHNAIT**, *'little prosperous one'; diminutive of* **REYNARD.** Used primarily for girls in Ireland, but sounds unisex to us. **Ren, Renn, Renne, Rennie.**

♂ **RENO.** *Place name.* Has a lively and swaggering sound and also some unfortunate associations with Reno, the American city of gambling and failed marriages. **Renos, Rino.**

RENON. *French, 'to make famous'.* Straightforward but very unusual choice, sometimes heard in Israel.

RENZO. *Diminutive of* **LORENZO.** Rakish nickname

able to stand on its own. **Renz, Renzy, Renzzo.**

REO. *See RIO.*

★**REUBEN.** *Hebrew, 'behold, a son'.* Rich and resonant Old Testament choice – Reuben founded one of the tribes of Israel – with a friendly down-home image. Maybe the current crowd of Jacobs will grow up and follow their biblical namesake by calling their own sons Reuben. It's recently entered the Top 100. **Reuban, Reubin, Reuvin, Rheuben, Rhuben, Ruban, Rube, Rubean, Ruben, Rubens, Rubey, Rubin, Rubino, Ruby, Rueban, Rueben, Ruebin, Ruvim. International: Reubén, Rubén** *(Spanish),* **Reuven, Rouben** *(Eastern European),* **Rouvin** *(Greek),* **Reuven** *(Hebrew).*

★**REX.** *Latin, 'king'.* Now that most dogs are named Max, it's safe to use this sleek, sexy regal name again for your child.

REY. *Spanish, 'king'.* Sounds exactly like Ray – for better or worse. **Reyes, Reyni.**

REYNARD. *German, 'powerful advice'.* Associated with Reynard the cunning fox in medieval European animal tales. **Rainart, Rainhard, Rainhardt, Rainhart, Ranard, Raynard, Raynarde, Reinard, Reinart, Reinhard, Reinhardt, Reinhart, Renard, Renardo, Renke, Rennard, Rey, Reynardo.**

REYNOLD, REYNOLDS. *English from German, 'counsel-power'.* Serious surname choices, the latter form known via award-winning author Reynolds Price. **Rainault, Rainhold, Ranald, Raynal, Raynald, Raynaldo, Raynold, Reinald, Reinaldos, Reinold, Reinwald, Renado, Renald, Renaldi, Renaldo, Renato, Renaud, Renauld, Renauldo, Renault, Renould, Rennold, Renold, Rey, Reynald, Reynaldo, Reynaldos, Reynauldo, Reynol, Rinald, Rinaldi, Ronald. International: Raghnall** *(Irish, Scottish),* **Ranald** *(Scottish),* **Rheinallt** *(Welsh),* **Renaud, Reynaud** *(French),* **Rinaldo** *(Italian),* **Reinaldo, Reynaldo** *(Spanish and Portuguese),* **Ronaldo** *(Portuguese),* **Reinhold** *(German),* **Ragnvald** *(Scandinavian),* **Reino** *(Finnish).*

RHETT. *Variation of* **RHYS.** More tied to *Gone with the Wind* than even Scarlett, but now sounds more girlish than gallant. **Rhet.**

RHODES. *Greek, 'where roses grow'.* A Greek island and a prestigious scholarship make an upper-class first name. **Rhoads, Rhodas. International: Rodas** *(Spanish).*

RHYS. *Welsh, 'fiery, zealous'.* This is the proper Welsh form, which is just entering the Top 50. Some parents now spell it as pronounced: Reese or Reece.

RIAN. *Irish, 'little king'.* More authentic and original form of Ryan. **Rhian, Rhyan.**

RICARDO. *Portuguese and Spanish variation of* **RICHARD.** Sexes up tired old standby Richard. **Racardo, Recard, Ricaldo, Ricard, Ricardoe, Ricardos, Riccardo, Riccarrdo, Ricciardo, Richardo.**

RICHARD. *German, 'dominant ruler'.* Far from stylish old Norman name, with a rich royal history. All the possible

nicknames – Richie, Ricky and especially Dick – are so over. **Dick, Dickie, Dicky, Raechard, Rashard, Ric, Ricard, Rich, Richar, Richardsen, Richardson, Richart, Richaud, Richer, Richerd, Richey, Richi, Richie, Richird, Richshard, Richy, Rick, Ricke, Rickee, Rickert, Rickey, Rickie, Ricky, Rishard, Rishi, Ritch, Ritchard, Ritcherd, Ritchie, Ritchy, Ritshard, Ritsherd, Ryk. International: Ristéard** *(Irish Gaelic),* **Riocard** *(Irish),* **Ruiseart** *(Scottish Gaelic),* **Rhisiart** *(Welsh),* **Ricardo** *(Italian, Spanish and Portuguese),* **Riccardo, Ricciardo, Ricco, Rico** *(Italian),* **Richi, Rico, Riqui** *(Spanish),* **Richart** *(German),* **Rickard, Rickert** *(Swedish),* **Rikard** *(Norwegian and Finnish),* **Reku** *(Finnish),* **Rye, Rysio, Ryszard** *(Polish),* **Riczi, Rikard** *(Hungarian),* **Dic** *(Romanian),* **Risa** *(Czech),* **Rostya, Slava, Slavik, Slavka** *(Russian),* **Richards, Rihards** *(Latvian),* **Arri, Juki, Riki, Riks, Rollo** *(Estonian),* **Rihardos** *(Greek).*

RICHMOND. *German, 'powerful protector'.* Place name – a town along the Thames here and the capital of Virginia in the

US – that makes a fresh way to honour an ancestral Richard. **Richman, Richmen, Richmon, Richmont, Richmound.**

RICK. *Diminutive of* **RICHARD, FREDERICK.** Last cool when Bogie roamed Casablanca. **Ric, Ricci, Ricke, Rickey, Rickie, Ricks, Ricky, Rik, Riki, Rikkey, Rikki, Rikky, Riks, Riky, Rykk.**

RICKY. *Diminutive of* **RICHARD, FREDERICK.** Gone with Richard and Rick. **Ricci, Rickey, Ricki, Rickie, Riczi, Riki, Rikki, Rikky, Riqui.**

RICO. *Spanish, diminutive of* **RICARDO.** Consider this short form for your little Richard. **Ric, Ricca, Ricci, Ricco.**

RIDER. *English, 'horseman'.* Rock-and-roll baby name. *See* **RYDER. Ridder, Ry, Rydder, Rye.**

RIDGE. *English word name.* Quintessential daytime drama name. **Ridgy, Rig, Rigg, Rigo, Rigs.**

RIDLEY. *English, 'cleared wood'.* Director Ridley Scott made this one known, but few parents would get beyond the negative first syllable. **Rhidley, Riddley, Ridlea, Ridleigh, Ridly.**

♂ **RILEY.** *Irish, 'courageous'.* Friendly, popular surname choice, quickly moving up the Top 100. **Reiley, Reilley, Reilly, Reily, Rhiley, Rhylee, Rhyley, Rieley, Rielly, Riely, Rilee, Rilley, Rillie, Rily, Rilye, Ryely, Rylee, Ryley, Rylie.**

RING. *Word name.* Cool and casual name.

RINGO. *English nickname.* Better to stick with John, Paul, or George.

♂ **RIO.** *Spanish, 'river'; Brazilian place name.* Seductive ranchero place name with an attractive Mexican lilt. **Reo.**

RIORDAN. *(REAR-den) Irish, 'bard, royal poet'.* Has a legitimate first name history in its native land and an appealing meaning, but pronunciation is far from obvious. **Rearden, Reardin, Reardon, Reerdan, Reerden, Reerdon, Riorden.**

RIP. *Dutch, 'ripe, full grown'.* The name of Rip Van Winkle –

the sleeping character in the story *Sleepy Hollow* – will probably never be ready for further consumption, if only because of the implications of R.I.P. **Ripp.**

♂ **RIPLEY.** *English, 'strip of clearing in the woods'.* The 'Believe It or Not' jokes will get old fast. **Rip, Ripleigh, Riply, Ripply.**

♂ **RISHI.** *Sanskrit, 'sage'.* In Hindu mythology, the Rishis are sages and seers; in modern times, Rishi Rich is a popular British-born musician and record producer.

RITTER. *German, 'knight, mounted warrior'.* Belittling kind of surname name, with rhymes like critter, fritter, bitter, litter, titter. **Rittner.**

♂ **RIVER.** *place name.* One of the first famous nature names, via the late actor River Phoenix and still muddied by his unfortunate fate. **Rivers, Riviera, Rivor.**

RIYAD. *Arabic place name, 'gardens'.* The capital of Saudi Arabia makes a difficult first

name. **Riad, Riyaad, Riyadh, Riyaz, Riyod.**

ROALD. *(RO-ahl) Norwegian, 'famous ruler'.* Intriguing Scandinavian name associated with Roald Dahl, author of the juvenile classics *James and the Giant Peach* and *Charlie and the Chocolate Factory.*

ROAN. *Spelling variation of* **ROWAN.** *See ROWAN.*

ROARK. *Irish, 'illustrious and mighty'.* Awkward surname choice. Keep looking. **Roarke, Rorke, Rourke, Ruark.**

ROB, ROBBIE. *English, diminutives of* **ROBERT.** Have claimed Bob's turf. **Robb, Robby, Robe.**

ROBERT. *English, 'bright fame'.* Slipping down the Top 100, Robert, though no longer stylish, is still widely used as a family name. Modern parents might sooner pick Robertson or Robinson. **Bert, Bertie, Bob, Bobbie, Bobby, Raby, Rhobbie, Rip, Rob, Roban, Robars, Robb, Robben, Robbey, Robbi, Robbie, Robbin, Robbins, Robbinson, Robby, Rober, Robers, Roberson,**

Names Dads Like More Than Mums

Ace

Austin

Brawley

Cash

Chance

Charlie

Cody

Dallas

Harry

Jack

Jake

Jesse

Jett

Junior

Luke

Maxwell

Nick

Rocco

Roman

Trey

Vincent

Roberte, Roberts, Robertson, Robeson, Robhy, Robi, Robie, Robin, Robinson, Robson, Roby, Robyn, Robynson, Rudbert, Rupert. International: Riobard, Riobart, Roibeard, Roibin *(Irish)*, Rab, Rabbie, Raibeart, Raibeartag, Roban *(Scottish)*, Robinet *(French)*, Roberto, Ruperto *(Italian)*, Roberto *(Spanish)*, **Rupert, Rupprecht, Ruprecht** *(German)*, **Pertti, Roope** *(Finnish)*, **Rubert** *(Czech)*.

ROBERTO. *Italian, Spanish and Portuguese variation of* **ROBERT.** Standard Latin classic. **Berto, Beto, Tito.**

ROBERTSON. *English, 'son of Robert'.* A better modern solution than Robert Jr; known to fiction readers via Canadian novelist Robertson Davies.

♂ **ROBIN.** *English, diminutive of* **ROBERT;** *also a bird name.* Now that it's no longer fashionable for girls, almost seems possible for boys again. **Roban, Robben, Robbin, Robbins, Robbyn, Roben, Robinet, Robinn, Robins, Robyn, Roibín.**

ROBINSON. *English, 'son of Robert'.* Cool and unusual way to honour your family Robert, though there could be some Robinson Crusoe joshing.

Robbinson, Robeson, Robinsen, Robson, Robynson.

ROC. *Irish, 'person with frizzy hair'.* Legendary Irish hero with rock star name. **Rock.**

ROCCO. *German and Italian, 'rest'.* Madonna did much to polish up the image of this old-neighbourhood Italian choice when she chose it for her son with British director Guy Ritchie. Also chosen for his son by Franklin Dettori. **Rocca, Roch, Roche, Rochus, Rocio, Rock, Rockey, Rockie, Rocko, Rocky, Roko, Roque.**

ROCHESTER. *English, 'stone camp or fortress'.* Calls to mind one of the most romantic fictional heroes, Jane Eyre's Mr Rochester. **Chester, Chet, Rock.**

ROCK. *Variation of* **ROCCO.** Faux macho name, à la Rock Hudson and The Rock; not recommended, despite rise of cousin Stone. **Roch, Rockey, Rockie, Rocky.**

ROCKET. *Word name.* Starbaby name that might prove too supercharged for real life.

ROCKWELL. *English, 'rock spring'.* Intriguing choice for an illustrator's child, thanks to Norman Rockwell and Rockwell Kent. **Rock, Rocky.**

ROD. *English, diminutive of* **RODERICK** *and* **RODNEY.** Macho-er than thou. **Rodd.**

RODERICK. *German, 'famous ruler'.* This kind of haughty masculine name, though it has many literary allusions, is far out of favour for modern boys. **Rhoderick, Rod, Rodd, Rodderick, Roddie, Roddrick, Roddy, Roderic, Roderich, Roderik, Roderrick, Roderyck, Rodgrick, Rodric, Rodrich, Rodrick, Rodrik, Rodrique, Rodryck, Rodryk, Rody.** International: **Rhydderch** *(Welsh),* **Rodrigue** *(French),* **Rodrigo** *(Italian),* **Roderigo, Rodrigo, Ruy** *(Spanish),* **Rodrigo, Rui** *(Portuguese),* **Rurik** *(Russian).*

RODMAN. *German, 'famous man, hero'.* Masculine in an outmoded, unappealing way. **Rodmond.**

RODNEY. *English, 'island near the clearing'.* Stereotyped, bratty rich-boy name. **Rhodney, Rod,** Rodnee, Rodnei, Rodni, Rodnie, Rodnne, Rodny.

RODOLFO. *Spanish, 'bold wolf'.* Romanticises Rudolph.

RODRIGO. *Spanish and Portuguese variation of* **RODERICK.** Rhythmically appealing international spin on the stiff original. **Gigo, Rodrego, Rui, Ruy.**

RODRIGUEZ. *Spanish, 'son of Rodrigo'.* Common Spanish surname that can work as a first. **Roddrigues, Rodrigquez, Rodrigues, Rodriques, Rodriquez, Rodriquiez.**

ROGAN. *Irish, 'redhead'.* Great, roguish alternative for overused Logan. **Rogein, Rogen.**

ROGELIO. *Spanish, 'famous warrior'.* Innovative twist on Roger. **Rojelio.** International: **Ruggiero** *(Italian),* **Rogerio** *(Spanish),* **Rutger** *(Dutch),* **Rüdiger** *(German),* **Rötger** *(Low German),* **Roar** *(Scandinavian).*

ROGER. *German, 'famous warrior'.* In the World War II era, Roger meant 'understood,' now it's on extended furlough.

Rodge, Rodger, Rodgy, Rog, Rogerick, Rogers. International: **Ruggero, Ruggiero** *(Italian),* **Rogerio** *(Portuguese),* **Rogier, Rutger** *(Dutch),* **Rüdiger** *(German),* **Roar** *(Norwegian).*

ROHAN. *Hindi, 'sandalwood'; also spelling variation of* **ROWAN.** From India, but feels like an Irish surname, so a possible cross-cultural choice.

ROJO. *(ROE-hoe) Spanish, 'red'.* Colourful middle name choice. **Rojay.**

ROLAND. *German, 'famous throughout the land'.* Chivalrous old name more widely heard in the US now in its Spanish form, Rolando. **Orlando, Rawlings, Rawlins, Rawlinson, Rawson, Rolan, Rolando, Roldan, Roley, Rolin, Rolla, Rolland, Rolli, Rollie, Rollin, Rollins, Rollo, Rolly, Rolo, Rowe, Rowland, Rowlando, Rowlands, Rowlandson, Rulan, Ruland, Rulon.** International: **Orlando** *(Italian),* **Rolando** *(Spanish, Portuguese),* **Roel, Roeland** *(Dutch),* **Rolle** *(Swedish),* **Loránd** *(Hungarian),* **Rolan** *(Russian).*

Hot Starbaby Names

August

Beau

Beckett

Dashiell

Finn

Henry

Holden

Homer

Hudson

Jackson

Julian

Mason

Miles

Milo

Oscar

Owen

Roman

Romeo

Ryder

ROLLO. *Variation of* **ROLAND.** Livelier, roly-poly *o*-ending version of Roland.

★**ROMAN.** *Latin, 'citizen of Rome'.* Surprise hit name of recent years, thanks to Cate Blanchett and Harvey Keitel who used it for their kids. **Roma, Romann, Romano, Romman, Rommie, Rommy, Romochka, Romy. International: Romain** *(French),* **Romano** *(Italian),* **Romanus** *(Latin),* **Romanos** *(Greek).*

♂ **ROMANY.** *English, 'gypsy'.* Fanciful name referring to Gypsies and their culture, with a definite feminine sound.

ROMEO. *Italian, 'pilgrim to Rome, Roman'.* Romantic, previously quasi-taboo Shakespearean name given new life by David and Victoria Beckham, who chose it for their second son, a path followed by Jon Bon Jovi. **Romar, Romario, Romarius, Romaro, Romarrio, Romeiro, Roméo, Romer, Romere, Romerio, Romeris, Romero, Romeryo.**

ROMNEY. *Welsh, 'winding river'.* With the fashion for all names *Rom,* this strong surname with ties to Old Master painter George has new possibilities.

ROMULUS. *Latin, 'citizen of Rome'.* The original Roman – he was Remus's twin and a founder of Rome – is one of the less user-friendly ancients. **Romel, Romele, Romell, Romello, Romelo, Rommel, Rommello, Romolo, Romono, Romulo.**

♂ **ROMY.** *German and English diminutive of* **ROMAN** *et al.* Best known as a feminine diminutive, but used now for boys too; has a lot of energy and bounce. **Romey.**

RONALD. *Norse, 'ruler's counselor'.* Ronald's off playing shuffleboard with Donald. **Ranald, Ron, Ronal, Roni, Ronie, Ronn, Ronnald, Ronney, Ronnie, Ronnold, Ronny. International: Raghnall** *(Irish),* **Naldo, Rainald, Ranaldo, Raynaldo, Reinaldo, Renaldo, Rey, Reynaldo** *(Spanish),* **Rinhaldo** *(Portuguese).*

★♂ **RONAN.** *Irish, 'little seal'.* Compelling, legendary name of ten Celtic saints that's now drawing some deserved attention; this cousin of the ascending Roman and Conan was chosen by actor Daniel

Day-Lewis and his writer-director wife Rebecca Miller. **Rónán.**

♂ **RONDEL.** *English from French, 'circle'.* The *-el* ending feels inevitably feminine; also a form of French poetry. **Rondal, Rondale, Rondall, Rondeal, Rondell, Rondey, Rondie, Rondrell, Rondy, Ronel, Ronell, Ronelle, Ronnel, Ronnell, Ronyell.**

RONI. *Hebrew, 'my song, my joy'.* Looks modern, but sounds like the dated Ronnie. **Rani, Roneet, Roney, Ronit, Ronli, Rony.**

RONSON. *Scottish, 'son of Ronald'.* Stronger and fresher than the original. **Ron, Ronaldson.**

★**ROONE.** *Irish, 'red-haired'.* Lively, attractive and unusual redhead entry.

ROONEY. *Irish, 'red-haired'.* Perfectly OK surname, but it does rhyme with goony and loony: stick with Roone.

ROOSEVELT. *Dutch, 'rose field'.* American presidential surname adopted as a first by numbers of mid-century parents. **Roosvelt, Rosevelt.**

ROPER. *English, 'rope-maker'.* Cowboyish occupational name sure to attract notice, but not necessarily the type your son would like – close to groper.

♂ **RORY.** *Irish, 'red king'.* Rory O'Connor was the last High King of Ireland in the twelfth century and his name makes an energetic choice for either sex. Skip baffling Gaelic spellings and stick with Rory. **Rorey, Rori, Rorrie, Rorry, Ruadhri, Ruadri, Ruaidhri, Ruaidhrigh, Ruaidri, Ruairi, Ruairidh, Ruaraí, Ruaraidh, Ruari, Ruaridh.**

★**ROSCOE.** *Norse, 'deer forest'.* Fairly popular a hundred years ago but out of sight now, the quirky Roscoe deserves a place on every adventurous baby namer's long list. **Rosco.**

ROSS. *Scottish, 'upland, peninsula'.* Like *Friends,* off the air and into syndication. **Rosse, Rossell, Rossi, Rossie, Rossy.**

ROTH. *German nickname for redhead.* There are lots more appealing redhead names.

★♂ **ROWAN.** *Irish, 'little redhead'; also name of a tree with red berries.* Strong surname choice deservedly growing in popularity. Sharon Stone chose the Roan spelling for her son. **Roan, Rohan, Rowe, Rowen, Rowney, Rowyn.** International: **Ruadhan** *(Gaelic).*

ROWLAND. *See ROLAND.* **Rowlando, Rowlands, Rowlandson.**

ROWLEY. *English, 'rough clearing'.* Rough-and-tumble surname with some degree of charm. **Rowlea, Rowlee, Rowleigh, Rowly.**

ROXBURY. *English, 'rook's town or fortress'.* The *x* gives it muscle, but the *bury* part buries it. **Roxburghe.**

ROY. *French, 'king'.* Country/cowboy name epitomised by Roys Rogers, Acuff and Clark, making it far from a modern baby name natural. **Rey, Roi, Roye, Ruy.**

ROYAL. *French, 'kingly, royal'.* A bit more subtle than Duke or Earl. **Roy, Royale, Royall, Royell.**

ROYCE. *English, 'son of the king'.* Make up your mind: Roy or Reece, but not both. **Roice, Roy, Royz.**

ROYDEN. *English, 'rye hill'.* One way to refer to an ancestral Roy, if not the most mellifluous. **Royd, Roydan.**

ROYSTON. *English, 'settlement of Royce'.* To honour Roy's son . . . or grandson.

RUDOLPH. *German, 'famous wolf'.* Unfortunately, still the red-nosed reindeer. Try Rudy. **Rodolf, Rudolf, Rudy.** International: **Rodolph, Rodolphe** *(French),* **Rodolfo, Rudolpho** *(Italian),* **Rodolfo, Rudi** *(Spanish),* **Ruud** *(Dutch),* **Rodolf** *(Dutch, German),* **Rudolf** *(German),* **Roffe** *(Swedish),* **Ruda** *(Czech),* **Rudi** *(Hungarian).*

♂**RUDY.** *German, diminutive of RUDOLF or RUDOLPH.* Some style currency, thanks to Giuliani, New York's mayor at the time of 9/11, and the fact that Jude Law used it for his son. **Roody, Ruda, Ruddy, Ruddie, Rude, Rudey, Rudi, Rudie, Ruedi.**

RUDYARD. *English, 'red enclosure'.* Not advised even for the most ardent Kipling admirers. **Rudd.**

RUE. *Nature name.* Botanical choice you may regret.

★**RUFUS.** *Latin, 'redhead'.* Rumpled, redheaded (it started as the nickname for red-haired King William) ancient Roman name popular with saints and singers (e.g., Rufus Wainwright), on the cutting edge of cool. **Rayfus, Rufe, Ruffis, Ruffus, Rufino, Rufo, Rufous.**

RUGBY. *English, 'rook fortress'.* Rough and sporty, but too specific.

RULE. *Word name.* Stricter than Peace or Justice.

RUMO. *Cornish, 'red'.* Ancient martyr name that sounds totally modern, but perhaps too close to rumour. **Rumon.**

RUNE. *German and Swedish, 'secret'.* Name with connotations both mystical and tragic, newly popular in Europe.

RUNYON. *Irish, 'son of a champion'.* Irish surname with considerable flair; some will connect it with *Guys and Dolls* writer Damon Runyon.

★RUPERT. *German variation of* ROBERT. Charming-yet-manly name popular over here (where it's attached to beloved Rupert Bear). **Ruperth, Ruperto, Ruprecht.**

RUSH. *English, 'someone who lives among rushes' or 'basket weaver'.* Might suggest speed, excitement, even danger, but also has an unsavoury drug culture connection. **Rushford, Rushi.**

RUSK. *Scottish, 'marsh, bog'.* Brisk.

RUSKIN. *Scottish, 'from a family of tanners'.* British-sounding literary surname choice. **Rush, Russ.**

RUSSELL. *French, 'redhead, fox-coloured'.* One of many names that started as a nickname for a redhead; this has lost its colour, except for one dynamic bearer, Russell Crowe. **Roussell, Rush, Russ, Russel, Russelle, Ruste, Rusten, Rustie, Rustin, Ruston, Rusty, Rustyn.**

RUTHERFORD. *English, 'cattle ford'.* Stuffy choice.

♂ RYAN. *Irish, 'little king'.* Extremely popular for several decades, with no sign of flagging from the Top 25, even though parents now have such a wide choice of Irish surnames, from Flynn to Finnigan and newer *Ry* names like Ryder. **Rayan, Rayaun, Rhyan, Rhyne, Ryane, Ryann, Ryein, Ryen, Ryian, Ryiann, Ryien, Ryin, Ryne, Rynn, Ryon, Ryuan, Ryun, Ryyan.**

RYDER. *Variation of* RIDER. In the spotlight since American actress Kate Hudson and her rocker husband chose it for their son.

RYE. *English, diminutive of* RYDER *or word name.* Ry when short for Ryder, is cool; Rye not so much. **Ry.**

RYLAN, RYLAND, RYKER. *English and Irish, 'island meadow'.* Parents seeking alternatives to the overused Ryan have used these fussier substitutes, but they lack the jaunty charm of the original – and Ryker could be associated with a prison in New York.

Occupational Names

Archer	Foster
Baird	Gardener
Baker	Miller
Baxter	Painter
Bishop	Pilot
Booker	Porter
Butler	Reeve
Carter	Roper
Collier	Ryder
Cooper	Sailor
Draper	Sawyer
Falkner	Sayer
Fisher	Shepherd
Fletcher	Taylor

S *boys*

SAAD. *Aramaic, 'help, support'.* Sounds too sad. **Saadia, Saadiah, Saadya, Saadyah.**

SAAR. *Hebrew, 'wind, tempest'; place name in Israel.* There is such a thing as a name that's too unusual.

Stellar Starbabies Beginning with R

Rafferty	Sadie Frost & Jude Law
Ralph	Matthew McFayden
Raymond	Jack Nicholson
Rebel	Robert Rodriguez
Rebop	Todd Rundgren
René-Charles	Celine Dion
Roan	Sharon Stone
Rocco	Madonna & Guy Ritchie, Frankie Dettori
Rocket	Robert Rodriguez
Rogue	Robert Rodriguez
Rohan	Bob Marley
Roman	Cate Blanchett, Harvey Keitel
Romeo	Victoria 'Posh Spice' & David Beckham, Jon Bon Jovi
Ronan	Rebecca Miller & Daniel Day-Lewis
Rory	Bill Gates
Rudy	Sadie Frost & Jude Law
Ryder	Kate Hudson & Chris Robinson

SABIN. *(SAY-bin) Latin, 'from the Sabines'.* Listed in the Koran as one of the 'People of the Book,' this male equivalent of Sabina is undiscovered and ripe for the adventurous baby namer. **Saban, Saben, Sabian, Sabien.** International: Saidhbhin *(Gaelic),* **Sabatay, Sabien, Sabinien, Sabinu, Saby, Savin,** *(French),* **Savino** *(Italian),* **Sabino** *(Spanish),* **Sabiny** *(Polish),* **Savin** *(Eastern European),* **Sabean, Sabian** *(Arabic and Persian).*

SABINO. *Latin, 'from the Sabines'; also Spanish, 'wise'.* This name of a famous ancient Roman jurist is sometimes heard in the Hispanic community. **Bino, Sabel, Sabí, Sabiniano, Sebelio.**

SABIR. *Arabic, 'patient'.* An Indian name that would have no trouble assimilating. **Saber.**

♂ **SACHA.** *French variation of* **SASHA.** *See* **SASHA.**

SACHEVERELL. *English, 'roebuck leap'.* Over the top, and playmates might shorten to Sac

– we don't think your son would like being called a bag. **Sachie.**

SADAKA. *Swahili, 'religious offering'.* This traditional Swahili folktale name could mark you as a Neil Sedaka fan.

SADIK. *Swahili, 'faithful'; Arabic, 'friend'.* Frequently found in all three forms: Sadik, Sadiki and Sadiq. **Saadiq, Sadeek, Sadek, Sadiki, Sadiq, Sadique.**

♂ **SAGE.** *Latin, 'wise and knowing'; also herb name.* Fits many criteria sought by modern parents: it's short and strong, with intimations of wisdom as well as fragrant herbal properties. **Sagan, Sagar, Sagen, Sager, Saige, Saje, Sayge. International: Salvio** *(Italian).*

SAHAJ. *(sah-haj) Hindi, 'natural'.* Soft and rhythmic.

SAHIL. *(sah-hil) Hindi, 'guide, leader'.* A name that could set an Indian boy on a path to leadership. **Saheel, Sahel.**

SAHIR. *Arabic, 'wakeful, charming'; Hindi, 'friend'.* Appealing Indian and Arabic choice. **Saahir, Saheer.**

SA'ID. *(sah-eed) Arabic, 'lucky, happy'.* A popular name in the Arab community, with an upbeat meaning. **Sa'ad, Saaid, Saed, Sa'eed, Saeed, Sahid, Said, Saide, Sa'ied, Saiyd, Saiyed, Saiyeed, Sayid.**

♂ **SAILOR.** *Occupational name.* Although this was used by model Christie Brinkley for her daughter, it would be even more appropriate for a boy. **Sailer, Sayler, Saylor.**

SAJAN. *Hindi, 'beloved'.* An attractive and exotic name for a cherished baby son. **Sajen.**

SAL. *English, diminutive of* **SALVADOR** *or* **SALVATORE.** The sidekick in almost every US film that has an Italo-American setting.

SALADIN. *Arabic, 'peace through faith'.* A name with considerable history, as the celebrated sultan of Egypt and Syria in the time of the Crusades.

SALĀH. *Arabic, 'peace through faith'.* Short form of the name Anglicised as Saladin, very popular throughout the Arab world. **Saleh.**

♂ **SALEM.** *Place name.* Several associations, but probably the strongest is the Salem witch trials in the US. **Shalom, Shelomi, Shlomi, Sholom.**

SALIM. *(sah-LEEM) Arabic 'secure'; also Swahili, 'peace'.* Distinguished by association with renowned African diplomat Salim Ahmed Salim. **Salam, Saleem, Saliym, Selim.**

SALINGER. *French literary name.* Fervent fans of *The Catcher in the Rye* might want to consider this as a literary tribute.

SALMAN. *Arabic, 'safety'.* Associated in this country with Anglo-Indian novelist Salman Rushdie. **Salmaan, Salmaine.**

♂ **SALMON.** *English from Latin, word name.* Nature names are in and even fish names like Pike and Salmon are open for consideration.

SALTON. *English, 'place in the willows'.* Stiff and sedate surname name, despite its salty start. **Salhtun, Salten, Saltin.**

SALVADOR. *Spanish from Latin* **SALVATOR,** *'savior'.* A common epithet of Christ, frequently heard in the Hispanic community. **Chavo, Sal, Salbador, Sallie, Sally, Salvado, Salvadore, Salvadro, Salvarado, Salvator, Salvidor, Salvodor. International: Sauveur** *(French),* **Salvatore, Salvatorio** *(Italian),* **Salbatore, Salvadore, Salvino, Xabat, Xalbador, Xalvador** *(Spanish),* **Xalbador** *(Basque),* **Salvator** *(Polish).*

SALVATORE. *Italian variation of* **SALVATOR.** For every Tío Salvador in a Latino family, there's a Zio Salvatore in an Italian one. **Sal, Sallie, Sally, Salvator, Salvatorio, Tore.**

♂ **SAM.** *English, diminutive of* **SAMUEL.** Long used on its own for boys and popular in the bohemian world for both sexes, but slipping in the Top 100. **Samm, Sammie, Sammy.**

SAMAL. *Aramaic, 'symbol, sign'.* Also a picturesque place name, referred to as the 'island garden city' of the Philippines.

♂ **SAMI.** *Arabic, 'exalted'; also diminutive of* **SAMUEL.**

Soundalike cousin of Sammy, cute but slight on its own. **Saami, Samie, Sammi, Sammie, Sammy, Samy.**

★**SAMIR.** *Arabic, 'a friend to talk with in the evening'.* Pleasing sound and has a lovely meaning. **Sameer.**

SAMMY. *Diminutive of* **SAMUEL.** You can call him Sammy, but don't put that on the birth certificate. **Sami, Sammi, Sammie, Samy.**

SAMO. *Czech variation of* **SAMUEL.** Energetic and bouncy, but keep it as a short form. **Samko.**

SAMSON. *Hebrew, 'sun'.* This name, once considered overly powerful due to the superhuman strength of the biblical figure, is now an option for parents in search of an unusual route to Sam. **Sampson, Sansom, Sanson. International: Samzun** *(Breton),* **Sansone** *(Italian),* **Sansón** *(Spanish),* **Samsó** *(Basque),* **Sansao** *(Portuguese),* **Simson** *(Swedish).*

SAMUEL. *Hebrew, 'told by God'.* Long a popular Old

Testament classic, Samuel is now in the Top 10. A cross-cultural, multi-nicknamed choice, which some see as overused and others think of as cool as Samuel L. Jackson. **Sam, Sami, Sammie, Sammy, Samual, Samualle, Samuele, Samuell, Samy. International: Somhairle** *(Irish),* **Sawyl** *(Welsh),* **Samuele** *(Italian),* **Samuelito** *(Spanish),* **Zamiel** *(German),* **Samuli** *(Finnish),* **Sami, Samu, Samuka** *(Hungarian),* **Samko, Samo** *(Czech),* **Samuelis** *(Lithuanian),* **Samuil** *(Bulgarian),* **Samoyla, Samuil, Samvel** *(Russian),* **Samouel** *(Greek),* **Shmuel** *(Hebrew),* **Schmuel, Shem, Shemuel** *(Yiddish),* **Samaru** *(Japanese).*

SANCHO. *Spanish variation of* **SANTOS.** Name of nine provincial Spanish kings, but more likely to conjure up Sancho Panza, the hapless squire of Don Quixote. **Sanchez, Sanctio, Sanctos, Santón, Sauncho.**

SANDER. *German, diminutive of* **ALEXANDER.** More conventional form of Zander or Xander. **Sanders, Sandor, Saunder, Saunders.**

SANDERSON. *English, 'Alexander's son'.* Possible alternative to Anderson.

SANDOR. *(SHAN-dor) Hungarian diminutive of* **ALEXANDER.** Despite a possible pronunciation problem, a pleasant, unusual choice. **Sanyi.**

SANDROS. *Greek, diminutive of* **ALEXANDROS.** Often given as an independent name in Greece.

♂ **SANDY.** *Scottish and English, diminutive, of* **ALEXANDER.** Like Red, Brownie and Blondie – rarely given on its own. **Sandey, Sandie.**

SANFORD. *English, 'sandy ford'.* Pretentious. **Sandford.**

SANJAY. *Sanskrit, 'triumphant'.* Historic and popular Indian name, borne by the son of Prime Minister Indira Gandhi. **Sanjaya, Sanje, Sanjeev, Sanjiv, Sanjo.**

SANJIRO. *Japanese, 'admired, praised'.* Interesting name that relates to those of Christian saints.

SANSONE. *(san-SO-nay) Italian variation of* **SAMSON.** Strong and seductive, would make an excellent import.

SANTIAGO. *Latin, 'Saint James' (Sant Iago); also capital of Chile.* Spirited Spanish name with great crossover potential: a place name, a surname and the patron saint of Spain. **Santago, Santeago, Santiaco, Santiego, Santigo. International: Antiago, Chago, Chano, Diago, Sandiago, Sandiego, Saniago, Santi, Tago, Vego, Yago, Yague** *(Spanish),* **Xanti** *(Basque),* **Tiago** *(Portuguese).*

SANTO. *Italian, 'saint, holy'.* Religious name long common in Italy, as is the diminutive Santino.

SANTOS. *Spanish, 'saint, holy'.* The Spanish and Portuguese variation of the all-saints name. **International: Santo, Sanzio** *(Italian),* **Sants** *(Catalan).*

SARAD. *Hindi, 'born in autumn'.* A pleasant seasonal name.

SARGENT. *Spelling variation of* **SERGEANT;** *also NCO in US Army.* One of the few military ranks used as a name. There's also an artistic association with painter John Singer Sargent. **Sarge, Sergeant, Sergent.**

SARKIS. *Armenian, 'protector, shepherd'.* Fairly common Armenian first and last name.

SAROYAN. *Armenian literary name.* Plausible literary name to honour upbeat Armenian-American playwright and prose writer William Saroyan.

SARTO. *Latin, 'mender'.* Associated with both Renaissance painter Andrea del Sarto and a contemporary brand of shoes, this Italian surname name has a stylish, artistic air.

♂ **SASHA.** *Russian, diminutive of* **ALEXANDER.** This Russian nickname name is being used increasingly on its own, though somewhat more for girls – chosen for its energy and ethnic flair. **Dacha, Sash, Sashka, Sashok, Sausha. International: Sacha** *(French),* **Sascha** *(German).*

♂ **SATCHEL.** *American nickname.* First Woody Allen, then Spike Lee named their children to honour the great black American pitcher, Leroy 'Satchel' Paige. Not, however, recommended for noncelebrity use. **Satch.**

SATURN. *Roman mythology name.* If you've rejected all the names on the earth, you might move on to the sixth planet from the sun, also the Roman god of agriculture. **Saturday, Saturnin. International: Saturni, Saturnino** *(Spanish),* **Satordi** *(Basque).*

SAUL. *Hebrew, 'asked for, desired, prayed for'.* Jewish parents in particular may be drawn to this quiet, composed name of the first king of Israel; also associated with novelist Saul Bellow. Its meaning makes it appropriate for a long-awaited child. **Shaul. International: Saúl, Saula** *(Spanish).*

SAVION. *Modern invented name, possibly derived from* **XAVIER.** Has lots of energy, perhaps due to its association with top tap dancer Savion

Glover. **Saveon, Savian, Savionn, Savo, Xavion.**

♂ **SAWYER.** *English, 'wood-cutter'.* A surname with a more relaxed and friendly feel than many others; would make a good choice for someone who works with wood.

SAX. *Diminutive of* **SAXON.** Rhythmic and sensual – maybe too sensual, in terms of playground teasing. **Saxe.**

SAXON. *German, 'people of the dagger'.* Feels as though it should be preceded by *Anglo*. **Sax, Saxe, Saxen, Saxony, Saxxen, Saxxon.**

♂ **SAYER.** *English, 'assayer of metals' or 'professional storyteller'.* A pleasant, open, last-name-first name, particularly apt for a family of writers. **Saer, Say, Saye, Sayers, Sayre, Sayres.**

♂ **SCHUYLER.** *Dutch, 'scholar'.* This worthy name, popular among the early Dutch colonists in North America, has been all but overpowered by the phonetic spellings – Skyler for boys and Skylar for girls.

Schuylar, Schylar, Schyler, Scy, Sky, Skyelar, Skylar, Skyler, Skylor.

SCIENCE. *Word name.* An American actress used this as the middle name for her son

Audio; one of the most do-not-try-this-at-home combos we've heard.

SCIPIO. *(SIP-ee-oh) Latin, 'staff or walking stick'.* This surname of an ancient Roman invader of Africa is an intriguing, undiscovered option.

SCORPIO. *Latin, 'scorpion'; zodiacal constellation.* Its overbearingly potent presence, combined with similarity to the word *scorpion,* could prove a burden to a young boy. **Scorpeo.**

SCOTT. *English, 'from Scotland'.* A cool, windswept, surfer babe-magnet in 1965, a nice dad – or even granddad – today, and now out of the Top 100. **Scot, Scottie, Scotto, Scotty.**

★♂ **SCOUT.** *Word name.* Chosen for their daughter by Bruce and Demi (inspired by the *To Kill a Mockingbird* character) this name can be an interesting choice for either sex, with overtones of a 'good scout' and the upstanding qualities of a Boy/Girl Scout.

♂ **SCULLY.** *Irish, 'herald or town crier'.* Relaxed, with an appealing touch of swagger.

♂ **SEAGULL.** *English word and nature name.* Hippy name of the *Jonathan Livingston Seagull* era.

♂ **SEAL.** *English word and nature name.* Projects the sleek and playful image of the aquatic mammal, plus that of the striking British-born Brazilian/Nigerian/Afro-Caribbean singer (born Sealhenry). **Seale, Seel, Seele.**

♂ **SEALEY.** *English, 'blessed'.* Has a nickname feel. **Sealy, Seeley, Seely.**

★**SEAMUS.** *(SHAY-muhs) Irish variation of* **JAMES.** Parents tiring of Sean are now contemplating this Irish form of James, which has more substance and verve. **Seumas, Shamus, Shay, Shemus.**

♂ **SEAN.** *Irish variation of* **JOHN.** After three decades as one of *the* Irish boys' name, Sean is now dropping in the Top 100 as parents look to fresher Irish choices, such as Aidan and Conor. **Eoin,**

Seaghan, Seanan, Seane, Seann, Shaan, Shain, Shaine, Shan, Shandon, Shandy, Shane, Shann, Shauden, Shaughan, Shaughn, Shaun, Shaundre, Shawn, Shayne, Shon, Shonn.

SEANÁN. *(SHAW-nan) Irish diminutive of* **SEAN.** This name of twenty early Irish saints sounds a little redundant.

♂ **SEATON.** *English, 'town by the sea'.* We'd prefer Keaton. **Seeton, Seton.**

SEB. *Egyptian, 'God of the earth'.* This name, also a short form of Sebastian, is conceivable for a full name, as is Bas.

★**SEBASTIAN.** *Latin from Greek, 'person from ancient city of Sebastia'.* This ancient martyr's name turned literary and *Little Mermaid* hero is steady in the Top 100 as a classic-yet-unconventional compatriot for fellow British favourites Colin and Oliver. **Bas, Basti, Bastian, Sabastian, Seb, Sebasten, Steb. International: Bastien, Sébastien** *(French),* **Bastiano, Sebastiano** *(Italian),* **Bastian, Bastien, Sebastian, Sebastiano, Sebo, Sevastian** *(Spanish),* **Bastiaio,**

Sebastiao *(Portuguese),* Sebestyen, Sebo *(Hungarian),* Sebastyen, Sevastian *(Russian).*

SEEGER. *English, 'seaman'.* Associated with archetypal American folk singer Pete Seeger. **Seager, Segar, Seger.**

SEGUNDO. *Spanish, 'second born'.* After your first little Primo, you could always call the next Segundo – though that's like naming them number one and number two.

SEIJI. *(SAY-jee) Japanese, 'lawful and just'.* Popular Japanese name exemplified by the distinguished conductor Seiji Ozawa.

♂ **SELBY.** *English, 'from the willow farm'.* British last name that, though rather gentle, still has more masculine drive than Shelby. **Selbey, Selbie, Shelby.**

SELDON. *English, 'from the house on the hill'.* Seldom heard as a first name. **Selden, Sellden.**

SELIG. *German, 'blessed, happy in life'.* Names ending in *ig* tend to sound – well – icky. **Saelig,** Sealey, Seeley, Seelig, Seely, Selik, Zelig, Zelik, Zeligman, Zelyg.

SELWYN. *Latin, 'sylvan, of the woods'.* Selwyn's not a wynner. **Selwin, Selwynn, Wyn.**

SEMAJ. *Meaning unknown, also James spelled backward.* Popular enough in the Indian community, possibly inspired by Jamaican activist Leachim Semaj (born Michael James).

♂ **SENECA.** *Latin surname and Native American, 'people of the standing rock'.* Its distinguished heritage as the name of the ancient Roman philosopher-playwright who tutored Nero and of an Iroquois tribe makes this an interesting choice for either sex. **Senyca.**

♂ **SENEGAL.** *African place name.* The name of this beautiful West African republic would make the epitome of exotic choices.

SENNETT. *English, 'bold in victory'.* New twist on Bennett. **Sennet, Sinnett, Sinnott.**

SEPTIMUS. *Latin, 'the seventh son'.* Even if you don't anticipate son number seven, you might be bold enough to consider this relic of Dickens and Virginia Woolf novels. Certainly preferable to sixth-son name Sextus.

♂ **SEQUOYAH.** *Native American, Cherokee, 'sparrow'.* A strong, meaningful name, associated with a famous Cherokee linguistic scholar; also suggests the magnificent California sequoia redwood trees. **Sequoia, Sequoiah.**

♂ **SERAPHIM.** *Hebrew, 'fiery'.* This ephemeral name of the loving angels surrounding the throne of God would not work out well in the playground. **Saraf, Saraph, Serafim. International: Seraffinu, Seraph, Séraphin, Xerafub** *(French),* **Serafino** *(Italian),* **Serafin, Serafito** *(Spanish),* **Serafí** *(Catalan).*

♂ **SEREN.** *(SER-en) Welsh, 'star'.* The name of an ancient goddess of hot springs sounds a bit soft for a boy.

SERENO. *Latin, 'calm'.* Appealingly peaceful and placid. **Serenus.**

SERGE. *French variation of ancient Roman family name* **SERGIUS**, 'servant'. Old saints' and popes' name that went to France in the 1920s with the Russian Ballets Russes; in its Russian form, Sergei, it retains an artistic, almost effete air.

SERGEANT. *Latin, 'to serve'.* See *SARGENT.* **Sargent, Sergent.**

SERGEI. *(sair-GAY) Russian variation of* **SERGIUS**. Common Russian name of one of that country's most beloved saints, known for his kindness and gentility. **Serezha, Sergay, Sergey, Sergi, Serguei, Serzh, Sirgio. International: Sergio** *(Italian),* **Cergio, Checho, Checo, Sergeo, Sergio, Serjio, Zergio** *(Spanish),* **Sergius** *(German),* **Serg, Sergiusz, Sewek** *(Polish),* **Serge, Sergey, Sergeyka, Sergi, Sergie, Sergo, Sergunya, Serhiy, Serhiyko** *(Russian).*

SERGIO. *Italian and Spanish variation of* **SERGIUS**. Widely heard in both Italian and Spanish households, most identified with spaghetti western director Sergio Leone.

Cergio, Seargeoh, Sergeo, Sergios, Serjio, Zergio.

♂ **SETH.** *Hebrew, 'appointed, placed'.* The long-neglected name of Adam and Eve's third son, Seth is a popular choice in Australia, increasingly appreciated for its gentle, understated presence. **Set, Sutekh.**

♂ **SEVEN** *English word and number name.* Only if your preceding children are one, two, three, four, five and six. Erykah Badu and Andre 3000 broke that rule when naming their son.

SEVERIN. *French variation of* **SEVERUS***; Latin, 'stern, serious'.* Ancient Roman name borne by several saints and still alive throughout Europe, ready for import here. **International: Sévère** *(French),* **Severino** *(Italian),* **Severin** *(German),* **Soren** *(Danish),* **Severi** *(Finnish),* **Seweryn** *(Polish),* **Szörény** *(Hungarian).*

SEVERO. *(say-VAY-ro) Italian and Spanish variation of* **SEVERUS**. An old Roman family name that could easily be mispronounced to make it supersevere. **Cevero, Saverio, Savero, Seve, Severano, Severeano, Severiano, Severino, Severito, Siverio, Sivero.**

SEWARD. *English, 'sea defender'.* Double whammy: the expression 'Seward's folly' and inevitable sewer jokes.

SEXTUS. *Latin, 'sixth born'.* Just think about those inescapable 'sexy' nicknames. **International: Sesto, Sisto** *(Italian).*

♂ **SEYMOUR.** *English, 'marshy land near the sea'.* Out playing shuffleboard and not expected back for several generations – unless it morphs into a girls' name, à la Sydney.

SHABAAN. *Arabic, 'coward'.* Despite its disagreeable meaning, this name has a distinctive literary heritage: the eminent Kiswahili writer Shabaan Roberts is called the Shakespeare of East Africa.

♂ **SHADE.** *English word name.* Nice sound, but double meaning – shady glen or shady character. **Shady.**

Names That Mean Peace

Absalom	Pacifica
Aerin	Paloma
Axel	Pax
Concord	Paz
Eir	Placida
Freda/	Salem
Frida/	Salome
Frieda	Serenity
Frederick	Shalom
Humphrey	Sheehan
Irene	Solomon
Malu	Uma
Manfred	Winifred
Milo	Zalman
Pace	

♂ **SHALOM.** *Hebrew, 'peace'.* Familiar as the most common form of greeting in Hebrew. **Shalem, Shalmiya, Shelemya, Shelemyahu, Shilem.**

SHAMAR. *Modern invented name, possible variation of* **SHAMIR.** This more exotic alternative to Omar is a popular choice in the US. **Shamaar, Shamare, Shamari.**

SHAMIR. *(SHAY-mir) Aramaic, 'a sharp thorn, flint'.* Traditional Jewish name and the implement said to have been used by Solomon to cut the huge stones for the building of the Temple. **Shahmir, Shamar, Shameer, Shamur.**

SHAMUS. *Anglicised spelling of Séamus. See SEAMUS.*

♂ **SHANAHAN.** *Irish, 'the wise one'.* Undiscovered Irish surname with a lot more bounce and masculine dash than Shannon.

SHANDAR. *Hindi, 'proud'.* Has a somewhat comic strip magician image.

♂ **SHANDY.** *English, 'boisterous'.* A jolly, bawdy image that recalls the hero of the eighteenth-century novel *Tristram Shandy;* also a drink in the pub. **Shandey, Shandie.**

♂ **SHANE.** *Irish variation of* **SEAN.** Shane ambled into the picture via the 1953 movie, adding a cowboy twist to its Irish essence; still used but feeling tired. **Shayne.**

SHANGO. *African, Yoruba, mythology name.* More substantial than it sounds: Shango was the god of thunder and legendary ancestor of the Yoruba people of Nigeria.

♂ **SHANNON.** *Irish, 'old and wise'; also river in Ireland.* The name of the longest river in the British Isles now has a distinctly feminine flavour. **Shannan, Shannen.**

SHAQIR. *Spelling variation of* **SHAKIR;** *Arabic, 'thankful'.* Shaquille O'Neal came as close as he could to naming his son after himself without using his own name.

SHAQUILLE. *(shah-KEEL) Arabic, 'well developed, handsome'.* No longer a one-person name, as a number of parents have been inspired by American basketball great Shaquille O'Neal to adopt it for their own future athletes. **Shakeel, Shakil, Shaq, Shaquil.**

SHARIF. *Arabic, 'the honourable one'.* Long associated with Egyptian-born actor/bridge expert Omar Sharif, also a title bestowed on descendants of

Muhammad. **Charif, Cherif, Shareef, Shereef, Sherif.**

♂ **SHAUN.** *Spelling variation of* **SEAN.** Very 1980s.

SHAVIV. *Hebrew, 'spark, ray of light'.* The *viv* syllable adds vitality.

♂ **SHAW.** *English, 'small wood, copse'.* With the current taste for last names first, this sounds a lot cooler than Shawn; it also has a creative connection to the great Irish playwright, George Bernard Shaw.

♂ **SHAWN.** *Spelling variation of* **SEAN.** Very 1970s. **DeShawn, Shaughan, Shaun, Shawon.**

♂ **SHAWNEL.** *Modern invented name.* Modern, none-too-classy elaboration of Shawn. **Shaunel, Shaunell, Shaunelle, Shawnell, Shawnelle.**

♂ **SHAY.** *Irish, diminutive of* **SEAMUS;** *spelling variation of* **SHEA.** Has an old-fashioned feel due to its association with the word for a kind of horse-drawn carriage.

♂ **SHAYNE.** *Spelling variation of* **SHANE.** Up 827% due to XFactor winner Shane Ward

♂ **SHEA.** *Irish, 'the stately, dauntless one'.* A common surname in Ireland that projects a complex image for a short-one-syllable name, combining spirit and substance. **Shae, Shai, Shay, Shaye, Shey.**

SHEEHAN. *Irish, 'peaceful'.* Has a decidedly Roman Catholic feel, thanks to the bishop. **Sheehn, Sheen.**

SHEFFIELD. *English, 'from the crooked field'.* One place name that doesn't make the cut as a person name, associated with several commercial enterprises. **Scaffeld.**

♂ **SHELBY.** *English, 'estate on the ledge'.* Southern name still occasionally heard in a male context (author Shelby Foote and the son of singer Reba McEntire), but it's much more associated with girls. **Selbey, Selby, Shel, Shelbey, Shell, Shellbey, Shellby, Shelny.**

SHELDON. *English, 'steep-sided valley'.* Like Marvin and Melvin,

about as far out as you can get, though there are very pretty towns in Devon and Derbyshire that inspired it. **Sheldan, Shelden, Sheldin, Sheldyn, Shelldon.**

♂ **SHELLEY.** *English, 'clearing on a bank'; also diminutive of* **SHELDON.** Despite its poetic associations, almost as dated as Sheldon and more feminine. **Shell, Shelly.**

SHELTON. *English, 'place on a ledge or bank'.* We're not too surprised that Shelton Lee changed his name to Spike.

SHEM. *Hebrew, 'renown'.* Now-obscure name of Noah's eldest son (born when Dad was around five hundred). **Shammai, Shemuel.**

SHEP. *Diminutive of* **SHEPHERD.** Three Stooges name (he's the one who wasn't Moe or Curly).

SHEPHERD. *Occupational name.* An occupational surname with a pleasant pastoral feel, chosen for their son by the Jerry Seinfelds, which might inspire others to follow their lead. **Shep,**

Shepard, Shephard, Sheppard, Shepperd.

♂ **SHERIDAN.** *Irish, 'wild one'.* The downside to this perfectly pleasant (except for its scary meaning) name is the feminine nickname Sherry, making it more appropriate for a girl. **Dan, Sheriden, Sheridon, Sherridan, Sherry.**

SHERLOCK. *English, 'fair-haired'.* If ever there was a one-person name . . . **Sherlocke, Shurlock, Shurlocke.**

SHERMAN. *English occupational name, 'shearer of woolen cloth'.* Not quite as over-the-hill as Herman, but not far behind. **Sherm, Shermann. International: Shermon** *(German).*

SHERWIN. *English, 'swift runner'.* You won't win with Sherwin. **Sherwen, Sherwinn, Sherwyn, Sherwynd, Sherwynn, Sherwynne, Win, Winn, Winnie, Winny, Wyn, Wynn, Wynne.**

SHERWOOD. *English, 'bright forest'.* Unfashionable surname, best left in the forest with Robin Hood and his Merry Men.

Sheriff, Sherlock, Sherman, Shermie, Shermy, Sherry, Shurwood, Wood, Woodie, Woody.

♂ **SHILOH.** *Hebrew, 'he who is to be sent'; biblical place name.* Haunting biblical and Civil War place name; now unisex – especially after the high-profile Brangelina couple picked it for their daughter. **Shilo, Shiloe, Shylo, Shyloh.**

SHIMON. *Hebrew, 'to be heard'; variation of* **SIMON.** Most parents would choose the more contemporary Simon. **Shimi, Shim'on.**

♂ **SHIRON.** *Hebrew, 'songfest'.* Associated with music; don't be surprised to see it on collections of Hebrew songs. **Sharone, Shir, Shiran.**

SHLOMO. *Hebrew, 'his peace'; variation of* **SOLOMON.** Schleppy. **Shelomi, Shelomo, Shlomi, Shlomot.**

SHMUEL. *(SHMUL) Hebrew variation of* **SAMUEL.** Less than zero chance of crossing into the mainstream.

International: Shem, Shemuel, Shmelke, Shmiel, Shmulke *(Yiddish).*

SHOLTO. *Scottish from the Gaelic, 'propagator'.* Though it doesn't sound particularly Scottish, a traditional first name in the Douglas clan.

SIÂM. *(SHAM) Welsh variation of* **JAMES.** We don't think a boy would want to be called a sham.

♂ **SIDNEY.** *French, 'Saint Denis'.* Since a number of little girls have been named Sydney in recent years, the male version has virtually lost what little testosterone it had. **Sid, Sidny, Syd, Sydney, Sydny. International: Sidonio** *(Spanish).*

SIEGFRIED. *German, 'victorious peace'.* Wagnerian. **Siegfred, Siegfried, Sig, Sigfrid, Sigfried, Sigfryd, Siggy, Sigo, Sikko, Sygfried, Szygfrid, Ziggy. International: Siffre, Sigfroi** *(French),* **Sigefriedo** *(Italian),* **Sigfrido, Sigifredo** *(Spanish),* **Fredo, Siguefredo** *(Portuguese),* **Seifert, Seifried, Siegfried** *(German),* **Zygfryd, Zygi** *(Polish),* **Szigfrid, Zigfrid** *(Hungarian),* **Zigfrids** *(Russian, Latvian).*

♂ SIERRA. *Spanish, 'saw-toothed'; also mountains in Spain and California.* Although used for a male character in an American TV soap, it is almost exclusively a feminine choice.

SIGMUND. *German, 'victorious protection'.* Only if you're a devout Freudian. **Siggy, Sigismund, Sigmond, Ziggy, Zsiga, Zsigmond. International: Siegmund** *(German)*, **Sigurd, Sigvard** *(Norse)*, **Zygmunt** *(Polish)*.

★SILAS. *Greek from Latin, 'wood'; Aramaic, 'to borrow'.* Once a folksy-sounding, rural New Testament name associated with George Eliot's Silas Marner, it's beginning to be reevaluated, à la similarly flavoured Caleb and Linus. Also associated with the indelible albino monk in *The Da Vinci Code*. **Cylas, Silo, Silus, Sylas.**

♂ SILVAIN. *(sil-VAYN) Latin, 'from the forest'.* Woodsy name referring to the Roman tree god Silvanus. **Sil, Sill, Silvanus, Silvius, Sylvan, Sylvanus. International: Selvyn, Silas, Sylvester** *(English)*, **Sylvain, Silvestre** *(French)*, **Silvano,**

Silvio *(Italian)*, **Silbanio, Silvanio, Silvano, Silviano** *(Spanish)*, **Silverio, Silvino** *(Portuguese)*, **Silvan, Silvester** *(German)*.

SILVANO. *(seel-BAH-no) Latin, 'from the forest'.* Has a nice Spanish swing. **Silbanio, Silván, Silvanio, Silviano.**

♂ SILVER. *English word name.* This shimmery Age of Aquarius unisex flower child name is making a comeback, along with metal and gem names like Steel, Jade and Ruby. **Sylver.**

SILVIO. *Italian, 'the man of the forest'.* Shiny and sylvan choice.

SIMBA. *Swahili, 'lion'.* Traditional African name made cartoonish by the Disney character in *The Lion King*.

♂ SIMCHA. *(seem-ca) Hebrew, 'gladness, mirth, festivity'.* Celebratory choice. **Semach, Simchai, Simchon. Simchoni.**

SIMEON. *Hebrew, 'harkening'.* Parents seeking a less simple form of Simon might consider

this biblical one. Caveat: it is undeniably similar to the word meaning 'ape-like'. **SIM, SIMM.**

★SIMON. *Hebrew, 'the listener'.* Simon pure and simple (not in the nursery rhyme sense), an appealingly genuine Old and New Testament name that's not overused, so it could make a stylish choice. **Si, Sim, Sime, Simeon, Sy, Syme, Symon. International: Simond, Síomón** *(Irish Gaelic)*, **Sim, Simidh** *(Scottish Gaelic)*, **Simeon, Simion** *(French)*, **Simone** *(Italian)*, **Ximen, Ximenes, Ximens** *(Spanish)*, **Ximun** *(Basque)*, **Simao** *(Portuguese)*, **Siemen** *(Dutch)*, **Simeon, Simmy** *(German)*, **Symon, Szmon, Szymon** *(Polish)*, **Simion** *(Romanian)*, **Šimon, Simunek, Šionek** *(Czech)*, **Semyon, Simeon** *(Russian)*, **Semon, Symeon** *(Greek)*, **Shimon, Siomon** *(Hebrew)*, **Samein** *(Arabic)*.

SINBAD. *Persian literary name.* Not one to consider – a name that is a combination of Sin and Bad could only lead to plenty of tough times in the playground.

Names Kids Consider Cool

Barnaby

Beau

Brady

Clancy

Dallas

Damian

Jake

Max

Oliver

Orion

Riley

Ryder

Shane

Sky

Taj

Wyatt

Zak

Zayden

Zeus

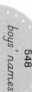

♂ SINCERE. *Word name.* An optimistic thought in this cynical world; could raise some eyebrows.

♂ SINCLAIR. *Scottish English, 'from the town of St. Clair'.* Could be a novel way for a boy's name to honour an ancestral Claire. **Sinclaire, Sinclare, Synclair.**

♂ SINDRI. *Norse, 'mythical dwarf'; also Indian place name.* Idiosyncratic Icelandic singer Björk chose this exotic name for her son.

SINJON. *English, phonetic spelling of* **ST JOHN.** *See ST JOHN.* **Sinjin, Sinjun.**

SIÔN. *(SHON) Welsh variation of* **JOHN.** A more authentic – and difficult – version of Sean. **Sioni, Sionyn.**

SIÔR. *(SHOR) Welsh variation of* **GEORGE.** A nice beachy name, but one that would require constant explanation.

SIRAJ. *(sir-rahj) Arabic, 'light, lamp'.* Exotic and evocative.

SIRIUS. *Latin from Greek, 'burning'.* Yes, it's the name of the brightest star in the sky, but can't you just hear people saying, 'Are you serious?'

Singer Erykah Badu used it as a middle name for son Seven.

SIRO. *Latin, 'from Syria'; Italian variation of* **CYRIL** *and* **SYRUS.** This Italian saint's name is one of the most unusual of the *o*-ending names. **Ciro.**

SISQÓ. *Spanish nickname.* Catchy stage name of popular R & B singer (born Mark – Sisqó was his childhood nickname). **Cisco, Cisqo, Sisco.**

SISYPHUS. *Greek, 'son of Aelous'.* One of the most severely punished characters in Greek mythology and completely sissified to boot.

SKEET. *English, 'swift'; form of trap-shooting.* Kind of a combination of scoot and fleet. **Skeat, Skete, Sketes.**

SKIPPER. *English, 'captain'; nickname.* Sure and we hope he has a good time playing with Buster and Buddy. **Skip.**

♂ SKY. *Nature name.* First legitimised as Sky Masterson in

Guys and Dolls, has a clear, wide-open feel.

♂ **SKYE.** *Scottish place name.* Referring to the Scottish Isle of Skye, brings Sky down to earth.

SKYLAR. *See SKYLER.*

♂ **SKYLER.** *Spelling variation of* **SCHUYLER.** A name very much in the air, for both boys and girls, often seen in the casts and character lists of American films and TV shows. The Skylar spelling is used more for females. **Schuyler, Schyler, Sky, Skyden, Skylar, Skyller, Skylor.**

♂ **SLADE.** *English, 'from the valley'.* Evoking the image of a shady glen, this could make a distinctive middle name. **Slaed, Slaid, Slayde.**

♂ **SLATE.** *Word name.* One of the more unusual of the current crop of strong, single-syllable boys' names, evoking the images of both old-fashioned chalkboards and modern stepping-stones.

SLATER. *English occupational name, 'maker of slates'.* Has a genial, friendly feel.

♂ **SLOAN.** *Irish, 'raider'.* A few decades back, this name – which hardly shows its Irish roots – evoked a man in a grey flannel suit or a Sloane Ranger; now, though still upscale, it's more likely to be attached to a female. **Sloane.**

SLY. *English word name, diminutive of* **SYLVESTER.** A bit too cunning.

♂ **SMITH.** *English occupational name, 'blacksmith'.* Even if it's not a family name, makes for a very cool middle. **Smitty, Smyth, Smythe.**

SOCRATES. *Greek philosopher; uncertain derivation.* Quite common in traditional Greek families, but for others, we think Plato might be easier to handle.

SOL. *(soul) Spanish, 'sun'; (sahl) Hebrew, diminutive of* **SOLOMON.** Although pinochle-playing partner Sam came out of retirement, we don't see it happening to Sol. Near soundalike Saul has more of a shot.

SOLOMON. *Hebrew, 'peace'.* Wise old biblical name that, along with other patriarchal classics, is finally beginning to shed its long white beard and step from the pages of the Old Testament. **Salman, Salmen, Salmon, Salo, Saloman, Salome, Salomone, Selman, Shelomo, Sol, Solamon, Sollie, Solly, Solmon, Soloman, Zalmen, Zalmon, Zelman, Zelmen, Zelmo, Zollie, Zolly. International: Solamh** *(Gaelic),* **Lasimonne, Salaun, Salomon** *(French),* **Salamone** *(Italian),* **Solomon** *(Spanish),* **Salomo** *(German),* **Salomon** *(Norwegian),* **Salamen** *(Polish),* **Salaman, Salamon** *(Hungarian),* **Salamun** *(Czech),* **Salamonas** *(Lithuanian),* **Shelomoh, Shlomo, Zalman** *(Yiddish),* **Suleiman** *(Arabic).*

SOLON. *Greek, 'the wise one'.* Despite the reputation of the sagacious ancient Greek lawmaker, this name hasn't moved to the modern world.

SONNY. *Nickname for 'son'.* Rarely heard since the *Godfather* films. **Son, Sonney, Sonnie, Sunnie, Sunny.**

SÖREN. *Danish variation of* **SEVERUS.** A gentle Danish name, soft and sensitive, but with more masculine punch than Loren.

♂ **SORLEY.** *Irish, 'a summer sailor'.* Ripe for sore and sore-loser teasing. **International: Somhairle** *(Irish Gaelic).*

♂ **SORRELL.** *French, 'reddish brown'; and botanical name.* Soft, amber-hued autumnal name that's used most often to describe the colour of a horse. **Sorel, Sorell, Soril, Sorrel, Sorril, Sorrill, Sorryl, Soryll, Soryl.**

♂ **SOUTINE.** *French artist name.* Creative choice relating to the Lithuanian-born expressionist painter known for his bold, vibrantly coloured canvases.

SPALDING. *English and Scottish, 'divided field'.* Has diverse links to a Groucho Marx character, a bouncing ball and performance artist Spalding Gray. **Spaulding, Spelding.**

SPECK. *English word name.* Not only did rocker John Mellencamp name his son Speck, but he appended the middle name Wildhorse to it.

★ ♂ **SPENCER.** *French, 'keeper of provisions'.* A name that briefly appeared in the Top 100 recently, it's both distinguished sounding and accessible, dignified but Spencer Tracy-like friendly. Picked by several celebrities (occasionally for girls), it's a recommended choice. **Spence, Spenser.**

SPIRO. *Greek, 'spirit'.* An Old Word name that is perhaps best left there.

♂ **SPRUCE.** *Nature name.* A handsome, spruced-up post-Bruce tree name.

SQUALL. *English word name.* A video-game name *(Final Fantasy VII)* with an unappealing sound and meaning.

SQUIRE. *French, 'esquire'.* Conjures up a tweedy English country gentleman with a large paunch. **Squier, Squiers, Squires.**

♂ **STACEY, STACY.** *Greek diminutive of* **EUSTACE.** Became completely feminised in the unisex name revolution of the 1970s.

STAFFORD. *English, 'from the ford by the landing place'.* Sounds like you should have a *shire* following it.

STAMOS. *Greek surname; variation of* **STEPHEN.** Has a dark, sexy image.

STANCIO. *(STAHN-see-o) Spanish variation of* **CONSTANTINE.** Unusual, with an energetic spirit.

STANFORD. *English, 'stony ford'.* Even if you're a loyal alumnus of the American college, consider something less ultra-upright, like Yale.

STANISLAV. *German, Slavic, 'glorious government'.* Long-haired classical conductor name. **Stan, Standa, Stanek, Staník, Stanislas, Stanislaus, Stanko, Stannes. International: Estamoslao** *(Spanish),* **Stanislaw, Stasiak** *(Polish),* **Stáňa** *(Czech),* **Stas** *(Russian).*

♂ **STANLEY.** *English, 'near the stony meadow'.* Although Stanley Kowalski in *A Streetcar Named Desire* personified brute force, most Stanleys have been portrayed as meek milquetoasts.

Could be a Sydney-like girls' choice. **Stan, Stanly.**

STANTON. *English, 'stony town'.* Seems to stand at attention and salute.

STAVROS. *Greek variation of* **STEPHEN.** Conjures up billionaire shipping magnates.

STEDMAN. *English, 'owner of a farmstead'.* Playmates could change the *e* to a *u*. **Steadman.**

♂ **STEEL, STEELE.** *Word name.* Hard and shiny, this surname projects an image that's smooth, macho . . . and cold.

STEFAN. *German, Scandinavian, Polish and Russian variation of* **STEPHEN.** An elegant, continental name for the post-Steve era. **Steffan, Steffel, Steffen, Steffon, Stenya, Stepa, Stepan.**

STEFANO. *Italian variation of* **STEPHEN.** As commonly heard in Rome, Italy, as Steve is in Bath (built in the English hills because they reminded the Romans of Rome).

★**STELLAN.** *Swedish, meaning unknown.* A Scandinavian-flavoured up-and-comer chosen by Jennifer Connelly and Paul Bettany for their son.

STEN. *Swedish, 'a stone'.* Once a short form of names containing this syllable, it is now used on its own, though we'd prefer Sven. **International: Steen** *(Danish),* **Stein** *(Norwegian).*

STEPHANOS. *(steh-FAH-nos) Greek, 'garland, crown'.* The original form of Stephen, a readily importable choice. **Istivan, Stefan, Stefanos, Stephanas, Stephanus.**

STEPHEN. *Greek, 'garland, crown'.* The likable nickname Steve has helped keep the classic Stephen/Steven very much alive; the name of the first Christian martyr is no longer fashionable, but still retains its strength, dignity and appeal. **Steafan, Stef, Steffen, Steffon, Steph, Stephanus, Stephon, Stevan, Steve, Steven, Stevenson, Stevey, Stevie, Stevin, Stevon, Stevy, Stevyn.**

♂ **STERLING.** *English, 'of the highest quality'.* A name with

some sterling qualities, but a slightly pretentious air. **Stirling.**

STETSON. *American surname.* Check the western millinery department.

STEVE. *Diminutive of* **STEPHEN** *or* **STEVEN.** Some parents just use Steve on the birth certificate, but it doesn't have the breezy charm of trendy short forms like Max, Sam and Jake.

STEVELAND. *Modern invented name.* Stevie Wonder was born Steveland, but it's not likely that many other babies will follow. **Steve, Stevie.**

STEVEN. *English variation of* **STEPHEN.** Phonetic and now predominant spelling of the classier Stephen. *See* *STEPHEN.*

STEWART. *Scottish, 'steward' See STUART.*

STIAN. *(STEE-an) Norse, 'wanderer'.* Popular in Norway, an interesting choice for anyone with northern European roots.

Stephen's International Variations

Irish Gaelic	Stiana, Stiofan
Irish	Steafan
Scottish Gaelic	Steaphan, Stiabhan
Welsh	Steffan, Steffen
French	Étienne, Stéphane
Provençal	Estéve
Italian	Stefano
Spanish	Estéban, Estebe, Estefan, Estevan, Estevon
Catalan	Esteve
Portuguese	Estefania, Estevão
German	Stefan, Steffen
Swedish	Staffan, Stefan
Norwegian	Steffen
Finnish	Tapani, Teppo
Polish	Stefan, Szczepan
Hungarian	Isti, István
Czech	Stepan, Stepka
Lithuanian	Steponas
Russian	Stefan, Stenya, Stepan
Latvian	Stefans
Greek	Stamos, Stavros, Stephanos
Armenian	Panos
Israeli	Tzefanyah
Maori	Tipene
Hawaiian	Kiwini

STIG. *Swedish, 'wanderer'.* Like Stian, a more manageable short form of the unwieldy Srigandr, but with a less euphonic sound.

ST JOHN. *(SIN-jin) English saint's name.* Mainly (but rarely) used by Catholics in England – there's one in *Jane Eyre* – this could be confused with the ambulance service. **Sinjin.**

STONE. *Word name.* Though some may find such names rather harsh and severe, increasing numbers of parents are gravitating toward this kind of flinty, steely, stony single-syllable name.

♂ **STORM.** *Word name.* Windswept and dramatic, but perhaps asking for trouble.

♂ **STORY.** *Word name.* A new name with a lot of charm, especially appropriate for the child of writers.

STREET. *Word name.* An unusual kind of place name, going beyond a country, state or city, it was used as a middle name for her son by American actress Elisabeth Shue.

STROM. *German, 'stream'.* Strom sounds like an anagram of Storm that's lost its strength. Storm, or maybe River, might make a better choice.

STUART. *Scottish, 'steward'.* This ancient royal Scottish name had been briefly in vogue in the USA in the 1950s, but it would be far from a fresh choice for a baby boy now. **Stew, Stewart, Stu.**

♂ **SUEDE.** *French, 'Swedish'; word name.* In the 1990s there was an American soap opera character named Suede, but few parents picked up on it; might be more appealing to today's generation of parents.

SUFJAN. *(SOOF-yahn), Armenian, 'comes with a sword'.* This name is growing in popularity, partly because of its tie to hipster musician Sufjan Stevens; is also related to Abu Sufyan, a figure from early Islamic history. **Sufyan.**

SULAIMAN. *(soo-lay-MAHN) Arabic variation of* **SOLOMON.** Muslim name very popular in North Africa. **Shelomon, Siliman, Sulaiman, Suleiman.**

SULIEN. *(SIL-yen) Welsh, 'sun born'; name of Celtic sun god.* Said to be the name of the most learned man in ancient Wales, elsewhere it would be open to mispronunciation, making it rhyme with Julien. **International: Silyen** *(Cornish).*

★♂ **SULLIVAN.** *Irish, 'dark eyes'.* Jaunty Celtic three-syllable name, with a real twinkle in its eye. **Sullavan, Sullevan, Sullie, Sully.**

SULLY. *French, 'stain'; English, 'from the south meadow'.* Jaunty but slightly muddied offshoot of Sullivan, associated by kids with the beloved character in *Monsters, Inc.*

SULTAN. *(sool-TAHN) Swahili, 'ruler'.* Passé pasha image.

SUTCLIFF. *English, 'from the southern cliff'.* Climbing a mountain somewhere with Radcliff and Heathcliff. **Sutcliffe, Sutclyf.**

♂ **SUTTON.** *English, 'from the southern homestead'.* Swanky via New York's ritzy Sutton Place – but not the Surrey town.

★**SVEN.** *Norse, 'youth'.* For non-football fans, a recommended import, with an appealing mix of strength and swagger. **Svevn, Sveyn, Swen, Swenson.**

Stellar Starbabies Beginning with *S*

Salvador	Ed *(Radiohead)* O'Brien
Sam	Tracy Pollan & Michael J. Fox
Samuel	Jack Black, Dave Steward & Siobhan Fahey
Sawyer	Kate Capshaw & Steven Spielberg
Sean	Britney Spears & Kevin Federline
Sebastian	James Spader
Seven	Erykah Badu & Andre *(Andre 3000)* Benjamin
Shane	Sinead O'Connor
Shaqir	Shaquille O'Neal
Shaqueel	Robin Van Persie
Shepherd	Jerry Seinfeld
Simeon	Wynton Marsalis
Sindri	Björk
Sonny	Sophie Ellis Bextor
Speck	John Mellencamp
Spencer	Cuba Gooding Jr, Cynthia McFadden, Gena Lee Nolin
Suleiman	Jemima Khan
Sullivan	Patrick Dempsey

International: Svend *(Danish)*, **Svens** *(Swedish)*, **Svein** *(Norwegian)*.

SWAIN. *English, 'knight's attendant'*. Old-fashioned, conjuring up an ardent suitor in a bow tie and straw boater. **Swaine, Swayn, Swayne.**

♂ **SWEDEN.** *Place name.* A pleasing place name that hasn't yet appeared in the baby name atlas. **Swede, Sweeden, Sweedon.**

♂ **SWEENEY.** *Irish, 'the little hero'.* The double *e* gives this Celtic surname a genial sound; only drawback is the association with Sweeney Todd, the bloodthirsty butcher of Sondheim stage-musical fame. **Sweeny.**

SWITHUN. *English, 'quick, strong'.* Obscure, obsolete saint's name. **Swithinn, Swithun.**

♂ **SYDNEY.** *Spelling variation of* **SIDNEY**. The Sydney spelling is most popular for girls. **Syd.**

SYLVESTER. *Latin, 'from the forest'.* This name of three early popes has been kept alive in recent years by the Italian Stallion hero of the *Rocky* and *Rambo* films; however it's not likely to be picked up on by many modern parents. **Silvester, Sly. International: Silvester** *(French)*, **Silvestro** *(Italian)*,

Silvestio, Silvestre, Sivestro (Spanish), Sylwester (Polish).

SYRUS. *Spelling variation of* **CYRUS.** This variation has one *s* too many, making it seem a bit sissified.

T boys

TAB. *Modern invented name.* A Hollywood agent created the name Tab Hunter and poof! – the former Arthur Gelien became a 1950s teen idol. We don't advise trying this at home. **Tabb, Tabbie, Tabby, Taber, Tabor.**

TABARI. *Arabic, 'he remembers'.* Has a haunting, rhythmic feel. **Tabahri, Tabares, Tabarious, Tabarius, Tabarus, Tabur.**

TABOR. *(TAH-bor) Hungarian, 'encampment'.* A common name in Hungary, rarely heard here. **Tabber, Taber, Taboras, Taibor, Taver, Tavor, Tayber, Taybor.**

TAD. *Diminutive of* **THADDEUS.** More than a tad meager. **Tadd, Taddy, Tade, Tadek, Tadey, Thad.** International: **Thadeo** *(Italian),* **Taddeo, Tadeo** *(Spanish).*

♂ **TADEN.** *Modern invented name.* One of the newer and fresher-sounding members of the Braeden, Jaden, Caden clan. **Tadin, Tadon, Tadyn, Taeden, Taedin, Taedon, Taedyn, Tayden, Taydin, Taydon.**

TADEO. *Spanish variation of* **THADDEUS.** Has a lot of energy and charm, as does the Italian form, Taddeo. **Tad, Taddeo, Tadzio.**

TAFT. *English, 'building site'.* A solid, brief but not brusque single-syllable surname. **Taffy, Tafton.**

TAGGART. *Irish, 'son of the priest'.* Not your typical jovial Irish surname; also has the danger of rhyming with braggart. **Tagart, Taggert.**

TAHMEL. *Nepalese place name.* This unusual geographic choice – Tahmel is an area of Katmandu – was selected for her son by singer Macy Gray.

♂ **TAHOE.** *Native American, 'big water' or 'edge of the lake'.* A unique natural-wonder option, conjuring up the beauty of the lake between California and Nevada that has become a popular tourist destination.

TAIDEN. *Modern invented name. See* **TADEN.**

TAIT. *(TITE or TATE) Norse, 'cheerful'.* Tate would be much more user-friendly in this country. **Taite, Taitt, Tate, Tayte.**

♂ **TAJ.** *(tahzh) Sanskrit, 'crown'.* Cool-sounding name reflecting the magnificence of the seventeenth-century Indian Taj Mahal, chosen by Aerosmith's Steven Tyler for his son. **Tahj, Taje, Tajee, Tajeh, Tajh, Taji.**

TAKEO. *Japanese, 'strong as bamboo'.* Well used in Japan, appreciated for its powerful meaning. **Takeyo.**

♂ **TAL.** *Hebrew, 'rain, dew'.* A unisex Hebrew name often found in combination with others, as in Tal-El and Tal-Or. **Tahl, Tali, Talley, Talor, Talya, Tatar.**

TALBOT. *English, 'command of the valley'.* Upscale and upstanding. **Talbert, Talbott, Tallbot, Tallbott, Tallie, Tally.**

TALCOTT. *English, 'cottage near the lake'.* A bit formal for our time, Alcott would be a bit less forbidding.

♂ **TALIESIN.** *(TAL-eh-sin) Welsh, 'shining brow'.* This unusual Welsh mythological name just might appeal to architect parents wishing to honour Frank Lloyd Wright, who called his two famous residences Taliesin and Taliesin West. **Tallas, Tallis.**

TALMAN. *Aramaic, 'injured, oppressed'.* Solemn. **Tal, Tallie, Tally, Talmai, Talmon.**

TALON. *French word name, 'large claw of a bird of prey'.* Despite its somewhat menacing meaning, this name has been chosen by hundreds of parents over the past few years, probably due to the appeal of its trendy *on* ending. **Taelon, Taelyn, Talen, Talin, Tallan, Tallen, Tallin, Tallon, Talyn.**

TAMARACK. *Nature name.* One of the clumsier nature names, that of a variety of pine tree; there's a potential that it will be rhymed with anorak.

♂ **TAMERLANE.** *Possibly 'Timur the Lame'.* This name of an ancient Mongol warrior, remembered primarily today through the works of Christopher Marlowe and Edgar Allan Poe, runs the risk of sounding pompous and pretentious. **Tamarlain, Tamarlayn, Tamberlaine, Tamberlan, Tamburlaine, Tamburlane, Tamurlaine, Tamurlayn, Tarnberlane.**

TAMIR. *Hebrew, 'erect, tall as a palm tree'; Arabic, 'owner of many palm trees'.* A Near Eastern favourite, with an agreeable, evocative sound. **Tamario, Tameer, Tamur.**

TANCREDO. *(ton-CRAY-dō) Italian from German, 'thoughtful counsel'.* A name rich in historic, poetic and operatic allusions and an interesting Italian alternative to the more ordinary Giovannis and Giorgios. **Tancredi. International: Tancréde** *(French),* **Tancred, Tancredo** *(Italian),* **Tancred** *(German).*

♂ **TANE.** *(TAH-NEH) Polynesian, mythology name.* The name of the powerful Polynesian sky god who set the sun and moon in place and studded the heavens with stars – a majestic legacy for a simple yet unusual name. **Tahnee, Tain, Taine, Tayn, Tayne.**

♂ **TANGIER.** *place name.* Exotic, unexplored Moroccan place name, conjuring up images of camels and palm trees and domed minarets. **Tangiers.**

TANGUY. *(tahn-guee) French, 'warrior'.* This engaging French saint's name also has a creative connection to French surrealist painter Yves Tanguy. **Tanghi, Tangi, Tangou, Tangui.**

TANNER. *English occupational name, 'leather tanner'.* One of the hot two-syllable *T* names of the 1990s (along with Tyler, Trevor and Taylor) and well represented on American soap operas; Tanner's popularity is declining. **Tan, Tanar, Taner, Tanery, Tann, Tannar, Tannen, Tannir, Tannis, Tannon, Tannor, Tanny, Tany.**

♂ **TAOS.** *American place name.* This beautiful New Mexican pueblo locale has long attracted artists and skiers and now may attract some baby namers as well.

TARAK. *Sanskrit, 'star, protector'.* Sci-fi vibe.

♂ **TARIAN.** *Modern invented name.* American country singer Travis Tritt is partial to the letter *t* for his sons' names, which includes a Tarian.

TARIQ. *(TAHR-ik) Arabic, 'the one who knocks at the door'.* A strong and confident name growing in popularity, in numerous spellings. **Tareck, Tareek, Tareeq, Tarek, Tareke, Tari, Taric, Tarick, Tariek, Tarik, Tarikh, Tariq, Tarique, Tarreq, Tarrick, Tarrik, Taryk, Tereik.**

♂ **TAROT.** *French, fortune-telling cards.* A psychic mystique clings to this name of cards used in fortune-telling.

★**TARQUIN.** *(TAR-kin) Roman clan name of uncertain meaning.* One of the few ancient Roman names that doesn't end in *us*, the rarely heard Tarquin has a decidedly creative, even dramatic flair, which could appeal to the parent looking for a strikingly original name. **Tarquinius, Tarquino.**

TASSO. *Italian, 'cup'.* A singular selection, noteworthy for its connection to the great sixteenth-century Italian epic poet, Torquato Tasso.

♂ **TATE.** *English from Norse, 'cheerful'.* A strong single-syllable surname with a joyful meaning – and the name of the modern art gallery – Tate is finding a place on more and more birth certificates. **Tah, Tait, Taitt, Tayte.**

TAURUS. *Latin, 'bull'; sign of the Zodiac.* His nickname would inevitably be Bull. **Taurean, Taurice, Tauris. International: Taurino, Tauro, Toro** *(Spanish).*

TAVISH. *Scottish variation of* **THOMAS.** This Scottish form of Thomas evokes images of men in plaid kilts playing the bagpipes and eating haggis. **Tav, Tavi, Tavis, Tavish, Tavon, Tevin, Tevis.**

♂ **TAY.** *Scottish place name.* This name of the largest river in Scotland, renowned for its salmon fishing, is usually thought of as a nickname for Taylor. **TAE.**

♂ **TAYE.** *African, Ethiopian, 'he has been seen'.* Taye, also seen as a short form of Taylor, is beginning to stand on its own.

♂ **TAYLOR.** *English occupational name.* The fact that Taylor was a popular girl's name in the 1990s might cause parents to consider Tyler, Tate or Taye instead, which might be why this popular name is dropping in the Top 100. **Taelor, Taelur, Tailer, Tailor, Talor, Taylar, Tayler, Tayller, Tayllor, Taylour, Taylr, Teyler, Teylor.**

TAYSON. *Modern invented name.* Parents wanting to move beyond Jason and Mason have created Tayson. **Tason, Taysen.**

♂ **TEAGAN.** *Irish, 'little poet'.* Increasingly used for boys, Teagan is probably riding in the slipstream of Reagan/Regan's popularity. **Teagon, Teegan, Teegon, Tegan, Tegon.**

TEAGUE. *Scottish, 'bard, poet'.* Might fit the bill if you're seeking a unique single-syllable first or middle name for your son.

♂ **TEAL.** *Bird and colour name.* This name of both a greyish-greenish-blue colour and a kind of wild duck can be used for both boys and girls. **Teale, Teel, Teele.**

TED. *Diminutive of* **THEODORE** *or* **EDWARD.** Like Teddy, Ed and Eddie, rarely used as an independent name. **Tedd, Teddey, Teddie, Teddy, Tedek, Tedik, Tedson.**

TEEL. *See* **TEAL.**

TEILO. *(TAY-lo) Welsh, meaning unknown.* Especially if you have Welsh roots, this prominent saint's name could be an interesting and more masculine alternative to Taylor.

TEMANI. *Hebrew, 'from the south'.* This biblical name is also a Hebrew term for someone from Yemen, since that country is south of Israel. **Teman, Temeni.**

♂ **TEMPLE.** *English, 'dweller near the temple'.* Rather formal word name that has been used occasionally over the years. **Templar, Templer.**

TEMPLETON. *English, 'temple settlement'.* Butler name and also that of the rat in *Charlotte's Web.* **Temp, Temple, Templeten.**

♂ **TENNESSEE.** *Native American, Cherokee, place name.* When playwright Thomas Lanier Williams adopted the pen name of Tennessee, he created a new possibility among American place names, although it's admittedly a bit bulky in size. **Tenn, Tenny, Tennesy, Tennysee.**

TENNYSON. *English, 'son of Dennis'.* The name of the famous Victorian poet would make a novel choice for the son of a Dennis; recently chosen by Russell Crowe. **Dennison, Tenison, Tenney, Tenneyson, Tennie, Tennis, Tennison, Tenny, Tenson.**

TERACH. *Hebrew, 'wild goat, silly old fool'.* A biblical name – he was the father of Abraham – but the father's name is much less appealing than the son's, in both sound and meaning. **Terah.**

TERENCE. *Latin clan name of uncertain meaning.* Out of style for several years – possibly because of the feminisation of nickname Terry – Terence might be due for a comeback, much like his Irish crony Patrick. One noble ancestor was the great ancient dramatist, once a North African slave. Spellings Terrance and Terrence now outperform the original. **Tarrance, Tarrants, Tarrenz, Tearance, Tearence, Tearnce, Tearrance, Teran, Terance, Teren, Terin, Terran, Terrance, Terren, Terrence, Terrey, Terri, Terriance, Terrien, Terrin, Terrious, Terris, Terrius, Terron, Terronce, Terry, Terryn, Teryn, Tiren, Torrence, Tyreas, Tyrease, Tyrece, Tyreece, Tyreese, Tyreice, Tyres, Tyrese, Tyresse, Tyrez, Tyreze, Tyrice, Tyriece, Tyriese.** International: **Terrance, Terrence, Theirry** *(French)*, **Terancio, Terenciano, Terencio** *(Italian)*, **Terencio** *(Spanish)*, **Terenz** *(German)*, **Tarantino, Terentilo, Terentino** *(Greek)*.

TERRANCE, TERRENCE. *See TERENCE.*

♂ **TERRE.** *(tair) French word name, 'earth'.* An intriguing but challenging choice, because of possible confusion with all the Terry-type names.

TERRELL. *Modern invented name.* Quite popular a few years ago, but gradually falling out of favour. **Tarel, Tarell, Tarelle, Tarrall, Tarrel, Tarrell, Taryl,** **Teral, Tereall, Terel, Terell, Terelle, Teriel, Teriell, Terrail, Terral, Terrale, Terrall, Terreal, Terrel, Terrelle, Terril, Terrill, Terron, Terryal, Terryel Terryl, Terryll, Teryl, Tirel, Tirell, Tirrel, Tirrell, Turrell, Tyrel, Tyrell, Tyrelle, Tyrill, Tyrrel, Tyrrell.**

♂ **TERRY.** *Diminutive of TERENCE.* One of the first breakaway unisex names, Terry, used independently since the days of *Terry and the Pirates,* has gradually become more feminine. **Tarry, Terrey, Terri, Terrie, Tery.**

TERTIUS. *(TER-shuss) Latin, 'third'.* Never as well known as that other Roman numeral name, Octavius, Tertius might just hold some appeal for the parent seeking a really obscure name with the patina of antiquity for her third son.

TETON. *(TEE-ton) Native American, Sioux tribe; also western American place name.* Rare and rugged.

♂ **TEVIN.** *Modern invented name.* This contemporary combo name is part Trevor, part

Kevin and thoroughly naff. **Tevan, Teven, Tevon, Tevvan, Tevvin, Tevvon.**

TEW. *Celtic, 'warrior god'.* Tew many conflicting word spellings. **Tewes.** International: **Tyw** *(Anglo-Saxon),* **Tyr** *(Scandinavian).*

TEX. *Place name, nickname for state of Texas resident.* Despite its rakish American West charm, still remains a cowboy costume without a real persona inside. **Tejas, Texas.**

THACKERAY. *English, 'place with thatching'.* The name of the famous British man of letters might just appeal to some English majors as a more interesting alternative to Zachary.

★**THADDEUS.** *Aramaic, meaning unclear.* This distinguished, long-neglected appellation has several areas of appeal: a solid New Testament legacy (it was another name for the Apostle Jude), a nice antique feel and the choice of several more modern nicknames and variations – we particularly like the Italian Taddeo. **Tad, Tadd, Taddeusz, Taddy, Tadio, Thad, Thadd, Thaddaeus, Thaddaios, Thaddaos, Thaddeau, Thaddeaus, Thaddeous, Thaddiaus, Thaddis, Thaddius, Thaddy, Thade, Thadeaou, Thadeaus, Thadee, Thadeous, Thadeus, Thadieus, Thadious, Thadius, Thadus, Thady.** International: **Thadee** (*French*), **Taddeo, Thaddeo** (*Italian*), **Tadeo** (*Spanish*), **Thaddaus** (*German*), **Tadek, Tadeuz, Tadzio** (*Polish*), **Tade** (*Hungarian*), **Tadeas, Tades** (*Czech*), **Faddei, Fadey, Tadey** (*Russian*), **Taddeus** (*Greek*).

♂ **THANE.** *Scottish, 'clan chieftain'.* This early Scottish title – known to us via Shakespeare's *Macbeth* – has recently surfaced as a baby name possibility, familiar sounding through its similarity to names like Zane and Wayne. **Thain, Thaine, Thayne.**

THANOS. *Greek, diminutive of* **ATHANASIOS,** *'immortality'.* Though this is a perfectly respectable Greek choice, be aware that Thanos the Mad

Titan is a sinister Marvel Comics villain. **Athanasios, Thanasios, Thanasis.**

♂ **THATCHER.** *English occupational name, 'roof thatcher'.* Fresher sounding than Tyler or Taylor, but forever linked with the former prime minister. **Thacher, Thatch, Thaxter.**

♂ **THAYER.** *French variation of* **TAYLOR.** An affable, less-used alternative to Taylor. **Thay.**

THELONIUS. *Latinised variation of* **TILLO,** *'lord'.* Forever cool, thanks to legendary jazz pianist T. Sphere Monk.

★**THEO.** *Diminutive of* **THEODORE.** Many modern parents – including such celebs as Cheryl Tiegs and the Steven Spielbergs – are bypassing the grandpa name Theodore and skipping to the hip nickname Theo – a cool, contemporary choice, now in the Top 100 thanks to young footballer Theo Walcott.

THEOBALD. *German, 'courageous people'.* Baby-naming rule Number 232: never give a

boy a name containing the syllable *bald*. **Dietbald, Dietbold, Ted, Teddy, Thebault, Theo, Theòbault, Thibaud, Tibalt, Tibold, Tiebold, Tiebout, Toiboid, Tybald, Tybalt, Tybault.** International: **Tiobóid** (*Irish Gaelic*), **Tiobaid** (*Scottish Gaelic*), **Thibault** (*French*), **Teobaldo** (*Spanish*).

THEODORE. *Greek, 'gift of God'.* One of the names last popular a century ago and now up for reconsideration. With Theo newly entered in the Top 100, granddaddy Theodore can't be far behind. **Tad, Teador, Ted, Teddie, Teddy, Tedor, Tedric, Tedrick, Teodoor, Teodore, Theo, Theodoras, Theodoros, Theodors, Theodorus, Tivadar.** International: **Teadoir** (*Gaelic*), **Tewdwr, Tudor** (*Welsh*), **Théodore** (*French*), **Teodoro, Teodosio** (*Italian*), **Feodor, Teodomiro, Teodoro** (*Spanish*), **Todor** (*Basque*), **Theodoor** (*Dutch*), **Tewdor, Theodor** (*German*), **Teodor** (*Swedish*), **Theodrekr** (*Norwegian*), **Dorek, Fedor, Tedorik, Teodor, Teodorek, Teos, Todor, Tolek** (*Polish*), **Tivadar, Todor** (*Hungarian*), **Bohdan, Fedor, Tedik, Teodor, Teodus** (*Czech*),

Fedar, Fedinka, Fedir, Fedor, Fedya, Feodor, Feodore, Fyodor, Todor, Todos (*Russian*), Thao, Theodosios (*Greek*).

THEODORIC. *German, 'people's ruler'; original form of* **DIETRICH.** Theodoric feels prehistoric. Derek, Derrick, Dieter, Dietrich, Dirck, Dirk, Rick, Ted, Thedric, Thedrick, Thilo, Til, Till, Tillman, Tillmann, Tilman, Tilson. International: Thierry (*French*).

THEOPHILOS. *Greek, 'loved by God'.* Multisyllabic New Testament relic dimly recalled from the Thornton Wilder novel *Theophilus North.* Teofil, Teofilo, Theophile, Theophilus, Theophlous, Theopolis. International: Théophile (*French*).

THESEUS. (*thee-see-us*) *Greek mythology name.* The name of the Greek mythological hero famous for slaying the Minotaur is also heard in Chaucer and Shakespeare, but would sound pretentious for a modern baby.

THIERRY. (*tyeh-REE*) *French variation of* **THEODORIC.** Very popular in France, this

would make an interesting import; it's somewhat familiar through designer Thierry Mugler and international football star Thierry Henry. Theirry, Theiry, Theory, Thery.

THOM. *Aramaic, 'twin'.* Pronounced like Tom, but not everyone will know that. Tom.

★**THOMAS.** *Aramaic, 'twin'.* One of the most commonly used classics. Thomas is steady in the Top 5 and has been used for males from the original apostle and several saints to Hardy and Edison, Hanks and the Tank Engine. Thomas is simple, straightforward and strong – all that a parent with a taste for the timeless could want. Thom, Thomason, Thomaz, Thomeson, Thomison, Thommas, Thompson, Thomsen, Thomson, Thomy, Tom, Tomah, Tomaisin, Tomie, Tomkin, Tomlin, Tomlinson, Tommas, Tommey, Tommy.

THOMPSON. *English, 'son of Tom'.* Not as popular as Jackson or Harrison, but a novel way to honour the son of a Thomas. Thomasen,

Thomason, Thompsen, Thomsen, Thomson, Tompsen, Tompson.

THOR. *Norse, 'thunder'.* The powerful name of the Norse god of thunder, strength and rain would make a bold statement. Thorald, Thorbert, Thordus, Thorin, Thorold, Thorvald, Thorwald, Tor, Torald, Torbert, Tore, Torin, Torre, Ty, Tyrell, Tyrus, Tyruss, Tyryss. International: Thoren, Thorian (*Scandinavian*).

THOREAU. *French literary name.* This distinctive possibility evokes the calm and tranquility of Henry David Thoreau's Walden Pond – but it could be seen as a bit feminine.

THORNE. *English, 'thorn thicket'.* Ouch! Call your daughter Rose, but don't name your son Thorne. Thorn, Thornie, Thorny.

THORNTON. *English, 'place in the thorns'.* Despite Thornton Wilder, playwright of the perennial *Our Town,* a bit lah-di-dah. Thorne.

Thomas's International Variations

Irish	Tomaisin, Tomás, Tomey
Scottish Gaelic	Tòmas, Támhas
Scottish	Tam, Tamas, Tamlane, Tammy, Tavis, Tavish, Tevis, Tevish
Welsh	Tomos
Italian	Maso, Tomasso, Tommaso
Spanish	Chumo, Tomás
Portuguese	Tomas, Tomaz, Tome
Dutch	Maas
German	Thoma, Tomas
Finnish	Tuomo
Eastern European	Tamás, Tamerlane
Polish	Tomasz, Tomaszy, Tomek, Tomislav, Tomislaw
Hungarian	Tamas, Tomi
Romanian	Foma, Toma
Estonian	Toomas
Russian	Foma, Fomka, Toma
Sumerian	Tammuz
Sanskrit	Tamas

THORPE. *English, 'farm, village'.* Brusque and charmless, two things you don't want your son to be. **Thorp.**

THURBER. *English literary name.* Pleasant surname connected to humourist James Thurber, with a sound as happy as a baby's gurgle.

THURGOOD. *Puritan virtue name.* This name probably originated as 'Thoroughgood' – quite a mouthful and a lot to live up to. **Thurloe.**

THURMAN. *Norse, 'defended by Thor'.* You may not want to name your daughter Uma, but you just might name your son Thurman. **Thurmon.**

THURSTON. *Scandinavian, 'Thor's stone'.* There's the posssibility that it might make someone think your son is thirsty when he tells them his name. **Thorstan, Thorstein, Thorsten, Thurstain, Thurstan, Thursten, Torsten, Torston.**

TIBOR. *(TEE-bore) Slavic, 'sacred place'.* Commonly heard in the Slavic countries; has a large measure of continental dash. **Tiburcio.**

♂ **TIDE.** *Nature name.* Referring to the rhythms of the ocean, but could be construed as wanting to be tied up. **Tyde.**

♂ **TIERNAN.** *Irish, 'son of a lord'.* Slightly edgier and more seductive cousin of Kiernan. **Tiarnan, Tiarney, Tiernen, Tierney, Tiernin, Tiernon.**

♂ **TIERNEY.** *Irish, 'descendant of a lord'.* Surname with an Irish twinkle, just waiting to be discovered. It has been occasionally used for girls. **Tiarnach, Tiernan, Tierny.**

TIGER. *Nature name.* If it's a choice between golf champ Woods's real name Eldrick or nickname Tiger, we'd have to go with the latter. **Ti, Tig, Tige, Tigger, Tighe, Ty, Tyg, Tygar, Tyge, Tyger, Tygh, Tyghe. International: Tigre** *(French, Italian, Spanish),* **Tigr, Tygr** *(German, Slavic),* **Tigris, Tygrys** *(Polish, Hungarian, Greek),* **Tighri** *(Ancient Persian),* **Harimau** *(Indonesian),* **Tora** *(Japanese).*

TILDEN. *English place name, 'fertile valley'.* Though it has some distinguished political and tennis world associations, most modern parents would go for the more contemporary sounding Holden. **Tildon, Tillden.**

TIM. *Greek, diminutive of* TIMOTHY. Boyish short form very rarely given on its own. **Timmie, Timmy.**

TIMBER. *Nature name.* Though some forward-looking parents are now choosing wood-related names like Oak, Pine and Ash, this generic option would be even more avant garde.

TIMON. *(tee-MONE) Greek, 'reward, honour'.* Kids would be more likely to associate this name with the hyperactive meercat in *The Lion King* than with the ancient Greek philosopher or Shakespearean character, which could cause playground problems. **Tymon.**

TIMOTHY. *Greek, 'honouring God'.* A second-tier classic, this New Testament name moves in and out of fashion more than the Johns and Jameses, but,

though it peaked in the 1960s, many modern parents still appreciate its familiarity and lively rhythm. **Tim, Timathy, Timethy, Timithy, Timkin, Timmathy, Timmie, Timmithy, Timmo, Timmothy, Timmoty, Timmthy, Timmy, Timoffey, Timon, Timontheo, Timonthy, Timote, Timoteus, Timothey, Timothi, Timothie, Timthie, Tomothy, Tymain, Tymaine, Tyman, Tymane, Tymeik, Tymen, Tymithy, Tymmothy, Tymothee, Tymothy. International: Tiomoid** *(Irish),* **Timotheus** *(Welsh),* **Timon, Timothé, Timothée** *(French),* **Timito, Timo, Timoteo** *(Spanish),* **Timotheus** *(German),* **Timoteus** *(Swedish, Norwegian),* **Timo** *(Finnish),* **Tymek, Tymon, Tymoteusz** *(Polish),* **Timot** *(Hungarian),* **Timotei** *(Bulgarian),* **Teemofe, Tima, Timka, Timofel, Timofey, Timok, Tiriro, Tisha, Tishka, Tyoma** *(Russian),* **Timotheos, Timun** *(Greek).*

TINO. *Spanish, diminutive of* AGOSTINO, JUSTINO, MARTINO, *et al.* This nickname name might be cute for a niño, but one of the full names ending in *tino* would make a more mature statement. **Teeno, Teino, Tion, Tyno.**

TIP. *American nickname.* It's usually best to leave names like Skip, Flip, Kip, Pip, Rip and Tip to the pets of the household. Sometimes a nickname for a third.

TITO. *Spanish variation of* TITUS. Has diverse associations: the long-term Communist head of Yugoslavia, one of Michael Jackson's older brothers and an animated Disney character – none of them a very strong recommendation.

TITUS. *Greek, 'to honour'.* Slightly forbidding Roman, New Testament and Shakespearean name that could possibly be swept along by the antiquity trend and brought back to life. **Titas, Titek, Titis, Titos, Tyus. International: Tite** *(French),* **Tiziano** *(Italian),* **Tito** *(Italian, Spanish),* **Titek, Tytus** *(Polish),* **Titos** *(Greek).*

TOBIAH. *Hebrew, 'the Lord is good'.* Extremely rare Old Testament name that could

make a distinctive alternative to Elijah or Tobias.

★**TOBIAS.** *Hebrew, 'the Lord is good'.* Friendly and appealing in an Old Testament/Dickensian kind of way. **International: Tevye** *(Hebrew),* **Teive, Tubia** *(Yiddish).*

♂ **TOBY.** *Diminutive of* TOBIAS. This jaunty unisex nickname name has recently been given a shot of testosterone via actor Tobey Maguire and is firmly in the Top 100. **Thobey, Thobie, Tobby, Tobe, Tobee, Tobey, Tobi, Tobie.**

TODD. *English, 'fox'.* A 1970s beach boy surfing buddy of Scott, Brad and Chad, Todd is given to relatively few babies these days. **Tod, Toddie, Toddy.**

TOLLIVER. *English occupational name, 'metal-worker'.* Tired of Oliver? Consider this energetic three-syllable surname instead.

TOM. *Diminutive of* THOMAS. It has recently slipped out of the Top 100, but like Sam and Ben, Tom remains

a simple, well-liked name on its own. **Teo, Thom, Tomm, Tommey, Tommie, Tommy.**

TOMÁS. *Variation of* THOMAS. The most popular version of Thomas worldwide – from Scandinavian to Latin to Slavic cultures. **International: Tòmag** *(Scottish),* **Tamás, Tamascio, Tomaso, Tomaz, Tomazcio, Tomi, Tomito** *(Spanish),* **Toman, Tománek, Tomášek, Tomik** *(Slavic).*

TOMMASO. *Italian variation of* THOMAS. *See THOMAS.*

TOMMY. *Diminutive of* THOMAS. A surprising number of parents choose to put the nickname Tommy on their sons' birth certificates. **Tommey, Tommie.**

TONIO. *Diminutive of* ANTONIO. This short form of Antonio has long been used as an independent name and would make a strong, slightly exotic choice. **Tono, Tonyo.**

TONY. *Diminutive of* ANTHONY. Tony, as in classy? Or To-nyyy, as yelled out a tenement window? **Tonee,**

Toney, Tonie, Tonik, Tonis, Tonnie, Tonny, Tono, Tonyo. International: **Tonio** *(Portuguese)*, **Toni** *(German)*, **Tonda, Tonek** *(Czech)*, **Toni** *(Slavic)*, **Toni** *(Greek)*.

TOPHER. *Diminutive of* **CHRISTOPHER.** The new kid on the block in terms of Christopher short forms, it was introduced into the mix by an American actor who didn't like Chris. **Tofer, Tophor.**

★TOR. *Variation of* **THOR**; *also, Hebrew for 'turtledove'.* An interesting and attractive bicultural choice – the Hebrew version is used for babies born in spring, when turtledoves arrive – especially as a middle name. **Thor, Torr.**

TORIN. *Irish, 'chief'.* Though it has a Scandinavian ring, this is an out-of-the-ordinary Irish family name. The hard *T* at the beginning saves it from sounding as feminine as, say, Loren. **Thorfin, Thorstein, Toran, Torean, Toren, Torian, Toriano, Toriaun, Torien, Torion, Torrian, Torrien, Torrin, Torryan, Toryn.**

TORQUIL. *(TOR-kill) Scottish from Norse, 'Thor's kettle'.* A quirky but intriguing option. **Thirkell, Thorkel, Torkili.** International: **Torcall** *(Gaelic)*, **Torkel** *(Swedish)*.

TOULOUSE. *(too-LOOSE) French place name and surname.* Creative choice, evoking the high-kicking can-can girls and other colourful figures in the works of Toulouse-Lautrec.

TOUSSAINT. *(too-SAHN) French, 'all saints'.* Has been used in the past by parents wishing to invoke the blessing and protection of all the saints, also given to boys born on 1 November, All Saints' Day.

♂ **TOVI.** *Hebrew, 'good'.* Pleasant, in a Bon Jovi kind of way. **Tov.**

TOWER. *Word name.* While nature names, even those of fierce animals and mountain peaks, are used for children these days, architectural features like this somehow seem a bit cold. **Towers.**

♂ **TRACE.** *Diminutive of* **TRACY.** Undoubtedly inspired by American country singer Trace Adkins, parents in the USA have chosen this name for their sons in recent years. **Trayce.**

♂ **TRACY.** *French, 'of Thracia'.* Almost always a girl's name now. **Trace, Tracey, Traci, Tracie, Treacy.**

TRAIL. *Word name.* Hiking enthusiasts might want to consider this nature name, though it also has the connotation of someone lagging behind. **Traill, Trale, Trayl, Trayle.**

♂ **TRAVELLER.** *Occupational name.* One of the less obvious newly plausible occupational names, could instill a sense of adventure in a child. **Traveler, Travellor, Travelor, Travler.**

TRAVIS. *French occupational name, 'tollgate-keeper'.* Has a laid-back rural feel; Kyra Sedgwick and Kevin Bacon chose it for their son. **Travais, Travees, Traver, Travers, Traves, Traveus, Travious, Traviss, Travius, Travous, Travus, Travys, Trayvis, Trevais, Treves, Trevez, Treveze, Trevis, Trevius.**

Trendier Than You Think

Ashton

Blake

Bryce

Caleb

Chase

Colin

Elijah

Henry

Isaiah

Jackson

Landon

Mason

Milo

Owen

Oscar

Sebastian

Trenton

Tristan

TRAVON *Modern invented name.* Typical of the kind of newly created combination names being increasingly used, Travon sounds strong and distinguished but has no real substance behind it. **Travan, Traven, Travin, Travyn.**

TREAT. *English word and nickname.* One of the magical words of childhood (and beyond), but most boys won't think it's a treat to be called by a name like Treat.

TRENNER. *Modern invented name.* One of the new two-syllable boys' names with more style than substance.

TRENT. *English, 'someone living on the river Trent'.* Strong single-syllable boy's name finding favour with many parents. **Trente, Trenten, Trentin, Trentino, Trento, Trenton, Trentonio.**

TRENTON. *English, place name, 'Trent's town'.* This name is rising in popularity in the US and may make inroads here as well. Trenten is another popular spelling. **Trendon, Trendun, Trenten, Trentin, Trentton, Trentyn, Trinten, Trintin, Trinton.**

TREVON. *Modern invented name.* Americanisation of Trevor that is catching on, as are other versions Trevion and Trevin. **Traevon, Traivon, Traven, Traveon, Travian, Travien, Travin, Travine, Travion, Travione, Travioun, Travon, Travone, Travonn, Travonne, Trayven, Tre, Treavan, Treavin, Treavion, Treavon, Trévan, Treveyon, Trevian, Trevien, Trevin, Trevine, Trevinne, Trevion, Trevione, Trevionne, Trevohn, Trevoine, Trévon, Trevone, Trevonn, Trevonne, Trevyn, Treyvan, Treyven, Treyvenn, Treyveon, Treyvin, Treyvion, Treyvon, Treyvone, Treyvonn, Treyvun.**

TREVOR. *Welsh, 'from the large village'.* Trevor, a British standard, retains its touch with representation provided by Sir Trevor McDonald, who has provided many years of news service. It's possible that Trevor could become popular again, as long as it's not seen as too clever. **Travor, Treavor, Trebor, Trev, Trevar, Trevares, Trevarious, Trevaris, Trevarius, Trevaros, Trevarus, Trever, Trevin, Trevion, Trevore, Trevores, Trevoris, Trevorus, Trevour, Trevyr, Treyvor. International: Trefor** *(Welsh).*

TREY. *English, 'three'.* Originally used as a nickname for a third-generation son, Trey is now being given to others and it has also expanded to Treynor and Treyton. **Trae, Trai, Traie, Tray, Traye, Tre, Trea, Treye, Treynor, Treyton, Tri, Trie.**

TRIP. *Word name.* This began as a nickname, but in an age where any noun goes, this could be thought of as representing a little voyager – hopefully not into psychedelic realms. **Tripp.**

★♂ **TRISTAN.** Celtic, 'riot; tumult'. This name, known through medieval legend and Wagnerian opera, has a slightly wistful, touching air, which, combined with the popular *an* ending, makes it very appealing to parents seeking a more original alternative to Christian. Tristen, Tristin and Triston are also often seen. **Trestan, Trestin, Treston, Trestton, Trestyn, Tris, Trisan, Trisden, Trissten, Tristain, Tristam, Tristen, Tristian, Tristin, Triston, Tristram, Tristyn, Tristynne, Tryistan, Trysten, Trystian, Trystin, Trystn, Tryston,**

Trystyn. *International: Trystan (Welsh),* **Tristano** *(Italian).*

TRISTIAN. *Variation of* **TRISTAN.** Combination of Tristan and Christian that is beginning to catch on.

TRISTRAM. *Welsh variation of* **TRISTAN.** This version of Tristan, known to English Lit students from the novel *Tristram Shandy,* is rarely used elsewhere and could prove confusing due to the popularity of its offshoot. **Tristam.**

TROUT. *Word name.* Yes, nature lovers are starting to name their children after all forms of life, including fish, but consider carefully before you cast your line into these tease-infested waters.

TROY. *Irish, 'descendant of foot soldier'; also Greek city.* Troy was a popular first name in the 1960s; its image has now, thanks in part to the Brad Pitt–starring epic, receded back to conjuring up the ancient site of the Trojan wars. **Troi, Troix, Troixe, Troixes, Troye, Troyton.**

♂ **TRUE.** *Word name.* Many parents seeking a return to more basic values and a simpler lifestyle are turning to such virtuous girls' names as Grace, Faith and Hope, but the few that can be used for boys as well, such as True, are more often seen as a middle name. **Tru, Truly, Truth.**

★**TRUMAN.** *English, 'loyal one'.* An American presidential name also identified with writer Truman Capote, Truman radiates an aura of integrity and truth, values any parent would want for her child. Tom Hanks and Rita Wilson chose it for their son. **Trueman, Trumain, Trumaine, Trumann, Trumen.**

TRUST. *Word name.* Like True, a virtuous word name, but a little more awkward. In Trust we trust?

♂ **TRUTH.** *Word name. See TRUE.*

♂ **TUCKER.** *English occupational name, 'fabric pleater'.* Tucker has more spunk than most last-name-first-names and also a positive, comforting ('Tuck me in, Mummy') feel.

Tuck, Tuckerman, Tuckie, Tucky, Tuckyr.

♂ **TUCSON.** *(too-sahn) American place name.* A southwestern American city name that could make a distinctive alternative to Dallas. **Tuson.**

TUDOR. *Welsh variation of* **THEODORE.** Known as a British royal family line as well as a style of architecture, this name has a forbidding solemnity; schoolmates might also confuse it with *tutor.* **Todor.**

TULIO. *Latin, 'lively'.* Heard in both Italy and Spain, this could make a more unusual alternative to Julio. **Tullio, Tullis, Tullius, Tullos, Tully.**

♂ **TULLY.** *Irish, 'ruler of the people'.* A relaxed, rarely used Irish surname possibility. **Tull, Tulley, Tullie, Tullio, Tullis.**

♂ **TURNER.** *English occupational name, 'woodworker'.* Preppy but painterly, recalling the exquisite watercolour seascapes of the painter J. M. W. Turner.

♂ **TWAIN.** *English, 'divided in two'.* Can be thought of as a modernisation (and possible namesake) of the dated Wayne, seasoned with the humour of Mark Twain, who adopted it from a river term. **Tawine, Trawyne, Twaine, Twan, Twane, Tway, Twayn.**

TY. *Diminutive of various Ty-beginning names.* As Tyler has risen in popularity, a number of parents, including the ice Hockey superstar Wayne Gretzky, have cut straight to the livelier short form. **Tye.**

♂ **TYLER.** *English occupational name, 'maker of tiles'.* Tyler has been rising up popularity charts and is in the Top 50, so if you're looking for a name to make your son stand out, be aware that there's a good chance he won't be the only Tyler in his class. **Tielar, Tieler, Tielor, Tielyr, Tilar, Tiler, Ty, Tyel, Tyelar, Tyeler, Tyelor, Tyhler, Tylar, Tylarr, Tyle, Tylee, Tylere, Tyller, Tylor, Tylour, Tylyr, Zyler.**

♂ **TYNAN.** *Irish, 'dark, dusty'.* A much fresher *Ty* name than Tyler or Tyson. **Tienan, Tinan, Ty, Tynell, Tynen, Tynin, Tynnen, Tynnin, Tynon.**

TYPHOON. *Chinese, 'great wind'.* Might be asking for trouble, especially when your son reaches the Terrible Twos.

TYREE. *Scottish, 'from Tyrie'.* Hundreds of families have adopted this Scottish name, attracted by its trendy *Ty* beginning and upbeat second syllable. (Tyrell and Tyrese are also increasing in popularity.) Tyree Glenn was a great jazz trombonist. **Tyra, Tyrae, Tyrai, Tyray, Tyre, Tyrea, Tyrée, Tyrell, Tyrese, Tyrey.**

TYRONE. *Irish, 'land of Owen'; a county in Ireland.* Forever a romantic name thanks to 1940s heartthrob superstar Tyrone Power . **Tayron, Tayrone, Teirone, Tereon, Terion, Terione, Teron, Terone, Terrion, Terrione, Terriyon, Terron, Terrone, Terronn, Terryon, Tiron, Tirone, Tirohn, Tirown, Ty, Tyran,.**

TYRUS. *Modern invented name.* This combination of Tyrone and Cyrus sounds too much like *virus* to hold much modern appeal. **Tyus.**

TYSON. *English, 'firebrand'.* As parents have begun to find too many Tylers at the neighbourhood playground, they have been looking to Tyson as an alternative, no longer concerned with any possible connections to boxer Mike Tyson. **Thyssen, Tiesen, Tison, Tiszon, Tyce, Tycen, Tyeson, Tysan, Tysen, Tysie, Tysin, Tysne, Tysone, Tyssen.**

U *boys*

UDELL. *English, 'yew-tree valley'.* Has a slightly feminine feel. **Del, Dell, Udale, Udall, Yudale, Yudell.**

UGO. *(OO-go) Italian variation of* **HUGH.** Very common in Italy, but here it might call to mind that little Yugoslavian car.

UILLEAM. *(WIL-lem) Scottish variation of* **WILLIAM.** Most parents would take the easy way out and spell it Willem, as in artist de Kooning.

UILLIAM. *(William) Irish variation of* **WILLIAM.** A spelling that would definitely attract a lot of attention – and a certain amount of confusion as well. **Liam.**

ULAN. *(oo-lahn) Sudan, 'firstborn twin'.* Twins Ulan and Mulan? We don't think so.

ULF. *Scandinavian, 'wolf'.* Commonly heard in Scandinavian, but hard to imagine it being used here. **International: Ulv** *(Norwegian).*

ULICK. *(OO-lik) Irish, 'little William'.* You lick? You like? We didn't think so.

ULL. *Norse, 'glory'.* This mythological name of the Norse god of winter sounds, uh, ill.

ULRIC. *English, 'wealthy, powerful ruler'.* Also related to the word for wolf, this name has a first syllable that's not appealing to the ear. Better *ic*-ending choices: Dominic, Frederic, Eric. **Alric, Ric, Rick, Ricki, Ricky, Ulf, Ulfa, Ull, Ulrick, Ulu. International:**

Ulrico *(Italian)*, **Alric, Uli, Ulrich, Ulz, Utz** *(German)*, **Ulrik** *(Scandinavian)*, **Ulryck** *(Polish)*.

ULTAN. *Irish, 'man from Ulster'.* This name of eighteen Irish saints of the past has no discernible future here.

ULYSSES. *Latin variation of the Greek* **ODYSSEUS.** One of the few *U* boys' names anyone knows – with heavy links to the Homeric hero, American president Grant (christened Hiram Ulysses) and the James Joyce novel – all of which makes it awfully weighty for a modern boy. **Uileos, Uley Uli, Ulick, Ulie, Uluxe. International: Ulysse, Ulisses** *(French)*, **Ulisse** *(Italian)*, **Ulises** *(Spanish)*, **Uleki, Ulesi** *(Hawaiian)*.

UMAR. *Arabic, 'flourishing, thriving'.* A possible alternative to the more popular (and attractive) Omar.

♂ **UMBER.** *Colour name.* Conjures up the rich brown colours of raw and burnt umber, but it may be too close to girls' Amber.

UMBERTO. *(oom-BAIR-toe) Italian variation of* **HUMBERT.** Not as euphonious as some Italian names, but definitely an improvement on Humbert. **Uberto.**

♂ **UNIKA.** *(oo-nee-kah) African, 'shining'.* Girlish, but has a nice feeling of uniqueness and unity.

♂ **UNIQUE.** *Word name.* Show, don't tell.

UPTON. *English, 'upper town'.* Uppity.

UPWOOD. *English, 'upper forest'.* Even more uppity.

♂ **URBAN.** *Latin, 'of the city'.* The name of several saints and seven popes and more commonly heard in its foreign versions, Urban could conceivably work for a city kid. **Orban, Urbane. International: Urbain, Urbaine** *(French)*, **Urbano** *(Italian, Spanish, Portuguese)*, **Urbanus** *(German)*, **Orban** *(Hungarian)*, **Ura, Urba, Urbek, Urek** *(Czech)*, **Urvan** *(Russian)*.

URI. *(YOOR-ee or OO-ree) Hebrew diminutive of* **URIAH** *and* **URIEL;** *also Swiss place name.* This short but strong name, commonly heard in Israel, has a lot more potential elsewhere than its long forms and is among the most usable on the minuscule menu of *U* names. **Uram, Urie, Uriya, Uriyahu, Uryan, Uryon.**

URIAH. *Hebrew, 'God is my light'.* A perfectly respectable Old Testament name ruined forever through its association with the odious Uriah Heep in *David Copperfield.* **Uria, Uriya.**

URIEL. *Hebrew, 'God is my light'; Israeli place name.* Rarely used name of an Old Testament archangel that's symbolically given to boys born on Chanukah, but the possibility of unsavoury nicknames down the line make the short form Uri a better bet. **Uram, Uriya, Uriyahu, Uryam, Uryan, Uryon.**

URIEN. *(yoo-RĪ-un) Welsh, 'of privileged birth'.* Too close to the name of a bodily fluid.

URSO. *(OOR-so) Italian from Latin, 'bear'.* Cool bear-like option, though Orson might be easier to like. **Ursel, Ursino, Ursinus, Ursus, Uslar.**

USHER. *English from French, 'doorkeeper'.* Associated with a popular single-named singer, it could start a fad.

USHI. *Chinese, 'the ox'.* In China, the ox represents patience and determination, a commendable combination.

♂ **UTAH.** *Place name.* This name for an American state would make a startling but likable choice; poet Dylan Thomas used it for a character in his play *Under Milk Wood*.

UZI. *Hebrew, 'Jehovah is my strength'.* Despite its biblical pedigree, it has far too many ties to the lethal submachine gun. **Uziel, Uziya, Uzzi.**

UZIAH. *Hebrew, 'Jehovah is my strength'.* One of the most unusual of the biblical *iah* options, this was the name of a king of Judah and might just appeal to the parent looking for a quasi-unique Old Testament choice. **Ozias, Uzia, Uziel, Uziya, Uzziah.**

V *boys*

VACHEL. *French, 'small cow'.* Odd name brought to the fore by poet Vachel Lindsay, too close to the feminine Rachel. **Vache, Vacheil, Vachelle.**

VÁCLAV. *Czech, 'wreath of glory'.* Notable name of Václav Havel, the heroic poet and playwright who became president of the Czech Republic. **Vasek.**

VADIM. *Russian, 'attractive'.* Shorter, more palatable form of Vladimir, best known as the surname of French director Roger.

♂ **VAIL.** *Place name, 'valley'.* Aspen's sibling, both cities in the US state Colorado. **Bail, Bale, Vaile, Vaill, Vale, Valle.**

♂ **VAL.** *Diminutive of* **VALENTINE.** Val Kilmer is so macho, you almost forget he bears this slight girls' nickname.

VALDEMAR. *Swedish variation of* **WALTER.** Walter is worlds

more acceptable to the British ear. **Valdamar, Waldemar.**

♂ **VALENTIN(E).** *Latin, 'healthy, strong'.* An attractive Shakespearean name via its romantic associations, but awkward for a modern British boy, as in 'Will you be my Valentine?' **Val, Valentinian, Valentinus, Valenton, Valentyn.** International: **Vailintín** *(Irish*

Gaelic), **Ualan**, **Uailean** *(Scottish Gaelic)*, **Folant** *(Welsh)*, **Valentin** *(French, German, Czech)*, **Valentino**, **Valentio** *(Italian)*, **Vale**, **Valencio**, **Valeno**, **Valentín**, **Valentiniano**, **Valentino** *(Spanish)*, **Valentim** *(Portuguese)*, **Valentijan** *(Dutch)*, **Velten** *(German)*, **Vanentin** *(Danish, Swedish)*, **Walenty** *(Polish)*, **Bálint**, **Valentyn** *(Hungarian)*.

VALERIAN. *Latin, 'potent'.* This name of a Roman emperor and of a sedating plant doesn't have much of a baby name future, unless you just like its strong, rhythmic sound. **Valeriano**, **Valerien**, **Valerii**, **Valerio**, **Valerius**, **Valery**, **Valeryan**, **Valeryn**. International: **Valerius** *(Latin)*, **Valerio** *(Italian, Spanish)*, **Valerii**, **Valery** *(Russian)*.

VALERIO. *Latin, 'strong' or 'healthy'.* The final *o* adds a macho touch. **Valerius**, **Valery**.

VALLIS. *French, 'from Wales'.* Intriguing way to signal Welsh ancestry; more unusual than Wallace. **Valis**.

VALO. *Finnish, 'light'.* Really offbeat, upbeat name with light sound and meaning.

VALOUR. *Word name.* Honour and bravery are certainly virtues any parent would want to encourage and the word itself is obscure enough that it manages to sound like a real name. **Valiant**.

VALTER. *German and Scandinavian variation of* **WALTER**. Vill always sound as if you're pronouncing Walter with an affected accent. **Valters**, **Valther**, **Valtr**.

★**VAN.** *Dutch, 'of'.* Whether it's used as a short form or on its own, this jazzy mid-century name is poised for a possible comeback along with brothers Ray and Walt. **Vander**, **Vane**, **Vann**, **Vanno**, **Von**, **Vonn**.

VANCE. *English and Irish, 'someone who lives near marshland'.* Short but sophisticated long-neglected name you might want to consider as an unusual choice that won't get competition in the classroom.

VANDYKE. *Dutch, 'of the dyke'.* Though it has worthy associations with the Old Master painter and singer-songwriter Van Dyke Parks, this would be tough on a child because of the slang meaning of the second syllable.

VANE. *English, 'banner'.* He'll have to prove his humility.

VANYA. *Russian, diminutive of* **JOHN**. This short form of Ivan just could join the other Russian nickname names coming into fashion and it does have the Chekhov connection. **Vanechka**, **Vanek**, **Vanja**, **Vanka**, **Vanusha**, **Wanya**.

VARAN. *Hindi, 'water god'.* Unusual and simple: a winning combination. But it was the name of a fifteen-thousand-tonne monster in a 1950s Godzilla movie. **Varoun**, **Varron**, **Varun**.

VARDON. *French, 'green knoll'.* Pleasant-sounding French surname. **Vardaan**, **Varden**, **Verdan**, **Verdon**, **Verdun**.

VASANT. *Sanskrit, 'spring'.* A name commonly used in India;

Vasant Panchami is a Hindu festival dedicated to the goddess of learning. **Vasanth.**

VASCO. *Spanish, 'someone from the Basque region'.* Schoolchildren might recognise this name via Portuguese explorer Vasco da Gama.

VASILI. *Greek, 'royal, kingly'.* Exotic form of Basil that might suit the adventurous. **Vas, Vasaya, Vaselios, Vashon, Vasil, Vasile, Vasilios, Vasilius, Vasiliy, Vasilos, Vasilus, Vasily, Vaso, Vazul, Wassily. International: Vasilik, Vasily, Vasya, Vasyenka** *(Russian),* **Vasilii** *(Slavic),* **Vasos** *(Greek).*

VAUGHAN, VAUGHN. *Welsh, 'small'.* This familiar but never popular name might be a good Sean alternative. **Vaughan, Vaughen, Vaun, Vaune, Von, Vougn.**

VED. *Sanskrit, 'sacred knowledge'.* Literary Indian choice, best known here via acclaimed writer Ved Mehta, who lost his sight at the age of four.

VEER. *Sanskrit, 'brave'.* Worth considering for the meaning.

♂ **VEGA.** *Arabic, 'swooping eagle'.* This name has a lot going for it: it's a self-confident Spanish surname, it identifies one of the most brilliant stars in the sky and it has a musical reference to singer-songwriter Suzanne Vega.

VENEDICTOS. *Greek variation of* **BENEDICT.** Though this one would be sure to inspire confusion, *Ven-* names can be an intriguing alternative to the *Ben-* group. **Ven, Venedict, Venediktos, Venka, Venya.**

VENEZIO. *Italian place name.* Venetia and even Venice are more common, though this could work. **Venetio, Venetziano, Veneziano.**

VENN. *English, 'from the marsh or fen'; Irish, 'fair'.* No, not Ben (you'll say a million times), not Van – Venn. **Ven.**

VENTURO. *Spanish, 'good fortune, good luck'.* Upbeat choice. **Venturio.**

VENYA. *Russian, diminutive of* **VENEDIKT,** *variation of* **BENEDICT.** Vanya is much more familiar. **Venedict, Venka.**

VERDI. *Italian, 'green'.* Outside possibility for opera-lovers.

VERE. *English from French, 'alder'.* Upper-class surname in England that might be prime for adoption elsewhere.

VERED. *Hebrew, 'rose'.* Has the ring of veracity, but not a very appealing sound.

♂ **VERMONT.** *French, 'green mountain'.* Place name of a US state waiting to be discovered.

VERNADOS. *Greek from German, 'courage of the bear'.* Rhythmic and powerful, if you don't mind the nickname Vern.

VERNON. *English, 'place of alders'.* A British surname that seems too outdated to be modern, as does its nickname, Vern. **Lavern, Varnan, Vern, Vernal, Verne, Vernen, Verney, Vernin.**

★**VERO.** *Latin, 'true'; Russian, 'faith'; Sanskrit, 'great hero'.* The *o* ending and the positive meaning in many languages makes this a winner. Only downside: sounds a bit like the old ladyish Vera. **International: Vereen, Veren** *(Scotch Irish),* **Verino** *(French),* **Vereno** *(Spanish, Portuguese),* **Verlin** *(German),* **Verlon** *(Swiss),* **Viro** *(Sanskrit).*

♂ **VERRILL.** *French, 'honest'.* Feminine, à la Beryl and Merrill. **Verill, Verrall, Verrell, Verroll, Veryl.**

VESUVIO. *Italian place name.* Volcano name for an active, bubbly child – but be careful – volcanoes do erupt. **Vesuvius.**

VICENTE. *(vee-CHEN-tay) Spanish variation of* **VINCENT.** Popular saint's name in Hispanic cultures, familiar enough to use elsewhere.

VICTOR. *Latin, 'conqueror'.* One of the earliest Christian names, borne by several saints and popes, this long-dormant name is being revived by fashionable parents in London and might be ripe for rediscovery elsewhere too. **Vic, Vick, Victa, Victer, Victorien, Victorin, Vitin. International: Victoir** *(French),* **Vittorio** *(Italian),* **Victoriano, Victorino, Victorio, Victoro** *(Spanish),* **Viktor** *(German, Swedish),* **Wictor** *(Polish),* **Vidor, Viktor** *(Hungarian),* **Viktor, Vitya** *(Russian).*

VIDAL. *Spanish from Latin, 'life, vital'.* Would be more usable if it wasn't so strongly associated with hairdresser Sassoon and his many hair products. **Bidal, Vida, Vidale, Vidall, Vidalo, Videl, Videlio, Videll.**

VIDAR. *Old Norse, 'quiet god'.* Mythological son of Odin, powerful and mute.

VIDOR. *(VEE-dore) Hungarian variation of* **HILARY.** Sounds a bit ominous, in a Transylvanian way.

★**VIGGO.** *Scandinavian, 'war'.* So far a one-person name: actor Mortensen (who shares his first name with his father), but it's so – well – vigorous, we think it might appeal to others as well.

VIJAY. *Sanskrit, 'conquering'.* Classic Indian name, but in this time and place it would be associated with a VJ or video disk jockey. **Bijay, Vijun.**

VIKRAM. *Hindi, 'valorous'.* Another traditional Indian name, best known elsewhere via novelist Vikram Seth. **Vikrum.**

VILHELM. *German variation of* **WILLIAM.** The way Wilhelm is pronounced anyway, so a pointless spelling variation. **Vilhelms, Vilho, Vili, Vilis, Viljo, Villem, Villy, Vilmos.**

VILIAM. *Czech variation of* **WILLIAM.** Substituting the *V* for the *W* sounds almost comedic to the British ear. **Vila, Vilek, Vilém, Viliami, Viliamu, Vilko, Vilous.**

VILJO. *(VEEL-yo) Finnish variation of* **WILLIAM.** Inventive nickname option, but with built-in pronunciation problems.

VILLARD. *(vee-YARD) French from German, 'battle fortress'.* Creative surname choice, associated with the great French postimpressionist artist Edouard Villard.

VILLIERS. *French, 'town-dweller'.* Name with aristrocratic overtones.

VIN. *Latin, diminutive of* **VINCENT.** Minimalist nickname. **Vinn.**

VINCENT. *Latin, 'conquering'.* One of those names that's so far out – as in out of style – it's coming back in. There may now be three kids named Oscar or Miles in many hip nursery schools, but we doubt you'll find another Vincent – yet. Even the nickname Vince has been given a reprieve via actor Vince Vaughn. **Vencent, Vin, Vince, Vincence, Vincentius. Vincents, Vinicent, Vinciente, Vincint, Vinnie, Vinny, Vinsent, Vinsint, Vyncent, Vyncint, Vyncynt.** International: **Uinseann** *(Gaelic),* **Vincenzio, Vicenzo, Vinci** *(Italian),* **Vicente** *(Spanish),* **Vicenç** *(Catalan),* **Vincentius** *(Dutch),* **Vincens, Vinzenz** *(German),* **Wicent, Wincenty, Wienczyslav, Wienczylaw** *(Polish),* **Vencel, Vince, Vinci, Vincien, Vinzenz** *(Hungarian),* **Vicenc** *(Czech).*

VINE. *English nature name.* Simple, strong, unique.

VING. *Diminutive of* **IRVING.** Imaginative shortening of the prosaic Irving, giving it new life and energy.

VINNY. *English, diminutive of* **VINCENT.** Yo, Vinny. **Vinnee, Vinney, Vinni, Vinnie.**

VINSON. *English, 'son of Vincent'.* For Grandpa Vincent. **Vinnis.**

♂ **VIREO.** *Nature name.* A vireo is a small green bird with a song as melodic as this highly unusual name, but it does sound a touch viral.

VIRGIL. *Latin, 'staff bearer'.* The name of the greatest Roman poet and an early Irish saint, Virgil is rarely heard nowadays, but it retains a certain likable twang. **Verge, Vergil, Vergitio, Virge, Virgial, Virgie, Virgilio.** International: **Virgile** *(French),* **Virgilio** *(Spanish).*

♂ **VIRIDIAN.** *Colour name.* Unusual and beautiful blue green colour and name possibility, à la Cerulean.

Italian Names Beyond Giovanni & Giuseppe

Alessio

Arrigo

Aurelio

Benedetto

Clemente

Dario

Ettore

Fabrizio

Gaetano

Luciano

Orlando

Paolo

Rafaele

Sansone

Taddeo

Ugo

VISCHER. *German, 'fisherman'.* If you're German and you love to fish – then *maybe.* **Visscher.**

VISHNU. *Hindi, 'protector'.* Name of one of the three main Hindu gods.

VITO. *(vee-to) Latin, 'alive'.* Old Italian name without much vigour. **Veit, Vital, Vitale, Vitas, Vitin, Vitis, Vitus, Vytas. International: Vidal, Viel, Vitalis** *(French),* **Videl** *(Spanish),* **Wit** *(Polish),* **Vitaly** *(Russian).*

★**VITTORIO.** *Italian variation of* **VICTOR.** Was there ever a name that rolled more appealingly off the tongue? **Vittore.**

VITUS. *Italian, 'life'.* No-no appelation of a child saint and martyr whose name is a term for the nervous condition known as Saint Vitus' Dance. **Vidal, Vitas. International: Veit** *(German),* **Wit** *(Polish),* **Vit** *(Czech).*

♂ **VIVIAN.** *Latin, 'alive'.* Though still occasionally used for boys in Britain, totally female elsewhere. **Viviani, Vivien, Vivyan, Vyvian, Vyvyan. International: Viviano** *(Spanish).*

VLAD. *Russian, 'to rule'.* The most famous Vlad was nicknamed 'the Impaler'. Enough said.

VLADIMIR. *Slavic, 'renowned prince'.* Musical prodigy name. **Bladimir, Dimka, Vimka, Vlad,**

Vladamir, Vladi, Vladik, Vladimar, Vladimeer, Vladimer, Vladimere, Vladimire, Vladimyr, Vladjimir, Vladka, Vladko, Vladlen, Vladmir, Vlady, Vladya, Volodimir, Volodya, Volya, Vova, Wladimyr, Wladunir. **International: Waldemar** *(Dutch, German),* **Waldemar, Valdemar** *(Scandinavian),* **Wlodzimirez** *(Polish),* **Vladimír** *(Czech).*

VLADISLAV. *Slavic, 'glorious rule'.* Sounds more like a city than a baby name. **Ladislav, Vlad, Vladik, Vladya, Vlas, Vlasislava, Vyacheslav, Wladislav. International: Vlas, Vyacheslav** *(Russian),* **Ladislas** *(Slavic).*

VOLANTE. *Latin, 'to fly'.* Soaring, speedy choice.

VOLNEY. *German, 'spirit of the people'.* Has a rather heavy surname feel.

VON. *Norse, 'hope'.* One of those mid-century shortenings that are starting to sound cool again, though we prefer Van. **Vonn.**

♂ **VRAI.** *French word name, 'true'.* Virtue, à la française.

VULCAN. *Latin, 'to flash'.* Vulcan was the Roman god of fire, but his name is now more familiar as the pointy-eared humanoids on *Star Trek,* represented by Mr Spock.

W *boys*

WADE. *English, 'at the river crossing'.* Grandpa of newer names like Cade and Slade. **Waed, Waid, Waide, Wayde.**

WAGNER. *German occupational name, 'wagon maker'.* Whether you pronounce this like the wag of a tail or in the correct German *VAHG-ner*, even a devoted opera buff probably would use this as a middle name, if at all.

WAINWRIGHT. *English occupational name, 'wagon maker'.* Some surnames should stay surnames. **Wain, Wainright, Wayne, Waynewright, Wright.**

WALDEMAR. *(VAHL-deh-mahr) German, 'famous ruler'.* The British child given this name of four kings of Denmark, not to mention one so similar to that of the Harry Potter archvillain Lord Voldemort, might have to pay a large emotional import tax. **International: Woldemar** *(German, Dutch, Danish),* **Valdemar, Waldemar, Woldemar** *(Scandinavian).*

♂ **WALDEN.** *German, 'to rule'; English, 'valley of the Welsh'.* A name that summons up placid images of Thoreau's Walden Pond. **Waldon.**

WALDO. *German, 'to rule'.* Its jaunty *o* ending makes this name more appealing than its Germanic brothers.

♂ **WALES.** *English place name.* Place names for boys are few and far between; this one would make a singular choice.

♂ **WALKER.** *English occupational name, 'worker in cloth, cloth-walker'.* The *W* in George W. Bush is one of the big surname names, but it also has a gentle ambling quality and a creative connection to such greats as writer Walker Percy and photographer Walker Evans.

WALLACE. *English from French, 'a Welshman, Celt'.* So square it could almost be ripe for a turnaround, especially with the hipness imparted by the British Claymation series *Wallace & Gromit.* **Wal, Wall, Wallache, Wallas, Wallie, Wallis, Wally, Walsh, Welch, Welsh.**

WALLY. *English, diminutive of* **WALTER** *or* **WALLACE.** An old-fashioned 1950s name, permanently vacationing. Possible hitch: although the craze is over, giggles could follow every asking of 'Where's Wally?' **Wallie.**

WALT. *German, diminutive of* **WALTER.** A straightforward, down-to-earth nickname many Walters, from Whitman to Disney, have chosen to go by.

WALTER. *German, 'powerful warrior'.* Seen as a noble name in the Sir Walter Raleigh era, long out of baby name favour. Now a few independent-minded parents are looking at it as a quirky classic, stronger and more distinctive than James or John. **Walt, Walten. International: Bhaltair Bhàtair** *(Scottish Gaelic),*

Gwallter *(Scottish),* **Gwallter** *(Welsh),* **Gauther, Gautier** *(French),* **Gualtiero** *(Italian),* **Gualterio, Gutierre** *(Spanish),* **Weit, Wolter, Wouter** *(Dutch),* **Walder, Walli, Walten, Walther, Waltili, Walton, Wolter** *(German),* **Valter, Wolter, Woulter** *(Scandinavian),* **Landislaus** *(Polish),* **Valtr, Vladko, Waltr** *(Czech),* **Waldemar** *(Lithuanian),* **Dima, Dimka, Vladimir, Volya, Vovka** *(Russian).*

WALTON. *English, 'fortified town'.* Slightly more modern than Walter, but only just.

WARD. *English occupational name, 'guard, watchman'; diminutive of* **EDWARD.** Until recently Ward was, like Wally, an old-fashioned name stuck in the 1950s, but today's parents are seeing it as a cooler nickname for Edward than Eddie and are also beginning to use it on its own. **Warde, Warden, Weard, Worden.**

WARNER. *English from German, 'army'.* Long-time connection to the film biz doesn't lend it any pizzazz.

WARREN. *French, 'park-keeper'.* Even back when Warren Beatty was a reigning Lothario, his name remained sombre and unromantic.

WARRICK. *English, 'fortress'.* Has recently come into the spotlight as a character on an American TV show, but we can't see it really catching on.

WASHINGTON. *English, 'home of the Wassa people'.* Of the American presidents, Lincoln, Tyler, Taylor, Jackson, Jefferson, Harrison, McKinley, Grant, Kennedy, Carter – yes. Washington? Probably not. **Wash.**

WATSON. *English, 'son of Wat' (a diminutive of Walter).* Only recommended for the most ardent Sherlock Holmes fan. **Watkins, Watsen, Watterkinson, Wattson.**

WAYLAND. *English, 'land beside the road'.* Way out. **Way, Walen, Weiland, Weyland.**

WAYLON. *English, 'land beside the road'.* American country singer Waylon Jennings bestowed a kind of outlaw image on his name. **Way,** Waylan, Waylen, Waylin, Weylan, Weylen, Weylin, Weylon.

WAYNE. *English occupational name, 'maker of wagons'.* When Marion Michael Morrison became John Wayne around 1930, his last name took on a tough air that lasted about thirty years, but now – even with the popularity of footballer Rooney – it's strictly a dad or even granddad name. **International: Vaino** *(Finnish).*

WEBB. *English occupational name, 'weaver'.* This otherwise perfectly usable single-syllable name has been ruined by the Internet. **Web, Webber, Weber.**

WEBSTER. *English occupational name, 'weaver'.* Might be appropriate for a son who likes spiders. **Web, Webb, Weeb.**

WELBY. *English, 'from farm by a spring'.* Although it connotes a sense of well-being, not likely to be a popular choice.

WENCZESLAW. *Polish, 'glory of the Wends' (old Slavic peoples).* Should only be used when singing Christmas carols. **Wencelas, Wenceslaus. International: Venceslao** *(Italian),* **Venceslao, Venceslás, Wenceslao,** *(Spanish),* **Venceslau** *(Portuguese),* **Wenzeslaus** *(German),* **Waclaw** *(Polish),* **Václav, Věnceslav** *(Czech),* **Vyacheslav** *(Russian).*

WENDELL. *German, 'to travel, to proceed'.* Has hardly been used since the 1940s.

WERNER. *(VER-ner) German, 'protecting army'.* Formal name lacking any sparkle or sheen. **Verner, Warner, Wernhar. International: Wessel** *(Dutch),* **Wetzel** *(German),* **Verner** *(Scandinavian).*

WERTHER. *(Ver-ther) German, 'worthy warrior'.* In literature identified with *The Sorrows of Young Werther* – not much to wish on a child.

WESLEY. *English, 'dweller near the western wood'.* Though not very fashionable – and with a feminine lilt thanks to its similarity to Lesley and Ashley – this surname of the founder of Methodism is still given to a number of baby boys each year. **Wes, Wesly, Wessley, West,**

Westbrook, Westcott, Westleigh, Westley, Weston, Wezley.

★ ♂ WEST. *Word name.* Names don't come any cooler than this.

WESTBROOK. *English, 'from the western brook'.* Pompous and pretentious.

WESTCOTT. *English, 'from the western cottage'.* Only slightly less pompous and pretentious than Westbrook. **Wes.**

WESTON. *English, 'from the western town'.* Has a glimmer of creative appeal via connection to poetic landscape photographer Edward Weston; Nicolas Cage chose it for his son. **Westan, Westen, Westin, Westyn.**

WHEELER. *English occupational name, 'wheel-maker'.* Has some potential in the company of the newly stylish occupational names, with its friendly, free-wheeling sound.

WHITFORD. *English, 'from the white ford'.* Quintessentially, stylelessly preppy.

♂ WHITNEY. *English, 'white island'.* Taken over by the girls in the 1970s, has virtually zero testosterone at this point.

WHITTAKER. *English, 'white field'.* Sort of posh. **Whitaker.**

WILBUR. *German, 'resolute, brilliant'.* If you had to pick a Wright brothers name, even Orville might be preferable. **Wilber, Wilbert, Wilburt. International: Wilbart** *(German).*

WILEY. *Spelling variation of* **WYLIE.** *See* **WYLIE.**

WILFRED. *English, 'desires peace'.* One of several *Wil-* starting names that are gone and best forgotten. **Wilford, Wilfried, Wilfryd, Will, Willfred, Willfredo, Willfrid, Willfried, Willfryd. International: Vilfredo, Vilfrido, Walfrido, Wilferdo, Wilfredo, Wilfrido** *(Spanish),* **Wilfrid, Willi, Willifred** *(German).*

WILHELM. *(vil-HELM) German variation of* **WILLIAM.** Since the World War I days of Kaiser Wilhelm, has been prohibitively heel clicking. **Wil, Willi, Willy, Wilm.**

WILKES. *English, a contraction of* **WILKINS.** Try Abraham or Lincoln instead. **Wilkie, Willkes, Willkie.**

★WILL. *Diminutive of* **WILLIAM.** Will has a nice old-fashioned down-home charm and with recent references such as Will Smith and *Good Will Hunting,* it has taken on an air of understated cool.

WILLARD. *English from German, 'resolutely brave'.* Unfortunate identification with an army of rats in the film of the same name. **Willerd.**

★WILLEM. *Dutch variation of* **WILLIAM.** Common in Holland, the appealing Willem (as in de Kooning and Dafoe) makes William fresh and distinctive.

WILLIAM. *English from German, 'resolute protection'.* Now solidly back in the Top 10, partially due to Britain's prince, this has been among the most enduring of classics, chosen in the last year counted by almost twenty thousand parents as being ideally conservative yet contemporary. Yesterday's Billys have given way to today's Wills

boys' names

William's International Variations

Irish Gaelic	Liam
Scottish Gaelic	Uilleam, Uilliam
Welsh	Gwilym
French	Guillaume
Italian	Guglielmo
Spanish	Giermo, Gigermo, Gillermo, Guilermo, Guillermino, Guillermo, Guillo,
Catalan	Guillem
Portuguese	Guilherme
Dutch	Willem
German	Wilhelm, Willem, Wim
Scandinavian	Vilhelm
Finnish	Viljami, Viljo, Vilppu
Hungarian	Vili, Vilmo
Czech	Vila, Vilek, Vilem, Viliam, Vilko, Vilous
Russian	Vasilak, Vasili, Vasiliy, Vaska, Vassili, Vassily
Greek	Vasilios, Vassos
Yiddish	Welfel, Wolf

– or Williams, no diminutive. **Bill, Bille, Billie, Billy, Pim, Wiley, Wilkes, Wilkie, Wilkinson, Will, Willi, Williamson, Willie, Willis, Wills, Willy, Wilmar, Wilson, Wim.**

WILLIE. *Diminutive of* **WILLIAM.** There have been many great Willies (Nelson, Wonka), but a boy with this name could never live it down in England. **Willey, Willi, Willy.**

WILLIS. *Diminutive of* **WILLIAM.** A common surname almost never used in recent times. **Willes, Willess, Williss, Williston.**

♂ **WILLOUGHBY.** *English, 'farm in the willows'.* An energetic last-name-first route to the popular short form Will. **Willoughbey, Willoughbie, Willughby.**

WILLY. *Diminutive of* **WILLIAM.** *See* **WILLIE.**

WILMER. *German, 'determined fame'.* Although the visibility of Spanish-born actor Wilmer Valderrama has highlighted this name in the US, it's not likely to spread because of its similarity to the feminine (and dated) Wilma. **Willmar, Willmer, Wilmar, Wylmer.**

WILSON. *English, 'son of Will'.* A new route to Will. **Willson, Wilsyn.**

WILTON. *English, 'place by a stream'.* As passé as Hilton and Milton.

WIM. *(vim) German, contracted form of* **WILHELM.** Film director Wim Wenders brought this to our attention; it certainly has vim and vigour.

♂ **WINDSOR.** *English, 'riverbank with a winch'.* Has a definite feminine feel, as in Windsor Rose. **Winsor, Wyndsor.**

WINSLOW. *English, 'friend's hill or burial mound'.* Creative reference to painter Winslow Homer doesn't take this name out of its sailor suit with short pants. **Win, Winslowe.**

WINSTON. *English, 'friend's town'.* Long associated with the Churchill family and common in the West Indies but neglected elsewhere. However it's John Lennon's middle name and is one British surname worthy of consideration. **Winnie, Winsten, Winstonn, Winton, Wynstan, Wynston, Wynstonn, Wynton.**

♂ **WINTER.** *Word name.* The girls have dibs on Spring, Summer and Autumn, leaving this name evocative of snowy landscapes as the one possible seasonal choice for boys. **Winters, Wynter, Wynters.**

WINTHROP. *English, 'friend's village'.* Proper Bostonian.

WINTON. *English, 'friend's farm'. See* **WYNTON.**

WOLCOTT. *English, 'cottage near a stream'.* One of many British *W* surnames that would subject a boy in the USA to years of teasing. If you chose it for your son, don't move across the Atlantic. **Woolcott, Woollcott.**

WOLF. *German, 'wolf'; diminutive of* **WOLFGANG.** It has a certain lupine appeal. **Wolfe, Wolff, Wolfhart,** **Woolf, Wulf, Wulfe. International:** Ulf *(Swedish),* Ulv *(Norwegian).*

WOLFGANG. *German, 'traveling wolf'.* Chef Wolfgang Puck has helped soften this thunderous Germanic name; music-lovers will appreciate its association with Mozart, though the composer's middle name Amadeus is more appealing. **International: Wolfgango** *(Spanish).*

WOODROW. *English, 'row of houses by a wood'.* Aside from Most Woodrows, including Herman, Guthrie and Harrelson, have chosen to be known as Woody, which says it all. **Woodroe, Woodrowe, Woody.**

WOODY. *Diminutive of* **WOODROW.** While Woodrow is too forbidding, its nickname Woody is a bit cartoonish, as in Woody Woodpecker and the animated cowboy character in *Toy Story*. Woody Allen was born Allen. **Woodey, Woodie.**

WORTH. *English, 'enclosure, homestead'; also word name.* No

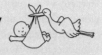
low self-esteem for this kid, or so his parents hope.

WORTHY. *English, 'valuable'.* Here too lies the danger of entitlement.

WRAY. *Scandinavian, 'dweller near the corner'.* Simplify life and call him Ray.

★**WYATT.** *English, 'guide'.* Hot – which is to say cool – for several years now in the US, which is a reflection of its easy Wyatt Earpish cowboy charm: it's relaxed but still highly respectable. **Wiatt.**

WYCLEF. *English, 'dweller at the white cliff'.* Haitian-born rap superstar and humanitarian Wyclef ('Fugees') Jean has lent

this name a powerful musical beat. **Wycleff, Wycleft, Wycliff, Wycliffe, Wyklef, Wykleff.**

★♂**WYLIE.** *Scottish diminutive of* **WILLIAM.** A friendly, nonchalant name with an almost irresistible charm; parents may pick up on its pleasant similarity to the more popular, unisex Riley. **Wiley, Wye.**

♂**WYN.** *Welsh, 'fair, blessed'.* Extremely popular in Wales, where it began as a nickname for someone who's fair, this name is winning but feels a bit close to the feminine Gwen and Winnie. **Win, Winn, Wyne, Wynn, Wynne.**

WYNDHAM. *English, 'from the windy village'.* This literary and

aristocratic surname would not blend in on most playgrounds – and Windy is not the choicest of nicknames. **Windham, Wynndham.**

WYNTON. *English, 'friend's farm'.* This spelling of Winton has gotten considerable buzz via jazz musician Wynton Marsalis.

WYSTAN. *English, 'battle stone'.* Prissy first name of poet W. H. Auden, whose surname is a new hottie.

X *boys*

Note: As a general rule, most names starting with X are pronounced with a Z sound.

XAN. *(zan) Diminutive of* **ALEXANDER.** With the plethora of Alexes around, Xan (and Xander) are emerging as the hot new nicknames for Alexander. It also stands well on its own. **Zan.**

XANDER. *(zander) Diminutive of* **ALEXANDER.** A spelling that first saw the spotlight via *Buffy the Vampire Slayer*, this newcomer is now quickly gaining in popularity in the US. **Xande, Xzander, Zander.**

XANTHOS. *(ZHAN-thos) Greek, 'golden-haired'.* This alternate name for Apollo has a noble sound and can always be shortened to Xan. **Xanthus.**

XAVIER. *(ex-AY-vee-er or ZAY-vee-er) Basque, 'new house'; Arabic, 'bright'.* The only *X* name most people know and use, often as a middle name following Francis, as in Saint Francis Xavier, cofounder of the Jesuit order. Today's parents are beginning to reassess Xavier, which was chosen by Donnie Wahlberg – as well as the Spanish classic Javier, pronounced *HAH-vee-ay.* **Javier, Saviero, Savion, Savyon, Xabier, Xaiver, Xavaeir, Xaver, Xavian, Xaviar, Xaviell, Xavior, Xavon, Xayver, Xayvion, Xever, Xzavier, Zavier.**

XENOPHON. *(ZEEN-oh-phon) Greek, 'foreign voice'.* This name of an ancient Greek historian sounds too

long-ago and faraway to consider for a modern child. **Xeno, Zennie.**

XENOS. *Greek, 'hospitality, guest'.* One of the more accessible *X* names, though Xeno or Zeno might sound more modern. **Xeno, Zeno, Zenos.**

XERXES. *(Zerks-eeze) Persian, 'monarch'.* The two *X*'s may be one too many for all but the most intrepid baby namer. **Zerk.**

XIMENES. *Spanish variation of* **SIMON.** The *J* spelling – both are pronounced as if they started with *H* – is more common, but the *X* has more flair. **Jimenes, Jimenez, Ximenez, Ximon, Ximun, Xymenes.**

Names That Sound Creative

Amedeo

Cerulean

Darius

Dmitri

Elia

Gulliver

Jasper

Joss

Merce

Misha

Ocean

Orion

Poe

Xan

Zeno

Stellar Starbabies Beginning with *X*

| Xavier | Donnie Wahlberg |

XYLON. *(ZEE-lawn) Greek, 'the forest'.* Sounds like the name of a new synthetic fabric.

Y *boys*

YAAKOV. *Hebrew, 'supplanting'.* The original Hebrew form of Jacob, it is still used in some religious families. **Kobi, Yaacob, Yaaqov, Yacov, Yago, Yaki. Yakob, Yakov. International: Yankel (Yiddish).**

YADA. *Hebrew, 'he knew'.* Anyone who ever saw *Seinfeld* wouldn't be able to resist adding a couple more 'yada's'. Also a bit too close to Yoda in the *Star Wars* films. **Yadael, Yadua, Yedaiah, Yedaya, Yediael.**

♂ **YAEL.** *Hebrew spelling variation of* **JAEL.** This phonetic form will help clarify the name.

YAKIM. *Hebrew, 'he will establish'.* One of many Hebrew *Y* names kept alive in Israel and in Jewish communities. **Jachim, Jakim, Yacheem, Yachim, Yakum, Yehoyakim, Yokim.**

YAKOV. *Russian variation of* **JACOB.** *See* **JACOB.** International: **Yasha** *(Russian).*

YALE. *Welsh, 'vigorous, fertile'.* Aspiring to the elite Ivy League colleges in the US.

YANAI. *Aramaic, 'he will answer'.* The biblical husband of the queen of Sheba; an unusual name with an interesting sound, rhyming with *lanai*. **Jania, Jannai, Yan, Yana, Yannai.**

♂ **YANCEY.** *Native American, 'Englishman'; from 'yankee'.* A fancy TV western name that didn't catch on like fellow cowboys Luke and Josh. **Yancy.**

YANN. *French/Breton variation of* **JOHN.** Might be a better choice than the similarly pronounced Jan, to avoid gender confusion. **Yannic, Yannick.**

YANNICK. *Extension of* **JANN** *or* **YANN.** Known through flamboyant French tennis star/singer Yannick Noah, a name not likely to appeal to many British ears. **Yanick.**

YANNIS. *Greek variation of* **JOHN.** As common in Greece as John is here. **Ioannis, Yannakis, Yanni.**

♂ **YARDEN.** *Hebrew, 'to flow down, descend'.* The name from which Jordan arose, Yarden has a nice combination of river imagery and a sound connoting a garden. Like Jordan, used for both sexes.

♂ **YARDLEY.** *English, 'fenced meadow'.* Sounds somewhat feminine and heavily perfumed. **Yardlee, Yardlea, Yardleigh, Yardly, Yarley, Yeardley.**

YARON. *(yah-ROHN) Hebrew, 'he will sing'.* Most modern parents would prefer Aaron. **Yoran.**

♂ **YARROW.** *English, 'rough stream'; also plant and herb name.* This plant whose pungent root is an old herbal cure, would make an unusual name.

♂ **YASHA.** *Russian, diminutive of* **YAKOV.** A less-known member of the Sasha-Misha family. **Jascha, Jasha.**

YASIR. *Arabic, 'wealthy, prosperous'.* In this country, very much tied to PLO leader Arafat. **Yaseer, Yasr, Yasser.**

♂ **YEATS.** *(yates) English, 'the gates'.* Admirers of the haunting works of esteemed Irish poet and playwright William Butler Yeats might consider this, especially as a middle name.

YEHUDA(H). *Hebrew, 'to praise'.* Anglicised as Judah, this name of a biblical patriarch is given symbolically to boys born on Hanukkah; a form of it was spotlighted by violin virtuoso Yehudi Menuhin. **Yechudi, Yechudit, Yehudi, Yehudit.**

YEVGENY. *Russian variation of* **EUGENE.** *See EUGENE.* **Yevgeni, Yevgeniy.**

YISRAEL. *Hebrew, 'contender with God'.* The name given to Jacob/Yaacov after wrestling with God's angel, most often used without the initial *Y.*

YITZHAK. *Hebrew variation of* **ISAAC.** Has taken on a musical tone via the great violinist, Itzhak Perlman. **Itzak, Itzhac, Itzik, Izaak, Yitzchak, Yizhac.**

YOEL. *Hebrew, 'Jehovah is his God'.* The Hebrew version of Joel has a pleasant, almost jolly sound. **Joel.**

YONAH. *Hebrew variation of* **JONAH.** This form of the stylish Old Testament name is too close to the feminine Yona. **Yonas.**

YORICK. *English literary name.* Alas! poor Yorick, your name is fated to remain locked forever as a skull in *Hamlet.*

♂ **YORK.** *English, 'from the yew estate'.* This British royal family name is rather formal and brusque. **Yorick, Yoricke, Yorke.**

YOSEF. *Hebrew, 'God shall add'.* A widely used form of Joseph, with a sophisticated continental air. **Seff, Sefi, Yehosef, Yosei, Yoseif, Yosi, Yosifel, Yosifya, Yossi, Yosufya.** International: **Yosel, Yossel, Yossil** *(Yiddish).*

♂ **YOSEMITE.** *Indian tribal name, 'those who kill'; California place name.* The evocative name of one of the most beautiful national parks in the US – yes, but also the bombastic cartoon character, Yosemite Sam.

Supermodel Babies

Alastair
Amael
Arpad/Arthur
Auden
Aurelius
Barron
Caspar
Finn
Hamzah
Henry
Lucas
Marcel
Mingus
Orson
Presley
Suhul
Tristan
Yannick

YOSHI. *Japanese, 'good, respectful'.* A classic Japanese name known to kids around the world as a Nintendo video-game character.

YU. *(yoo) Chinese, 'shining brightly'.* Yu the Great founded China's first dynasty, but elsewhere 'Hey, you!' would make this name utterly confusing.

YUKIO. *Japanese, 'snow boy'.* In the Japanese culture, this name, often used for boys born in December, suggests a sense of independence. **Yuki, Yukie, Yukiko.**

YUL. *Mongolian, 'beyond the horizon'.* Russian-born actor Yul (christened either Youl or Taidje) Brynner gave this name a bald-headed king of Siam image.

YULE. *English, 'winter solstice'.* A possibility for a Christmas baby, if you find Noel too mundane. **Euell, Ewell, Yul.**

♂ **YUMA.** *North American Indian, 'son of a chief'; Arizona place name.* The *a* ending gives it a feminine feel.

YURI. *(YOOR-ee) Russian variation of* **GEORGE.** Common Russian name familiarised elsewhere via cosmonaut Yury Gagarin and a character in *Dr Zhivago,* but we don't see it ever gaining permanent resident status. **Yore,**

Yorii, Yura, Yurick, Yurii, Yurochka, Yury. International: Juri *(Polish).*

YŪSUF. *Arabic variation of* **JOSEPH.** Closer to the original in sound than in looks. **Yazid, Yousef, Youssef, Yousuf, Yusef.**

YVES. *(eve) French variation of* **IVES,** *'yew wood'.* On paper, with its stylish ties to fashion legend Yves Saint-Laurent *(born Henri),* Yves looks great, but the pronunciation could lead to gender confusion. **Evo, Ives, Yvo, Yvon. International: Ivo** *(German),* **Iwo** *(Polish).*

Z boys

ZABE. *Modern invented name.* Parents with a penchant for inventing names seem especially enamoured of the letter *Z,* maybe for its counterculture feel and its extra zip.

ZAC. *Diminutive of* **ZACHARIAH/ZACHARY.** A popular nickname that, over the past few decades, has acquired enough standing to work on its own, à la earlier equivalents such

as Jack and Max; an alternative to Zach/Zack. **Zacc, Zach, Zack, Zacky, Zak.**

ZACCHEUS. *Variation of* **ZACHARIAH.** A New Testament tax collector was called Zaccheus, the freshest spin on this biblical favourite. **Zacceus, Zacchaeus, Zacchious, Zachaios.**

ZACH, ZACK. *See* **Zac.**

ZACHALIE. *French variation of* **ZACHARY.** This is one you will get tired of explaining.

ZACHARIAH. *Hebrew, 'the Lord has remembered'.* This distinguished name still feels a bit ancient, but with the rise of such former greybeards as Moses and Elijah, it also sounds child-friendly again, as does the Latin-Greek form Zacharias. **Zac, Zacaria, Zacarias, Zacarius, Zacary, Zaccaria, Zaccariah, Zaccheus, Zach, Zacharia, Zacharias, Zacharie, Zachary, Zacharyah, Zacheriah, Zachery, Zacheus, Zachory, Zachury, Zack, Zackariah, Zackerias, Zackery, Zak, Zakaria, Zakarias, Zakarie, Zakariyyah, Zakery, Zako,**

Zecharia, Zechariah, Zecharya, Zeggery, Zekariah, Zeke, Zekeriah, Zhachory.

ZACHARY. *Hebrew, 'the Lord has remembered'.* Staying at the bottom of the Top 100 in recent years, Zachary's best style days are behind it. But with its ancient roots and modern feel, you can understand why it's been such a longtime winner. **Xachary, Zac, Zacary, Zaccary, Zaccery, Zach, Zacha, Zachaery, Zachaios, Zacharay, Zacharey, Zachari, Zacharia, Zacharias, Zacharie, Zacharry, Zachaury, Zachery, Zachory, Zachrey, Zachry, Zachuery, Zachury, Zack, Zackarey, Zackary, Zackery, Zackory, Zak, Zakaria, Zakary, Zakery, Zakkary, Zechary, Zechery, Zeke.**

ZADE. *Modern invented name.* Zesty brother of Cade and Slade.

ZADEN. *Modern invented name.* A nouveau member of the Aidan/Braden/Jaden group. Yet another variation on a too-trendy genre – never the most original way to go, even if there aren't yet many Zadens on your street. **Zadan, Zadin, Zadon,** Zadun, Zaedan, Zaeden, Zaedin, Zaedon, Zaedun, Zaidan, Zaiden, Zaidin, Zaidon, Zaidun, Zaydan, Zayden, Zaydin, Zaydon, Zaydun.

ZADOCK. *Hebrew, 'fair, righteous'.* A biblical name that was used centuries ago, but which has an unpleasant sound to the modern ear. **Zadok, Zaddik, Zadik, Zadoc, Zaydok.**

ZADORNIN. *Basque, 'Saturn'.* If you want something truly different that also has an interesting origin and meaning, this is a far-out – if not unlikely – possibility.

ZAFAR. *Arabic, 'victory'.* A strong name with a strong meaning, like its cousin Zafir. **Zafeer, Zafer, Zaffar, Zafir, Zaphar.**

ZAHAVI. *Hebrew, 'gold'.* A Middle Eastern name rarely heard elsewhere, but with a certain swashbuckling charm. **Zehavi.**

ZAHIR. *Arabic, 'flourishing, brilliant'; Hebrew, 'shining'.* A popular name in the Middle East and one of the most evocative choices of its genre. **Zahair, Zahar, Zaheer, Zahi, Zahur, Zair, Zaire, Zayyir.**

ZAHN. *German or Ashkenazic Jewish, 'tooth'.* this makes a dramatic, unusual Zane alternative – though you may not want to enlighten your child as to its prosaic meaning.

ZAILEY. *Modern invented name.* Zee-ifying Bailey. **Zaley, Zalley, Zally, Zaily.**

If You Like Zachary, *You Might Love . . .*

Barnaby
Gabriel
Jackson
Mack
Malachi
Nathaniel
Nickolai
Zachariah
Zane
Zebedee

ZAIRE. *Place name*. African-Caribbean parents have been especially interested in adopting African place names for their children.

ZAK. *Diminutive of* Zachery. This popular and zippy short form has been added to many birth certificates recently and has made a brief apperance in the Top 100.

ZAKI. *Arabic, 'full of virtue, pure'*. Not related to Zack, Zacky, Zachary or Zachariah – but everyone will think it is.

ZAKO. *Hungarian variation of* **ZACHARIAH**. If for whatever reason you're wed to the whole Zachary concept, this variation – either as a proper name or a nickname – is one way to make it new. **Zacco, Zacko.**

ZALE. *Greek, 'sea-strength'*. Appealing sound and meaning, but not one to be too zealous about. **Zayle.**

ZALMAI. *Afghan, 'young'*. Not many Afghan names make it into the Western culture, but this one stands a slim chance.

ZALMAN. *Variation of* **SOLOMON**. More familiar now via its Salman form, thanks to author Rushdie; this is an unusual biblical alternative. **Salman, Zalomon.**

ZAMIEL. *German variation of* **SAMUEL**. For Sam-lovers who want to make a slight detour off that well-travelled road. **Zamal, Zamuel.**

ZAMIR. *Hebrew, 'song, bird'*. An interesting choice if you want a nonbiblical Hebrew name. **Zameer.**

ZAN. *Diminutive of* **ALEXANDER**. Xan for those who like to say it as it is. **Xan, Zander, Zandro, Zandros, Zann.**

ZANDER. *Diminutive of* **ALEXANDER**. On the rise as an independent name: Zander and Xander are both becoming more popular in the US and can be found as characters in American films. **Zandore, Zandra, Zandrae, Zandy.**

ZANDY. *Greek, meaning unknown*. Like Gandy, a rarely heard name (there was a 1970s movie called *Zandy's Bride*) that has a lot more energy and charm than its commoner cousins Andy, Randy and Sandy.

ZANE. *Variation of* **JOHN**. Western novelist Zane (born Pearl!) Grey made this name famous. Now, it's in tune with the style of the times, while retaining that cowboy image. **Zain, Zayne.**

ZARED. *Hebrew, 'trap'*. If there are too many Jareds in your neighbourhood, you might want to consider this Hebrew alternative. **Zarod.**

ZARNEY. *Modern invented name*. We can't believe we're saying this, but we'd even prefer Arnie or Barney.

ZARREN. *Modern invented name*. On the other hand, Zarren is an improvement on Darren. **Zaren, Zarin, Zarrin, Zarron, Zarryn, Zaryn.**

ZAVID. *Russian, meaning unknown*. This Old Russian name is mentioned in several genealogical sources, but few modern name books. Pronounced either to rhyme with David, or as *zah-VEED*, it can be a highly unusual alternative.

ZAVIER. *Arabic variation of* **XAVIER.** This phonetic version is occasionally used. **Zavair, Zaverie, Zavery, Zavierre, Zavior, Zavyr, Zayvius, Zxavian.**

ZAYD. *(zah-eed) Arabic, 'increase, growth'.* Zayd (or its most common variant Zaid), an old and still well used Arabic name, was a slave whom Muhammad adopted as his son. **Zahid, Zaid, Zaied, Zaiid, Ziyad, Ziyyad.**

ZBIGNIEW. *(zeh-big-new) Polish, 'to dispel anger'.* One of the first authentically Slavic names heard elsewhere, via 1960s to 70s former presidential advisor Zbigniew Brzezinski. Even after all these years, pronunciation is problematic.

ZEB. *Diminutive of* **ZEBEDIAH** *or* **ZEBULON.** Short and to-the-point, it turns an ancient biblical name into a friendly cowboy. **Zev.**

★**ZEBEDEE.** *Variation of* **ZEBEDIAH.** Adorable and unusual name from the Bible. The Jeremy of the future? **Zebadee, Zebedy.**

ZEBEDIAH. *Hebrew, 'gift of Jehovah'.* The New Testament father of apostles John and James – definitely a biblical choice that still has some life left in it. **Zeb, Zebedee, Zebedijah.**

ZEBULON. *Hebrew, 'to give honour to'.* An Old Testament name with a Puritan feel and post-Zachary possibilities. **Zabulon, Zeb, Zebulan, Zebulen, Zebulin, Zebulun, Zebulyn, Zev, Zevulon, Zevulun, Zhebulen, Zubin.**

★**ZED.** Diminutive of **ZEDEKIAH.** Newer than Zac, cooler than Ed, Ned or Ted.

ZEDEKIAH. *(zeh-deh-KY-uh) Hebrew, 'the Lord is just'.* The name of an Old Testament king and yet another *Z* choice from the Bible that still retains some zip, especially with the appealing nickname Zed. **Zed, Zedechiah, Zedekias, Zedikiah.**

Clunky but Cool

Abner

Angus

Augustus

Caspar

Conrad

Cornelius

Digby

Fergus

Frank

George

Harvey

Hiram

Hugo

Leopold

Louis

Orson

Oscar

Raymond

Rufus

Rupert

Vincent

Zebediah

ZEÉV. *Hebrew, 'wolf'.* Sharp and sleek, it refers to Benjamin being compared to a wolf in Genesis. **Zeévi, Zeff, Zif.**

ZEKE. *Diminutive of* **EZEKIEL.** Casual form of the name of an important prophet. How well this name holds up depends on the boy: it could be a cooler alternative of Zack, or it could prove too close to 'geek'.

ZEKI. *Turkish, 'clever, intelligent'.* Cute but slight. **Zeky.**

ZELIG. *Yiddish variation of* **SELIG,** *'blessed, happy'.* Forever Woody's name. **Selig, Zeligman, Zelik, Zetik.**

ZELL. *Modern invented name.* Here's one Zell of note: video-game character Zell, a hero of Final Fantasy. **Zel.**

ZELMO. *Athlete name.* Zelmo Beaty was a noted basketball player in the 1960s and 1970s. Elmo not wacky enough for you? – choose Zelmo.

♂ **ZEN.** *Japanese, form of Buddhism.* A spiritual word name well-suited for these serenity-seeking times.

ZENO. *Greek, 'a stranger'.* This name of an ancient philosopher has a muscular dynamism that's lightened by its cheerful final vowel, resulting in a kind of offbeat sci-fi feel. **Zenan, Zenas, Zenon, Zino, Zinon.**

ZENOBIOS. *Greek, 'life of Zeus'.* Zealous and noble, an unusual and strong choice – and if the original is too much of a mouthful, you can always call him Zen. **International: Zenobio, Zenobius** *(Spanish),* **Zinov, Zinoviy** *(Russian).*

ZEO. *Modern invented name.* Neo, but maybe less than zero – name heard in the Power Rangers film title *Power Rangers Zeo.* **Zio.**

♂ **ZEPHYR.** *Greek, 'west wind'.* A name from mythology with many European variations. The Babar books feature a monkey named Zephyr – and it does have a pet-like quality. **Zayfeer, Zayfir, Zayphir, Zefir, Zeferino, Zeffrey, Zephery, Zephir, Zephire, Zephiros, Zephirus, Zephram, Zephran, Zephrin, Zephyrus.**

ZEPHYRIN. *French variation of* **ZEPHYR.** This name feels warmer and more human-appropriate in its longer version. Fun fact: Zephyrinus was a Jewish pope. **Zephirin, Zephyrinus.**

ZERO. *Arabic, 'void'.* Zero Mostel took on this name for its comedic value, but there would be nothing funny about giving it to an unfortunate child.

ZERRICK. *Modern invented name.* Updates the tired Derek or Eric. **Zerek, Zeric, Zerick, Zerok, Zerreck, Zerroch, Zerrock.**

ZESIRO. *Luganda, 'older of twins'.* Unusual and exotic name, might be worth consideration if you're expecting twins.

ZEUS. *Greek, 'living'.* The supreme Olympian god and a mighty image for a little fella to live up to, but more and more parents are beginning to consider it seriously.

ZEVI. *Hebrew variation of* **ZVI.** More distinctive than Levi. **Zhvie, Zhvy, Zvi.**

ZEVON. *Musician name.* The late great singer-songwriter Warren Zevon would make a worthy namesake.

ZHIVAGO. *Russian literary name, 'life'.* For lovers of Pasternak's great doctor, a lively middle name choice, one made by actress Nia Long.

ZIA. *Hebrew, 'trembling, moving'; Arabic, 'light'.* While this is an ancient male name, it's too similar to modern girls' choices like Mia and Pia to work for a boy today. **Ziah.**

ZIGGY. *German, diminutive of* SIEGFRIED *and* SIGMUND. The ultimate jokey name, à la Ziggy Stardust or the comic-strip character Ziggy. Then again, there's Ziggy Marley and most anything Marley is cool. **Ziggie.**

ZIKOMO. *Ngono (Malawi), 'thank you'.* Gracious African choice.

ZIMRAN. *Hebrew, 'song'.* In the Bible, a son of Abraham and Keturah; this ancient and musical name nonetheless

sounds like a character in a 1950s science fiction movie.

ZINC. *Colour or mineral name.* Extreme cool possibilities in either of these modern categories, like a postmodern Linc.

ZINEDINE. *Arabic, 'beauty of the faith'.* Zinedine Zidane is France's biggest football star, spawning a legion of little Zinedines in that country. **Zinnedine.**

♂ **ZION.** *Hebrew, 'highest point'.* Zion has taken off in recent years, especially after singer Lauryn Hill used it for her son. It combines a user-friendly Ryan-Brian sound with the gravitas of religious significance. **Sion.**

ZIV. *Hebrew, 'full of life, glorious, splendid'.* The ebullient

meaning enlightens this rather constricted name. **Ziven, Zivon.**

ZIVEN. *Slavic, 'vigorous, lively'.* This version is a bit more in tune with modern tastes. **Zev, Ziv, Zivka, Zivon.**

ZOILO. *Spanish derivation of Greek, 'life'.* A male take on the feminine name Zoe, it's hard to give an attractive pronunciation.

♂ **ZOLA.** *Literary name.* Authors or Francophiles – or both – may want to use this as a middle name to honour French writer Émile Zola. Warning: as a first name, it is frequently female.

ZOLTAN. *Hungarian, 'life'.* Though a common name in Hungary, it has a bit of Mandrake the Magician exoticism here. It was also the name of Dracula's dog. **Zolfen.**

ZORION. *Basque variation of* **ORION.** Cosmic. **Zoran, Zoren, Zorian, Zoron, Zorrine, Zorrion.**

ZUBIN. *Hebrew, 'to honour'.* Most familiar here as a musical name, via conductor Zubin Mehta, but it certainly could be used by others.

ZURI. *African, Kiswahili, 'good, beautiful'.* Singular, strong and exotic.

ZVI. *Hebrew, 'deer'.* Although there are only three letters, it's still a mouthful.

ZYLER. *Modern invented name.* Tyler, with zest.

About the Authors

Pamela Redmond Satran, who has been collaborating with Linda Rosenkrantz on baby name books for more than twenty years, is also the author of five novels: *The Home for Wayward Supermodels, Suburbanistas, Younger, Babes in Captivity* and *The Man I Should Have Married.* A contributing editor for *Parenting* magazine, she cowrites the popular Glamour List column for *Glamour* magazine and contributes frequently to such publications as *The New York Times, Bon Appétit* and *Good Housekeeping.* Pam lives with her husband and three children near New York City. You can visit her Web site at www .pamelaredmondsatran.com.

Linda Rosenkrantz is the author of several non-name books, including *Telegram! Modern History As Told Through More Than 400 Witty, Poignant and Revealing Telegrams* and the memoir, *My Life As a List: 207 Things About My (Bronx) Childhood;* and coauthor (with her husband, Christopher Finch) of *Gone Hollywood* and *Sotheby's Guide to Animation Art.* In addition to contributing articles to numerous magazines, she writes a nationally syndicated column on collectables. She lives in Los Angeles and named her daughter Chloe.